Manual of Diagnostic Antibodies for Immunohistology

2nd Edition

To Wendy and Nimmie, for their love, strength and support

Manual of Diagnostic Antibodies for Immunohistology

2nd Edition

Anthony S-Y Leong

MBBS, MD, FRCPA, FRCPath, FCAP, FASCP,
FHKAM (Pathol), Honorary FHKCPath, Honorary FRCPath (Thailand)

Medical Director,
Hunter Area Pathology Service, Newcastle
Professor and Head,
Discipline of Anatomical Pathology, University of Newcastle, Australia,
Medical Director,
Australia ImmunoPathology Laboratories, Newcastle, Australia

Kumarasen Cooper

BSc (Hons), MBChB, DPhil (Oxon), FFPath, FRCPath

Director of Anatomical Pathology, University of Vermont/Fletcher
Allen Health Care, Burlington, Vermont, USA.
Professor of Pathology, University of Vermont, Burlington, Vermont, USA

F Joel W-M Leong

MBBS, DPhil (Oxon)

Clinical Lecturer in Pathology, Nuffield Department of Clinical Laboratory Sciences,
University of Oxford, United Kingdom

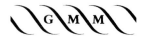

© 2003
Greenwich Medical Media Ltd.
137 Euston Road
London
NW1 2AA

ISBN 1 84110 100 1

First Published 2003

A catalogue record for this book is available from the British Library

Project Manager
Gavin Smith

Production and Design by
Saxon Graphics Limited, Derby

Printed in Great Britain by
William Clowes, Beccles, Suffolk

Preface to the First Edition

The rapid acceptance and entrenchment of immunohistochemistry as an important and, in some cases, indispensable adjunct to morphological examination and diagnosis has imposed the necessity for anatomical pathology laboratories to be proficient in immunostaining procedures. However, for immunohistochemical stains to be meaningful, technical competence must be accompanied by a familiarity with the characteristics and specificities of the reagents employed. In particular, the medical technologist and pathologist must have knowledge of the sensitivity and specificity of the primary antibody employed, the nature of the epitope demonstrated by each antibody and its sensitivity to common fixatives. They should be equally conversant with protocols for tissue processing as well as the various methods of antigen/epitope retrieval which are appropriate for the demonstration of the specific protein sought for in the tissue section or cell preparation.

The versatility and contributions of immunohistochemistry to diagnostic pathology, particularly in the areas of tumor diagnosis, lineage identification, prognostication and therapy are largely dependent on the ever-increasing range of antisera and monoclonal antibodies that are commercially available. However, this latter feature is a two-edged sword. While the extensive spectrum of antibodies allows the identification of a wider and wider range of cellular antigens, the user must also be familiar with the properties and characteristics of each of these many antibodies.

This book provides a comprehensive list of antisera and monoclonal antibodies that have useful diagnostic applications in tissue sections and cell preparations. Various clones, which are commercially available to detect the same antigen, are listed and the sensitivities and specificities of the antibodies are discussed. Importantly, our own experience with these reagents is provided together with pertinent references. While as many available sources of antibodies are provided, it is acknowledged that the listing cannot be exhaustive and only major sources are covered. A brief coverage of the diagnostic approach to the general categories of the poorly differentiated round cell and spindle cell tumors in various anatomical sites using panels of selected antibodies is provided in the form of tables. Staining protocols and antigen/epitope retrieval procedures including those employing enzymes, microwaves and heat are also given in detail.

It is hoped that this compendium will provide a source of useful and practical information to both the diagnostic as well as research laboratory.

Anthony S-Y Leong, MBBS, MD
Shatin, Hong Kong

Kumarasen Cooper, MBBCh, DPhil
Johannesburg, South Africa

F Joel W-M Leong, MBBS
Oxford, England

Preface to the Second Edition

Since the publication of the 1st edition of this book in 1999, the role of immunohistology in diagnostic pathology has consolidated further and continued to expand. Immunohistology has rapidly become an integral part of microscopic examination and diagnosis, occupying a position of importance only next to the hematoxylin and eosin section and usurping many of the diagnostic roles of histochemical stains and electron microscopy. There is widespread use of immunohistology in diagnostic services throughout the world and in the field of oncologic pathology and as many as 25% of tumors require immunostaining for accurate diagnosis. The percentage is considerably higher in the case of anaplastic and pleomorphic tumors where morphologic features to allow accurate typing of the tumor are absent. With the introduction of Herceptin as the first antibody treatment for cancer, immunolabelling for the Herceptin or cerbB-2 antigen has empowered immunostaining even further. The detection of other antigens such as CD117 (*c-kit*) provides equally important information that predicts response to the specific therapeutic agent SYT-571. Immunostaining is a requirement for the examination of sentinel node biopsies in most treatment protocols. The role of immunostaining in cancer pathology continues to increase so that it now is employed not only for diagnosis but also for other parameters including prognosis, microscopic tumor staging, prediction of response to therapy, and for the selection of specific therapeutic agents. Immunostaining also provides invaluable information for the understanding of tumorigenesis and the identification of carrier states through the identification of gene products.

Automation in immunohistology is well established with a variety of machines employing a number of different patented techniques for antibody incubation. Such instruments have the main advantage of consistency over manual techniques rather than cost or labor savings. Many autoimmunostainers suffer from the disadvantage of rigid incubation times so that overnight incubation of primary antibodies at room temperature or at 4°C is impossible or difficult to perform as an automated procedure. Optimal conditions for antigen detection have thus given way to expediency.

The threshold of antigen detection continues to be lowered as more sensitive detection methods are developed, the tyramide signal amplification or catalysed reporter deposition system being a notable example. Modifications of amplification systems that employ multiple antibody layers such as the mirror image complementary antibody (MICA) detection system also continue to be introduced. Such systems increase the cost of the procedure making it prohibitive to use routinely or in high volumes. Furthermore, they sometimes produce undesirable background staining if not optimally employed.

Undoubtedly, a major milestone in immunohistology was the introduction of heat-induced antigen retrieval, which lowered antigen detection thresholds sufficiently that most proteins of diagnostic interest could be demonstrated with standard detection systems. A variety of methods to generate heat for retrieval have been introduced with minor differences in efficacy so that the method of choice has been very much influenced by familiarity or convenience of use. This was so until the recent demonstration that superheating to 120°C, attained under pressure, appeared to lower detection thresholds further than conventional methods. This is in keeping with the concept that both time and temperature are major influences in heat-induced antigen retrieval. The pH of the retrieval solution is another major factor and it has been demonstrated that the majority of antigens are better enhanced following retrieval at alkaline pH. The breaking of protein cross linkages induced by aldehyde fixatives is the prevalent concept heat-induced antigen retrieval. However, the true mechanism of antigen retrieval continues elude us particularly as it has been shown that ultrasound, which generates negligible heat, can be an effective form of antigen

retrieval. Furthermore, microwave heating also enhances immunostaining of tissues fixed in a non-cross linking fixative such as ethanol suggesting that heating may unmask epitopes by mechanisms other than through the breakage of cross-linkages.

While the great majority of diagnostic antibodies are highly sensitive, highly specific antibodies are few and far between. Other than those raised to specific gene products most antibodies, at best, are only tissue-selective and their effective usage is, to some extent dependant on knowledge the range of tissues that the reagent may label, specific or otherwise. As often is the case, with the progression of time and usage, newly developed antibodies are found to stain an increasing range of cells besides what they were intended for. Much of this

2nd edition is devoted to this aspect of antibody properties as well as to newer applications. Pertinent references are updated and new diagnostic panels are provided. Also, newly produced antibodies are discussed particularly as there are now a number of antibodies available that have been raised against specific gene or fusion gene products that are of diagnostic importance.

Anthony S-Y Leong, MB, BS, MD
(UAdelaide)
Newcastle, Australia

Kumarasen Cooper, MB, BCh, DPhil
(Oxon)
Vermont, USA

F Joel W-M Leong, MB, BS, DPhil
(Oxon)
Oxford, United Kingdom

October 2002

Contents

SECTION 2 Appendices

Contents

xi

SECTION 3 Suppliers

Introduction

This book discusses diagnostic antibodies and antisera in alphabetical order and provides the background, applications and diagnostic pitfalls of each reagent, together with pertinent references. Common clones of diagnostic relevance and some sources are listed but this is not purported to be exhaustive; furthermore, mainly antibodies shown to be immunoreactive in fixed paraffin-embedded tissue sections are discussed, as paraffin sections remain the mainstay of diagnostic histopathology.

Diagnostic Approach

Diagnostic antibodies should not be employed in isolation but always as part of a panel of antibodies directed to the entities considered in differential diagnosis. As the latter is derived from the cytomorphologic appearances of the tumor, it is clearly evident that immunohistochemical diagnosis is morphology based. For this reason we favor "immunohistology" over the more-established term "immunohistochemistry" as it emphasizes the relationship of immunostaining to morphology and that immunostaining is not a test procedure but an integral component of microscopic diagnosis. To assist with the diagnostic process, both antibodies to markers recognized as being expressed by the tumor in question as well as those associated with entities considered in differential diagnoses should make up the panel. As markers are almost never tissue-specific, the application of a panel of antibodies will generate an immunophenotypic profile comprising both positive and negative findings which, in combination, produce the most accurate results. By defining the immunophenotype of the tissue tested, the errors of false positive and false negative staining will be reduced and the highest diagnostic yield obtained (Leong & Gown, 1993; Gown & Leong, 1993). For example, anaplastic large cell lymphoma has carcinoma and melanoma as morphologic mimics. Anaplastic large cell lymphoma may express epithelial membrane antigen (EMA) in about 45% of cases, and may fail to stain for CD45 (leukocyte common antigen) in as many cases. These findings, taken in isolation, may be mistaken for that of a carcinoma. However, if antibodies to vimentin, broad spectrum cytokeratin, S100 and HMB45 (melanoma-associated antigen) are also employed, the error will be averted as the profile of EMA+, CD45-, VIM+, CK-, S100-, HMB45- fits best with that of anaplastic large cell lymphoma, in the context of the differential diagnoses. In some situations it may be necessary to perform the immunostaining in two stages. A primary panel of antibodies provides the major categorization of the tumor and a secondary panel allows further subtyping. For example, positivity for CD30 will be useful for the confirmation of the diagnosis of anaplastic large cell lymphoma and lineage typing can be further performed.

As an alternative, the algorithmic approach may be adopted (Leong et at, 1997) but whichever approach is favored, it is important that antibodies directed to all entities considered in differential diagnosis be employed. Of course, exceptions to this rule include the application of immunostaining for prognostic markers and the identification of infectious agents in tissue sections.

Standardization and Optimization of Immunostaining

Much has been discussed in recent times about standardization in immunohistology (Taylor 1993), but this goal is difficult or impossible to achieve simply because fixatives, durations of fixation, and methods of tissue processing employed by laboratories are different. The ability to demonstrate various tissue antigens is very much dependant on their preservation and therefore on the method of fixation and processing employed. With the vastly different practices in laboratories throughout the world, is clear that standardization as a goal may be impossible to achieve.

It would be more appropriate to aim for optimization of immunostaining within the individual laboratory. This means consistency, reproducibility and the ability to obtain the optimal results with the method of fixation and processing employed. To this end, it is necessary for each laboratory to adopt a method of fixation and tissue processing which will allow the optimal antigen preservation and yet not compromise cytomorphological preservation. It may be appropriate to examine each fixation and processing step and adjust for optimization, remembering that antigen preservation may also be influenced by the surgeon or physician who has responsibility for placing the excised specimen into the fixative.

Antigen Retrieval

It is imperative to test every new antibody on tissue blocks processed in the your own laboratory. While reagent dilutions and tissue preparation instructions provided by the manufacturers are useful guides, they are universal recommendations and not individualized. It is necessary evaluate various methods of antigen retrieval and to determine, by titration, antibody concentrations that are optimal for tissue processed in your laboratory. The introduction of the heat-induced epitope retrieval (HIER) procedure (Shi et al, 1993) has contributed significantly to our ability to optimize immunostaining procedures and HIER must be evaluated for each new antibody used. With very rare exceptions, we have not found HIER to be deleterious to the majority of diagnostic antigens and recommend that it be applied as a routine before any immunostaining be performed (Leong et al, 1993; Gown et al, 1993). The combination of HIER with enzymatic digestion should also be explored for some antigens. A protocol for HIER employing microwaves is provided in Appendix II. A variety of methods for HIER have become popular including the use of microwave irradiation, pressure cooker heating, steaming, wet autoclaving and simple boiling. While there continues to be debate on the actual mechanism of antigen retrieval induced by heating of deparaffinised tissue sections and the role of microwave irradiation, there is general agreement that the threshold of antigen staining is largely dependent on both temperature and the duration of heating. Recent work from our laboratory indicates that superheating to 120°C, attained under pressure, produces the most effective antigen retrieval (Leong et al, 2002).

Controls

Diagnostic interpretation in immunohistology includes the assessment of internal positive control cells or tissues. Many test sections contain normal tissue, which express the antigen being tested. Positive controls should also be used routinely in each antibody staining run, remembering that it is more appropriate to employ neoplastic tissues known to express equivalent amounts of the antigen tested rather than non-lesional tissues that may express much higher levels of antigen. A negative control of tissues known not to express the antigen should also be employed. In addition, a nonspecific negative reagent control should be employed in place of the primary antibody to evaluate nonspecific staining. Ideally, a negative reagent control contains the same isotype as the primary antibody but exhibits no specific reactivity with human tissues in the same matrix or solutions as the primary antibody. All control tissues should be fixed, processed and embedded in a manner identical to the test sample.

In addition to these technical aspects, consideration should also be given to the nature of the diagnostic specificity of the antibodies used and the properties of the target antigen. Much of this information is theoretical and beyond the control of the diagnostic laboratory. Nonetheless, you should have some familiarity with this aspect of the reagents and the information is often available in the literature and may be available in the product profiles provided by the manufacturer.

It is clear from the foregoing that immunohistology is not a simple matter of a positive or negative stain. While it is a powerful diagnostic tool, immunostaining is only an adjunct to histologic examination and requires careful optimization if it is intended to produce the highest diagnostic yield (Leong 1992).

This book contains antibodies and antisera which we consider to be of diagnostic relevance. Except for some antibodies such as the cytokeratins, pituitary and pancreatic hormones, the antibodies are discussed separately and listed in alphabetical order for easy reference. The antibodies are listed by their main and alternate names but specific clone numbers are not indexed.

References

Gown AM, Leong AS-Y: Immunohistochemistry of "solid" tumors: poorly differentiated round cell and spindle cell tumors II. IN: Leong AS-Y (ed) Applied immunohistochemistry for the surgical pathologist. London: Edward Arnold, 1993, pp 73–108.

Gown AM, de Wever HT, Battifora H. Microwave-based antigenic unmasking: a revolutionary new technique for routine immunohistochemistry. Applied Immunohistochemistry 1993; 1:256–231.

Leong AS-Y. Commentary: Diagnostic immunohistochemistry – problems and solutions. Pathology 1992; 24:1–4.

Leong AS-Y, Gown AM. Immunohistochemistry of "solid" tumors: poorly differentiated round cell and spindle cell tumors I. IN: Leong AS-Y (ed) Applied immunohistochemistry for the surgical pathologist. London: Edward Arnold, 1993, pp 23–72.

Leong AS-Y, Milios J. An assessment of the efficacy of the microwave antigen-retrieval procedure on a range of tissue antigens. Applied Immunohistochemistry 1993; 1:267–74.

Leong AS-Y, Wick MR, Swanson PE. Chapter 6: Immunohistology and ultrastructural features in site-specific epithelial neoplasm – an algorithmic approach. IN: Immunohistology and electron microscopy of anaplastic and pleomorphic tumors. Cambridge: Cambridge University Press, 1997, pp 209–40.

Leong AS-Y, Haffajee Z, Lee ES, Kear M, Pepperral D. Superheating antigen retrieval. Applied Immunohistochemistry and Molecular Morphology 2002; 10:263–8.

Shi S-R, Key ME, Kalra KL. Antigen retrieval in formalin-fixed, paraffin-embedded tissues: an enhancement method for immunohistochemical staining based on microwave oven heating of tissue sections. Journal of Histochemistry and Cytochemistry 1991; 39:741–8.

Taylor CR. An exaltation of experts: concerted efforts in the standardization of immunohistochemistry. Applied Immunohistochemistry 1993; 1:232–43.

Antibodies

α-Smooth Muscle Actin (α-SMA)

Sources/clones

Accurate (1A4), Biodesign (asm-1, A4), Biogenex (1A4), Cymbus Bioscience (asm-1), Dako (1A4), Enzo (CGA7), ICN (1A4), Immunotech (1A4), Medac (TCS), Novocastra (asm1), RDI (asm-1), Sigma (1A4) and Zymed (Z060).

Fixation/preparation

Several of the antibody clones to α-smooth muscle actin (α-SMA) are immunoreactive in fixed paraffin-embedded sections. HIER at 120°C enhances immunolabelling.

Background

Cytoplasmic actins vary in amino acid sequences and can be separated by electrophoresis into six different isotopes, all having the same molecular weight of 42 kD. Alpha actins are found in muscle cells, beta and gamma actins may be present in muscle cells as well as most other cell types in the body including non-muscle cells. Both striated and smooth muscle fibers differ in their expression of actin isotypes and this has formed the basis for the generation of antibodies directed at muscle-specific actin subtypes. HHF35 (muscle specific actin) identifies all four actin isoforms present in smooth muscle as well as skeletal muscle cells, pericytes, myoepithelial cells and myofibroblasts. In contrast, antibodies to α-SMA specifically identify the single alpha isoform characteristic of smooth muscle cells and those cells with myofibroblastic differentiation.

Applications

Antibodies to α-SMA are used in several diagnostic situations. These include the identification of myoepithelial cells, which are admixed, with epithelial cells in benign proliferative lesions of the breast, allowing their distinction from neoplastic proliferations. Myoepithelial cells also line benign ductules of the breast compared to their absence in neoplastic tubules (Raymond & Leong, 1991). α-SMA is also a useful marker to identify myofibroblastic differentiation and has been used in studies of idiopathic pulmonary fibrosis (Ohta et al, 1995) and of the fibrogenic Ito cells in the liver (Enzan et al, 1994). In diagnostic pathology, α-SMA is used mostly as a discriminator of smooth muscle tumors in the identification of spindled and pleomorphic tumors (Jones et al, 1990). It is important to emphasize that this marker should not be used in isolation (Leong et al, 1997a). Because myogenic determinants are not always synthesized by normal and neoplastic cells simultaneously, the highest diagnostic yield is obtained with a panel of antibodies that include α-SMA, desmin and muscle-specific actin (Appendix 1.23 and 1.24). In the diagnostic context of the morphologically indeterminate spindle cell tumor, it should also be remembered that myofibroblasts might express these myogenic markers. However, expression of desmin tends to be focal and within scattered cells in myofibroblastic proliferations and these cell types show a thin and fragmented basal lamina compared to the thick, irregular and long runs of basal lamina around smooth muscle tumors (Leong et al, 1997b). Myofibroblastic proliferations may display a characteristic "tram track" pattern of distribution of muscle actins distributed in a subplasmmalemal location. Furthermore, smooth muscle cells may express low molecular weight cytokeratin. α-SMA positivity is also observed in adult and juvenile granulosa cell tumors, and in the theca externa and focally in the cortex-medulla of the ovary (Santini et al, 1995). Myofibroblastic differentiation is not uncommon in malignant fibrous histiocytoma so that "pleomorphic myofibrosarcoma" has been suggested as an alternative name for this tumor (Montgomery & Fisher, 2001). α-SMA is a useful marker to identify myoepithelial cells and was used to show the presence of myoepitheliomas in several extra-salivary sites such as the breast, larynx, retroperitoneum and more recently, the skin (Kutzner et al, 2001).

Some melanomas may exhibit an aberrant immunophenotype that includes contractile proteins α-SMA and desmin (Banerjee & Harris, 2000). SMA-positive cells have been suggested to play a role in the pathogenesis of tubulointerstitial damage in the kidney (Ranieri et al, 2001). The significance of muscle actin expression observed in mesotheliomas is presently unknown (Kung et al, 1995). α-SMA expression and staining has recently been demonstrated in articular chondrocytes (Kinner & Spector, 2001).

Comments

Clone 1A4 produces the best results in our hands. Immunoreactivity appears not to be enhanced by boiling or proteolytic digestion and is best demonstrated following retrieval at 120°C in citrate buffer at pH6.0.

References

Banerjee SS, Harris M. Morphological and immunophenotypic variations in malignant melanoma. Histopathology 2000;36:387–402.

Enzan H, Himeno H, Iwamura S, et al. Immunohistochemical identification of Ito cells and their myofibroblastic transformation in adult human liver. Virchows Archives 1994;424:249–56.

Jones H, Steart PV, DuBoulay CE, Roche WR. Alpha-smooth muscle actin as a marker of soft tissue tumors: a comparison with desmin. Journal of Pathology 1990;162:29–33.

Kinner B, Spector M. Smooth muscle actin expression by human articular chondrocytes and their contraction of a collagen-glycoasaminoglycan matrix in vitro. Journal of Orthopedic Research 2001;19:233–41.

Kung IT, Thallas V, Spencer EJ, Wilson SM. Expression of muscle actins in diffuse mesothelioma. Human Pathology 1995;26:565–70.

Kutzner H, Mentzel T, Kaddu S, et al. Cutaneous myoepithelioma: an under-recognised cutaneous neoplasm composed of myoepithelial cells. American Journal of Surgical Pathology 2001;25:348–55.

Leong AS-Y, Wick MR, Swanson PE. Immunohistology and electron microscopy of anaplastic and pleomorphic tumors.
Cambridge: Cambridge University Press, 1997a, pp 64–8.

Leong AS-Y, Milios J, Leong FJ. Patterns of basal lamina immunostaining in soft-tissue and bony tumors. Applied Immunohistochemistry 1997b;5:1–7.

Montgomery E, Fisher C. Myofibroblastic differentiation in malignant fibrous histiocytoma (pleomorphic myofibrosarcoma): a clinicopathological study. Histopathology 2001;38:499–509.

Ohta K, Mortenson RL, Clark RA, et al. Immunohistochemical identification and characterization of smooth muscle-like cells in idiopathic pulmonary fibrosis. American Journal of Respiratory & Critical Care Medicine 1995;152:1659–65.

Ranieri E, Gesualdo L, Grandaliano G, et al. The role of alpha-smooth muscle actin and platelet-derived growth factor-beta receptor in the progression of renal damage in human IgA nephropathy. Journal of Nephrology 2001;14:253–62.

Raymond WA, Leong AS-Y. Assessment of invasion in breast lesions using antibodies to basement membrane component and myoepithelial cells. Pathology 1991;23:291–7.

Santini D, Ceccarelli C, Leone O, et al. Smooth muscle differentiation in normal human ovaries, ovarian stromal hyperplasia and ovarian granulosa-stromal cell tumors. Modern Pathology 1995;8:25–30.

α-1-antichymotrypsin

Sources/clones

Biodesign (8E6, polyclonal),
Biogenesis (polyclonal),
Calbiochem/Novocastra
(monoclonal), Dako (polyclonal),
Fitzgerald (polyclonal).

Fixation/preparation

The antibodies are
immunoreactive in fixed,
paraffin-embedded tissues.
Immunoreactivity is increased
following proteolytic digestion.

Background

α-1-antichymotrypsin (AACT), a
68 kD glycoprotein, is a serum
protease inhibitor which is
synthesized mainly by cells of the
mononuclear phagocytic system.
AACT was initially employed as a
marker of histiocytes
(monocytes/macrophages) but
the demonstration of this enzyme
in a large variety of normal and
neoplastic tissues of both
epithelial and mesenchymal
derivation has resulted in only
restricted use in diagnostic
immunohistology. It most likely
identifies cells that are rich in
phagolysosomes and has no tissue
specificity. Within restricted
settings, AACT can be of value in
diagnostic immunohistology
although, to a large extent, more
specific markers of
histiocytes/macrophages have
replaced this marker.

(See discussion on α-1-
antitrypsin)

NOTES

α-1-antitrypsin

Sources/clones

Axcel/Accurate (polyclonal), Biodesign (1101, 1103), Biogenesis (polyclonal), Biogenex, Biomeda (polyclonal), Chemicon (monoclonal), Calbiochem/Novocastra, Dako (polyclonal), Fitzgerald (polyclonal), Sanbio (F50.4.1, F43.8.1), Sera-Lab (polyclonal), Serotec (polyclonal), Zymed (ZMAAT3).

Fixation/preparation

The antigen is preserved in formalin fixed, paraffin-embedded tissue. Proteolytic digestion increases immunoreactivity but HIER appears unhelpful.

Background

α-1-antitrypsin (AAT), a 51 kD glycoprotein, is mainly synthesized in the liver, where a pair of at least 24 possible codominant alleles, which belong to the protease inhibitor (Pi) locus on chromosome 2, determine production. It functions as an inhibitor of proteases, especially elastase, collagenase and chymotrypsin. Individual homozygous of Pi M produce normal quantities of functionally normal AAT whereas, individuals with abnormal Pi genes such as those designated ZZ, SZ, and PS, have serum concentrations of AAT that are, 40% of normal. Such individuals are at risk for hepatic cirrhosis in childhood or pulmonary emphysema as young adults.

Interest in AAT as an immunohistochemical marker arose in the early 1980s because of the search for a marker of histiocytes (monocytes/macrophages). AAT, α-1-antichymotrypsin (AACT) and muramidase (lysozyme) were touted as specific markers of histiocytes (Isaacson et al, 1981), launching their use as a marker of such cells and malignant tumors derived from them. Monocytes have recently been shown to be another site of synthesis of AAT, short-term cultures of plastic-adherent peripheral blood cells releasing isotopically labeled AAT into the supernatant. AAT was used to distinguish histiocytic from lymphoid neoplasms (Isaacson et al, 1983). In particular, this enzyme was used to characterize a large pleomorphic lymphoma of the intestine as "malignant histiocytosis" (Isaacson et al, 1982). Many studies employed AAT to support the histiocytic differentiation of malignant fibrous histiocytoma and other so-called "fibrohistiocytic" tumors (Meister & Nathrath, 1981; du Boulay 1982; Kindblom et al, 1982; Roholl et al, 1985). As with many previous claims in immunohistochemistry of "specific markers", the initial enthusiasm was soon tempered by caution when it was shown that AAT, AACT and lysozyme immunoreactivity can be commonly found in a large variety of tumors of both epithelial and mesenchymal differentiation. These included carcinoid tumors, malignant melanomas, schwannomas (Permanetter & Meister, 1984; Soini & Miettinen, 1989), islet cell tumors of the pancreas (Ordonez et al, 1983), mixed mesodermal tumor of the ovary (Dictor 1981), uterine sarcomas (Marshall & Braye 1985) and ameloblastoma (Takahashi et al, 1995). The enthusiasm for AAT, AACT and lysozyme as immunohistochemical markers fell off rapidly as this information became more widely known (Dar et al, 1992). Interestingly, the entity of so-called "malignant histiocytosis" in the intestine was soon shown to be of T cell lineage (Isaacson et al, 1985).

Immunoreactivity for this group of proteolytic enzymes may well be a reflection of the intracytoplasmic accumulation of phagolysosomes and do imply histiocytic differentiation.

Applications

AAT, AACT and lysozyme can still provide useful diagnostic information but they have to be used in the context of a panel of antibodies directed to the diagnostic entities considered in differential diagnosis. For example, in pleomorphic tumors of the skin, these markers are useful for the separation of atypical fibroxanthoma from its mimics (Leong & Milios, 1987), although other markers can provide more relevant information to separate such entities (Appendix 1.23), and in identifying tumors rich in phagolysosomes such as granular cell tumors. Immunolabelling for AAT remains an important way of demonstrating the presence of accumulated enzyme within hepatocytes in AAT deficiency (Palmer et al, 1978). Interestingly, it was recently demonstrated that the hepatocyte globules characteristically associated with AAT deficiency may be mimicked by AACT deficiency and distinctinction can only be made by immunolabelling (Thomas et al, 2000); there was not a good correlation between serum levels of these protease inhibitors and the hepatocyte globules. AACT globules should be included in the differential diagnosis of PAS/D-positive hepatocyte inclusions. It has been suggested that the presence of this protease inhibitor is found in thyroid papillary carcinoma but not in normal thyroid tissue, a finding confirmed by Western blotting and immunoprinting (Poblete et al, 1996). Given the elusive nature of specific markers of histiocytes/macrophage differentiation, AAT has still limited application and may be useful in the appropriate histological context.

References

Dar AU, Hird PM, Wagner BE, Underwood JC. Relative usefulness of electron microscopy and immunocytochemistry in tumour diagnosis: 10 years of retrospective analysis. Journal of Clinical Pathology 1992;45:693–6.

Dictor M. alpha-1-antitrypsin in a malignant mixed mesodermal tumor of the ovary. American Journal of surgical Pathology 1981;5:543–50.

Du Boulay. Demonstration of alpha-1-antitrypsin and alpha-1-antichymotrypsin in fibrous histiocytomas using the immunoperoxidase technique. American Journal of Surgical Pathology 19812;6:559–64.

Isaacson PG, Jones DB, Millward-Sadler GH, et al. Alpha-1-antitrypsin in human macrophages. Journal of Clinical Pathology 1981;34:982–90.

Isaacson PG, Jones DB, Sworn MJ, Wright DH. Malignant Histiocytosis of the intestine: report of three cases with immunological and cytochemical analysis. Journal of Clinical Pathology 1982;35:510–16.

Isaacson PG, Jones DB. Immunohistochemical differentiation between histiocytic and lymphoid neoplasms. Histochemical Journal 1983;15:621–35.

Isaacson PG, Spencer J, Connolly CH, et al. Malignant histiocytosis of the intestine: a T cell lymphoma. Lancet 1985;1:688–91.

Kindblom LG, Jacobsen GK, Jacobsen M. Immunohistochemical investigations of tumors of supposed fibroblastic-histiocytic origin. Human Pathology 1982;13:834–40.

Leong AS-Y, Milios J. Atypical fibroxanthoma of the skin: a clinicopathological and immunohistochemical study and a discussion of its histogenesis. Histopathology 1987;11:463–75.

Marshall RJ, Braye SG. Alpha-1-antitrypsin, alpha-1-antichymotrypsin, actin and myosin in uterine sarcomas. International Journal of Gynecological Pathology 1985;4:346–54.

Meister P, Nathrath W. Immunohistochemical characterization of histiocytic tumors. Diagnostic Histopathology 1981;4:79–87.

Ordonez NG, Manning JTJr, Hanssen G. Alpha-1-antitrypsin in islet cell tumors of the pancreas. American Journal of Clinical Pathology 1983;80:277–82.

Palmer PE, Wolfe HJ, Dayal Y, Gang DL. Immunocytochemical diagnosis of alpha-1-antitrypsin deficiency. American Journal of surgical Pathology 1978;2:275–81.

Permanetter W, Meister P. distribution of lysozyme (muramidase) and alpha-1-antichymotrypsin in normal and neoplastic epithelial tissues: a survey. Acta Histochemia 1984;74:173–9.

Poblete MT, Nualart F, del Pozo M, et al. Alpha-1-antitrypsin expression in human thyroid papillary carcinoma. American Journal of Surgical Pathology 1996;20:956–63.

Roholl PJ, Kleyne J, Pijpers HW, van Unnik JA. Comparative immunohistochemical investigation of markers for malignant histiocytes. Human Pathology 1985;16:763–71.

Soini Y, Miettinen M. Alpha-1-antitrypsin and lysozyme. Their limited significance in fibrohistiocytic tumors. American Journal of Clinical Pathology 1989: 91:515–21.

Takahashi H, Tsuda N, Yamabe S, et al. Immunohistochemical detection of alpha 1-antitrypsin, alpha 1-antichymotrypsin, transferrin and ferritin in ameloblastoma. Annals of Cellular Pathology 1995;9:135–50.

Thomas RM, Schiano TD, Kueppers F, Black M. Alpha-1-antichymotrypsin globules within hepatocytes in patients with chronic hepatitis C and cirrhosis. Human Pathology 2000;31:575–57.

NOTES

α-Fetoprotein (AFP)

Source/clones

Accurate, Biodesign (polyclonal), Biogenesis (219–2, BIOAFP003, polyclonal), Biogenex (A-013–01), Bioprobe (F2, C3), Cymbus Bioscience (946.11), Dako (polyclonal), Immunotech (IC5, C3), Pierce (ZGAFP1), Sigma (C3), Zymed (ZSA06, ZMAF2, polyclonal).

Fixation/preparation

The antibody is immunoreactive in routinely prepared sections. HIER enhances staining.

Background

α fetoprotein (AFP) is a glycoprotein composed of 590 amino acid residues. Cells of the embryonic yolk sac, fetal liver and intestinal tract synthesize this glycoprotein. By immunostaining, the antigen is detectable in hepatocellular carcinoma, and gonadal and extragonadal germ cell tumors including yolk sac tumors. It is otherwise not present in adult tissues.

Applications

Staining for AFP is largely used for the identification of the glycoprotein in germ cell tumors and in the separation of hepatocellular carcinoma (HCC) from its mimics such as cholangiocarcinoma and metastatic carcinoma in the liver (Appendix 1.8). Unfortunately, although specific, AFP is of low sensitivity and estimated to be present in no more than 44% of hepatocellular carcinomas (Chedid et al, 1990). Other antibodies employed in a panel may be useful in this context. They include anti-albumin (specific to HCC but not a sensitive marker), cytokeratin 19 (expressed by bile duct epithelium and cholangiocarcinoma), cytokeratin 20 (expressed by both cholangiocarcinoma and gastrointestinal tract tumors), polyclonal CEA (highlights bile canaliculi in HCC but stains the cytoplasm of cholangiocarcinoma and metastatic adenocarcinoma diffusely), alpha-1-antitrypsin (found in HCC but is of low specificity being expressed in various carcinomas) (Leong et al, 1998), sialoglycoproteins such as B72.3 and Leu M1 (found in some metastatic adenocarcinomas) (Fucich et al, 1994; Guindi et al, 1994). Another mimic of HCC is the recently described hepatoid tumor that has immunophenotypic characteristics similar to that of HCC including staining for AFP, canalicular staining for CEA and alpha-1 antitrypsin. Such tumors have been described in the urinary bladder, lung, gastrointestinal tract and focally in germ cells tumors Ishikura, et al, 1990; Sinard et al, 1994) and represent areas of true hepatocellular differentiation.

Comments

We employ clone A-013–01, routinely following HIER.

References

Chedid A, Chejfec G, Eichorst M, et al. Antigenic markers for hepatocellular carcinoma. Cancer 1990;65:84–7.

Fucich LF, Cheles MK, Thung SN, et al. Primary versus metastatic hepatic carcinoma. An immunohistochemical study of 34 cases. Archives of Pathology and Laboratory Medicine 1994;118:927–30.

Guindi M, Yazdi HM, Gilliatt MA. Fine needle aspiration biopsy of hepatocellular carcinoma. Value of immunocytochemical and ultrastructural studies. Acta Cytologica 1994;38:385–91.

Ishikura H, Kanda M, Ito M, et al. Hepatoid adenocarcinoma: a distinctive histological subtype of alpha-fetoprotein producing lung tumor. Virchows Archives A Pathology, Anatomy and Histopathology 1990;417:73–80.

Leong AS-Y, Sormunen RT, Tsui WM-S, Liew CT. Immunostaining for liver cancers. Histopathology 1998;33:318–24.

Leong AS-Y, Liew CT. Needle biopsy diagnosis of hepatocellular carcinoma. In: Hepatocellular carcinoma. Diagnosis, investigation and management. Leong AS-Y, Liew CT, Lau JWY, Johnson PJ (eds). London: Arnold, 1999, pp107–26.

Sinard J, Macleay LJR, Melamed J. Hepatoid adenocarcinoma in the urinary bladder. Unusual localization of a newly recognized tumor type. Cancer 1994;73:1919–25.

Amyloid

Sources/clones

Amyloid-A (AA)

Dako (mc1), polyclonal anti-AA, Calbiochem/Novocastra (polyclonal), Axcel/Accurate (mc1), American Research Products (REU86.2), Biogenesis (polyclonal), Biosource (5G6), Sanbio/Monosan/Accurate (REU86.2)

Transthyretin (ATTR/pre-albumin)

Axcel/Accurate (polyclonal), Biodesign (polyclonal), Biogenesis (polyclonal), Dako (polyclonal).

β2-microglobulin (Aβ2M)

Accurate (FMC16, polyclonal), Accurate/Sigma Chemical (BM63), Advanced Immunochemical (1F10, 2G3, 6G12), American Research Products (1672–18), Biodesign (GJ14, polyclonal), Biogenesis (B2M01), Biosource (MIG-85), Cymbus Bioscience (GJ14, polyclonal), Pharmingen (TU99), Sanbio/Monsan (B2M01), Zymed (Z022).

Amyloid β precursor protein (βAPP)

Boehringer Mannheim (polyclonal), Dako (6F/3D), Zymed (LN27)

Fixation/preparation

These antibodies are applicable to formalin-fixed paraffin-embedded tissue sections.

Background

The amyloidoses are characterized by local, organ-limited or generalized proteinaceous deposits of autologous origin (Glenner, 1980a,1980b). The pattern of distribution, progress of disease and complications are dependent on the fibril protein. Amyloid is characterized by the following: (I) a typical green birefringence with polarized light after Congo red staining, (ii) non-branching linear fibrils with a diameter of 10–12 nm and (iii) an X-ray diffraction pattern which is consistent with Pauling's model of a cross-β fibril (Lansbury, 1992). The diagnosis and classification of amyloidosis requires both histological proof and detection of the amyloid fibril: histochemical confirmation of amyloid deposits using Congo red evaluation in polarized light followed by identification of the fibril protein by immunostaining, thereby revealing the probable underlying disease. Apart from the rare familial syndromes, localized forms of amyloid affect certain organs or lesions (Aβ in brain; calcitonin in medullary carcinoma; islet amyloid polypeptide in insulinomas or islets of Langerhans). The five major different fibril proteins are usually associated with the most common generalized amyloid syndromes: amyloid A (AA), amyloid of λ- (Aλ) and κ- (Aκ) light chains, of transthyretin (ATTR) and β2-microglobulin origin. These fibril proteins may be deposited in a wide variety of tissues and organs (Glenner, 1980a,1980b). They therefore have to be considered in the investigation of any biopsy considered to be amyloidogenic.

Applications

In most instances good correlation is achieved between the immunohistochemical classification of amyloid and the underlying diseases (Röcken et al, 1996). AA-amyloidosis is commonly associated with chronic inflammatory disorders. AL-amyloidosis (either λ- or κ-light chain origin) is linked mainly to the plasma cell dyscrasias or interpreted as being idiopathic. ATTR-amyloidosis is found in cases with familial amyloidosis. AβM-amyloidosis is associated with long-term hemodialysis.

However, a critical issue in the clinicopathological typing of amyloidosis is the interpretation of the immunostaining (Röcken et al, 1996). Occasionally, more than one antibody may show immunostaining of amyloid deposits. Immunohistochemistry detects any associated contaminating component in the amyloid deposit (amyloid P component, apolipoprotein E and glycosaminoglycans) and not merely the currently known obligate fibril proteins. Further, the five syndromic fibril proteins originate from plasma proteins (Glenner, 1980a, 1980b), which may themselves 'contaminate' amyloid deposits. The most critical of these are the immunoglobulin light chains (Röcken et al, 1996). Based on these aberrant staining patterns, Röcken et al have proposed that the identification of a fibril protein with a single antibody, demonstrate an even and homogeneous immunostaining for the entire amyloid deposit; whilst staining of the contaminant protein remains uneven. Instances also arise where two immunoreactive antibodies demonstrate similar uneven staining patterns, interpreted as being due to the irregular presentation of the epitope of the fibril protein resulting in a similar staining pattern as contaminating proteins. These workers strongly recommend testing an additional specimen or biopsy to determine the causative fibril protein. In addition, the correlation of immunohistopathological observations and the clinical diagnosis is also mandatory to arrive at the correct classification of the amyloid fibril.

Another problem area is the false negative detection of amyloid. This can be avoided by increasing the sensitivity of detection by using both immuno- and Congo red-staining methods (Röcken et al, 1996). The latter method of detection is also influenced by the sample quality. It has long been recognized that the diagnostic yield of gastrointestinal biopsies (especially rectal) is extremely high, but should contain submucosa. Other recommended sites include subcutaneous fat, sural nerve, heart, kidney and bone marrow. Whilst AA-amyloidosis is commonly detected in rectal biopsies; any involved organ or tissue is suitable for identification/classification of AL-amyloidosis. Interestingly, a recent study has shown that long-term hemodialysis-associated $\beta 2$-microglobulin amyloid may also involve the gastrointestinal and reproductive systems (Mount et al, 2002) in addition to the usual osteoarticular involvement (Shimizu et al, 1997).

The distinction and classification of amyloidosis has major therapeutic implications, as studies have recommended that AL-amyloidosis be treated with cytotoxic drugs (melphalan and prednisolone), whilst AA-amyloidosis responds better to colchicine and dimethylsulphoxide (Kyle et al, 1985; Ravid et al, 1982).

The role of antibodies against amyloid β precursor protein has assisted in the diagnosis of Alzheimer's disease (Iwamoto et al, 1997) and early detection of axonal injury (Sherriff et al, 1994) in the brain. Antibodies to transthyretin amyloid protein are useful in the diagnosis of cardiac amyloidosis (Jacobson et al, 1997) and familial amyloidotic polyneuropathy (Sousa et al, 2001).

References

Glenner GG. Amyloid deposits and amyloidosis. The β-fibrilloses. New England Journal of Medicine 1980a;302:1283–92.

Glenner GG. Amyloid deposits and amyloidosis. The β-fibrilloses. New England Journal of Medicine 1980b;302:1333–43.

Iwamoto N, Nishiyama E, Ohwada J, Arai H. Distribution of amyloid deposits in the cerebral white matter of the Alzheimer's disease brain: relationship to blood vessels. Acta Neuropathologica (Berlin) 1997;93:334–40.

Jacobson DR, Pastore RD, Yaghoubian R et al. Variant-sequence transthyretin (isoleucine 122) in late-onset cardiac amyloidosis in Black Americans. New England Journal of Medicine 1997;336:466–73.

Kyle RA, Greipp RP, Garton JP et al. Primary systemic amyloidosis: Comparison of melphalan/prednisolone versus colchicine. American Journal of Medicine 1985;79:708–16.

Lansbury PT Jr. In pursuit of the molecular structure of amyloid plaque: New technology provides unexpected and critical information. Biochemistry 1992;31:6865–70.

Mount SL, Eltabbakh GH, Hardin NJ. Beta-2 microglobulin amyloidosis presenting as bilateral ovarian masses: a case report and review of the literature. American Journal of Surgical Pathology 2002;26:130–3.

Sousa MM, Cardoso I, Fernandes R, et al. Deposition of transthyretin in early stages of familial amyloidotic polyneuropathy: evidence for toxicity of non fibrillar aggregates. American Journal of Pathology 2001;159:1993–2000.

Ravid M, Shapiro J, Lang R et al. Prolonged dimethylsulphoxide treatment in 13 patients with systemic amyloidosis. Annals of Rheumatic Diseases 1982;41:587–92.

Röcken C, Schwotzer EB, Linke RP, Saeger W. The classification of amyloid deposits in clinicopathological practice. Histopathology 1996;29:325–35.

Sherriff FE, Bridges LR, Sivaloganathan S. Early detection of axonal injury after human head trauma using immunocytochemistry for beta-amyloid precursor protein. Acta Neuropathologica (Berlin) 1994;87:55–62.

Shimizu M, Manabe T, Matsumoto T et al. β_2 Microglobulin haemodialysis related amyloidosis: distinctive gross features of gastrointestinal involvement. Journal of Clinical Pathology 1997;50:873–5.

Androgen receptor

Sources/clones

Accurate (polyclonal), Biogenex (F39.4.1), Novocastra (2F12, polyclonal), Pharmingen (G122–25.3, G122–434, G122–77.14, AN1–15), Sanbio/Monosan (F39.4.1).

Fixation/preparation

The antibodies are immunoreactive in frozen sections, cell preparations and paraffin-embedded sections; HIER enhances the latter.

Background

The intracellular action of androgens is mediated by the androgen receptor, which is a key element of the androgen signal transduction cascade and a target of endocrine therapy for prostatic carcinoma. Qualitative and quantitative alterations of androgen receptor expression in prostatic carcinomas and their possible implications for tumor progression and treatment are therefore of diagnostic and research interest. Findings in prostatic tumor cell lines of rat and human origin suggest that reduction of androgen receptor protein expression is accompanied by an increase in tumor aggressiveness. However, immunohistochemical analysis and binding assays have demonstrated the presence of androgen receptors in all histological types of prostatic carcinoma and in both therapy-responsive and well as therapy-unresponsive tumors

Applications

Much of the immunohistochemical studies of androgen receptors have been related to prostatic carcinoma and experimental animals. The androgen receptor content of prostatic carcinoma has been inversely correlated to Gleason grade in stage D2 carcinomas, although it was unrelated to extent of disease and response to hormonal therapy at three months. Patients with 48% or more androgen receptor-positive cells had statistically significant better outcome in terms of both progression-free and cause-specific survival (Takeda et al, 1996). Another study suggested that pretreatment androgen receptor expression alone is not related to prognosis of hormonally treated prostate cancer; however, when combined with bcl-2 expression, it acts as an independent prognostic factor for clinical progression (Noordzij et al, 1997). One explanation for the discrepancy in findings may relate to the mutations that occur in the androgen receptor, which account for the variable response to hormonal therapy. These mutations produce broadened ligand specificity so that transcriptional-factor activity of the receptor can be stimulated not just by dihydrotestosterone but also by estradiol and other androgen metabolites. Such activation of mutant androgen receptors by estrogen and weak androgens could confer on prostate cancer cells an ability to survive testicular androgen ablation through the activation of the androgen receptor by adrenal androgens or exogenous estrogen. Thus, mutated androgen receptors that occur prior to therapy may characterize a more aggressive disease (Hakimi et al, 1996).

The variability of androgen receptor protein content per unit nuclear area has been shown to increase with increasing histological grade, suggesting that this variability might account for the variable response to endocrine therapy in high grade tumors (Magi-Galluzzi et al, 1997). The extent of heterogeneity of androgen receptor expression may be a useful indicator of response to hormonal therapy (Klocker et al, 1994).

Immunostaining for androgen receptor expression has been studied in other cell types including endometrium (Mettens et al, 1996), genital melanocytes (Tadokoro et al, 1997), meningiomas (Carroll et al, 1995), most bone marrow cells other than erythroid and lymphoid cells (Mantalaris et al, 2001) and urinary bladder carcinomas (Zhuang et al, 1997). Salivary duct carcinoma, a rare aggressive tumor that bears resemblance to invasive ductal carcinoma of the breast shows frequent staining for androgen receptor making this a possible diagnostic discriminator (Hoang et al, 2001; Moriki et al, 2001). Androgen receptor staining has been demonstrated in 45% of adenocarcinomas and 21% of squamous carcinomas of the esophagus. There was no suggestion of difference between male and female patients (Tihan et al, 2001). These findings raise the possibility of anti-androgen therapy in such tumors.

Comments

The receptor is intra-nuclear in location. A cut-off of 10% androgen receptor-positive cells has been suggested to maximize assay prognostic efficiency with 48% positivity showing

significant correlation with response, time to progression and survival, but not with grade or stage of prostatic cancer (Pertschuk et al, 1994). Clone G122–25 is immunoreactive in fixed, paraffin-embedded tissue sections and does not appear to cross-react with estrogen or progesterone receptors.

References

Carroll RS, Zhang J, Dashmner K, et al. Androgen receptor expression in meningiomas. Journal Neurosurgery 1995;82:453–60.

Hakimi JM, Rondinelli RH, Schoenberg MP, Barrack ER. Androgen-receptor gene structure and function in prostate cancer. World Journal of Urology 1996;14:329–37.

Hoang MP, Callender DL, Sola Gallego JJ, et al. Molecular and biomarker analyses of salivary duct carcinomas: comparison with mammary duct carcinoma. International Journal of Oncology 2001;19:865–71.

Kloker H, Culig Z, Hobisch A, et al. Androgen receptor alterations in prostatic carcinoma. Prostate 1994;25:266–73.

Magi-Galluzzi C, Xu X, Hlatky L, et al. Heterogeneity of androgen receptro content in advanced prostate cancer. Modern Pathology 1997;10:839–45.

Mantalaris A, Panoskaltsis N, Sakai Y, et al. Localization of androgen receptor expression in human bone marrow. Journal of Pathology 2001;193:361–6.

Mertens HJ, Heineman MJ, Koudstaal J, et al. Androgen receptor content in human endometrium.

European Journal of Obstetrics, Gynecology and Reproductive Biology 1996;70:11–13.

Moriki T, Ueta S, Takashi T, et al. Salivary duct carcinoma: cytologic characteristics and application of androgen receptor immunostaining for diagnosis. Cancer 2001;93:344–50.

Noordzij MA, Bogdanowicz JF, van Krimpen C, et al. The prognostic value of pretreatment expression of androgen receptor and bcl-2 in hormonally treated prostate cancer patients. Journal of Urology 1997;158:1880–4.

Pertschuk LP, Macchia RJ, Feldman JG, et al. Immunocytochemical assay for androgen receptors in prostate cancer: a prospective study of 63 cases with long-term follow-up. Annals of Surgical Oncology 1994;1:495–503.

Tadokoro T, Itami S, Hosokawa K, et al. Human genital melanocytes as androgen target cells. Journal of Investigative Dermatology 1997;109:513–7.

Takeda H, Akakura K, Masai M, et al. Androgen receptor content of prostate carcinoma cells estimated by immunohistochemistry is related to prognosis of patients with stage D2 prostate carcinoma. Cancer 1996;77:934–40.

Tihan T, Harmon JW, Wan X, et al. Evidence of androgen receptor expression in squamous and adenocarcinoma of the esophagus. Anticancer Research 2001;21:3107–14.

Zhuang YH, Blauer M, Tammela T, Tuohimaa P. Immunodetection of androgen receptor in human urinary bladder cancer. Histopathology 1997;30:556–62.

Anti-apoptosis

Sources/clones

Dako (BM-1), Oncor (Apop Tag), Monosan (Annexin V – polyclonal), Pharmingen (APO-BRDU, Annexin V-FITC).

Fixation/preparation

Various methods of detection of apoptotic bodies are available. All methods can be used on formalin-fixed, paraffin-embedded tissue sections. Some require proteolytic digestion. Acetone-fixed cryostat sections and fixed cell smears may also be used.

Background

Cell death may occur by necrosis or apoptosis. Necrosis results from direct physical or chemical damage to the plasma membrane or disturbances in the osmotic balance of a cell (Wyllie et al, 1980). With the entrance of extracellular fluid into the cell, resultant cell swelling and lysis precedes a subsequent inflammatory response. Furthermore, necrosis affects groups of cells, with consequent disruption of normal tissue architecture.

In contrast to necrosis, apoptotic cell death is a highly regulated physiologic process. The balance between apoptosis and cell proliferation results in the maintenance of cell homeostasis (Kerr et al, 1972). Apoptotic bodies are rapidly engulfed by neighboring cells or macrophages, without an inflammatory response being elicited. The nuclear structure alteration in apoptotic cells is induced by endonuclease DNA cleavage that results in the generation of large 50–300 kb fragments. This produces the characteristic DNA "ladders" of apoptosis as viewed on agarose gel electrophoresis (Oberhammer et al, 1993).

Recently, reliable methods have been developed that enable the rapid assessment of apoptosis on sections prepared from paraffin-embedded material, e.g., the TUNEL method for TdT-mediated dUTP-biotin nick end labeling (Sarkiss et al, 1996). The APO-BRDU kit utilizes the same principle. The enzyme TdT is used to catalyze a template independent addition of bromolated deoxyribonucleotide triphosphates (Br-dUTP) to the 3'-hydroxyl ends of the numerous fragments of double- and single-stranded DNA present in apoptotic cells. This allows the labeling of the very high concentrations of 3'-OH ends that are localized in apoptotic bodies. Br-dUTP is claimed to be more readily incorporated into the genome of apoptotic cells than are deoxyribonucleotide triphosphates complexed to larger ligands like fluorescein, biotin or digoxigenin (Nagata & Golstein, 1995). Although rather specific for cells undergoing apoptosis, these techniques may also label cells undergoing necrosis. However, this is seldom a problem since the distinction between focal apoptotic events and necrosis is fairly clear. The histologic features of apoptosis include cell shrinkage and loss of junctional contact resulting in a "halo" around the cell. The nucleus shows condensation and margination of the chromatin. This is followed by the fragmentation or "pinching off" of pieces of nuclear material, which are surrounded by cytoplasm with intact cytoplasmic organelles as shown at ultrastructural level, These apoptotic fragments of pyknotic nuclear material and cytoplasm are phagocytosed by adjacent cells or macrophages. Apoptotic cells have been called by various names in different tissues and include "Councilman bodies", "Civatte bodies", "necrobiotic cells" and "nuclear dust".

The BM-1 antibody is directed to the Lewis[y] antigen, which has been identified phenotypically as a marker of specific types of cells, and possibly specific stages of differentiation. Lewis[y] is totally absent at the morula stage, but is highly expressed on the blastocyst surface and has been shown to play a role in the implantation process (Fenderson et al, 1991). Recently, Lewis[y] has been identified as a characteristic of cells undergoing apoptosis (Hiraishi et al, 1993). In Lewis[y] positive areas of tissue sections, typical apoptotic morphological changes and DNA fragmentation were frequently observed in certain loci, although not all Lewis[y] positive cells showed such signs of apoptosis. Although the BM-1 antibody against the Lewis[y] antigen is reputed to detect apoptotic cells, further studies to test its efficacy, including a comparative analysis with the in-situ end labeling techniques, is awaited.

Another method of detection of apoptotic bodies is the use of Annexin V, which is a 35–36 kD Ca^{2+}-dependent phospholipid-binding protein that has a high affinity for the membrane phospholipid phosphatidylserine (PS). In apoptotic cells, PS is translocated from the inner to the outer leaflet of the plasma membrane, thereby exposing PS to the external cellular environment allowing its binding to Annexin V. Binding to a signal system such as fluorescein isothiocyanate allows the easy identification of apoptotic cells (in frozen sections and cell preparations). Annexin V is thought to identify cells at an earlier stage of apoptosis than assays based on DNA fragmentation because externalization of PS occurs earlier than the nuclear changes associated with apoptosis (Raynal & Pollard, 1994).

Applications

BM-1 antibody may be applied to neoplasms in general to assess the apoptotic index, e.g., endometrial adenocarcinoma (Kuwashima et al, 1995). Recently, apoptosis has been considered to be a key event in oncogenesis, e.g., apoptosis has been reported to be promoted by tumor-suppressor gene p53 and inhibited by oncogene *bcl-2* (Arends & Wyllie, 1991). Although apparent cell loss by apoptosis occurs in carcinomatous tissue (Hiraishi et al, 1993), the physiological significance is unclear (Umansky 1982). BM-1 positivity has been found to be as high as 25–35% in T cells of lymph nodes of patients with AIDS-related complex (ARC), in contrast to healthy controls that were less than 5% (Adachi et al, 1988).

Comments

Strong BM-1 immunoreactivity is observed in the apical surface of tubular urothelium, basal cells (glandular foveoli) of gastric and esophageal mucosa, and these tissues may be employed as controls.

The optimal method for the identification of apoptotic cells depends on the experimental system and the mode of induction of apoptosis. The degree of DNA degradation can vary according to the cell type, the nature of the inducing agent and the stage of apoptosis.

Several other methods of assessing apoptosis in paraffin-embedded sections are available and they include cyclin D1, bcl-2, MDM2, p53, Fas (CD95), c-kit (CD117), and CD40L, some of these being of relevance as prognostic markers (Bukholm et al, 2002). Antibodies to all of these proteins are separately discussed under their respective headings. In addition, antibodies to Bcl-X, Bax and Bak can also be used to study apoptosis.

Bcl-X protein is a member of the Bcl-2 oncoprotein family that functions as apoptosis protective proteins (Chao & Korsmeyer, 1998) and is overexpressed in 60% of carcinomas and 50% of adenomas compared to normal epithelial cells of adjacent mucosa (Krajewska et al, 1996). The polyclonal antibody to Bcl-X is available through Dako (A3535).

The Bax protein belongs to a family of proteins that share homology with Bcl-2 oncoprotein in several highly conserved regions. Overexpression of Bax functions to promote cell death through apoptosis. It has been suggested that the relative expression of the different Bcl-2 family proteins controls the sensitivity of cells to apoptotic stimuli. A polyclonal anti-Bax is available through Dako (A3533) and is immunoreactive in paraffin sections following HIER. The protein is located in the cytoplasm and stains a granular, punctate pattern. The Bak protein is another member of the Bcl-2 family that functions in the regulation of apoptosis. The Bak protein binds Bcl-x and Bcl-2 and is thought to induce apoptosis by counteracting the apoptotic protective effects of

Bcl-x and Bcl-2. Altered levels of Bak expression have been reported in *H. pylori* infected tissues and may have a role in the development of gastric mucosa-associated lymphoid tissue (MALT) lymphoma through its interaction with helicobacter-induced expression of Bcl-x (Morgner et al, 2001). Anti-Bak is available through Dako (A3538). These Bcl-2 family proteins have been employed as prognostic markers in a variety of epithelial (Trask et al, 2002; Schelweiss et al, 2002; Sjostrom et al, 2002; Hsia et al, 2001; Evans et al, 2001; and soft tissue tumors (Dan'ura et al, 2002) with varying degrees of success.

The application of multiple methods, each based on a different feature of the apoptotic process, may provide more information about the cell population than any one method would give alone.

References:

Adachi M, Hayami M, Kashlwagi N, et al. Expression of le^y antigen in human immunodeficiency virus-infected human T cell lines and in peripheral lymphocytes of patients with acquired immune deficiency syndrome (AIDS) and AIDS-related complex (ARC). Journal of Experimental Medicine 1988;167:233–331.

Arends MJ, Wyllie AH. Apoptosis: mechanism and roles in pathology. International Reviews in Experimental Pathology 1991;32:223–54.

Bukholm IR, Bukholm G, Nesland JM. Reduced expression of both Bax abd Bcl-2 is independently associated with lymph node metastasis in human breast carcinomas. APMIS 2002;110:214–20.

Chao DT, Korsmeyer SJ. Bcl-2 family: regulators of cell death. Annual Reviews in Immunology 1998;16:395–419.

Dan'ura T, Kawai A, Morimoto Y, et al. Apoptosis and expression of its regulatory proteins in soft tissue sarcomas. Cancer Letters 2002;178:167–74.

Evans JD, Cornford PA, Dodson A, et al. Detailed tissue expression of bcl-2, bax, bak, and bcl-x in the normal human pancreas and in chronic pancreatitis, ampullary and prancreatic ductal adenocarcinomas. Pancreatology 2001;1:254–62.

Fenderson BA, Killma N, Stroud MR, et al. Specific interaction between Le^y and H as a possible basis for trophectoderm-endometrium recognition during implantation. Glycoconjugate Journal 1991;8:179 (Abstract 8.5).

Hiraishi K, Suzuki K, Hakomori S, Adachi M. Le^y antigen expression is correlated with apoptosis (programmed cell death). Glycobiology 1993;3:381–90.

Hsia JY, Chen CY, Hsu CP, et al. Expression of apoptosis-regulating proteins p53, Bcl-2, and Bax in primary resected esophageal squamous cell carcinoma. Neoplasma 2001;48:483–8.

Kerr JFR, Wyllie AH, Currie AR. Apoptosis: a basic biological phenomenon with wider ranging implications in tissue kinetics. British Journal of Cancer 1972;26:239–57.

Krajewska M, Moss SF, Krajewski S, et al. Elevated expression of bcl-x and reduced Bak in primary colorectal adenocarcinomas. Cancer Research 1996;56:2422–7.

Kuwashima Y, Uehara T, Kishi K, et al. Proliferative and apoptotic status in endometrial adenocarcinoma. International Journal of Gynecological Pathology 1995;14:45–9.

Morgner A, Sutton P, O'Rourke JL, et al. Helicobacter-induced expression of Bcl-X(L) in B lymphocytes in the mouse model: a possible step in the development of gastric mucosa-associated lymphoid tissue (MALT) lymphoma. International Journal of Cancer 2001;92:634–40.

Nagata S, Golstein P. The Fas death factor. Science 1995;267:1445–9.

Oberhammer F, Wilson JW, Dive C, et al. Apoptotic death in epithelial cells: cleavage of DNA to 300 and/or kb fragments prior to or in the absence of internucleosomal fragmentation. EMBO Journal 1993;12:679–84.

Raynal P, Pollard HB. Annexins. The problem of assessing the biological role for a gene family of multifunctional calcium and phospholipid-binding proteins. Journal of Biological Chemistry 1994;265:4923–8.

Sarkiss M, Hsu B, El-Naggar AK, McDonnell TJ. The clinical relevance and assessment of apoptotic cell death. Advances in Anatomical Pathology 1996;3:205–11.

Schelwies K, Sturm I, Grabowski P, et al. Analysis of p53/BAX in primary colorectal carcinoma: low BAX protein expression is a negative prognostic factor in UICC stage III tumors. International Journal of Cancer 2002;99:589–96.

Sjostrom J, Blomqvist C, von Boguslawski K, et al. The predictive value of bcl-2, bax, bcl-xL, bag-1, fas, and fasL for chemotherapy response in advanced breast cancer. Clinical Cancer Research 2002;8:811–6.

Trask DK, Wolf GT, Bradford CR, et al. Expression of Bcl-2 family proteins in advanced laryngeal squamous cell carcinoma: correlation with response to chemotherapy and organ preservation. Laryngoscope 2002;112:638–44.

Umansky SR. The genetic program of cell death: Hypothesis and some applications: transformation, carcinogenesis, and aging. Journal of Theoretical Biology 1982;97:591–602.

Wyllie AH, Kerr JFR, Currie AR. Cell death: the significance of apoptosis. International Reviews in Cytology 1980;68:251–306.

NOTES

Anti-p80 (ALK-NMP fusion protein)

Sources/clones

Dako (monoclonal antibody ALK1, ALKc, polyclonal p80).

Fixation/preparation

All three antibodies are reactive in routine formalin-fixed, paraffin-embedded tissues and work best with heat-induced epitope retrieval systems.

Background

Anaplastic large cell lymphoma (ALCL) is characterized by a proliferation of predominantly large lymphoid cells infiltrating in a distinctive pattern and with strong expression of CD30 a cytokine receptor. Three types of ALCL are now recognized based on the expression of the anaplastic lymphoma kinase (ALK) protein, namely ALK+ primary systemic ALCL, ALK– primary systemic ALCL and ALK–primary cutaneous ALCL. ALK expression is characterized by chromosomal translocations, the most common of which is t(2;5) (p23;q35). The cloned gene, located at the breakpoint on chromosome 2p23, was named "anaplastic lymphoma kinase" (ALK) after the tumor type from which it was discovered (Morris et al, 1994). ALK is closely related to leukocyte receptor tyrosine kinase, but is not expressed in normal lymphoid cells (Morris et al, 1997). The t(2;5) results in the fusion of the *ALK* and *NPM* genes, producing a chimeric protein comprising the amino-terminal of *NPM* linked to the entire intracytoplasmic domain of *ALK*. As a result of the gene fusion, the *NPM* gene forces the expression of *ALK*.

The ALK1 antibody is raised against a fragment of the cytoplasmic portion of ALK protein (Pulford et al, 1997). The ALKc antibody is raised against the full-length NPM-ALK chimeric protein, but reacts specifically with the intracytoplasmic region of ALK. ALK1, ALKc and p80 antiserum all react with both the ALK protein and the NPM-ALK fusion protein expressed by t(2;5)-positive ALCL. Normal cells consistently lack immunohistochemical expression of ALK, with the exception of occasional cells in the central nervous system. Hence, a positive ALK immunoreactivity strongly correlates with the presence of t(2;5) translocation. ALK expression is highly restricted in lymphomas, observed in two types: ALCL with t(2;5) or variant translocation, and a rare large B-cell lymphoma expressing the full-length ALK protein (staining in the form of coarse cytoplasmic granules, but not in the nuclei) in the absence of t(2;5) (Chan, 1998). Staining for ALK in ALCL should be observed in both the nuclei and cytoplasm of neoplastic lymphoid cells. In approximately 15–28% of ALK-positive ALCL, the staining is confined to the cytoplasm and/or cell membrane. This abnormal pattern of staining represents variant translocations in which the *ALK* gene fuses to a partner other than *NMP* to produce variant X-ALK+ proteins (Stein et al, 2000)). Such variants include t(1;2), t(2;3), t(2;22) and inv (2). It is of pathogenic significance that all chimeric ALK variants contain the same functional domain of ALK as that present in the NPM-ALK protein. The lack of nuclear localisation signals in all fusion proteins other than NPM-ALK accounts for the absence of these proteins in the nucleus and their cytoplasmic distribution only. Patients with ALK+ ALCL appear to benefit from chemotherapy more than those with ALK- forms of systemic ALCL.

Although various carcinomas, sarcomas and miscellaneous tumors have tested negative for

ALK (Pulford et al, 1997), recent evidence has shown ALK to be implicated in the genesis of inflammatory myofibroblastic tumors (IMT). The recurrent involvement of chromosome 2p22–24 in approximately 50% of reported cases led to fluorescence in situ hybridization studies confirming involvement of the *ALK* gene (Griffin et al, 1999). The spindle cells were further demonstrated to be immunoreactive for ALK protein. These findings have been confirmed in a subsequent study (Coffin et al, 2001) showing abnormalities of *ALK* and p80 (with chromosomal rearrangements of 2p23) in a significant proportion of IMTs (about 40%) involving the abdomen and lung in the first decade of life and associated with a higher frequency of recurrence. An independent study (Chan et al, 2001) also implicated ALK in a proportion of IMT but associated with a favorable outcome. The latter study also showed ALK to be negative in pulmonary and lymph node IMTs and the rare EBV-positive and hepatosplenic IMT with follicular dendritic cells. Rhabdomyosarcoma and neuroblastoma have, to date, been the only other tumors that displayed immunoexpression of the ALK protein (Morris et al, 1994; Lamant et al, 2000), the latter tumor showing rearrangement of the 2p23 region where the *ALK* gene is located (Lamant et al, 2000)

Applications

Identification of the ALK+ ALCL recognizes a subgroup of ALCL with a highly favorable prognosis, eminently curable by chemotherapy. The ALK-positive immunoreaction also helps distinguish a subset ALCL from peripheral T-cell lymphomas and Hodgkin's lymphoma. It is also useful to identify early or subtle relapse of ALK-positive lymphomas. Primary cutaneous ALCLs are ALK-negative, helping to distinguish from primary systemic ALCL presenting in the skin (Chan, 1998).

ALK staining can also potentially be used in the differential diagnosis of IMT from mimics such as leiomyosarcoma and nodular fasciitis, which are both negative for ALK (Lawrence et al, 2000).

Comments

Although ALK1 and ALKc antibodies appear to react with different epitopes of the ALK protein, they produce an identical immunoreaction (Chan, 1998). Normal and reactive lymphocytes consistently lack immunoreactivity for ALK, resulting in the absence of an internal positive control.

Immunolocalisation of ALK protein is in the nucleus and cytoplasm. Other sites of localisation such as the cytoplasm alone suggest a variant translocation of the *ALK* gene.

References

Chan JKC. Anaplastic large cell lymphoma: redefining its morphologic spectrum and importance of recognition of the ALK-positive subset. Advances in Anatomical Pathology 1998;5:281–313.

Chan JKC, Cheuk W, Shimizu M. Anaplastic lymphoma kinase expression in inflammatory pseudotumors. American Journal of Surgical Pathology 2001;25:761–8.

Cheuk W, Chan JKC. Timely topic: Anaplastic lymphoma kinase (ALK) spreads its influence. Pathology 2001;33:7–12.

Coffin CM, Patel A, Perkins S, et al. ALK2 and p80 expression and chromosomal rearrangements involving 2p23 in inflammatory myofibroblastic tumor. Modern Pathology 2001;14:569–76.

Griffin CA, Hawkins AL, Dvorak C, et al. Recurrent involvement of 2p23 in inflammatory myofibroblastic tumors. Cancer Research 1999;59:2776–80.

Lamant L, Pulford K, Bischof D, et al. Expression of the ALK tyrosine kinase gene in neuroblastoma. American Journal of Pathology 2000;156:1711–21.

Lawrence B, Perez-Atayde A, Hibbard MK, et al. TPM3-ALK and TPM4-ALK oncogenes in inflammatory myofibroblastic tumors. American Journal of Pathology 2000;157:377–84.

Morris SW, Kirstein MN, Valentine MB, et al. Fusion of a kinase gene, ALK, to a nucleolar protein gene, NPM, in non-Hodgkin's lymphoma. Science 1994;63:1281–4.

Morris SW, Naeve C, Matthew P, et al. ALK, the chromosome 2 gene locus altered by the t(2;5) in non-Hodgkin's lymphoma, encodes a novel neural receptor tyrosine kinase that is highly related to leukocyte tyrosine kinase (LTK). Oncogene 1997;14:2175–88.

Pulford K, Lamant L, Morris SW, et al: Detection of anaplastic lymphoma kinase (ALK) and nucleolar protein nucleophosmin (NPM)-ALK proteins in normal and neoplastic cells with the monoclonal antibody ALK1. Blood 1997;9:1394–04.

Stein H, Foss HD, Durkop H, et al, CD30(+) anaplastic large cell lymphoma: a review of its histopathologic, genetic, and clinical features. Blood 2000;96:3681–95.

Bcl-2

Sources/clones

Dako (124), Immunotech (124), Zymed (BCL2–100).

Fixation/preparation

Antibodies to bcl-2 are reasonably robust and work very well on paraffin-embedded tissue. Staining is not too dependent on fixation protocols and good results may be obtained with formalin-fixed, B5-fixed, methacarn-fixed and fresh frozen tissues. Staining is significantly enhanced by the use of antigen retrieval with either microwave or pressure-cooking pretreatment. The bcl-2 antibody may be used for labeling acetone-fixed cryostat sections or fixed cell smears.

Background

The bcl-2 gene was identified more than a decade ago with the discovery and analysis of the t(14; 18) (q32; q21) translocation (Bakhshi et al, 1985). This translocation occurs in 70–80% of follicular lymphoma, comprising juxtaposition of the bcl-2 gene with the immunoglobulin heavy chain (IgH) gene on chromosome 14q32 (Chen–Levy et al, 1989). This results in an overexpression of the translocated bcl-2 allele induced by enhancers in the IgH region; although the translocation is not a prerequisite for bcl-2 protein expression, since this occurs in many cases without this rearrangement (Pezzella et al, 1990). The bcl-2 polypeptide is a 26 kD protein that is found on intracellular (mitochondrial and nuclear) membranes and in the cytosol (on the smooth endoplasmic reticulum), rather than on the cell surface. bcl-2 is not an oncogene and has no effect on cell replication. bcl-2 protein does however, prevent cells from undergoing apoptosis conferring a survival advantage on cell harbouring the t(14; 18) translocation. In normal lymphoid tissue, bcl-2 antibody reacts with small B lymphocytes in the mantle zone and many cells within T cell areas. In the thymus many cells in the medulla are stained, with weak/negative reaction in the cortex (Chetty et al, 1997).

Applications

The initial diagnostic application of bcl-2 immunostaining was for the distinction of reactive follicular lymphoid hyperplasia from follicular lymphoma (Cooper & Haffajee, 1996; Veloso et al, 1995). Positive staining is cytoplasmic in location. Follicular lymphomas show striking bcl-2 expression in neoplastic follicles, whilst only isolated individual cells within the reactive follicle centers are positive (mostly T-cells). This difference in staining pattern is not due to down regulation or decreased bcl-2 mRNA, but largely to a post-translational mechanism that results in decreased protein levels. Furthermore, bcl-2 protein expression is demonstrated in all grades of follicle center cell lymphomas in both small and large cells (Cooper & Haffajee, 1997). Strongly bcl-2 positive lymphoid aggregates in the bone marrow of patients previously diagnosed with nodal follicular lymphoma are indicative of lymphoma involvement (Chetty et al, 1995). However, there is no practical value of applying the bcl-2 antibody for classification of a malignant lymphoid infiltrate, since many different lymphoma types can be bcl-2 positive. Nevertheless, it has been demonstrated that non-Hodgkin's lymphoma with bcl-2 expression had a significantly higher relapse rate and a lower cause-specific survival than in those without (Hill et al, 1996). Bcl-2 immunostaining together with

CD10, CD5, CD20 and CD23 has been shown to be useful in identifying follicular lymphoma in bone marrow biopsies (West et al, 2002)

Expression of bcl-2 has been studied in many epithelial neoplasms (Graflund et al, 2002; Uchida et al, 2002) and attempts have been made to correlate bcl-2 expression with survival. In general, better prognoses accompany bcl-2 positive neoplasms than negative ones, with some prostatic cancers being the exception to the rule (Colombel et al, 1993; Banerjee et al, 2002). A reciprocal relationship has been demonstrated between bcl-2 reactivity and p53 overexpression in 65% of colorectal neoplasia, with a bcl-2 +ve/p53 -ve subgroup showing a strong correlation with negative lymph node status, implying a less aggressive pathway of neoplastic transformation (Kaklamanis et al, 1996). A similar reciprocal relationship was shown in acute leukemias (Klobusicka et al, 2001); whereas, a dissociated immunoexpression of bcl-2 and Ki-67 was demonstrated in endometrial benign and malignant lesions (Risberg et al, 2002). Bcl-2 protein was also detected in all grades of cervical intraepithelial neoplasia, with a striking increase in the number of positive cells with increasing severity of CIN, in combination with a mild increase in staining intensity (Harmsel et al, 1996).

Bcl-2 expression has been demonstrated in 79 per cent (15 of 19 cases) of synovial sarcoma (Hirakawa et al, 1996), but was negative in 20 leiomyosarcomas, 4 malignant peripheral nerve sheath tumors and 4 fibrosarcomas.

However, in another study, bcl-2 protein was expressed in 7 rhabdomyosarcomas and 5/7 leiomyosarcomas, 4 epithelioid leiomyomas and 6/14 leiomyomas (Soini et al, 1996). Bcl-2 family proteins have been shown to modulate radiosensitivity in malignant glioma cells (Streffer et al, 2002)

References

Bakhshi A, Jensen JP, Goldman P, et al. Cloning the chromosomal breakpoint of t(14; 18) human lymphomas: clustering around J_H on chromosome 14 near a transcriptional unit on chromosome 18. Cell 1985;41:899–906.

Banerjee PP, Banerjee S, Brown TR. Bcl-2 protein expression correlates with cell survival and androgen independence in rat prostatic lobes. Endocrinology 2002;143:1825–32.

Chen-Levy Z, Nourse J, Cleary ML. The bcl-2 candidate protooncogene is a 24 kilodalton integral-membrane protein highly expressed in lymphoid cell lines and lymphomas carrying the t(14; 18) translocation. Molecular and Cell Biology 1989;9:701–10.

Chetty R, Echezarreta G, Comley M, Gatter K. Immunohistochemistry in apparently normal bone marrow trephine specimens from patients with nodal follicular lymphoma. Journal of Clinical Pathology 1995;48:1035–38.

Chetty R, Dada MA, Gatter KC. bcl-2: Longevity personified. Advances in Anatomic Pathology 1997;4:134–8.

Colombel M, Symmans F, Gill S, et al. Detection of the apoptosis-suppressing oncoprotein bcl-2 in hormone refractory human prostate cancer. American Journal of Pathology 1993;143:390–400.

Cooper K, Haffajee Z. bcl-2 Immunohistochemistry distinguishes follicular lymphoma from follicular hyperplasia in formalin-fixed tissue with microwave antigen retrieval. Journal of Cellular Pathology 1996;1:52–6.

Cooper K, Haffajee Z. bcl-2 and p53 protein expression in follicular lymphoma. Journal of Pathology 1997;182:307–10.

Graflund M, Sorbe B, Karlsson M. MIB-1, p53, bcl-2 and WAF-1 expression in pelvic lymph nodes and primary tumors in early stage cervical carcinomas. Correlation with clinical outcome. International Journal of Oncology 2002;20:1041–7.

Harmsel BT, Smedts F, Kruijpers J, Jeunink M, Trimbos B, Ramaekers F. bcl-2 immunoreactivity increases with severity of CIN: a study of normal cervical epithelia, CIN, and cervical carcinoma. Journal of Pathology 1996;179:26–30.

Hill ME, MacLennan KA, Cunningham DC, et al. Prognostic significance of BCL-2 expression and bcl-2 major breakpoint region rearrangement in diffuse large cell non-Hodgkin's lymphoma: A British National Lymphoma investigation study. Blood 1996;88:1046–51.

Hirakawa N, Naka T, Yamamoto I, Fukuda T, Tsuneyoshi M. Overexpression of bcl-2 protein in synovial sarcomas. Human Pathology 1996;27:1060–5.

Kaklamanis L, Savage A, Mortensen N, et al. Early expression of bcl-2 protein in the adenoma-carcinoma sequence of colorectal neoplasia. Journal of Pathology 1996;179:10–14.

Kl0busicka M, Kusenda J, Babusikova O. Expression of p53 and bcl-2 proteins in acute leukemias: an immunocytochemical study. Neoplasma 2002;48:489–95.

Pezzella F, Tse AGD, Cordell JL, Pulford KAF, Gatter KC, Mason DY. Expression of the bcl-2 oncogene protein is not specific for the 14;18 chromosomal translocation. American Journal of Pathology 1990;137:225–32.

Pezzella F, Gatter K. What is the value of bcl-2 protein detection for the histopathologist? Histopathology 1995;26:89–93.

Risberg B, Karlsson K, Abeler V, et al. Dissociated expression of bcl-2 and Ki-67 in endometrial lesions: Diagnostic and histogenetic implications. International Journal of Gynecological Pathology 2002;21:155–60.

Soini Y, Pääkkö P. bcl-2 is preferentially expressed in tumours of muscle origin but is not related to p53 expression.

Histopathology 1996;28:141–5.

Streffer JR, Rimmer A, Rieger J, et al. Bcl-2 family proteins modulate radiosensitivity in human malignant glioma cells. Journal of Neurooncology 2002;56:43–9.

Uchida T, Gao JP, Wang C, et al. Clinical significance of p53, mdm2, and bcl-2 proteins in renal cell carcinoma. Urology 2002;59:615–20.

Veloso JD, Rezuke WN, Cartun RW, Abernathy EC, Pastuszak WT. Immunohistochemical distinction of follicular lymphoma from follicular hyperplasia in formalin-fixed tissues using monoclonal antibodies MT2 and bcl-2. Applied Immunohistochemistry 1995;3:153–9.

West RB, Warnke RA, Natkunam Y. The usefulness of immunohistochemistry in the diagnosis of follicular lymphoma in bone marrow specimens. American Journal of Clinical Pathology 2002;117:636–43.

NOTES

Bcl-6

Sources/clones

Dako (PG-B6p), Novocastra (P1F6), Santa Cruz (C-19, N-3)

Fixation/preparation

The antibodies are applicable to formalin-fixed paraffin-embedded or frozen tissues. Pretreatment with EDTA and heat-induced epitope retrieval is recommended.

Background

Bcl-6 gene was identified from translocations involving the 3q27 locus in diffuse large B-cell lymphomas (Baron et al, 1993; Ye et al, 1993). The *bcl-6* gene product is a 92–98kD nuclear phosphoprotein that is highly expressed in germinal centre B-cells and their neoplastic counterparts (Onizuka et al, 1995). Hence, bcl-6 protein is expressed exclusively by follicular centre B-cells in reactive lymphoid tissue and lymphomas which are thought to rise from follicular centre cells, namely, follicular lymphoma, Burkitt's lymphoma, some diffuse large B-cell lymphomas and nodular lymphocyte predominant Hodgkin's disease (NLPHD) (Dogan et al, 2000). Whilst the bcl-6 protein was expressed in the L&H cells of NLPHD in the majority of cases, half of the cases of classic Hodgkin's disease were also immunopositive for bcl-6. Cases of primary cutaneous follicular lymphoma have also been characterized by expression of bcl-6 (Franco et al, 2001). Marginal zone/MALT lymphomas and mantle cell lymphomas are negative. However, 50% of high-grade MALT lymphomas demonstrate bcl-6 immunoreaction (Omonishi et al, 1998) similar to systemic diffuse large B-cell lymphoma.

All primary mediastinal large B-cell lymphomas have been demonstrated to express bcl-6 protein, supporting a germinal centre derivation (de Leval et al, 2001). However, only 40% of T-cell rich B-cell lymphomas were immunoreactive with bcl-6 (Kraus and Haley, 2000). The diffuse large B-cell cutaneous lymphomas that are AIDS-related have also been shown to express bcl-6 in 50% of cases (Beylot-Barry et al, 1999).

Applications

Bcl-6 in conjunction with CDw75 and CD10 is a reliable marker of follicular centre B-cell derivation with a sensitivity of 100% (Dunphy et al, 2001).

Immunoexpression of bcl-6 may be a useful marker to distinguish follicular center cell lymphoma from other diffuse small lymphocytic lymphomas. In follicular lymphoma, bcl-6 is expressed in both the follicular and interfollicular neoplastic B-cells; whilst in reactive lymphoid hyperplasia bcl-6 expression is confined exclusively to the germinal centres. The combination of bcl-6 and bcl-2 immunostaining can help in distinguishing neoplastic from reactive follicles as they stain bcl-6+bcl-2+ and bcl-6+bcl-2- respectively. Also bcl-6 provides distinction between pseudo-growth centers and entrapped germinal centres, which are bcl-6- and bcl-6+ respectively. bcl-6 expression may also be helpful in identifying main subsets of diffuse large B-cell lymphomas, those of follicular center cell origin showing bcl-6 immunoexpression.

References

Baron BW, Nucifora G, McCabe N, et al. Identification of the gene associated with the recurring chromosomal translocations t(3;14)(q27;q32) and t(3;22)(q27;q11) in B-cell lymphomas. Proceedings of the National Academy of Science USA 1993;90:5262–6.

Beylot-Barry M, Vergier B, Masquelier B, et al. The spectrum of cutaneous lymphomas in HIV infection: a study of 21 cases. American Journal of Surgical Pathology 1999;23:1208–16.

de Leval LD, Ferry JA, Falini B, et al. Expression of bcl-6 and CD10 in primary mediastinal large B-cell lymphoma: evidence for derivation from germinal center B cells? American Journal of Surgical Pathology 2001;25:1277–82.

Dogan A, Bagdi E, Munson P, Isaacson PG. CD10 and BCL-6 expression in paraffin sections of normal lymphoid tissue and B-cell lymphomas. American Journal of Surgical Pathology 2000;24:846–52.

Dunphy CH, Polski JM, Lance Evans H, Gardner LJ. Paraffin immunoreactivity of CD10, CDw75, and bcl-6 in follicle center cell lymphoma. Leukemia and Lymphoma 2001;41:585–92.

Franco R, Fernandez-Vazquez A, Rodriguez-Peralto JL, et al. Cutaneous follicular B-cell lymphoma: description of a series of 18 cases. American Journal of Surgical Pathology 2001;25:875–83.

Kraus HJ: Lymphocyte predominant Hodgkin's disease: the use of bcl-6 and CD57 in diagnosis and differential diagnosis. American Journal of Surgical Pathology 2000;24:1068–78.

Omonishi K, Yoshino T, Sakuma I, et al. bcl-6 protein is identified in high-grade but not low-grade mucosa-associated lymphoid tissue lymphomas of the stomach. Modern Pathology 1998;11:181–5.

Onizuka T, Moriyama M, Yamochi T, et al: BCL-6 gene product, a 92- to 98-kD nuclear phosphoprotein, is highly expressed in germinal center B cells and their neoplastic counterparts. Blood 1995;86:28–37.

Ye BH, Rao PH, Chaganti RS, Dalla-Favera R: Cloning of BCL-6, the locus involved in chromosome translocations affecting band 3q27 in B-cell lymphoma. Cancer Research 1993;53:2732–5.

Ber-EP4

Sources/clones

Axcel/Accurate, Dako, Diagnostic Bioscience.

Fixation/preparation

Ber-EP4 can be used on formalin-fixed, paraffin-embedded tissue sections. Prolonged formalin-fixation can be deleterious to immunoreactivity, which is enhanced by HIER or by enzymatic predigestion with proteolytic enzymes such as trypsin and pronase. Ber-EP4 may also be used to label acetone-fixed cryostat sections and fixed cell smears. A major advantage of this antibody is the high sensitivity allowing use at high dilutions.

Background

Ber-EP4 was raised against MCF-7 cells and is directed against two glycoproteins of 34 and 49 kD present on the surface and in the cytoplasm of all epithelial cells with the exception of the superficial layers of squamous epithelia, hepatocytes and parietal cells (Latza et al, 1990). Although it is not yet clear what antigen is recognized by the antibody, an absence of reactivity

to keratins was found in immunoblotting experiments. A positive reaction is seen in epithelial cells known to contain large amounts of the Ber-EP4 antigen, e.g., epithelial cells in the bile ducts and ducts of the epididymis.

Applications

Ber-EP4 shows a broad pattern of reactivity with human epithelial tissues from simple epithelia to basal layers of stratified non-keratinized squamous epithelium and epidermis (Appendix 1.20). In addition most cases of carcinoma demonstrated immunoreaction with this antibody (Latza et al, 1990). However, two cases of malignant mesothelioma studied reacted negatively. In a separate study (Sheibani et al, 1992), 87% of 83 adenocarcinomas were found to express Ber-EP4. The only adenocarcinomas that failed to react were of breast origin (8 of 25 cases non-reactive) and kidney (all 3 cases non-reactive). In contrast, only one of 115 mesotheliomas studied showed positivity. The morphologic similarity between mesothelioma and synovial sarcoma poses a uncommon diagnostic dilemma which may be resolved by

staining for BerEP4 which showed a sensitivities of 90% for biphasic synovial sarcoma versus 13% for epithelial mesothelioma (Miettinen et al, 2001).

Focal expression of Ber-EP4 in the mesothelium of the peritoneum and the ovarian surface epithelium adjacent to endometriotic lesions suggest that the mesothelium possibly acquires characteristics of epithelial nature, supporting a metaplastic process of the peritoneal mesothelium in the pathogenesis of endometriosis (Nakayama et al, 1994).

Comments

Any attempt to use Ber-EP4 to help distinguish epithelial mesothelioma from adenocarcinoma should be accompanied by a panel of antibodies (Appendix 1.17) including CEA, Leu-M1, B72.3 (all 3 antibodies in combination were reported to distinguish over 90% pulmonary adenocarcinomas from pleural mesotheliomas) (Sheibani et al, 1992) and more recent additions to the panel include calretinin, cadherin, WT1 and CK 5/6. In addition anti-EMA has been shown to produce a distinctive pattern of membrane staining corresponding to the circumferential long microvilli which are pathognomonic of malignant mesothelial cells (Leong et al, 1990).

References

Latza U, Niedobitek G, Schwarting R, et al. Ber-EP4: New monoclonal antibody which distinguishes epithelia from mesothelia. Journal of Clinical Pathology 1990;43:213–9.

Leong AS-Y, Parkinson R, Milios J. "Thick" cell membranes revealed by immunocytochemical staining: A clue to the diagnosis of mesothelioma. Diagnostic Cytopathology 1990;6:9–13.

Miettinen M, Limon J, Niezabitowski A, Lasota J. Calretinin and other mesothelioma markers in synovial sarcoma: analysis of antigenic similarities and differences with malignant mesothelioma. American Journal of Surgical Pathology 2001;25:610–7.

Nakayama K, Masuzawa H, Shuan-Fang L, et al. Immunohistochemical analysis of the peritoneum adjacent to endometriotic lesions using antibodies for Ber-EP4 antigen, estrogen receptors and progesterone receptors: Implication of peritoneal metaplasia in the pathogenesis of endometriosis. International Journal of Gynecologic Pathology 1994;13:348–58.

Sheibani K, Shin S, Kezirian J, et al. Ber-EP4 antibody as a discriminant in the differential diagnosis of malignant mesothelioma versus adenocarcinomas. American Journal of Surgical Pathology 1991;15:779–84.

Sheibani K, Esteban JM, Bailey A, Battifora H, Weiss L. Immunologic and molecular studies as an aid to the diagnosis of malignant mesothelioma. Human Pathology 1992;23:107–16.

β-hCG (Human Chorionic Gonadotropin)

Sources/clones

Biodesign ([427,681], [812,813], [827,829,830], [827,31], 2B1–3, ME.1, ME.106, ME.108, polyclonal), Biogenesis (2F4/3, BIO-BCG-001, BIO-BCG-005, BHCG-010, polyclonal), Biogenex (D7), Caltag Laboratories (2092), Dako, Fitzgerald (M15292, M15294, M94138, M94139, M94140, M94141, polyclonal), Immunotech (2B1.3), Sanbio/Monosan (2092), Zymed (ZMCG13, ZSH17).

Fixation/preparation

These antibodies are applicable to both formalin-fixed paraffin-embedded sections and to frozen sections. Both enzyme digestion and HIER do not appear to enhance immunoreactivity.

Background

Human chorionic gonadotropin (hCG) is a glycoprotein (40 kD) comprising a protein core and a carbohydrate side chain (Bellisario et al, 1973). The molecule is composed of two dissimilar subunits – α and β. The α subunit is indistinguishable immunologically from the α subunit of pituitary glycoprotein hormones: luteinizing hormone (LH), follicle stimulating hormone (FSH) and thyroid stimulating hormone (TSH). The β subunits are different from each other and confer specificity. hCG, secreted in large quantities by the placenta, normally circulates at readily detectable levels only during gestation (Braunstein et al, 1976).

The monoclonal antibody (IgG[1]) to βhCG was produced by immunization with pure chorionic gonadotropin beta subunit. βhCG is demonstrable in syncytiotrophoblasts of normal human placenta.

Applications

hCG is the most important marker of gestational trophoblastic cells, being present in syncytiotrophoblastic cells and cells of the intermediate trophoblast but absent in cytotrophoblast (Appendix 1.33, 34). In syncytiotrophoblast cells, hCG is demonstrable from the 12th day of gestation, reaches a peak at six weeks and decreases thereafter; at term hCG is present only focally in these cells. In choriocarcinoma strong diffuse immunostaining for hCG occurs in syncytiotrophoblastic cells (and focal immunostaining for human placental lactogen). In contrast, placental site trophoblastic tumor shows focal hCG immunopositivity (and diffuse human placental lactogen immunoreaction) (Appendix 1.34).

βhCG expression in non-trophoblastic tumors may indicate aggressive behavior of the tumor. It is worth noting that hCG may be demonstrated in 14% of patients with hepatocellular carcinoma (Braunstein et al, 1973). hCG may be demonstrated in the trophoblast-like cells which develop in undifferentiated carcinoma of the endometrium (Pesce et al, 1991); however, the presence of recognizable glandular structures and the lack of the biphasic pattern of alternating rows of syncytial and cytotrophoblasts rule out the possibility of choriocarcinoma.

hCG has also been demonstrated in poorly differentiated areas with cells resembling syncytiotrophoblasts in three women with serous papillary or mucinous adenocarcinomas of the ovary (Civantos & Rywlin, 1972). In 6–8% of dysgerminomas, there are individual or collections of syncytiotrophoblastic giant cells that contain/produce hCG.

Serum hCG is a promising tumor marker of gastrointestinal malignancies and a monoclonal antibody applied to 107 cases of gastrointestinal malignancies showed staining in 24%, the most frequent tumors showing immunoreactivity being gastric (60%), Pancreatic (56%) carcinomas and extrahepatic cholangiocarcinomas (36%). By comparison a polyclonal antibody showed a higher frequency of positivity but the staining was diffuse (Louhimo et al, 2001). Positive immunostaining for beta-hCG with a monoclonal antibody has also been suggested to be of prognostic relevance in colorectal carcinoma especially when employed in combination with serum levels of the hormone (Lundin et al, 2001).

References

Bellisario R, Carlsen RB, Bahl Om P. Human chorionic gonadotropin. Linear amino acid sequence of the α subunit. Journal of Biology and Chemistry 1973;248:6796–809.

Braunstein GD, Vogel CL, Vaitukaitis JL, Ross G. Ectopic production of hCG in Ugandan patients with hepatocellular carcinoma. Cancer 1973;32:223–6.

Braunstein GD, Rasor J, Adler, et al. Serum human chorionic gonadotropin levels throughout normal pregnancy. American Journal of Obstetrics and Gynecology 1976;126:678–81.

Civantos F, Rwylin AM. Carcinomas with trophoblastic differentiation and secretion of chorionic gonadotrophins. Cancer 1972;29:789–98.

Louhima J, Nordling S, Alfthan H, et al. Specific staining of human chorionic gonadotropin beta in benign and malignant gastrointestinal tissues with monoclonal antibodies. Histopathology 2001;38:418–24.

Lundin M, Nordling S, Lundin J, et al. Tissue expression of human chorionic gonadotropin beta predicts outcome in colorectal cancer: a comparison with serum expression. International Journal of Cancer 2001;95:18–22.

Pesce C, Merino MJ, Chambers JT, Nogales F. Endometrial carcinoma with trophoblastic differentiation: an aggressive form of uterine cancer. Cancer 1991;68:1799–1802.

CA 125

Sources/clones

Dako (OC125), Immunotech (Ov185).

Fixation/preparation

Monoclonal anti-CA 125 (M11) can be used on formalin-fixed, paraffin-embedded tissue sections. The deparaffinised tissue sections must be treated with heat (in citrate buffer or Dako Target Retrieval Solution) prior to the immunohistochemical staining procedure.

Background

CA 125 was discovered with a monoclonal screen for tumor-specific antigens of hybridomas derived from mouse lymphocytes immunized to an ovarian cell culture line, OVCA433 (Bast et al, 1981). The MUC16 gene is a strong candidate for the CA 125 antigen and a partial cDNA was recently cloned. Transfection of thism partial cDNA into two CA 125-negative cell lines resulted in synthesis of CA 125 (Yin et al, 2002). The antigen is located on the surface of ovarian tumor cells with essentially no expression in normal adult ovarian tissue (Kabawat et al,

1983). Significantly, CA 125 is also found in sera of patients with ovarian, pancreatic (about 50%), liver, colon and other (22% to 32%) adenocarcinomas (Kuzuya et al, 1986). Although CA 125 is not specific for ovarian carcinoma, it nevertheless does correlate directly with disease status (Bast et al, 1983). Similar to other tumor markers, CA 125 is also expressed normally in fetal development: the antigen has been localized to the amnion celomic epithelium and derivatives of Müllerian epithelium (Hardardottir et al, 1990). In adult tissue, the monoclonal antibody OC 125 reacted with the epithelium of the fallopian tube, endometrium, endocervix, apocrine sweat glands and mammary glands (Hardardottir et al, 1990; Kabawat et al, 1983).

Presently, little is known of the structure of this extracellular matrix molecule, nor is there any indication of its function. It appears to be part of a large molecular weight mucin-like glycoprotein complex that can be resolved to a 200 to 250 kD species on gel electrophoresis. Although the antigen is thought to contain a carbohydrate component, the antigenic epitope

recognized by OC 125 is considered to be peptide in nature (Davis et al, 1986).

Applications

The most important property of CA 125 is that it is regularly expressed on the tumor cell surface of serous cystadenocarcinoma of the ovary (>95%), whilst no expression is detected in mucinous cystadenocarcinomas. Although only a small number of tumors were examined, the following were also found to stain positively with CA 125: colonic adenocarcinoma (1/2), breast carcinoma (3/8), uterine papillary serous carcinoma (1/1), thyroid follicular adenoma (1/1), transitional cell carcinoma of the bladder (2/3), uterine adenomatoid tumor (1/1), lung bronchoalveolar carcinoma (1/1), endometrioid carcinoma of the ovary (2/2) and squamous cell carcinoma of the penis (1/1) (Dako specifications). Employed in an appropriate panel, CA125 is useful for the separation of colonic carcinoma from ovarian endometrioid carcinoma in the pelvis (Appendix 1.14). Similarly, when used with other markers may be useful in distinguishing renal clear cell carcinoma from clear cell carcinomas of the ovary and other Mullerian tumors, the latter being CA 125 positive (McCluggage, 2000; Nolan & Heatley, 2001).

Recently, a mesothelioma which demonstrated both serum and immunohistochemical positivity with CA 125 was reported (Almudévar Bercero et al, 1997). This indicates that CA 125 cannot reliably distinguish between metastatic serous epithelial tumors of the peritoneum and mesothelioma, an observation more recently confirmed in a study which demonstrated positivity for the antigen in 95% of serous papillary peritoneal carcinomas, 67% ovarian and peritoneal carcinomas and 25% of peritoneal mesotheliomas (Attanoos et al, 2002). In a study of occult nodal metastasis in endometrial carcinoma, CA125 was found on macrophages in the lymph nodes raising doubts as to the specificity of some antibodies to CA125 (Yabushita et al, 2001)

Comments

The major role of CA 125 in immunohistology is in the identification of metastatic serous carcinoma of the ovary. Primary serous cystadenocarcinoma of the ovary is the recommended positive control tissue for optimization of CA 125.

References

Almudévar Bercero E, García-Rostan Y Pérez GM, F García Bragado, Jiménez C. Prognostic value of high serum levels of CA-125 in malignant secretory peritoneal mesotheliomas affecting young women. A case report with differential diagnosis and review of the literature. Histopathology 1997;31:267–73.

Attanoos RL, Webb R, Dojcinov SD, Gibbs AR. Value of mesothelial and epithelial antibodies in distinguishing diffuse peritoneal mesothelioma in females from serous papillary carcinoma of the ovary and peritoneum. Histopathology 2002;40:237–44.

Bast RC Jr, Feeney M, Lazarus H, et al. Reactivity of a monoclonal antibody with human ovarian carcinoma. Journal of Clinical Investigation 1981;68:1331–7.

Bast RC, Lug TL, St John E et al. A radioimmunoassay using a monoclonal antibody to monitor the course of epithelial ovarian cancer. New England Journal of Medicine 1983;309:883–7.

Davis AM, Zurawski VR, Bast RC, Klug TL. Characterization of the CA 125 antigen associated with human epithelial ovarian carcinomas. Cancer Research 1986;46:6143–8.

Hardardottir H, Parmley TH, Quirk JG, et al. Distribution of CA 125 in embryonic tissues and adult derivatives of fetal periderm.

American Journal of Obstetrics and Gynecology 1990;163:1925–31.

Kabawat SE, Bast RC, Bhan AK, et al. Tissue distribution of a coelomic-epithelium-related antigen recognized by the monoclonal antibody OC 125. International Journal of Gynecologic Pathology 1983;2:275–85.

Kuzuya K, Nozaki M, Chihara T. Evaluation of CA 125 as a circulating tumor marker for ovarian cancer. Acta Obstetric et Gynecologica Japan. 1986;38:949–57.

McCluggage WG. Recent advances in immunohistochemistry in the diagnosis of ovarian neoplasms. Journal of Clinical Pathology 2000;53:327–34.

O'Brien TJ, Raymond LM, Bannon GA, et al. New monoclonal antibodies identify the glycoprotein carrying the CA 125 epitope. American Journal of Obstetrics and Gynecology 1991;165:1857–64.

Yabushita H, Shimazu M, Yamada H, et al. Occult lymph node metastases detected by cytokeratins immunohistochemistry predict recurrence in node-negative endometrial cancer. Gynecological Oncology 2001;80:139–44.

Yin BW, Dnistrian A, Lloyd KO. Ovarian cancer antigen CA125 is encoded by the MUC16 mucin gene. International Journal of Cancer 2002;98:737–40.

N/97-Cadherin / E-Cadherin

Sources/clones

Monoclonal antibody anti-N-cadherin (clone 13A9) and anti-E-cadherin (clone E9) (Soler et al, 1995). Accurate (6F9), American Research Products (6F9), Calbiochem (HybEcad#1), Eurodiagnostica/Accurate (5H9), Immunotech (67A4), Sanbio/Monosan/Accurate (5H9), Urodiagnostica/Accurate (5H9), Zymed (HECD1, ECCD1, ECCD2, SHE78–7).

Fixation/preparation

Initially applied primarily to frozen sections, both antibodies are now applicable to formalin-fixed paraffin-embedded tissue with heat pretreatment in citrate buffer.

Background

It has long been recognized that cancer cells have differences in their adhesive properties when compared with nontransformed cells (Hedrick et al, 1993). There is evidence that among the different cell adhesion molecules, the cadherin family of calcium-dependent cell-cell adhesion molecules and their associated proteins are indeed tumor suppressors. The cadherin family includes several distinctive members, two of which include E (epithelial)-cadherin (Gumbiner and Simons, 1986), a 120 kD protein expressed in epithelial cells and concentrated in cell-cell adherens junctions and N (nerve)-cadherin (Redies et al, 1993), a 135 kD protein expressed in nerve cells, developing skeletal muscle (Knudsen et al, 1990), embryonic and mature cardiac muscle cells (Solar et al, 1994) and pleural mesothelial cells (Hatta et al, 1987). The E-cadherin gene (CDH1) is located on chromosome 16q22.1, a region frequently affected with loss of heterozygosity in sporadic breast carcinoma. During embryonic development, expression of distinctive members of the cadherin family determines the aggregation of cells into specialized tissues as they interact with identical cadherins within the same tissue. Hence, the mesoderm-derived mesothelial cells that form the pleura express N-cadherin, whilst epithelial cells of the lung express E-cadherin (Hatta et al, 1987). Therefore, the development of well-characterized monoclonal antibodies that recognize N-cadherin without cross-reactivity with E-cadherin provided an opportunity for its application to immunohistology.

Applications

In 1995, Soler et al found a high level of expression of N-cadherin in all mesotheliomas and E-cadherin in all pulmonary adenocarcinomas on fresh frozen sections. The same group of investigators recently confirmed these findings using antibodies to N-cadherin and E-cadherin that reacted with fixation and paraffin-embedding resistant epitopes in a series of malignant mesotheliomas and adenocarcinomas (Han et al, 1997). Although one case of mesothelioma was negative for N-cadherin and one adenocarcinoma was weakly positive for N-cadherin (but strongly positive for E-cadherin), these antibodies appeared to offer a sufficient degree of sensitivity and specificity for use in the differential diagnosis of mesothelioma and adenocarcinoma.

The application of antibodies to N- and E-cadherin to ovarian epithelial tumors has revealed interesting findings (Soler et al, 1997). Both E- and N-cadherins were expressed in serous and endometrioid tumors, whilst mucinous tumors strongly expressed E-cadherin only. The expression of N-cadherin in serous and endometrioid tumors traces their origin to the mesoderm-derived ovarian surface epithelium. Another recent study (Daraï et al, 1997) demonstrated both E- and N-cadherins in benign but not malignant ovarian tumors, whilst only N-cadherin was present in borderline tumors. Further, negative E-cadherin ovarian carcinomas presented a shorter survival. These workers suggest that the E- and N-cadherin differential expression may be involved in ovarian carcinogenesis and may have diagnostic and prognostic value.

Reduction in E-cadherin expression has been associated with lack of cohesiveness, high malignant potential and invasiveness in epithelial neoplasms of the colon (Kinsella et al, 1993), ovary (Hashimoto et al, 1989), stomach (Matsuura et al, 1992), pancreas (Moller et al, 1992), lung (Williams et al, 1993), breast (Gamallo et al, 1993; Sormunen et al, 1999) and head/neck (Schipper et al, 1991). In contrast, N-cadherin has also been demonstrated in astrocytomas/glioblastomas (Shinoura et al, 1995) and rhabdomyosarcomas (Soler et al, 1993). We have shown that the loss of E-cadherin, demonstrated by immunostaining, is associated with a loss of staining for beta-catenin in infiltrating ductal carcinoma of the breast and in src cell lines heralds a change from epithelial shapes to spindle forms (Sormunen et al, 1999). Down-regulation of E-and P-cadherin was suggested to be predictive markers of nodal metastasis in

breast cancer (Madhavan et al, 2001) and loss of E-cadherin is considered to be fundamental defect in diffuse-type gastric carcinoma and infiltrating lobular carcinoma of the breast (Chan and Wong, 2001). Invasive lobular breast carcinomas, which are typically completely E-cadherin negative, often show inactivating mutations in combination with loss of heterozygosity of the wild type CDH1 allele. Mutations were found at early noninvasive stages, thus associating E-cadherin mutations with loss of cell growth control and defining CDH1 as the tumor suppressor for the lobular breast carcinoma subtype. Ductal breast carcinoma in general show heterogenous loss of E-cadherin expression, associated with epigenetic transcriptional downregulation (Berx and van Roy, 2001).

Comments

Malignant mesothelioma and colonic adenocarcinoma tissue are recommended for use as positive controls for N- and E-cadherin respectively. We have found trypsin predigestion followed by HIER to produce the greatest immunoreactivity for these antigens, particularly E-cadherin.

References

Berx G, van Roy F. The E-cadherin/catenin complex: an important gatekeeper in breast cancer tumorigenesis and malignant progression. Breast Cancer Research 2001;3:289–93.

Chan JK, Wong CS. Loss of E-cadherin is the fundamental defect in diffuse-type gastric carcinoma and infiltrating lobular carcinoma of the breast. Advances in Anatomical Pathology 2001;8:165–72.

Daraï E, Scoazec Y-Y, Walker-Combrouze F et al. Expression of cadherins in benign, borderline, and malignant ovarian epithelial tumors: a clinicopathologic study of 60 cases. Human Pathology 1997;28:922–8.

Gamallo C, Palacios J, Suarez A, et al. Correlation of E-cadherin expression with differentiation grade and histological type in breast carcinoma. American Journal of Pathology 1993;142:987–93.

Han AC, Soler AP, Knudsen KA, et al. Differential expression of N-cadherin in pleural mesotheliomas and E-cadherin in lung adenocarcinomas in formalin-fixed, paraffin-embedded tissues. Human Pathology 1997;28:641–5.

Hedrick L, Cho KR, Vogelstein B. Cell adhesion molecules as tumor suppressors. Trends in Cell Biology 1993;3:36–9.

Gumbiner B, Simons K. A functional assay for proteins involved in establishing an epithelial occluding barrier: Identification of a uyomorulin-like peptide. Journal of Cell Biology 1986;102:457–68.

Hashimoto M, Niwa O, Nitta Y, et al. Unstable expression of E-cadherin adhesion molecules in metastatic ovarian tumor cells. Japanese Journal of Cancer Research 1989;80:459–63.

Hatta K, Takgari S, Fujisawa H, et al. Spatial and temporal expression pattern of N-cadherin cell adhesion molecules correlated with morphogenetic processes of chicken embryos. Developmental Biology 1987;120:215–27.

Kinsella AR, Green B, Lepts GC, et al. The role of the cell-cell adhesion molecule E-cadherin in large bowel tumor cell invasion and metastasis. British Journal of Cancer 1993;67:904–9.

Knudsen KA, Myers L, McElwee SA. A role for the Ca²⁺-dependent adhesion molecule, N-cadherin in myoblast interaction during myogenesis. Experimental Cell Research 1990;188:175–84.

Madhavan M, Srinivas P, Abraham E, et al. Cadherins as predictive markers of nodal metastasis in breast cancer. Modern Pathology 2001;14:423–7.

Matsuura K, Kawanishi J, Jujii S et al. Altered expression of E-cadherin in gastric cancer tissues and carcinomatous fluid. British Journal of Cancer 1992;66:1122–30.

Moller CJ, Christgau S, Williamson MR et al. Differential expression of neural cell adhesion molecules and cadherins in pancreatic islets, glucagonomas, and insulinomas. Molecular Endocrinology. 1992;6:1332–42.

Redies C, Engelhardt K, Takeichi M. Differential expression of N-and R-cadherin in functional neuronal systems and other structures of the developing chicken brain. Journal of Comparative Neurology 1993;333:398–416.

Schipper JH, Frixen UH, Behrens J et al. E-cadherin expression in squamous cell carcinoma of head and neck: Inverse correlation with differentiation and lymph node metastasis. Cancer Research 1991;51:6328–37.

Shinoura N, Paradies NE, Warnick RE, et al. Expression of N-cadherin and α-catenin in astrocytomas and glioblastomas. British Journal of Cancer 1995;72:627–33.

Soler AP, Johnson KR, Wheelock MJ, et al. Rhabdomyosarcoma-derived cell lines exhibit aberrant expression of the cell-cell adhesion molecules N-CAM, N-cadherin, and cadherin-associated proteins. Experimental Cell Research 1993;208:84–93.

Soler AP, Knudsen KA. N-cadherin involvement in cardiac myocyte interaction and myofibrillogenesis. Developmental Biology 1994;162:9–17.

Soler AP, Knudsen A, Jaurand M-C, et al. The differential expression of N-cadherin and E-cadherin distinguishes pleural mesotheliomas from lung adenocarcinomas. Human Pathology 1995;26:1363–9.

Soler AP, Knudsen KA, Tecson-Miguel A. Expression of E-cadherin and N-cadherin in surface epithelial-stromal tumors of the ovary distinguishes mucinous from serous and endometrioid tumors. Human Pathology 1997;28:734–9.

Sormunen RT, Leong AS-Y, Varaaniemi JP, et al. Fodrin, E-cadherin and β-catenin immunolocalization in infiltrating ductal carcinoma of the breast correlated with selected prognostic indices. Journal of Pathology 1999;187:417–26.

Williams CL, Hayes VY, Hummel AM et al. Regulation of E-cadherin-mediated adhesion by muscarinic acetylcholine receptors in small cell lung carcinoma. Journal of Cell Biology 1993;121:643–54.

NOTES

Calcitonin

Sources/clones

Axcel/Accurate (polyclonal), Biodesign (polyclonal), Biogenesis (polyclonal, 1I5), Biogenex (polyclonal), Chemicon (polyclonal), Dako (polyclonal, CAL-3-F5), Fitzgerald (polyclonal), Immunotech (polyclonal), Sanbio/Monosan (polyclonal), Seralab (polyclonal), Zymed (polyclonal).

Fixation/preparation

These antibodies are applicable to formalin-fixed paraffin sections. HIER does not appear to enhance immunoreactivity but is not deleterious.

Background

CAL-3-F5 was raised against the synthetic peptide corresponding to C-terminal portion of human calcitonin (aa 24–32). The polyclonal antibodies were raised in rabbits using synthetic human calcitonin (35 kD). Molecular biology studies have shown that most regulatory peptides are cleavage products of larger precursor molecules (Sikri et al, 1985). The structure of the calcitonin precursor was predicted from the nucleotide sequence of cloned cDNA prepared from the mRNA obtained from medullary thyroid carcinoma (Allison et al, 1981; Amara et al, 1982a). In the human calcitonin precursor, calcitonin is flanked by two molecules: PDN (peptide-aspartic acid-asparagine) a 21- amino acid C-terminal flanking peptide, and a larger N-terminal peptide. Calcitonin gene-related peptide (CGRP) alpha is also encoded by the calcitonin gene and is produced as a result of differential RNA processing (Amara et al, 1982b). The differential production of CGRP and calcitonin from the calcitonin gene is regulated in a tissue specific manner, with CGRP being produced in nervous tissue and calcitonin in thyroid C-cells. However, both CGRP and calcitonin is found in normal, hyperplastic, and neoplastic C-cells in man, although the immunohistochemical pattern of localization is different for individual antigens.

Applications

Antibodies to calcitonin are useful to identify normal, hyperplastic and neoplastic C-cells. Medullary thyroid carcinoma (MTC) occurs both in a sporadic and inherited form, with a biological behavior between that of anaplastic and differentiated thyroid carcinomas. Given the morphologic heterogeneity of MTC, both in histological structure (solid, trabecular, or insular) and cellular patterns (spindle, polyhedral, angular or round) as well as the description of papillary, follicular, clear cell and anaplastic variants (Schröeder et al, 1988), the role of antibodies to calcitonin becomes crucial in making the correct diagnosis. All MTC in a series of 60 (Schröeder et al, 1988) and 25 (Sikri et al, 1985) cases demonstrated immunoreaction with antibodies to calcitonin. It has also been suggested that calcitonin-rich tumors appeared to have a better prognosis than calcitonin-poor neoplasms (Saad et al, 1984). However, subsequent studies were at a variance with these observations (Schröeder et al, 1988). Studies have also shown sporadic MTC to be a more life-threatening neoplasm than MTC occurring in the setting of MFN IIa syndrome, whilst those in MEN IIb syndrome were most aggressive.

Antibodies to calcitonin are also useful to identify the concept of C-cell hyperplasia in benign and malignant thyroid glands

(Santeusanio et al, 1997). Recently, a novel application of immunostaining in forensic science was proposed. Immunoreactivity for calcitonin in thyroid C-cells was consistently lost 13 days following death allowing this finding to delimit the time of death (Wehner et al, 2001).

Comments

Antibody to calcitonin is a compulsory addition to any immunohistochemical histopathology laboratory for the diagnosis of MTC. Normal parafollicular C-cells are suitable as positive control tissue.

References

Allison J, Hall L, MacIntyre I, Craig RK. The construction and partial characterisation of plasmids containing complementary DNA sequences to human calcitonin precursor polyprotein. Biochemistry Journal 1981;199:725–31.

Amara SG, Jonas V, O'Neil JA et al. Calcitonin COOH-terminal cleavage peptide as a model for identification of novel neuropeptides predicted by recombinant DNA analysis. Journal of Biology and Chemistry 1982a;257:2129–32.

Amara SG, Jonas V, Rosenfeld MG, Ong ES, Evans RM. Alternative RNA processing in calcitonin gene expression generates mRNAs encoding different polypeptide produces. Nature 1982b;298:240–4.

Saad MF, Ordonez NG, Guido JJ, Samaan NA. The prognostic value of calcitonin immunostaining in medullary carcinoma of the thyroid. Journal of Clinical Endocrinology and Metabolism 1984;59:850–6.

Santeusanio G, Iafrate E, Partenzi A, et al. A critical reassessment of the concept of C-cell hyperplasia of the thyroid. Applied Immunohistochemistry 1997;5:160–72.

Schröeder S, Böcker W, Baisch H, et al. Prognostic factors in medullary thyroid carcinomas. Survival in relation to age, sex, stage, histology, immunocytochemistry, and DNA content. Cancer 1988;61:806–16.

Sikri KL, Varndell IM, Hamid QA, et al. Medullary carcinoma of the thyroid. An immunocytochemical and histochemical study of 25 cases using eight separate markers. Cancer 1985;56:2481–91.

Wehner F, Wehner HD, Subke J. Delimitation of the time of death by immunohistochemical detection of calcitonin. Forensic Science International 2001;122:89–94.

Calponin

Sources/clones

Accurate (CP-93), Dako (Calponin, N3), Novocastra (CALP), Sigma (CP-93).

Fixation/preparation

These antibodies are applicable to formalin-fixed paraffin-embedded tissue sections. A heat-induced epitope retrieval system with additional enzyme digestion is required.

Background

Calponin is a 34kDa, smooth muscle-specific protein implicated in the regulation of smooth contraction as a result of its ability to inhibit actin-activated MgATPase of smooth muscle myosin (Carmichael et al, 1994). Calponin is a calmodulin negative, F-actin negative and tropomyosin negative binding protein (Takahashi et al, 1986).

Calponin has been demonstrated in all periacinar and periductal myoepithelial cells of normal salivary glands, being negative in acinar/ductal epithelial cells (Savera et al, 1997). This study also found calponin immunoexpression in 98% of pleomorphic adenomas, reacting to almost all myoepithelial cells, including 60% of modified and 30% of transformed myoepithelial cells. These authors concluded that calponin was the most sensitive marker of neoplastic myoepithelium. This sensitivity has also been demonstrated in myoepithelial carcinomas with up to 75% calponin immunopositivity (Savera et al, 2000).

In mesenchymal tumors, calponin immunoexpression has been demonstrated in benign smooth muscle tumors from various locations and retroperitoneal and uterine leiomyosarcomas (Miettinen et al, 1999). However, caution is advised as calponin also reacted with myofibroblasts, both reactive and in myofibroblastic lesions.

Myofibrosarcomas may also be highlighted with calponin (Watanabe et al, 2001). The demonstration of calponin in 85% of angiomatoid fibrous histiocytomas is further confirmation of the myoid phenotype of these tumors (Fanburg-Smith & Miettinen, 1999). About 80% of neurothekeomas, including cellular and mixed variants, have been shown to express calponin (Laskin et al, 2000).

Applications

Within the established panel of muscle markers, including S-100 protein, calponin is probably the most sensitive marker for myoepithelial cells. However, caution is advised, as myofibroblasts may also be immunopositive.

References

Fanburg-Smith JC, Miettinen M. Angiomatoid "malignant" fibrous histiocytoma: a clinicopathologic study of 158 cases and further exploration of the myoid phenotype. Human Pathology 1999;30:1336–43.

Laskin WB, Fetsch JF, Miettinen M. The "neurothekoma": immunohistochemical analysis distinguishes the true nerve sheath myxoma from its mimics. Human Pathology 2000;31:1230–41.

Miettinen MM, Sarloma-Rikala M, Kovatich AJ, Lasota J. Calponin and h-Caldesmon in soft tissue tumors: Consistent h-Caldesmon immunoreactivity in gastrointestinal stromal tumors indicates traits of smooth muscle differentiation. Modern Pathology 1999;12:756–62.

Nagao T, Sugano I, Ishida Y, Tajima Y, et al. Salivary gland malignant myoepithelioma: a clinicopathologic and immunohistochemical study of ten cases. Cancer 1998;83:1292–9.

Savera AT, Gown AM, Zarbo RJ. Immunolocalization of three novel smooth muscle-specific proteins in salivary gland pleomorphic adenoma: assessment of the morphogenetic role of myoepithelium. Modern Pathology 1997;10:1093–100.

Savera AT, Sloman A, Huvos AG, Klimstra DS. Myoepithelial carcinoma of the salivary glands: a clinicopathologic study of 25 patients. American Journal of Surgical Pathology 2000;24:761–74.

Takahashi K, Hiwada K, Kokubu T. Isolation and characterization of a 34,000 dalton calmodulin- and F-actin binding protein from chicken gizzard smooth muscle. Biochemical and Biophysical Research Communications 1986;141:20–6.

Watanabe K, Ogura G, Tajino T, et al. Myofibrosarcoma of the bone: a clinicopathologic study. American Journal of Surgical Pathology 2001;25:1501–7.

Calretinin

Sources/clones

Biogenesis (polyclonal),
Chemicon (polyclonal AB149),
Novocastra (mouse anti-human
1568), Swart (7696 raised against
human recombinant calretinin),
Zymed (pre-diluted polyclonal)

Fixation/preparation

These antibodies are applicable to
formalin-fixed paraffin sections.
Pretreatment of tissue sections
with citrate buffer in a microwave
oven or with 0.01% pronase in
phosphate-buffered saline at
room temperature increases
calretinin immunoreactivity
(Doglioni et al, 1996).

Background

Calretinin is a calcium-binding
protein of 29 kD. It is a member
of the large family of EF-hand
proteins, to which the S-100
protein also belongs. EF – hand
proteins are characterized by a
peculiar amino acid sequence that
folds up into a helix-loop-helix
that acts as a calcium-binding
site. Calretinin contains six such
EF- hand stretches (Schwaller et
al, 1995). The calretinin gene was
initially isolated from a cDNA
clone from the chick retina
(Rogers et al, 1990) and is

abundantly expressed in central
and peripheral neural tissues,
particularly in the retina and in
neurons of the sensory pathways.
Although the function of
calretinin is unknown, a possible
role as a calcium buffer has been
postulated. Consistent calretinin
immunoreactivity has been found
in a variety of normal tissues
including mesothelial cell lining
of all serosal membranes, eccrine
glands of skin, convoluted tubules
of kidney, Leydig and Sertoli cells
of the testis, epithelium of rete
testis, endometrium and ovarian
stromal cells and adrenal cortical
cells.

The consistent calretinin
immunoreactivity (using Ab
7696) in normal and hyperplastic
mesothelial cells led to its
establishment as a reliable positive
marker for mesothelial
differentiation (Doglioni et al,
1996). Exhibiting a sensitivity
close to 100%, immunoreactivity
was observed in the majority of
tumor cells in epithelioid,
biphasic and sarcomatoid
mesotheliomas, with focal
positivity in about 10% of
adenocarcinomas metastatic to
serous membranes (Dei Tos &
Doglioni, 1998). At variance, a
study published in abstract form,
using an alternative antibody to
calretinin (AB149) demonstrated

calretinin immunopositivity in
both mesotheliomas and
adenocarcinomas following a
heat-induced antigen retrieval
system (Folpe & Gown, 1997).
Using the same antibody to
calretinin, another group
demonstrated immunopositivity
in about 42% of mesotheliomas
with a diffuse distribution in the
majority of cases but only
approximately 6% of
adenocarcinomas with a weak or
moderate staining pattern (Riera
et al, 1997). Hence, while
specificity with the calretinin
antibody AB149 was high,
sensitivity was low; in contrast to
the anti-calretinin antibody 7696,
which demonstrated both high
specificity and sensitivity. Similar
findings have also been
demonstrated with the anti-
calretinin polyclonal antibody
from Zymed (Ordonez, 1998).

Immunocytochemical analysis
of cytologic specimens from
serous effusions demonstrated
positive immunoreaction in all
cases of mesothelioma (Doglioni
et al, 1997). These findings were
confirmed in an independent
study (Barberis et al, 1997).

As calretinin is expressed
abundantly in neurons of the
central and peripheral nervous
system, neoplasms exhibiting
neuronal differentiation also

demonstrated immunoreactivity with calretinin (Doglioni et al, 1996).

Applications

Calretinin represents one of the more sensitive and specific markers for mesothelial differentiation available to date. Applicable to both histologic and cytologic material, it is recommended for inclusion in a panel of antibodies when investigating the differential diagnosis between epithelioid mesothelioma and adenocarcinoma. The E-cadherin/calretinin combination has been shown to demonstrate both a high specificity and sensitivity in distinguishing between mesothelioma and metastatic adenocarcinoma with E-cadherin highlighting the latter (Leers et al, 1998). A note of caution is that calretinin decorates both normal/hyperplastic and neoplastic mesothelial cells and therefore does not distinguish between reactive and neoplastic mesothelial cells.

Calretinin is particularly useful for distinguishing central neurocytoma from oligodendroglioma, being negative in the latter. It has a wider potential application in distinguishing between brain tumors with glial and neuronal differentiation (Appendix 1.17).

Calretinin is a sensitive marker of ovarian sex cord-stromal tumors and may be of value in this diagnostic setting as part of a larger panel (McCluggage & Maxwell, 2001). In ovarian sex cord-stromal tumors, strong calretinin immunostaining was seen in all hilus cell tumors and

Leydig cell component of Sertoli-Leydig cell tumors; and absent staining in fibrothecomas and granulosa cell tumor (Cao et al, 2001).

Recently, calretinin was shown to be an important diagnostic marker for both solid and cystic ameloblastomas (Altini et al, 2000) and helpful in the differential diagnosis of unicystic ameloblastomas (Coleman et al, 2001). Although immunopositivity was demonstrated in mast cell lesions of the skin, the cost-effectiveness has been questioned in view of the availability of less expensive special stains (Mangini et al, 2000). Demonstration of calretinin-positive cells in biphasic synovial sarcomas has been largely confirmed to the spindle cells with a focal distribution (Miettinen et al, 2001), raising a cautionary note in the differential diagnosis of pleural-based malignancies and underscoring the role of an antibody panel in such investigations. Positive expression of calretinin in neoplastic cells of cardiac myxoma supports the concept that myxoma cells may originate from endocardial sensory nerve tissue (Terracciano et al, 2000).

Comments

Calretinin immunoexpression involves both the nucleus and cytoplasm. An often useful "built-in" positive control in test sections is adipocytes. Purkinje cells of mature cerebellum may be used as controls. Biogenesis polyclonal antiserum (1741–1007) cross reacts with rat, monkey, guinea pig, cow, mouse and chick calretinin.

References

Altini M, Coleman H, Doglioni C, Favia G, Maiorano E: Calretinin expression in ameloblastomas. Histopathology 2000;37:27–32.

Barberis MCP, Faleri M, Veronese S, et al: Calretinin: A selective marker of normal and neoplastic mesothelial cells in serous effusions. Acta Cytologica 1997;41:1757–61.

Cao QJ, Jones JG, Li M: Expression of calretinin in human ovary, testis, and ovarian sex cord-stromal tumors. International Journal of Gynecologic Pathology 2001;20:346–52.

Coleman H, Altini M, Ali H, Doglioni C, Favia G, Maiorano E: Use of calretinin in the differential diagnosis of unicystic ameloblastomas. Histopathology 2001;38:312–7.

Dei Tos AP, Doglioni C: Calretinin: A novel tool for diagnostic immunohistochemistry. Advances in Anatomical Pathology 1998;5:61–6.

Doglioni C, Chiodera PL, Furlanetto A, Vecchiato N, Macri E, Dei Tos AP: Calretinin: a specific mesothelial marker for evaluation of serous effusions (abstract). Laboratory Investigation 1997;76:33A.

Doglioni C, Dei Tos AP, Furlanetto A, et al: Calretinin: a novel immunocytochemical marker of neuronal differentiation in tumors of the brain (abstract). Mod Pathol 1996;9:140A.

Doglioni C, Dei Tos AP, Laurino L, et al: Calretinin: a novel immunocytochemical marker for mesothelioma. American Jouranl of Surgical Pathology 1996;20:1037–46.

Folpe AL, Gown AM: Calretinin, a mesothelioma-associated protein, is a sensitive marker of ovarian serous carcinoma (abstract). Laboratory Investigation 1997;76:100A.

Leers MPG, Aarts MMJ, Theunissen PHMH: E-cadherin and calretinin: A useful combination of immunochemical markers for differentiation between mesothelioma and metastatic adenocarcinoma. Histopathology 1998;32:209–16.

Mangini J, Silverman JF, Dabbs DJ, Tung MY, Silverman AR: Diagnostic value of calretinin in mast cell lesions of the skin. International Journal of Surgical Pathology 2000;8:119–22.

McCluggage WG, Maxwell P: Immunohistochemical staining for calretinin is useful in the diagnosis of ovarian sex cord-stromal tumours. Histopathology 2001;38:403–8.

Miettinen M, Limon J, Niezabitowski A, Lasota J: Calretinin and other mesothelioma markers in synovial sarcoma: Analysis of antigenic similarities and differences with malignant mesothelioma. American Journal of Surgical Pathology 2001;25:610–7.

Ordonez NG: Value of calretinin immunostaining in differentiating epithelial mesothelioma from lung adenocarcinoma. Modern Pathology 1998;10:929–33.

Reifegerste R, Grimm S, Albert S, et al: An invertebrate calcium-binding protein of the calbindin subfamily: protein structure, genomic organization and expression pattern of the calbindin-32 gene of Drosophilia. Journal of Neurosciences 1998;13:2186–98.

Riera JR, Astengo-Osuna C, Longmate JA, Battifora H: The immunohistochemical diagnostic panel for epithelial mesothelioma: A reevaluation after heat-induced epitope retrieval. American Jouranal of Surgical Pathology 1997;21:1409–19.

Rogers J, Khan M, Ellis J. Calretinin and other CaBPs in the nervous system. Advances in Experimental Medicine and Biology 1990;269:195–203.

Schwaller B, Buchwald P, Blumcke I, Celio MR, Hunziker W. Characterization of a polyclonal antiserum against purified human recombinant calcium binding protein calretinin. Cell Calcium 1993;14:639–48.

Schwaller B, Celio MR, Hunziker W: Alternative splicing of calretinin mRNA leads to different forms of calretinin. European Journal of Biochemistry 1995;230:424–30.

Terracciano LM, Mhawech P, Suess K, et al: Calretinin as a marker for cardiac myxoma: Diagnostic and histogenetic considerations. American Journal of Clinical Pathology 2000;114:754–9.

NOTES

Candida Albicans

Sources/clones

Biogenex (monoclonal antibody 1B12)

Fixation/preparation

Antigen retrieval involving microwave treatment of specimens in citrate buffer is required for formalin-fixed paraffin-embedded tissue sections.

Background

The diagnosis of oral candidiasis requires the sampling of the mucosal surface for the culture and identification of *Candida* spp. In chronic hyperplastic candidiasis, the fungal hyphae of *Candida* spp invade the superficial layers of the epithelium, making diagnosis difficult on candidal culture alone. Hence, biopsy of such lesions for microscopic examination is essential for diagnosis. Staining with periodic acid-Schiff (PAS) or methenamine-silver stains detect hyphal structures consistent with *Candida* spp in formalin-fixed tissue sections. However, these stains do not permit identification of individual candida species. Further, the variable sensitivity of *Candida* spp to antifungal agents makes identification of the infecting species important (Williams et al, 1998).

The mouse monoclonal antibody (1B12) was raised against the high molecular weight mannoproteins of *Candida albicans* (BioGenex). This antibody is species specific and suitable for use with formalin-fixed, paraffin-embedded material (Monteagudo et al, 1995).

In a study using 20 strains of seven *Candida* species suspended in agarose blocks, fixed in formalin and embedded in paraffin wax (FFPE), only *Candida albicans* was 1B12 immunopositive (Williams et al, 1998), ruling out cross reactivity with other *Candida* spp. In addition, 16 blocks of FFPE known to contain PAS-positive fungal hyphae, also proved to be immunopositive with 1B12 antibody.

Identification of the infecting species is not only important for therapeutic purposes, but may help clarify the association of chronic hyperplastic candidiasis with the development of squamous cell carcinoma (Banoczy, 1977).

Applications

The ability of monoclonal antibody 1B12 to identify candida hyphae penetrating lesional tissue in chronic candidiasis provides an opportunity to enhance our understanding of the role of *Candida* spp in this form of oral candidiasis.

References

Banoczy J. Follow-up studies in oral leukoplakia. Journal of Maxillofacial Surgery 1977;5:69–75.

Monteagudo C, Marcilla A, Mormeneo S, et al. Specific immunohistochemical identification of Candida albicans in paraffin-embedded tissue with a new monoclonal antibody (1B12). American Journal of Clinical Pathology 1995;103:130–5.

Williams DW, Jones HS, Allison RT, et al. Immunocytochemical detection of *Candida albicans* in formalin fixed, paraffin embedded material. Journal of Clinical Pathology 1998;51:857–9.

NOTES

Carcinoembryonic Antigen (CEA)

Sources/clones

Accurate (C234, 12–140–10, MIC0101), Axcel/Accurate (A5B7, polyclonal), Biodesign (ME.104, CEJ 065, MAM6, 9207, 9201, 9203, polyclonal), Biogenesis (6.2, 1G9/9, 10, MAC601, polyclonal), Biogenex (SP-651, TF3H8–1), Biosource, Calbiochem, Caltag Laboratories (CEA6.2), Cymbus Bioscience (85A12), Dako (11–7, polyclonal), E-Y Labs, Fitzgerald (M94129, M94130, M94131, M94132, M 2103124, M2103125, polyclonal), Immunotech Inc (FJ95, CEJ 065), Immunotech SA (F023C5), Novocastra (85A12, 12–140–10), Oncogene (TF3H8), Shandon Lipshaw (CEJ065), Sigma Chemical (C6G9), Zymed (ZCEA1, COL-1).

Fixation/preparation

This antibody can be used on formalin-fixed paraffin-embedded tissue sections. Prolonged fixation in buffered formalin may destroy the epitope. Antibody to CEA may also be used for frozen sections. Trypsinization is essential for antigen unmasking. HIER does not appear to enhance staining.

Background

CEA consists of a heterogeneous family of related oncofetal glycoproteins (approximately 200 kD molecular weight) which is secreted into the glycocalyx surface of gastrointestinal cells. CEA was first described in 1965 as a specific antigen for adenocarcinoma of the colon and the digestive tract of a 2–6 month old fetus (Gold et al, 1965). The monoclonal antibody to CEA was raised using tumor cells derived from a hepatic metastasis of colonic carcinoma (Rogers et al, 1976). CEA is a complex glycoprotein; hence, even after purification some degree of molecular heterogeneity exists (Sheibani et al, 1992). Therefore antibodies to CEA, particularly polyclonal, commonly react against a nonspecific cross-reactive antigen (NCA) located in normal colon and granulocytes. Because of the cross-reactivity of most heterologous anti-CEA antisera with NCA, the results obtained when polyclonal anti-CEA antibody was used, have been recently questioned (Whitaker et al, 1982). The anti-NCA reactivity of anti-CEA antibody is demonstrated with positive immunoreaction in polymorphonuclear leukocytes and macrophages since the cells lack CEA antigen, but contain NCA. Therefore it is recommended that positive results obtained with a polyclonal anti-CEA antibody without preabsorption with NCA, be interpreted as being nonspecific (Sheibani et al, 1992). Even monoclonal antibodies to CEA may cross-react with other molecules of the CEA family, including NCA (Sheibani et al, 1992). Therefore, each antibody needs to be evaluated to avoid nonspecific results.

Applications

CEA is found in several adenocarcinomas, such as colon, lung, breast, stomach and pancreas. Some studies have found over 70% of adenocarcinomas from a variety of organs to be positive, with no evidence of expression of CEA by neoplastic cells in several hundred cases of malignant mesothelioma (Shebani et al, 1986, 1988). Hence, in these studies expression of CEA by adenocarcinomas and their absence in mesothelioma represents a valuable marker in the discrimination of mesotheliomas from morphologically similar adenocarcinomas involving any organ (Sheibani et al, 1992). However, it should be stressed that such results are dependent on the antibody evaluation and one study obtained cytoplasmic or membrane-related staining in five of 45 cases of mesothelioma studied (Stirling et al, 1990). Occasional hyaluronate-rich epithelial mesotheliomas may produce false positivity with CEA, although this staining can be abolished by hyaluronidase digestion prior to immunoprocessing (Robb et al 1989). In a study examining multiple-marker immunohistochemical phenotypes to distinguish between malignant pleural mesothelioma from pulmonary adenocarcinoma, demonstrated CEA to be the best single marker (Brown et al, 1992): positive: 97% specific and sensitive for adenocarcinoma; negative: 97% specific and sensitive for mesothelioma (Appendix 1.17). Polyclonal CEA is also useful for the demonstration of bile canaliculi in hepatocytes and the cells of hepatocellular carcinoma both in cytologic preparations and tissue sections (Appendix 1.8). Although the presence of bile canaliculi is specific for hepatocytes, its sensitivity is low.

Comments

The fact that no single antibody is sufficiently specific and sensitive for the distinction of mesothelioma from

adenocarcinoma (Roberts et al, 2001) necessitates the use of a panel of antibodies comprising a broad spectrum cytokeratin, monoclonal CEA, Leu M1 and BER-EP4, which allows for confident differentiation of these tumors in approximately 90% of cases (Leong & Vermin-Roberts, 1994; Attanoos et al, 1996). The addition of calretinin, CK 5/6 and WT1 to the panel increases the diagnostic accuracy. Colonic carcinoma is the favored positive control tissue for antibodies against CEA.

References

Attanoos RL, Goddard H, Gibbs AR. Mesothelioma-binding antibodies: thrombomodulin, OV632 and HBME-1 and their use in the diagnosis of malignant mesothelioma. Histopathology 1996;29:209–15.

Brown RW, Clark GM, Tandon AK, Allred DC. Multiple-marker immunohistochemical phenotypes distinguishing malignant pleural mesothelioma from pulmonary adenocarcinoma. Human Pathology 1993;24:347–54.

Leong AS-Y, Vermin-Roberts E. The immunohistochemistry of malignant mesothelioma. Pathology Annual 1994;29:157–79.

Robb JA. Mesothelioma versus adenocarcinoma: false positive CEA and Leu-M1 staining due to hyaluronic acid (Letter). Human Pathology 1989;20:400.

Roberts F, Harper CM, Downie I, Burnett RA.

Immunohistochemical analysis still has a limited role in the diagnosis of malignant mesothelioma. A study of thirteen antibodies. American Journal of Clinical Pathology 2001;116:253–62.

Sheibani K, Battifora H, Burke JJ. Antigenic phenotype of malignant mesotheliomas and pulmonary adenocarcinomas. An immunohistologic analysis demonstrating the value of the Leu M1 antigen. American Journal of Pathology 1986;123:212–9.

Sheibani K, Azumi N, Battifora H. Further evidence demonstrating the value of Leu-M1 antigen in differential diagnosis of malignant mesothelioma and adenocarcinoma: An immunohistologic evaluation of 395 cases. Laboratory Investigation 1988;58:84A.

Sheibani K, Esteban JM, Bailey A, Battifora H, Weiss LM. Immunopathologic and molecular studies as an aid to the diagnosis of malignant mesothelioma. Human Pathology 1992;23:107–16.

Stirling JW, Henderson DW, Spagnolo DV, et al. Unusual granular reactivity for carcinoembryonic antigen in malignant mesothelioma. Human Pathology 1990;21:678–9.

Whitaker D, Sterrett GF, Shilkin KB. Detection of tissue CEA-like substance as an aid in the differential diagnosis of malignant mesothelioma. Pathology 1982;14:255–8.

Catenins, α, β, γ

Sources/clones

α-catenin: Becton Dickinson (1G5), Transduction Laboratories
β-catenin: Transduction Laboratories, Zymed (5H10)
γ-catenin: Becton Dickinson (10C4), Transduction Laboratories

Fixation/preparation

HIER is necessary for the immunoreactivity of these antibodies in fixed paraffin-embedded sections. Immunoreactivity is preserved in frozen sections and cell preparations.

Background

There is currently a great deal of interest in the adhesion molecules and their expression and localization. Cell-to-cell adhesion not only plays a major role in embryogenesis but also in the intercellular adhesion of cancer cells and hence their motility and metastasis (Jiang 1996; Ilyas & Tomlinson, 1997). The transmembrane molecule E-cadherin is considered to be one of the key molecules in the formation of the intercellular junctional complex and establishment of polarity in epithelial cells. The cytoplasmic domain of E-cadherin in adherens junctions interacts via intracellular catenins with the actin-based cytoskeleton and includes fodrin, whereas the extracellular domain is involved in homotypic cell-to-cell adhesion through the formation of a molecular zipper complex. The integrity of the E-cadherin adhesion system has been shown to be disturbed or disrupted in experimental and human carcinomas and reduced expression of E-cadherin induces dedifferentiation and invasiveness in tumor cells (Tsukita et al, 1992; Birchmeier & Behrens, 1994; Ilyas & Tomlinson, 1997; Sormunen et al, 1999).

Catenins, the α-subunit (102 kD), β-subunit (88 kD) and γ-subunit (82 kD), are a group of proteins that interact with the intercellular domain of E-cadherin, resulting in complexes of E-cadherin/β-catenin/α-catenin or E-cadherin/γ-catenin/α-catenin (Hinck et al, 1994). α-catenin shows sequence homology to vinculin and interacts with the actin cytoskeleton, either directly or indirectly via α-actinin, β-catenin is the vertebrate homologue of the *Drosophila* segment polarity gene armadillo, and γ-catenin, which is identical to plakoglobin and is also found in desmosomes (Jiang 1996). The regions of both α- and β-catenin, located on 5q21–22 and 3p21 have been shown to be involved in the development of certain tumors (see Jiang 1996) and reduced expressions of both α- and β-catenin have been described in various tumors including breast carcinoma (Hashizume et al, 1996). Besides adhesion functions, β-catenin binds to APC (adenomatous polyposis coli) protein, a putative tumor suppressor. APC mutation disturbs the equilibrium and levels of free β-catenin level in the cell and may have a role in tumorigenesis. β-catenin has recently been shown to have a function in signal transduction when bound with members of the Tcf-LEF family of DNA-binding proteins (Behrens et al, 1996). In src cell line, the loss of E-cadherin is associated with loss of immunostaining for β-catenin and heralds a change in morphology from epithelial to spindled shapes (Sormunen et al, 1999). Recently, it was demonstrated that somatic mutations of the β-catenin and adenosis polyposis coli (APC) genes with resultant nuclear translocation of β-catenin in both sporadic and familial adenomatous polyposis- (FAP) associated breast fibromatosis (Abraham et al,

2001). The nuclear accumulation of β-catenin has also been shown in sporadic basal cell carcinoma (Yamazaki et al, 2001) and pancreatic solid-pseudopapillary neoplasm (Tanaka et al, 2001).

Applications

Although currently not of diagnostic importance, the expression of the catenin proteins and their localization are potentially important markers to predict motility and invasiveness of epithelial neoplasms (Sormunen et al, 1998). Our studies suggest that the detachment of β-catenin from the cell membrane heralds the breakdown of the cadherin-catenin-fodrin-cytoskeletal complex both in vitro and in vivo. The loss of cell-to-cell adhesion is concomitant with a change in cell shape, from epithelioid to fibroblastoid (Sormunen et al, 1998).

Comments

The monoclonal antibodies from Transduction Laboratories are immunoreactive in routinely fixed, paraffin-embedded tissue section but only following HIER in citrate buffer.

References

Berhens J, von Kries JP, Kuhl M, et al. Functional interaction of beta-catenin with the transcriptional factor LEF-1. Nature 1996;384:638–42.

Birchmeier W, Behrens J. Cadherin expression in carcinomas: role in the formation of cell junctions and the prevention of invasiveness. Biochemia Biophysiology Acta 1994;1198:11–26.

Hashizume R, Koizumi H, Ihara A, et al. Expression of beta-catenin in normal breast tissue and breast carcinoma: a comparative study with epithelial cadherin and alpha-catenin. Histopathology 1996;29:139–46.

Hinck L, Nathke IS, Papkoff J, Nelson WJ. Dynamics of cadherin/catenin complex formation: Novel protein interactions and pathways of complex assembly. Journal of Cell Biology 1994;125:1327–40.

Jiang WG. E-cadherin and its associated protein catenins, cancer invasion and metastasis. British Journal of Surgery 1996;83:437–446.

Ilyas M, Tomlinson IPM. The interactions of APC, E-cadherin and β-catenin in tumour development and progression. Journal of Pathology 1997;182:128–37.

Sormunen RT, Leong AS-Y, Vaaraniemi JP, et al. Fodrin, E-cadherin and β-catenin immunolocalization in infiltrating ductal carcinoma of the breast correlated with selected prognostic indices. Journal of Pathology 199;187:416–23.

Tanaka Y, Kato K, Notohara K, et al. Frequent beta-catenin mutation and cytoplasmic/nuclear accumulation in pancreatic solid-pseudopapillary neoplasm. Cancer Research 2001;61:8401–4.

Tsukita S, Nagafuchi A, Yonemura S. Molecular linkage between cadherins and actin filaments in cell-cell adherens junctions. Current Opinion in Cell Biology 1992;4:834–39.

Yamazaki F, Aragane Y, Kawada A, Tezuka T. Immunohistochemical detection for nuclear beta-catenin in sporadic basal cell carcinoma. British Journal of Dermatology 2001;145:771–7.

Cathepsin D

Sources/clones

Accurate (polyclonal), Axcel/Accurate (polyclonal), Biodesign (polyclonal), Biogenesis/Novocastra (C5, polyclonal), Biogenex (C5, M1G8, polyclonal), Calbiochem (polyclonal), Caltag Laboratories (NCL-CDm), Chemicon (polyclonal), Dako (polyclonal), Immunotech (C5), Lab Vision Corp (C5), Novocastra (polyclonal), Oncogene (OS13A), Zymed (polyclonal).

Fixation/preparation

The antigen is immunoreactive in fixed, paraffin-embedded tissue sections only following HIER. Staining can also be performed on frozen sections and cell preparations.

Background

The cathepsins are ubiquitous lysosomal proteases and are classified both functionally and according to their active site. Cathepsin D, cathepsin B and to a lesser extent other cathepsins have been described as prognostic markers in cancer. Cathepsin D is the most widely studied of the cathepsins. It is an estrogen-regulated protease. A precursor form of 52 kD is processed in lysosomes into the mature 14 kD and 34 kD forms. This enzyme is thought to have proteolytic activity, which may facilitate the spread of neoplastic cells through different mechanisms and at different levels of the metastatic cascade. Cathepsin D is thought to promote tumor cell proliferation by acting as an autocrine mitogen through the activation of latent forms of growth factors or by interacting with growth factor receptors. The enzyme has also been shown, in vitro, to be able to degrade extracellular matrix and to activate latent precursor forms of other proteinases involved in the invasive steps of the cancer metastasis. Although its active role in promoting these processes in vivo has yet to be proven, recent clinical observations which show a positive correlation between levels of cathepsin D activity and malignant progression of some human neoplasms, further supports this hypothesis (Duffy 1992; Leto et al, 1992). Cathepsin B, which catalyzes the degradation of laminin, may also play a role in the rupture of the basal membrane and may be of relevance in colorectal and pancreatic cancer (Schwartz 1995).

Immunohistochemical studies in breast cancer have found that cathepsin D expression was significantly associated with poor overall survival in node-positive (Aaltonen et al, 1995) and node-negative patients (Isola et al, 1993). Recent observations that high levels of cathepsin D activity may be observed in macrophage-like stromal cells may account for some of the previous apparently conflicting reports concerning the prognostic relevance of biochemical and immunohistochemical estimations of cathepsin D in breast cancers. Cytosol assays measured total cathepsin D levels, whereas, the immunohistochemical assessment was restricted to enzyme expression within tumor cells (Razumovic et al, 1997). When stromal cathepsin D levels were taken into account in immunohistochemical studies, significant associations were found with high tumor grade, increased tendency to local recurrence, regional recurrence, poorer disease free survival and poorer overall patient survival (O'Donoghue et al, 1993; Joensuu et al, 1995; Charpin et al, 1997).

Cathepsin D expression has been studied in a variety of other tumors with variable results. Tumors studied include carcinomas of the lung (Sloman et al, 1996; Higashiyama et al, 1997), stomach (Allgayer et al, 1997), uterine cervix (Kristensen et al, 1996), endometrium (Losch et al, 1996; Saygili et al, 2001) and urinary bladder (Dickinson et al, 1995), medullary carcinoma of the thyroid (Holm et al 1995) and colorectal cancer (Theodoropoulos et al, 1997). In gastric adenocarcinoma the percentage of cathepsin-positive tumors cells appeared to correlate with depth of invasion (Ikeguchi et al, 2001) and with nodal micrometastasis (Ikeguchi et al, 2001).

Comments

Cathepsin D has recently been advocated as a marker of immature ganglion cells in suspected cases of Hirschsprung's disease, the intense granular cytoplasmic reactivity for the enzyme forming a collarette around the nucleus (Abu-Alfa et al, 1997).

References

Aaltonen M, Lipponen P, Kosma VM, et al. Prognostic value of cathepsin-D expression in female breast cancer. Anticancer Research 1995;15:1033–37.

Abu-Alfa AK, Kuan SF, West AB, Reyes-Mugica M. Cathepsin D in intestinal ganglion cells. A potential aid to diagnosis in suspected Hirschsprung's disease. American Journal of Surgical Pathology 1997;21:201–5.

Allgayer H, Babic R, Grutzner KU, et al. An immunohistochemical assessment of cathepsin D in gastric carcinoma: its impact on clinical prognosis. Cancer 1997;80:179–87.

Charpin C, Garcia S, Bouvier C, et al. Cathepsin D detected by automated and quantative immunohistochemistry in breast carcinomas: correlation with overall and disease free survival. Journal of Clinical Pathology 1997;50:586–90.

Dickinson AJ, Fox SB, Newcomb PV, et al. An immunohistochemical and prognostic evaluation of cathepsin D expression in 105 bladder carcinomas. Journal of Urology 1995;154:237–41.

Duffy MJ. The role of proteolytic enzymes in cancer invasion and metastasis. Clinical and Experimental Metastasis 1992;10:145–55.

Higashiyama M, Doi O, KodamaK, et al. Influence of cathepsin D expression in lung adenocarcinoma on prognosis: possible importance of its expression in tumor cells and stromal cells, and its intracellular polarization in tumor cells. Journal of Surgical Oncology 1997;65:10–19.

Holm R, Hoie J, Kaalhus O, Nesland JM. Immunohistochemical detection of nm23/NDP kinase and cathepsin D in medullary carcinomas of the thyroid gland. Virchows Archives 1995;427:289–94.

Ikeguchi M, Fukuda K, Oka S, et al. Clinicaopathological significance of cahtepsin D expression in gastric adenocarcinoma. Oncology 2001;61:71–8.

Okeguchi M, Fukuda K, Oka S, et al. Micro-lymph node metastasis and its correlation with cathepsin D expression in early gastric cancer. Journal of Surgical Oncology 2001;77:188–94.

Isola J, Weitz S, Visakorpi T, et al. Cathepsin D expression detected by immunohistochemistry has independent prognostic value in node-negative breast cancer. Journal of Clinical Oncology 1993;11:36–43.

Joensuu H, Toikkanen S, Isola J. Stromal cell cathepsin D expression and long-term survival in breast cancer. British Journal of Cancer 1995;71:155–9.

Kristensen GB, Holm R, Abeler VM, Trope CG. Evaluation of the prognostic significance of cathepsin D, epidermal growth factor receptor, and c-erB-2 in early cervical squamous cell carcinoma. An immunohistochemical study. Cancer 1996;78:433–40.

Leto G, Gebbia N, Rausa L, Tumminello FM. Cathepsin D in the malignant progression of neoplastic diseases (review). Anticancer Research 1992;12:235–40.

Losch A, Kohlberger P, Gitsch G, et al. Lysosomal protease cathepsin D is a prognostic marker in endometrial cancer. British Journal of Cancer 1996;73:1525–8.

O'Donoghue AE, Poller DN, Bell JA, et al. Cathepsin D in primary breast carcinoma: adverse prognosis is associated with expression of cathepsin D in stromal cells. Breast Cancer Research and Treatment 1995;33:137–45.

Razumoviv JJ, Stojkovic RR, Petrovecki M, Gamulin S. Correlation of two methods for determination of cathepsin D in breast carcinoma (immunohistochemistry and ELIZA in cytosol). Breast Cancer Research and Treatment 1997;43:117–22.

Saygili U, Koyuncuoglu M, Altunyurt S, et al. May cathepsin D immunoreactivity be used as a prognostic factor in endometrial carcinomas? A comparative immunohistochemical study. Gynecologic Oncology 2001;83:20–4.

Schwartz MK. Tissue cathepsins as tumor markers. Clinical Chimia Acta 1995;237:67–78.

Sloman A, D'Amico F, Yousem SA. Immunohistochemical markers of prolonged survival in small cell carcinoma of the lung. An immunohistochemical study. Archives of Pathology and Laboratory Medicine 1996;120:465–72.

Theodoropoulos GE, Panoussopoulos D, Lazaris AC, Golematis BC. Evaluation of cathepsin D immunostaining in colorectal adenocarcinoma. Journal of Surgical Oncology 1997;65:242–8.

NOTES

CD 1

Sources/clones

Accurate (WM35–1a), Becton-Dickinson (Leu5), Biogenesis (DMC1), Biogenex (T6–1a), Bioprobe, Biosource (BB5), Boehringer Mannheim (YIT6), Coulter (T6), Cymbus Bioscience (CBNT6–1a), Dako (NA1/34), Immunotech (010), Oncogene, Sanbio (66–11-C7), Serotec (4A76, NAI-34–1a), and Sera-Lab (CD 1), and Immunotech (CD 1a).

Fixation/preparation

Fresh frozen tissues. CD 1a (clone 010) is effective in paraffin-embedded tissues, immunoreactivity enhanced by HIER.

Background

Human CD1 genes are a family of five non-polymorphic genes that, although homologous to both class I and II major histocompatibility complex genes, map to chromosome 1. Four isoforms of the CD 1 proteins have been clustered, namely, CD 1a, -b, -c and -d and are expressed on the surface of cells in association with beta 2-microglobulin and may function as nonclassical antigen-presenting

molecules. While CD 1 genes have been found in a wide variety of vertebrates, they have shown differences in size and complexity in different mammals. Most CD 1 molecules can be separated into two groups based mainly on homology of nucleotide and amino acid sequences. Group 1 includes the human CD 1a, -b, and -c proteins, which are the classic CD 1 antigens first identified on human thymocytes and now recognized on a variety of specialized Ag-presenting cells, including dendritic cells in lymphoid and non-lymphoid tissues. These proteins can also be induced in vitro on virtually all circulating human monocytes by exposure to granulocyte-macrophage-CSF, suggesting that they might be up-regulated on tissue macrophages in many inflammatory lesions. The Group 2 CD 1 proteins include the human CD 1d and mouse CD 1, which so far have been found to be most prominently expressed by gastrointestinal epithelia and B lymphocytes (Boumsell, 1989).

CD 1a, -b, and -c are expressed in about 70% of all thymocytes, predominantly the cortical thymocytes. CD 1 is not expressed early thymocytes or by mature resting or activated T

lymphocytes. This distribution is reflected by neoplastic populations of T cells in that precursor T-ALL/LBLs expressing cortical or immature phenotypes are CD1 positive, in contrast to those with prothymocyte or medullary thymocyte phenotypes. All post-thymic or Tdt-negative T cell neoplasms such as T-CLL, T-PLL, Tγ-lymphoproliferative disorder, Sézary syndrome, cutaneous T cell lymphoma and node-based T cell lymphoma are consistently negative for CD 1 (Porcelli & Modlin, 1995).

Applications

CD 1a, CD 1b and CD 1c antigens are membrane glycoproteins with MWs of 49 kDa, 45 kDa and 43 kDa, respectively. Their expression on thymocytes and also on a variety of antigen presenting cells including Langerhans' cells and interdigitating dendritic cells make detection, particularly of CD 1a, useful in the diagnosis of Langerhans' cell histiocytosis, and the classification of thymomas and malignancies of T-cell precursors.

CD 1a is a specific marker for Langerhans' cells (Shinzato et al, 1995). Thymic lymphocytes that are CD 1-positive represent cortical thymocytes. Myeloid leukemias, some B cell malignancies and dendritic cells in most peripheral cutaneous T cell lymphomas are also positive (Schmuth et al, 2001).

Comments

Antibodies to CD1a are useful in diagnosis of Langerhans' cell histiocytosis, in the classification of thymomas especially when used in combination with the PE-35 antibody that reacts with a variety of epithelia including the medullary epithelium of the thymus (Hattori et al, 2000) and malignancies of T-cell precursors. While most of the antibodies available are only reactive in fresh frozen tissues, clone 010, is reactive in paraffin sections following heat-induced epitope retrieval, is available through Immunotech (Krenacs et al, 1993). S100 positivity has been employed as the conventional marker to distinguish between Langerhans histiocytosis and non-Langerhans histiocytosis but it is now clearly recognized that abnormal histiocytes may stain for this marker (Tomaszewski & Lupton, 1998; Lu et al, 2000) so that CD1a staining becomes an important diagnostic discriminator.

References

Boumsell L. Cluster report: CD1. In: Knapp W, Dorken B, Reiber EP, et al. (eds). Leucocyte Typing IV: White Cell Differentiation Antigens. Oxford: Oxford University Press. 1989:251–4.

Hattori H, Tateyama H, Tada T, et al. PE-35-related antigen expression and CD1a-positive lymphocytes in thymoma subtypes based on Muller-Hermelink classification. An immunohistochemical study using catalyzed signal amplification. Virchows Archives 2000;436:20–7.

Krenacs L, Tiszalvicz LT, Krenacs T, Boumsell L: Immunohistochemical detection of CD1a antigen in formalin-fixed and paraffin-embedded tissue sections with monoclonal antibody 010. Journal of Pathology 1993;171:99–104.

Lu D, Estalilla OC, Manning JTJr, Medeiros LJ. Sinus histiocytosis with massive lymphadenopathy and malignant lymphoma involving the same lymph node: a report of four cases and review of the literature. Modern Pathology 2000;13:414–9.

Porcelli SA, Modlin RL. CD 1 and the expanding universe of T cell antigens. Journal of Immunology 1995;55:709–10.

Schmuth M, Sidoroff A, Danner B, et al. Reduced numbers f CD1a+ cells in cutaneous B cell lymphoma. American Journal of Clinical Pathology 2001;116:72–8.

Shinzato M, Shamoto M, Hosokawa S et al. Differentiation of Langerhans cells from interdigitating cells using CD1a and S-100 protein antibodies. Biotechnology and Histochemistry 1995;70:114–8.

Tomaszewski MM, Lupton GP. Unusual expression of S100 protein in histiocytic neoplasms. Journal of Cutaneous Pathology 1998;25:129–35.

CD 2

Sources/clones

Becton Dickinson (Leu 5, S5.2), Biodesign (BH1), Boehringer Mannheim (MT26), Caltag Labs (G11), Coulter (6F10.3, T11, 39C15), Cymbus Bioscience (GJ12), Dako (MT910), Immunotech (39C1.5), Novocastra (X1X8), Ortho (OKT2), Pharmingen (RPA2.10), Sanbio (MEM65), Serotec (MCA651), Zymed (RPA2.10).

Fixation/preparation

Fresh frozen tissue, fresh air-dried cell preparations.

Background

Human T lymphocytes were initially distinguished from B lymphocytes by their ability to produce spontaneous rosettes with sheep red blood cells, a phenomenon mediated by the CD2 molecule, a glycosylated transmembrane receptor molecule also referred to as T11 antigen or LFA-3 antigen (leukocyte function associated antigen -3). Three functionally important epitope groups have been defined on the human CD2 molecule, designated $T11_1$, $T11_2$ and $T11_3$ (CD2R). $T11_1$ is the epitope responsible for E-rosetting and

T cell stimulation through this epitope is mediated by an IL-2 dependent pathway. Stimulation of the $T11_2$ and $T11_3$ epitopes occurs via an alternative pathway (Meur et al, 1984; Knowles, 1984).

CD2 is one of the earliest T cell lineage restricted antigens to appear during T cell differentiation and only rare CD2+ cell can be found in the bone marrow. It is found in all T-lymphocytes and natural killer cells but not in B cells or any other cell population. CD2 binds to its counter receptor CD-58 (LFA-3), a member of the Ig gene superfamily, which locates on the surface of target cells. CD2 binding to LFA-3 activates T cells and may also have a role in prothymocyte homing as it is known to mediate thymocyte-thymic epithelium adhesion. Although it is known that CD2 appears after CD7 but before CD1, its temporal relationship with CD3 is less definite, with some recent evidence suggesting that CD3 appears in the cytoplasm before CD2 (Osborn et al, 1995)

Applications

CD2 can be considered a pan-T cell antigen and is therefore useful for the identification of

virtually all normal T lymphocytes. It is also very useful in the assessment of lymphoid malignancies as it is expressed in the majority of precursor and post-thymic lymphomas and leukemias and is not expressed by B neoplasms (Foon & Todd, 1986). As with other pan-T cell antigens, CD2 may be aberrantly deleted in some neoplastic T cell populations, especially peripheral T cell lymphomas. Rarely, sIg+ B cell neoplasms have been described to form spontaneous E-rosettes but these reactions are not mediated via the CD2 receptor (Knowles, 1989).

Comments

CD2 antibodies can be used for identification of lymphomas and leukemias of T-cell origin. Positive staining cells include thymocytes (95%), mature peripheral T cells (almost all), NK cells (80–90%) and thymic B cells (50%). Currently, the majority of monoclonal antibodies available are reactive only in fresh frozen tissue. Clones MCA651 (Serotec) and 6F10.3 (Beckman/Coulter) are claimed to be immunoreactive in fixed sections and it has been shown that some of the other antibody clones may be reactive in tissues fixed with special fixatives such as non-aldehyde, zinc salts-containing fixatives (Gonzalez et al, 2001) or formal dichromate and with appropriate antigen retrieval and signal amplification system (Gutierrez et al, 1999).

References

Foon KA, Todd RF. Immunologic classification of leukemia and lymphoma. Blood 1986;68:1–31.

Gonzalez L, Anderson I, Deane D, et al. Detection of immune system cells in paraffin wax-embedded ovine tissues. Journal of comparative Pathology 2001;125:41–7.

Gutierrez M, Forster FI, McConnell SA, et al. The dection of CD2+, CD4+, CD8+, and WC1+ T lymphocytes, B cell and macrophages in fixed and paraffin embedded boving tissue using a range of antigen recovery and signal amplification techniques. Veterinary Immunology and Immunopathology 1999;71:321–34.

Knowles DM. Lymphoid cell markers: their distribution and usefulness in the immunophenotypic analyses of lymphoid neoplasms. American Journal of Surgical Pathology 1985;9 (suppl): 85–108

Knowles DM. Immunophenotypic and antigen receptor gene rearrangement analysis in T cell neoplasia. American Journal of Pathology 1989;134:761–85.

Meuer SC, Hussey RE, Fabbi M, et al. An alternative pathway of T cell activation: a functional role for the 50 kd T11 sheep erythrocyte receptor protein. Cell 1984;36:897–906.

Osborn L, Day ES, Miller GT, Karpusas M, Tizard R, Meuer R, Hochman PS. Amino acid residues required for binding of lymphocyte function-associated antigen 3 (CD58) to its counter-receptor CD2. Journal of Experimental Medicine 1995;181:429–34.

CD 3

Sources/clones

Accurate (CLBT3, T3, UCHT1), Becton-Dickinson (Leu 4), Biodesign, Biogenex (CD3, 12F6), Bioprobe, Boehringer Mannheim (4B5), Coulter (T3, CD3), Dako (T3–4B5, UCHT1), Novocastra (UCHT1) Ortho (OKT3), Pharmingen (HIT3A), Sanbio (MEM57), Serotec, and Zymed (SPV-T36) and polyclonal CD3 antisera from Dako, Serotec and Bioprobe/Tha.

Fixation/preparation

The monoclonal antibodies are immunoreactive only in fresh frozen section and cell preparations, whereas polyclonal antisera will react in fixed paraffin-embedded tissue, but only following HIER or prolonged enzyme digestion.

Background

The CD3 antigen consists of five structurally distinct membrane glycoproteins of molecular weight 20–28 kD assembled as a complex comprising extracellular, transmembrane and intracellular domains, is noncovalently associated with the polymorphic TCR α/β or, alternatively, the TCR γ/δ heterodimer.

Stimulation of the CD3 complex results in T cell proliferation, release of cytokines and display of non-specific cytotoxicity, properties requiring the participation of accessory cells. It is believed that the CD3 complex is responsible for mediating signal transduction to the internal environment upon antigenic recognition by the TCR although the actual mechanisms of T cell activation following antigen binding to the TCR are not known (Campana et al, 1987).

CD3 is present in the cytoplasm prior to its detection on the cell surface of thymocytes and more than 95% of thymocytes bear surface and/or cytoplasmic CD3. The antigen is one of the earliest to be expressed in T cell differentiation and begins during the prothymocyte stage prior to entrance into the thymus. It is a T-cell specific surface marker normally present in resting and activated T lymphocytes. Cytoplasmic CD3 expression is lost as common thymocytes differentiate into medullary thymocytes and the antigen is found only on the cell surface in post-cortical T-cells but not in B cells, monocytes/macrophages, myeloid cells or any other cell type except for weak expression

in Purkinje cells of the cerebellum. CD3δ and CD3[epsilon] proteins are detectable in the cytoplasm of virtually all surface CD3-negative ALLs, including those that have not yet rearranged their TCR β genes (van Dongen et al, 1887, 1988), supporting the contention that CD3 gene transcription is one of the earliest events to occur in T cell ontogeny, beginning prior to its entrance into the thymus. The polyclonal anti-CD3 may produce weak staining of squamous epithelium and Hassal's corpuscles in the thymus but this lacks the distinct membrane ring-like pattern seen in T cells and may represent weak cross reactivity (Campana et al, 1989).

Applications

CD3 is the most specific T cell antibody. It is therefore a useful marker to distinguish precursor T cell acute lymphoblastic leukemia/lymphoblastic lymphoma from their B cell counterparts and acute myeloid leukemia (Chetty & Gatter, 1994). CD3 is a pan-T cell lineage-restricted antigen, which is useful for labeling both neoplastic and non-neoplastic T cells and surface CD3 is expressed by all categories of post-thymic T cell lymphomas as well as lymphoblastic lymphoma but not lymphomas of B cell lineage. CD3 may be aberrantly deleted in some peripheral T cell lymphomas (Van Dongen et al, 1988; Cabecadas & Isaacson, 1991). The majority of antyi-CD3 monoclonal antibodies including Leu4 and UCHT1 recognize epitopes mapping to the CD3[epsilon] subunit. Positive staining cells are thymocytes, peripheral T cells, NK cells and also Purkinje cells of the cerebellum.

Comments

The appropriate antibody should be used for cytocentrifuge preparations as MoAb OKT3 (Ortho) detects surface CD3 but not the cytoplasmic antigen in cytocentrifuge preparations. MoAbs Leu 4 (Becton-Dickinson) and UCHT1 (Ancell, Immunotech, Sera Lab, Biodesign) detect cytoplasmic CD3 in cytocentrifuge preparations and many other antibodies are not reactive at all in such preparations. The polyclonal CD3 antibody is a useful reagent for paraffin embedded sections as well cytocentrifuge smear especially following heat-induced epitope retrieval. It is reactive against both normal and neoplastic T cells. CD3 is absent in a subpopulation of T cell neoplasms including cases of mycosis fungoides, pleomorphic small cell lymphoma, pleomorphic medium and large cell lymphoma and anaplastic large cell lymphoma. This may reflect aberrant gene expression by the malignant T cells with loss of the antigen at the outset; alternatively, deletion may occur during the process of large cell transformation as seen in anaplastic large cell lymphoma (Picker et al, 1987).

A recently developed monoclonal anti-CD3 (clone NCL-CD3-PS1) generated to a recombinant fusion protein representing the epsilon subunit of the CD3 molecule is reactive in paraffin embedded sections and promises to be very useful but is currently not commercially available (Steward et al, 1997).

References

Cabecadas JM, Isaacson PG. Phenotyping of T cell lymphomas in paraffin sections – which antibodies? Histopathology 1991;19:419–24.

Campana D, Thompson JS, Amlot P, et al. The cytoplasmic expression of CD3 antigen in normal and malignant cells of the T lymphoid lineage. Journal of Immunology 1987;138:648–55.

Campana D, Janossy G, Coustan-Smith, et al. The expression of T cell receptor-associated proteins during T cell ontogeny in Man. Journal of Immunology 1989;142:57–66.

Chetty R, Gatter K. CD3 structure, function, and role of immunostaining in clinical practice. Journal of Pathology 1994:173;303–7.

Picker LJ, Weiss LM, Medeiros JL, et al. Immunophenotypic criteria for the diagnosis of non-Hodgkin's lymphoma. American Journal of Pathology 1987;128:181–201.

Steward M, Bishop R, Piggott NH, et al. Production and characterization of a new monoclonal antibody effective in recognizing the CD3 T-cell associated antigen in formalin-fixed embedded tissue. Histopathology 1997;30:16–22.

Van Dongen JJM, Quertermous T, Bartram CR, et al. T cell receptor-CD3 complex during early T cell differentiation: analysis of immature T cell acute lymphoblastic leukemias (T-ALL) at DNA, RNA and cell membrane level. Journal of Immunology 1987;138:1260–69.

Van Dongen JJM, Krissansen GE, Wolvers-Tettero ILM, et al. Cytoplasmic expression of the CD3 antigen as a diagnostic marker for immature T-cell malignancies. Blood 1988;71:603–12.

CD 4

Sources/clones

Becton-Dickinson (Leu3), Biotest (T4, TT1), Dako (MT310), Immunotech (BL4, 13B8.2), Novocastra (IF6), Sanbio (BL-TH4, MEM115), Sera-Lab, Serotec (B-A1, B-F5, B-B14, 13B8.2), Pharmingen (RM-4–4, RM-4–5), Zymed (IF6).

Fixation/preparation

Paraffin-embedded sections, fresh frozen tissue and cell preparations.

Background

After the discovery that lymphocytes could be divided into B cells and T cells, discrete subsets of T cells, which function as helper, suppressor and cytotoxic cells were recognized. The CD4 molecule is a nonpolymorphic glycoprotein belonging to the Ig gene superfamily that is expressed on the surface membrane of functionally distinct subpopulation of T cells, mutually exclusive of the CD8 molecule (Maddon et al, 1985). The CD4 molecule is a 55 kd glycoprotein with five external domains, each homologous to an Ig light chain variable region, a transmembrane domain, and a highly conserved intracellular domain. The CD4 gene has been mapped to the short arm of chromosome 12 (Isobe et al, 1986; Brady & Barclay, 1996).

The CD4 molecule acts as a co-receptor with the TCR complex and appears to bind to the nonpolymorphic region of the MHC class II molecule and may serve to increase the avidity of cell-to-cell interactions. The CD4 molecule also serves as a receptor for the human immunodeficiency virus on T cells, monocytes/macrophages and in some neural cells (Dalgleish et al, 1984; Doyle & Strominger, 1987).

The CD4 antigen, like CD8, appears at the common thymocyte stage of T cell differentiation and is expressed in about 80–90% of normal thymocytes. CD4 thus marks helper/inducer T cell and is expressed in 55–65% of mature peripheral T cell. It should be noted that the phenotype-functional association of CD4 to helper and CD8 to suppressor/cytotoxic function is not universal. Subpopulations of suppressor or cytotoxic T cells can be identified among CD4-positive T cells. Although also expressed on monocytes/macrophages, Langerhans' cells and other dendritic cells, B cells do not express CD4.

Applications

The CD4 antibody is useful for the identification of T helper/inducer cells and plays an important role in the immunophenotyping of reactive lymphocytes and in lymphoproliferative disorders. The majority of peripheral T cell lymphomas are derived from the helper T cell subset so that most post-thymic T cell neoplasms are CD4+CD8-. Tγ lymphoproliferative disease is an exception where the proliferative cells are CD4-CD8+. As with other T cell antigens, CD4 may be aberrantly deleted in neoplastic T cells so that the evaluation of such tumors requires the application of a panel of markers in order to identify tumors with such anomalous antigenic expression. CD4 immunostaining is seen in thymocytes (80–90%), mature T cells (65%, T helper and CD4/CD8 thymocytes), macrophages, Langerhans cells, dendritic cells, granulocytes and acute myeloid leukemia cells.

Comments

Anti-CD4 antibodies are mostly immunoreactive only in fresh frozen tissue sections and fresh cytologic preparations. In the latter preparations, fixation in 10% buffered formalin or in 0.1% formal saline produces consistent immunostaining especially if heat induced epitope retrieval is employed. As many phagocytic histiocytes and dendritic cells are also CD4 positive, frozen section staining interpretation is difficult.

Clone 1F6 is immunoreactive in fixed paraffin-embedded sections (Lugovic et al, 2001;Izban et al, 1998) but the use of 1% or greater of hydrogen peroxide to block endogenous peroxidase is detrimental to staining with this antibody and if blocking is necessary it should be done before unmasking with 0.5% H_2O_2/methanol for 10 minutes. Fixation in formal dichromate was claimed to improve immunoreactivity in paraffin sections of bovine tissue (Gutierrez et al, 1999).

OPD4 (CD45RA) was initially claimed to be specific for CD4-positive T cells, but this has not been proven to be so and OPD4 labels both CD4- and CD8-positive cells.

References

Brady RL, Barclay AN. The structure of CD4. Current Topics in Microbiology and Immunology 1996;205:1–18.

Dalgleish AG, Beverley PLC, Clamham PR, et al. The CD4 (T4) antigen is an essential component of the receptor for the AIDS retrovirus. Nature 1984;312:763–6.

Doyle C, Strominger JL. Interaction between CD4 and Class II MHC molecules mediates cell adhesion. Nature 1987;330:256–9.

Isobe M, Huebner K, Maddon PJ, et al. The gene encoding the T cell surface protein T4 is located on human chromosome 12. Proceedings of the National Academy of Science USA 1986;83:4399–402.

Izban KF, His ED, Alkan S. Immunohistochemical analysis of mycosis fungoides on paraffin-embedded tissue sections. Modern Pathology 1998;11:978–82.

Lugovic L, Lipozenocic J, Jakic-Razumovic J. Atopic dermatitis: immunophennotyping of inflammatory cells in skin lesions. International Journal of Deromatology 2001;40:489–94.

Maddon PJ, Littman DR, Godfrey M, et al. The isolation and nucleotide sequence of a cDNA encoding the T cell surface protein T4: a new member of the immunoglobulin gene family. Cell 1985;42:93–104.

CD 5

Sources/clones

Ancell (UCHT2), Becton-Dickinson (Leu1), Biodesign (BL1a, UCHT2), Biogenex (T1), Bioprobe (T1), Coulter (T1), Cymbus Bioscience (UCHT2), Dako (DK23), Novocastra (NCL-CD5, NCL-CD5–4C7), Oncogene (UCHT2), Sanbio (BL-TP), Sera-Lab (UCHT2), Serotec, Sigma and Pharmingen (UCHT2).

Fixation/preparation

Fresh or frozen tissue for most antibodies. Clone NCL-CD5–4C7 is immunoreactive in fixed paraffin-embedded sections following antigen retrieval at 98°C.

Background

The CD5 molecule is a transmembrane glycoprotein of 67 kD, with the typical tripartite structure of a signal peptide. The human CD5 has a sequence similar to that of the Ly-1 antigen in mouse and both are distantly related members of the immunoglobulin super family of genes. CD5 is expressed on both T and some B-lymphocytes. It is weakly positive in the most immature T-cell precursors which are CD34-positive, with the intensity of expression increasing with maturation. CD5 expression is first seen in intra-thymic T-cell progenitors (CD5+/CD34+) which differentiate into CD3+/CD4+/CD8+ T-cells. This antigen is expressed in the majority of T-cells with only as many as 11% of CD4+ lymphocytes being CD5-negative. Two-thirds of these CD5-negative cells are αβ T-cell receptor-positive cells and one-third are γδ T-cells. Anti-CD5 antibodies have been shown to prolong the proliferative response of anti-CD3 activated T-lymphocytes by enhancing signal transduction by the T-cell receptor antigen, a process associated with increased IL-2 production and increased IL-2 receptor expression by the T-cells. The CD5 antigen may also act as a signal transducing molecule in a manner independent of CD3. It has also been suggested that the B-cell surface protein CD72 (Lyb-2) is the ligand or counterstructure for CD5 and occupancy of CD72 by anti-CD72 antibodies, and possibly CD5-positive T-cells, enhances IL-4-dependent CD23 expression on resting B-lymphocytes.

When CD5 is expressed on B-lymphocytes, it is usually weakly staining compared to the strong expression of mature T-lymphocytes. This weak expression makes precise identification of the CD5-positive and CD5-negative B-cell populations difficult. CD5-positive B-cells (B-1 cells) are first seen in the peritoneal and pleural cavities of the foetus at gestation week 15. The cells become prominent in the foetal spleen with 60% or more of splenic B-cells expressing the antigen. At birth, about 68% of cord blood B-cells and approximately half of the peripheral blood B-lymphocytes are CD5 positive and this level drops dramatically in the peripheral blood, to near adult levels, within the first year of life. Fifteen to twenty-five percent of peripheral blood B-lymphocytes in adults are positive for CD5.

There is some suggestion that CD5-positive B-lymphocytes represent a distinct sub-population. Although both CD5-positive and CD5-negative B-cells produce immunoglobulin, upon activation CD5-positive cells selectively produce primarily IgM antibodies, while CD5-negative B-cells make primarily IgG antibodies, an observation made in cord blood. CD-positive B-cells have also been reported to be associated with usually low affinity, polyreactive antibody production, often called auto-antibodies. About 50% of auto-antibody-associated cross-reactive idiotype-bearing B-lymphocytes are CD5-positive. It is possible that some of these differences may be due to lineage differences or simply secondary to some type of B-cell activation and require further investigation (Arber & Weiss, 1995).

Applications

CD 5 is a fairly specific and sensitive marker of T-cell lineage. Almost 85% of T-cell acute lymphoblastic leukemias are CD5-positive and lack of CD5 expression in T-ALL in patients with a white cell count of less than 50,000/ml is reported to be associated with a worse prognosis than corresponding patients with CD5-positive T-cells. CD5 expression has been reported in 3–10% of cases of acute myeloid leukemia. As CD5 is a pan T-cell marker, it is not surprising that the majority of T-cell malignancies (76%) are CD5-positive (Shuster et al, 1990). In peripheral T-cell lymphomas including cutaneous T-cell lymphomas, the loss of CD5 expression can be employed to support a diagnosis of malignancy. In cutaneous T-cell lymphoma, CD5 is not as frequently lost when compared to loss of CD7.

With B-cell neoplasms, CD5 expression has been considered an almost defining characteristic of many entities. Chronic lymphocytic leukemia (CLL) is the most common CD5-positive B-cell malignancy. It is assumed that the small population of

CD5-positive B-cells found in normal healthy adults and prominent in cord blood, is the non-neoplastic counterpart of this type of CLL. B-cell CLL is also associated with poly-specific antibodies or auto-antibodies, and frequently express cross-reactive idiotypes. Over 90% of cases of typical CLL are CD5 positive. CD5 expression may be lost when the large cell lymphoma of Richter's syndrome supervenes in CD5-positive CLL (Matutes & Catovsky, 1991).

Unlike small lymphocytic lymphoma (chronic lymphocytic leukemia) and mantle cell lymphoma, with rare exceptions, monocytoid B-cell lymphoma and low-grade B-cell lymphoma of mucosa-associated lymphoid tissue are usually CD5-negative, a feature which can be employed to distinguish the small B cell lymphoid neoplasms (Chen et al, 2000) (Appendix 2.9). CD5-positive B-cells have been reported to be increased in some patients with monoclonal gammopathy of undetermined significance and in cases of multiple myeloma. De novo expression of CD5 in diffuse large B cell lymphoma was shown to be an indicator of poor prognosis associated with a centroblastic phenotype, interfollicular growth pattern and intravascular or sinusoidal infiltration (Yamaguchi et al, 2002).

CD5-positive neoplastic cells have been found in cases of thymic carcinomas and some cases of atypical thymomas but not in typical thymomas (Hishima et al, 1994). Carcinomas of the lung, breast, oesophagus, stomach, colon, and uterine cervix have been reported to be all CD5-negative.

Positive staining for CD5 is seen in almost all T cells and most T cell malignancies, B cells of the mantle zone of the spleen and lymph node and the corresponding mantle cell lymphomas, B cells in peritoneal and pleural cavities, B cell small cell lymphomas and hairy cell leukemia.

Comments

Most publications indicate that the CD5 antigen is only demonstrable in fresh and frozen tissues but we have successfully demonstrated CD5 using Leu1 antibody following MW epitope retrieval with TUR (Leong et al, 1996). A recently produced antibody to CD5 (clone NCL-CD5) was claimed to be immunoreactive in paraffin-embedded tissues following steam-heat induced antigen retrieval but in a study of 12 CD5+ malignancies, only one, a small cell lymphoma was positive in fixed tissues (Ben-Ezra et al, 1996). Clone NCL-CD5–4C7 shows good immunoreactivity in fixed paraffin-embedded sections following antigen retrieval at 98°C (Dorfman et al, 1997).

References

Arber DA, Weiss LM. CD5. A review. Applied Immunohistochemistry 1995;3:1–22.
Ben-Ezra JM, Kornstein MJ. Antibody NCL-CD5 fails to detect neoplastic CD5+ cells in paraffin sections. American Journal of Clinical Pathology 1996;106:370–373.
Chen CC, Raikow RB, Sonmez-Alpan E, Swerdlow SH. Classification of small B cell lymphoid neoplasms using a paraffin section immunohistochemical panel.

Applied Immunohistochemistry and Molecular Morphology 2000;8:1–11.

Dorfmann DM, Shaksafei A. Usefullness of a new CD5 antibody for the diagnosis of T and B cell lymphoproliferative disorders in paraffin embedded sections. Modern Pathology 1997;10:859–63.

Hishima T, Fukayama M, Fujisawa M, et al. CD5 expression in thymic carcinoma. American Journal of Pathology 1994;145:268–75.

Leong AS-Y, Milios J, Leong FJ. Epitope retrieval with microwaves. A comparison of cirtrate buffer and EDTA with three commercial retrieval solutions. Applied Immunohistochemistry 1996;4:201–7.

Matutes E, Catovsky D. Mature T-cell leukaemias and leukaemia/lymphoma syndromes. Review of our experience in 175 cases. Leukaemia and Lymphoma 1991;4:81–91.

Shuster JJ, Falletta JM, Pullen J, et al. Prognostic factors in childhood T-cell acute lymphoblastic leukaemia: a paediatric oncology group study. Blood 1990;95:116–73.

Yamaguchi M, Seto M, Okamoto M, et al. De novo CD5+ diffuse large B cell lymphoma: a clinicopathologic study of 109 patients. Blood 2002;99:815–21.

NOTES

CD 7

Sources/clones

Becton-Dickinson (Leu 9), Biodesign (WT1, WM31, 8H8.1), Biogenesis (WM31), Coulter (3A1), Cymbus Bioscience (WM31), Dako (DK24), GenTrak, Immunotech, Oncogene U3A1E), Sanbio (WT1), Sera-Lab and Serotec (B-F12, B-5, HNE51).

Fixation/preparation

Fresh frozen tissue and fresh cytologic preparations.

Background

CD 7 antigen is a cell surface glycoprotein of 40 kd expressed on the surface of immature and mature T cells, and natural killer cells. It is the member of immunoglobulin gene superfamily and is the first T cell lineage associated antigen to appear in T cell ontogeny, being expressed in pre-thymic T cell precursors (preceding CD2 expression), and in myeloid precursors in fetal liver and bone marrow, and persisting in circulating T cells. While its precise function is not known, there is recent suggestion that the molecule functions as an Fc receptor for IgM (Lazarovits et al, 1994).

Applications

CD7 is the most consistently expressed T cell antigen in lymphoblastic lymphomas and leukemias, and is specific for T cell lineage and is therefore a useful marker in the identification of such neoplastic proliferations. In mature post-thymic T cell neoplasms, it is the most common pan-T antigen to be aberrantly absent and its absence in a T cell population is a useful pointer to a neoplastic conversion.

CD7 is immunoexpressed on 85% of mature peripheral T cells, the majority of post-thymic T cells, NK cells, some myeloid cells, T cell acute lymphoblastic leukemia/lymphoma, acute myelogenous leukemia (especially M4/5) and chronic myelogenous leukemia. Interestingly, CD7 is conspicuously absent in adult T cell leukemia/lymphoma (Chadburn et al, 1991) and is not expressed in Sezary cells.

Comments

Current antibodies are not immunoreactive in fixed tissues. A recently described antibody to CD7 (clone CBC.37) was reported to be immunoreactive in fixed, paraffin-embedded sections (Saati et al, 2001).

References

Chadburn A, Athan E, Wieczorek R, et al. Detection and characterization of human T cell lymphotropic virus type 1 (HTLV-1) associated T cell neoplasms in an HTLV-1 nonendemic region by polymerase chain reaction. Blood 1991;77:2419–30.

Lazarovits AI, Osman N, Le Feuvre CE, et al. CD7 is associated with CD3 and CD 45 in human T cells. Journal of Immunology 1994;153;3956–66.

Saati TA, Alibaud L, Lamant L, et al. A new monoclonal anti-CD7 antibody reactive in paraffin sections. Applied Immunohistochemistry and Molecular Morphology 2001;9:289–96.

NOTES

CD 8

Sources/clones

Becton-Dickinson (Leu2), Biodesign (UCHT4, CD8.C12, B9.11, B9.2), Biogenex (T8), Biotest (Tu102), Biogenesis (T80C), Dako (DK25, C8/144B), Novocastra (1A5, 4B11), Pharmingen (RPA-Y8), Research Diagnostics (CLB-T8/4, UCHT4), Sanbio (MEM31, BL-T58/2), Sera-Lab (UCHT4) and Serotec (BHT, MF8).

Fixation/preparation

Fresh frozen section and fresh cytological preparations. Clones C8/144B and 1A5 are immunoreactive in fixed paraffin-embedded tissue sections following HIER.

Background

Like CD4, the CD8 molecule is composed of nonpolymorphic glycoproteins, belonging to the Ig superfamily, that are expressed on the surface membrane of mutually exclusive, functionally distinct T cell populations. The CD8 molecule is a 34 kD glycoprotein that forms disulfide-linked homodimers and homomultimers on the cell surface of peripheral T cells; the CD8 gene being linked to the κ locus on chromosome 2. The CD8 molecule comprises an external domain and highly conserved transmembrane and intracellular domains; the external domain showing striking homology with other members of the Ig gene superfamily (Eichmann et al, 1989). The CD8 molecule functions as a TCR co-receptor on suppressor/cytotoxic T cells and recognizes foreign antigens as peptides presented by MHC Class I molecules. In the thymus, the CD8 molecule forms complexes with the CD1 glycoprotein, an MHC class I-like molecule. CD8 appears to bind to the non-polymorphic regions of MHC class I molecules and may thus serve to enhance the avidity of cell-to-cell interactions (Christinck et al, 1991). Both CD4 and CD8 antigens appear during the common thymocyte stage of T cell differentiation and CD8 is expressed by about 80% of normal thymocytes. Thereafter, CD4 and CD8 are retained by those maturing thymocytes destined to become helper/inducer and suppressor/cytotoxic T cells respectively, CD8 being expressed by about 25–35% of peripheral T cells, specifically of the suppressor/cytotoxic subset (Martz et al, 1982). In addition, about 30% of NK cells express low levels of CD8. This phenotypic-functional association is not universal and subpopulations of suppressor/cytotoxic T cells can be identified among CD4-positive cells (Parnes 1989).

Applications

As with the CD4 marker, CD8 has an important role in the immunophenotypic analysis of reactive and neoplastic populations of T cells, being used to identify a mature T cell subset with suppressor/cytotoxic function. Like the CD4 marker, CD8 may also be aberrantly deleted from neoplastic T cells. The CD8 antigen is expressed on T cell lymphoblastic lymphomas (Picker et al, 1987).

A hypopigmented form of mycosis fungoides has been shown to frequently express CD8+ phenotype (El-Shabrawi-Caelen et al, 2002).

25–35% of mature peripheral T cells stain for CD8, these mostly being cytotoxic T cells, CD8 positivity is also seen in NK cells including 30% that are CD3 negative and 70–80% of cortical thymocytes.

Comments

The development of clones C8/144B and 1A5 that are immunoreactive in fixed, paraffin-embedded sections has allowed the study of CD8+ T cells in a variety of diseases including the inflammatory dermatoses (Deguchi et al, 2001; Akiba et al, 2002), cutaneous T cell lymphomas (Jones et al, 2002), gastrointestinal diseases and colorectal carcinoma (Honma et al, 2001; Suzuki et al, 2002), and neuronal destruction (Bien et al, 2002).

References

Akiba H, Kehren J, Ducluzeau MT, et al. Skin inflammation during contact hypersensitivity is mediated by early recruitment of CD8+ T cytotoxic 1 cells inducing keratinocyte apoptosis. Journal of Immunology 2002;168:3079–87.

Bien CG, Bauer J, Deckwerth TL, et al. Destruction of neurons by cytotoxic T cells: a new pathogenic mechanism in Rasmussen's encephalitis. Annals of Neurology 2002;51:311–8.

Christinck ER, Luscher MA, Barber BH, Williams DB. Peptide binding class I MHC on living cells and quantitation of complexes required for CTL lysis. Nature 1991;352:67–70.

Deguchi M, Ohtani H, Sato E, et al. Proliferative activity of CD8+ T cells as an important clue to analyze T cell-mediated inflammatory dermatoses. Archives of Dermatology 2001;293:442–7.

Eichmann K, Boyce NW, Schmidt UR, Jonsson JI. Distinct functions of CD8 (CD4) are utilised at different stages of T lymphocyte differentiation. Immunological Reviews 1989;109:39–75.

El-Shabrawi-Caelen L, Cerroni L, Medeiros LJ, McCalmont TH. Hypopigmented mycosis fungoides: frequent expression of a CD8+ T cell phenotype. American Journal of Surgical Pathology 2002;26:450–7.

Honma J, Mitomi H, Murakami K, et al. Nodular duodenitis involving CD8+ cell infiltration in patients with ulcerative colitis. Hepatogastroenterology 2001;48:1604–10.

Jones D, Vega F, Sarris AH, Medeiros LJ. CD4-CD8- "Double-negative" cutaneous T cell lymphomas share common histologic features and an aggressive clinical course. American Journal of Surgical Pathology 2002;26:225–31.

Martz E, Davignon D, Kurzinger K, Springer TA. The molecular basis for cytotoxic T lymphocyte function: analysis with blocking monoclonal antibodies. Advances in Experimental Medicine and Biology 1982;146:447–465.

Parnes JR. Molecular biology and function of CD4 and CD8. Advances in Immunology 1989;44:265–311.

Picker LJ, Weiss LM, Medeiros JL et al. Immunophenotypic criteria for the diagnosis of non-Hodgkin's lymphoma. American Journal of Pathology 1987;128:181–201.

Suzuki A, Masuda A, Nagata H, et al. Mature dendritic cells make clusters with T cells in the invasive margin of colorectal carcinoma. Journal of Pathology 2002;196:37–43.

CD 9

Sources/clones

Biodesign (ALB6, MM2/57),
Cymbus Bioscience (MM2/57),
GenTrak, Immunotech (ALB6),
Novocastra (72F6), Research
Diagnostics (MM2/57), Sanbio
(CLB/CD9), Sera-Lab (FMC56,
FMC8), Serotec (MM 2/57)

Fixation/preparation

Fresh frozen tissue and cytologic
preparations, and formalin-fixed
paraffin-embedded tissue.

Background

The CD 9 antigen is a cell
surface glycoprotein (p24) of
MW 24 kDa belonging to the
tetra-membrane-spanning protein
family (tetraspanins), coded by
chromosome 12. The antigen is
present on pre-B cells, monocytes
and platelets and has protein
kinase activity. The majority of
mature peripheral blood or
lymphoid tissue B cells or other
normal circulating hematopoietic
cells other than platelets does not
express it. It is present on
activated T cells, mast cells and
some dendritic reticulum cells
(Kersey et al, 1981; Ash et al,
1982; Carbone et al, 1987). CD9
also regulates motility in a variety
of cell lines and appears to be an
important regulator of Schwann
cell behavior in the peripheral
nervous system.

Applications

The expression of CD9 in
malignant cells is complex and not
strictly lineage, activation or
differentiation associated. It is
found in >75% of precursor B cell
ALL/LBL, about 50% of B cell
CLL and some better
differentiated B cell neoplasms
such as prolymphocytic leukemia
and multiple myeloma as well as
some T cell lymphomas and
acute myeloid leukemias. Other
B cell lymphomas including
centrocytic lymphoma, follicle
center cell lymphoma and
Burkitt's lymphoma may also
express this antigen and there is
also variable expression on
neuroblastomas and some
epithelial tumors (Komada et al,
1983; San Miguel et al, 1986;
Lardelli et al, 1990). CD9
immunoexpression has been
claimed to indicate a favourable
prognosis in breast carcinoma
although a recent study showed no
benefit (Jamil et al, 2001). Anti-
CD9 antibodies were found to
specifically inhibit the
transendothelial migration of
melanoma cells (Longo et al, 2001)
and the protein immunostaining
was suggested to be useful in the
differential diagnosis papillary renal
cell carcinoma dn collecting duct
carcinomas and also between
chromophobe and conventional
renal cell carcinomas, being
consistently positive in papillary
and chromophobe carcinomas
(Kuroda et al, 2001).

Comments

Expressed on pre-B cells, B cell
subset, T cells, macrophages,
platelets, eosinophils, basophils,
megakaryocytes, endothelial cells,
brains, peripheral nerves, vascular
smooth muscle, cardiac muscle
and epithelial cells. Because of its
expression by a wide spectrum of
B and T cell neoplasms, this
marker has limited application in
the phenotypic analysis of
hematopoietic neoplasms. It may
have other diagnostic applications
in non-hematopoietic tumors
discussed above. We employ the
Novocastra 72F6 clone in
paraffin-embedded sections with
retrieval in EDTA at pH8.0.

References

Ash RC, Jansen J, Kersey JH, et al.
Normal human pluripotential and
committed hematopoietic
progenitors do not express the
p24 antigen detected by
monoclonal antibody BA-2;
implication for immunotherapy of

lymphocytic leukemia. Blood 1982;60:1310–6.

Carbone A, Poletti A, Manconi R, et al. Heterogenous in situ immunotyping of follicular dendritic reticulum cells in malignant lymphomas of B cell origin. Cancer 1987;60:2919–26.

Jamil F, Preston D, Shousha S. CD9 immunohistochemical staining of breast carcinoma: unlikely to provide useful prognostic information for routine use. Histopathology 2001;39:572–7.

Kersey JH, LeBien TW, Abramson CS, et al. P24: A human leukemia associated and lymphohemopoietic progenitor cell surface structure identified with monoclonal antibody.

Journal of Experimental Medicine 1981;153;726–31.

Komada Y, Peiper SC, Melvin, et al. A monoclonal antibody (SJ-9A4) to p24 present on common ALLs, neuroblastoma and platelets. I. Characterization and development of a unique radioimmunometric assay. Leukemia Research 1983;7:487–98.

Kuroda N, Inoue K, Guo L, et al. Expression of CD9/motility-related protein 1 (MRP-1) in renal parenchymal neoplasms: consistent expression in papillary and chromophobe renal cell carcinomas. Human Pathology 2001;32:1071–7.

Lardelli P, Bookman MA, Sundeen J, et al. Lymphocytic lymphoma of

intermediate differentiation: Morphologic and immunophenotypic spectrum and clinical correlations. American Journal of Surgical Pathology 1990;14:752–63.

Longo N, Yanez-Mo M, Mittelbrunn M, et al. Regulatory role of tetraspanin CD9 in tumor-endothelial cell interaction during transendothelial invasion of melanoma cells. Blood 2001;98:3717–26.

San Miguel JF, Caballero MD, Gonzalez M, et al. Immunological phenotype of neoplasms involving the B cell in the last step of differentiation. British Journal of Haematology 1986;62:75–83.

CD 10 (CALLA)

Sources/clones

Accurate, Biodesign (ALB1, ALB2), Coulter (J5), Cymbus Bioscience (Mem 78), Dako (SS2/36), GenTrak, Immunotech (ALB1, ALB2), Novocastra (56C6), Research Diagnostics (MEM 78, J-149), Sanbio (MEM 78, BFA.11), Sera-Lab (B-E3) and Serotec.

Fixation/preparation

With the exception of clone 56C6, current antibodies are mostly immunoreactive only in fresh frozen tissue.

Background

The common acute lymphoblastic leukemia antigen (CALLA) is a 100 kD single chain glycoprotein whose sequence is virtually identical to that of neutral endopeptidase (NEP-24.11 enkephalinase). It is a metalloenzyme that requires zinc as a cofactor and is thought to inactivate regulatory peptides favoring cell differentiation. It was originally defined by hetero-antiserum raised in rabbits by immunization with cells of a "non-B, non-T" cell acute lymphoblastic leukemia. CD10 is present on the cell surface of stem cells in the bone marrow and fetal liver that are also TdT and HLA-DR antigen positive (Anderson et al, 1984; Letarte et al, 1988).

Applications

CD10 was originally used as a specific marker for non-B, non-T cell ALL. It is expressed in approximately 75% of precursor B cell ALL and more than 90% of cases of myelogenous leukemia in lymphoid blast crisis, but CD10 is not a leukemia-specific antigen nor is it B or T cell lineage restricted (Carrel et al, 1983). The antigen is found on variable proportions of cells making up T cell ALL/LBL, Burkitt's lymphoma, follicular lymphoma and multiple myeloma (Durie & Grogan, 1985; Ruiz-Arguelles, 1994). In addition, CD10 is expressed on the renal glomerular and tubular cells, fibroblasts, bile canaliculi, melanoma cell lines and various other epithelial cells. More recent applications of CD10 include the staining of endometrial stroma including endometrial stromal nodules and endometrial stromal sarcoma so that it can be used as a discriminator from histologic mimics such as uterine cellular leiomyoma and leiomyosarcoma,

adult granulosa cell tumor and undifferentiated endometrial carcinoma (McCluggage et al, 2001), the latter staining diffusely for alpha smooth muscle actin and desmin, alpha-inhibin, and cytokeratins respectively.

There is recent suggestion that CD10 immunostaining in large B cell lymphoma correlates with prognosis (Ohshima et al, 2001). CD10 immunoreactivity is significantly stronger in follicular lymphoma compared to hyperplastic follicles so that this antigen has been used to distinguish the two forms of lymphoid nodules (Barcus et al, 2000). Interestingly, CD10 positivity has been demonstrated in the neoplastic T cells of 90% of cases of angioimmunoblastic lymphoma but not in other peripheral T cell lymphomas (Attygalle et al, 2002). The antigen has also been shown in melanoma cells (Carrel, 1993), renal cell carcinoma (Chu & Arber, 2000) and mesenchymal cells of the skin (Kanitakis et al, 2000) including tumors like dermatofibroma, dermatofibrosarcoma protuberans, neurofibromas and as many as 47% of malignant melanoma cases (Kanitakis, 2001). The recent demonstration of CD10 immunoexpression in myoepithelial cells of the breast suggested that it might be an alternative to smooth muscle actin as a marker of such cells particularly as the latter stains normal vessels and spindled stromal cells (Moritani et al, 2002). CD10 immunoexpression has also been employed to stain the canaliculi in 60% (of 15 cases) of hepatocellular carcinomas studied but were not seen in cholangiocarcinomas or metastatic carcinoma (Xiao al, 2001).

Comments

Clone 56C6 is the most immunoreactive antibody for paraffin sections and requires HIER for enhancement. Paraffin section immunostaining correlates well with flow cytometric analysis and decalcification did not appear to affect immunoreactivity (Chu et al, 2000). Retrieval at 120°C produces the best results. While CD10 is neither lineage specific nor tumor restricted, it remains a useful marker, especially in the analysis of childhood ALL/LBL and follicular lymphomas (Greeves et al 1975; 1983).

CD10 is localized to cell membranes and cytoplasm of hematolymphoid cells and rarely Golgi staining is seen.

References

Anderson KC, Bates MP, Slaughtenhoupt BL, et al. Expression of human B cell associated antigens on leukemias and lymphomas: a model of B cell differentiation. Blood 1984;63:1424–33.

Attygalle A, Al-Jehani R, Diss TC, et al. Neoplastic T cells in angioimmunoblastic T cell lymphoma express CD10. Blood 2002;99:627–33.

Barcus ME, Karageorge LS, Veloso YL, Krostein MJ. CD10 expression in follicular lymphoma versus reactive follicular hyperplasia. Evaluation in paraffin-embedded tissue. Applied Immunohistochemistry and Molecular Morphology 2000;8:263–6.

Carrel S, Schmidt-Kessen A, Mach J-P, et al. Expression of common acute lymphoblastic leukemia (cALLa) by lymphomas of B cell and T cell lineage. Journal of Immunology 1983;130:2456–60.

Carrel S, Zografos L, Schreyer M, et al. Expression of CALLA/CD10 on human melanoma cells. Melanoma Research 1993;3:319–23.

Chu P, chang KL, Weiss LM, Arber DA. Immunohistochemical detection of CD10 in paraffin sections of hematopoietic neoplasms. A comparison with flow cytometry detection in 56 cases. Applied Immunohistochemistry and Molecular Morphology 2000;8:257–62.

Chu P, Arber D. Paraffin section detection of CD10 in 505 non-hematopoietic neoplasms: frequent expression in renal cell carcinoma and endometrial stromal sarcoma. American Journal of Clinical Pathology 2000;113:374–82.

Durie BGM, Grogan TM. CALLA-positive myeloma: an aggressive subtype with poor survival. Blood 1985;66:229–32.

Greeves MF, Brown G, Rapson NT, Lister TA. Antisera to acute lymphoblastic leukemia cells. Clinical Immunology and Immunopathology 1975;4:67–84.

Greeves MF, Hariri G, Newman RA, et al. Selective expression of the common acute lymphoblastic leukemia (gp 100) antigen on immature lymphoid cells and their malignant counterparts. Blood 1983;61:628–39.

Kanitakis J. Usefullness of CD10 antigen detection in paraffin-embedded tissue specimens (letter). American Journal of Clinical Pathology 2001;115:466

Kanitakis J, Bourchany D, Claudy A. Expression of CD10 antigen by mesenchymal tumors of the skin. Anticancer Research 2000;20:3539–44.

McCluggage WG, Sumathi VP, Maxwell P. CD10 is a sensitive and diagnostically useful immnohistochemical marker of normal endometrial stroma and of endometrial stromal neoplasms. Histopathology 2001;39:273–78.

Moritani S, Kushima R, Sugihara H, et al. Availability of CD10 immunohistochemistry as a marker of breast myoepithelial cells on paraffin sections. Modern Pathology 2002;15:397–405.

Letarte M, Vera S, Tran R, et al. Common acute lymphocytic leukemia antigen is identical to neutral endopeptidase. Journal of Experimental Medicine 1988;168:1247–53.

Ohshima K, Kawasaki C, Muta H, et al. CD10 and Bcl10 expression in diffuse large B cell lymphoma: CD10 is a marker of improved prognosis. Histopathology 2001;39:156–62.

Ruiz-Arguelles GJ, San Miguel JF. Cell surface markers in multiple myeloma. Mayo Clinic Proceedings 1994;69;684–90.

Xiao SY, Wang HL, Hart J, et al. cDNA arrays and immunohistochemistry identification of CD10/CALLA expression in hepatocellular carcinoma. American Journal of Pathology 2001;159:1415–21.

CD 103

Sources/clones

Biogenex (2G5), Coulter (2G5), Dako (Ber-ACT8), Immunotech (2G5), Serotec (295.1).

Fixation/preparation

The antibodies are mainly immunoreactive in cryostat sections of fresh frozen tissue. Immunoreactivity in fixed paraffin-embedded sections has not been reported.

Background

The antibody to CD 103, also known as anti-Human Mucosal Lymphocyte 1 antigen (HML-1) and integrin alphaE chain, recognizes a T cell associated trimeric protein of 150, 125 and 105 kD (Falini et al, 1991), which is expressed on 95% of intraepithelial lymphocytes and only on 1–2% of peripheral blood lymphocytes (Spencer et al, 1988, Kruschwitz et al, 1991). CD 103 (alpha E integrin) antigen is part of the family of beta 7 integrins on human mucosal lymphocytes which play a specific role in mucosal localization or adhesion (Parker et al, 1992). CD 103 is a receptor for the epithelial cell-specific ligand E-cadherin and is expressed by a major subset of CD3+, CD8+, CD4- lymphocytes present in the intestinal mucosa. About 40% of isolated intestinal lamina propria lymphocytes (LPL) expressed HML-1, the majority being CD8+. Virtually all LPL expressed CD45RO, whereas only about 50% were CD29+, a percentage similar to that in peripheral blood lymphocytes. HML-1+ cells were almost exclusively CD45RA- and the in vitro expression of HML-1 was inducible on T cells by mitogen (Schieferdecker et al, 1990). CD103+ CD8+ T lymphocytes have also been demonstrated in the bladder urothelium and their corresponding tumors (Cresswell et al, 2001), the epidermis in inflammatory skin disorders (Pauls et al, 2001), pancreas in chronic pancreatisis (Ebert et al, 1998) and graft epithelium during renal allograft rejection (Hadley et al, 2001).

Applications

Antibodies to CD 103 are used for the diagnosis of intestinal T cell lymphoma (Schmitt-Graff et al, 1996). CD103 has been found to be a useful marker of B cell hairy cell leukemia which shows strong reactivity for CD 22, CD 25, CD 103, DBA.44 as well as immunoglobulin light chain restriction (Harris et al, 1994; Cordone et al, 1995). The abnormal coexpression of CD103, CD25, and intense CD11c and CD20 on monomorphic, slightly large B lymphocytes has been shown to be highly characteristic of hairy cell leukemia (Cornfield et al, 2001; Wu et al, 2000). The antigen may be occasionally expressed by some B cell lymphomas (Moller et al, 1990). The antigen has also been demonstrated in T lymphoblastic lymphoma (Falini et al, 1991).

Comments

Current diagnostic applications of antibodies to CD 103 are restricted by their immunoreactivity only in fresh cell preparations and cryostat sections. CD103 may be employed as a marker of intraepithelial lymphocytes and activated lymphocytes. It is positive in B hairy cell leukemia, acute myeloid leukemia, enteropathy-associated T cell lymphoma, adult HTLV-1 associated T cell leukemia.

References

Cordone I, Annino L, Masi S, et al. Diagnostic relevance of peripheral blood immunocytochemistry in hairy cell leukemia. Journal of Clinical Pathology 1995;48:955–60.

Cornfield DB, Mitchell Nelson DM, Rimsza LM, et al. The diagnosis of hairy cell leukemia can be established by flow cytometric analysis of peripheral blood, even in patients with low levels of circulating malignant cells. American Journal of Hematology 2001;67:223–6.

Cresswell J, Robertson H, Neal DE, et al. Distribution of lymphocytes of the alpha(E)beta(7) phenotype and E-cadherin in normal urothelium and bladder carcinomas. Clinical and ExperimentalImmunology 2001;126:397–402.

Ebert MP, Ademmer K, Muller-Ostermeyer F, et al. CD8+CD103+ T cells analogous to interstinal intraepithelial lymphocytes infiltrate the pancreas in chronic pancreatitis. American Journal of Gastroenterology 1998;934:2141–7.

Falini B, Flenghi L, Fagioli M, et al. Expression of the intestinal T-lymphocyte associated molecule HML-1; analysis of 75 non-Hodgkin's lymphomas and description of the first HML-1 positive T-lymphoblastic lymphoma. Histopathology 1991;18:421–6.

Hadley GA, Charandee C, Weir MR, et al. CD103+ CTL accumulate within the graft epithelium during clinical renal allograft rejection Transplantation 2001;72:1548–55.

Harris NL, Jaffe ES, Stein H, et al. A revised European-American classification of lymphoid neoplasms: a proposal from the International Lymphoma Study Group. Blood 1994;84:1361–92.

Kruschwitz M, Fritzsche G, Schwarting M, et al. Ber-ACT8: new monoclonal antibody to the mucosa lymphocyte antigen. Journal of Clinical Pathology 1991;44:636–45.

Moller P, Mielke B, Moldenhauer G. Monoclonal antibody HML-1, a marker for intraepithelial T cells and lymphomas derived thereof, also recognizes hairy cell leukemia and some B cell lymphomas. American Journal of Pathology 1990;136:509–12.

Parker CM, Cepek KL, Russell GJ, et al. A family of beta 7 integrins on human mucosal lymphocytes. Proceedings of the National Academy of Sciences USA 1992;89:1924–8.

Pauls K, Schon M, Kubitza RC, et al. Role of integrin alphaE (CD103) beta 7 for tissue-specific epidermal localization of CD8+ T lymphocytes. Journal Investigative Dermatology 2001;117:569–75.

Schieferdecker HL, Ullrich R, Weiss-Breckwoldt AN, et al. The HML-1 antigen of interstinal lymphocytes is an activation antigen. Journal of Immunology 1990;144:2541–9.

Schmitt-Graff A, Hummel M, Zemlin M, et al. Intestinal T-cell lymphoma: a reassessment of cytomorphological and phenotypic features in relation to patterns of small bowel remodelling. Virchows Archives 1996;429:27–36.

Spencer J, Cerf-Bensussan N, Jarry A, et al. Enteropathy associated T cell lymphoma (malignant histiocytosis of the intestine) is recognized by a monoclonal antibody (HML1) that defines a membrane molecule on human lymphocytes. American Journal of Pathology 1988;132:1–5.

Wu ML, Kwaan HC, Goolsby CL. Atypical hairy cell leukemia. Archives of Pathology and Laboratory Medicine 2000;124:1710–3.

CD 11

Sources/clones

CD 11a

Ancell (38), Biodesign (MEM 25, SPV-L7), Cymbus Bioscience (38), Dako (MHM24), GenTrak, Immunotech (25.3), Sanbio (MEM 25), Serotec (B-B15) and Pharmingen (2D7).

CD11b

Ancell (44), Biodesign (44, Bear-1), Biogenex, Boehringer Mannheim, Cymbus Bioscience, Dako (2LPM19c), GenTrak, Immunotech (Bear-1), JapanTanner, Research Diagnostics (CD 44), Sanbio (Bear-1), Sera Lab (44), Serotec (ED7) and Pharmingen (M1/70).

CD 11c

Ancell (3.9), Becton Dickinson (Leu M5), Biodesign (FK24, BU15), Cymbus Bioscience, Dako (KB90), GenTrak, Immunotech (BU15), Oncogene (3.9), Research Diagnostics (CD39), Sanbio (FK24), Serotec (3.9) and Sera-Lab (FK24).

Fixation/preparation

Current antibodies are only immunoreactive in fresh frozen tissue.

Background

Each of the CD11 subtypes represents a different α chain which forms one of the $\beta 2$ family of integrin adhesion receptors when linked non-covalently to $\beta 2$ (CD18) to form a heterodimer. CD11a, leukocyte function-associated protein (LFA-1), with a MW 180 kD is present on B cells, T cells, NK cells, monocytes, granulocytes, megakaryocytes and activated platelets. CD11b (Mac-1), the C3bi receptor, has a MW of 165 kD and it is present on granulocytes, monocytes and some histiocytes. CD11c, which has a MW of 150 kD, is present on monocytes, tissue macrophages, granulocytes, some suppressor/cytotoxic T cells and a subset of B cells. It is usually positive on true histiocytic malignancies and some B cell lymphomas including hairy cell leukemia and monocytoid B cell lymphoma (Chadburn et al, 1990).

CD11/CD18 integrins have a function in intercellular communication between lymphocytes and between lymphocytes and endothelial cells. The interaction between leukocytes and endothelial cells involves CD11/CD18 integrins which bind to intercellular adhesion molecules ICAM-1 (CD-45) and ICAM-2 (Albelda et al, 1994).

Applications

Currently, the diagnostic applications for this marker are very limited and available antibodies are reactive only in frozen sections. Differential expression of CD11a (LFA-1) has been described in small cell lymphocytic lymphoma and CLL and has been used to account for the difference in peripheral blood involvement in these entities but the findings require confirmation. In the immunophenotypic separation of monocytoid B cell lymphoma from other small cell lymphomas such as plasmacytoid small cell lymphoma, CLL and mantle cell lymphoma, CD11c has been suggested to be a useful discriminant, being more frequently expressed in monocytoid lymphoma.

CD11a is found on all leukocytes. CD11b is found on granulocytes, macrophages, NK cells, follicular dendritic cells, myeloid cells and some B and T lymphocytes. Hairy cell leukemia expresses this antigen. CD11c stains 50% of activated CD4/8+ T cells, granulocytes, lymphocytes, macrophages, NK cells. In B-CLL expression is associated with good prognosis and it is expressed in virtually all cases of hairy cell leukemia.

References

lbelda SM, Smith CW, Ward PA. Adhesion molecules and inflammatory injury. FASEB Journal 1994:8;504–12.

Chadburn A, Inghirami G, Knowles DM. Hairy cell leukemia-associated antigen Leu M5 (CD 11c) is preferentially expressed by benign activated and neoplastic CD8 cells. American Journal of Pathology 1990;136:29–37.

CD 15

Sources/clones

Accurate (C3D-1), Becton-Dickinson (Leu M1), Biodesign (B428, 80H5, G15), Biogenex (Tu9), Cymbus Bioscience (28), Dako (C3D-1), Immunotech (80H5), Novocastra, Research Diagnostics (28), Sanbio (BL-G15), Sera-Lab (MC-1), Serotec (NH6, B-H8).

Fixation/preparation

Fresh frozen tissue and formalin fixed paraffin-embedded tissue. Muramidase pre-treatment increases reactivity, particularly in acute myeloid leukemia.

Background

A variety of antibodies to CD15 has been generated in different ways but appears to have similar immunoreactivity patterns. Some antibodies were developed by immunization and screening against human hematopoietic cell lines and were originally felt to be specific for myeloid leukemias, while other antibodies were developed from specific human and mouse carcinoma cell lines and were later found to react with granulocytes and a variety of human carcinomas. The antibodies are mostly of IgM

isotype and have the common property of being able to recognize a specific sugar sequence that occurs in the glycolipid lacto-N-fucopentaose III ceramide and is also found in several glycolipids such as glycoproteins. The sugar sequence is referred to as X hapten or Le^x and its highly immunogenic nature in mice has led to the production of several IgM monoclonal antibodies to the CD15 cluster. The lacto-N-fucopentaose III has been identified in human milk and is virtually absent in benign human epithelium. A related substance lacto-N-fucopentaose II is present in many benign human epithelial cells. The glycolipid lacto-N-fucopentaose III has a structure similar to the Lewis blood group antigens. The CD15 antigen exists in a sialylated or un-sialylated form, the former requiring prior digestion with muramidase to enable detection. Mature granulocytes and monocytes express the un-sialylated molecule (Aber & Weiss, 1993).

Applications

CD15 antibodies react with mature neutrophils, generally the reactivity is less with the less

mature forms of the granulocyte series. Normal bone marrow myeloblasts are negative and some promyelocytes may not stain. Paraffin-embedded cells show both membrane and cytoplasmic staining. Normal platelets, red blood cells and B-lymphocytes are routinely negative as are the vast majority of T-lymphocytes. Mitogen activated lymphocytes show positivity with the Leu M1 antibody and these are mostly T-lymphocytes of the T4 subset. While some T8-positive cells also express the antigen, a longer period of stimulation was needed to induce this finding.

In leukemia, CD15 antibodies react with all neoplastic myeloid and monocytic proliferations although there is a variable pattern with different antibodies (Appendix 2.5). CD15 positivity is reported to be lost in cases of relapsed acute myeloid leukemia, correlating with a poorer survival. Almost all cases of chronic myelogenous leukemia have demonstrated the presence of CD15 while in chronic phase. Approximately 16% of cases of acute lymphoblastic leukemia demonstrate the co-expression of at least one myeloid antigen and up to 50% of such cases are reportedly CD15 positive although the range of positivity is between 2–6%. CD15 expression is highest in common acute lymphoblastic leukemia antigen (CALLA)-negative cases, which generally have a worse prognosis than cases of CALLA-positive ALL (Bernstein, 1982).

CD15 expression is very helpful in the diagnosis of Hodgkin's disease as almost all the CD15 antibodies available react with Reed-Sternberg cells and the mononuclear variants (Appendix 2.3, 2.10). Characteristically, the staining is membranous with globular, juxta-nuclear staining of the Golgi complex. The cytoplasmic membrane staining has been confirmed by ultrastructural studies and lysosomal granules contiguous with perinuclear vesicles representing the Golgi apparatus are also stained. Reed-Sternberg cells and atypical mononuclear variants in Hodgkin's disease of mixed cellularity type, nodular sclerosing and lymphocyte depleted type show staining with CD15 antibodies. However, lymphocyte predominant Hodgkin's disease is CD15-negative particularly in the nodular and in some cases of the diffuse subtype (Stein et al, 1986) (Appendix 2.10). Digestion with neuraminidase has been reported to result in staining of the L & H cells in lymphocyte predominant Hodgkin's disease although the staining has been described to be less intense and predominantly cytoplasmic in distribution. Similarly, enzyme pre-treatment has been reported to produce positivity in T-cell lymphomas mostly of the mature phenotype, particularly in advanced stage mycosis fungoides. A smaller percentage of low-grade B-cell lymphomas have also been

reported to be CD15 positive. CD15 is a useful marker for granulocytic sarcoma, staining the majority of cases. (Swerdlow & Wright, 1986).

While CD15 expression has been widely employed for the confirmation of the diagnosis of Hodgkin's disease, little is known of the role of the CD15 antigen in the pathobiology of the disease and its prognostic relevance, if any. It has been shown that CD15 expressed in its non-sialylated form (clones LeuM1 and 80H5) and the absence of sialylated CD15 (FH6 and CSLEX1) expression on Reed Sternberg cells correlated with favourable outcome. There was also preferential expression of sialyl-CD15, notably in bone marrow metastases so that it was suggested that in the progression of Hodgkin's disease towards a widely disseminated form, the LewisX moiety of the antigen acquires sialyl-group, conferring on the tumor cells the capacity to metastaze (Benharroch et al, 2000)

Strong CD15 positivity has been found in carcinomas from a wide variety of sites. It is employed in a panel for the discrimination of adenocarcinoma from malignant mesothelioma, the latter being generally CD15-negative. However, it should be noted that this is not an absolute discriminator as CD15 may be immunoexpressed in as many as 6% of mesotheliomas (Roberts et al, 2001). Cytomegalovirus infected cells have also been found to react with CD15 antibodies, predominantly with cytoplasmic staining. The combination of immunostaining with cytokeratin, HBME, CD57

or (CD15) is said to be a sensitive and specific test for papillary thyroid carcinoma, allowing separation from reactive thyroid nodules (Mai et al, 2000).

Comments

CD15 antibodies are particularly useful for the identification of Reed-Sternberg cells especially when they are employed in a panel that includes CD45 (LCA), Reed-Sternberg cells showing the characteristic membranous and Golgi staining for CD15 and negative staining for CD45 (Appendix 2.3; 2.10). It is also a useful discriminant when used in an appropriate panel for the separation of adenocarcinoma from malignant mesothelioma, adenocarcinomas and the antibodies label the myeloid cells of granulocytic sarcoma CD15 being mostly negative in mesothelioma (Sewell et al, 1987). Staining is enhanced with microwave epitope retrieval using citrate buffer and enzyme digestion should not be performed when employed for the identification of Reed-Sternberg cells and adenocarcinomas.

Positive staining is seen in myeloid cells (90%), activated B and T cells (including infectious mononucleosis), Reed Sternberg cells, 20% of T cell lymphomas, 5% of B cell lymphomas and 50% of carcinomas. No staining is seen in erythroid cells, platelets or acute lymphocytic leukemia.

References:
Aber DA, Weiss LM. CD15: A review. Applied Immunohistochemistry 1993;1:17–30.
Benharroch D, Dima E, Levy A, et al. Differential expression of sialyl and non-sialyl CD15 antigens on

Hodgkin-Reed Sternberg cells: significance in Hodgkin's disease. Leukemia and Lymphoma 2000;39:185–94.

Bernstein ID, Andrews RG, Cohen SF, McMaster BE. Normal and malignant human myelocytic and monocytic cells identified by monoclonal antibodies. Journal of Immunology 1982;128:876–81.

Mai KT, Ford JC, Yazdi HM, et al Immunohistochenical study of papillary thyroid carcinoma and possible papillary thyroid carcinoma-related benign thyroid nodules. Pathology Research and Practice 2000;196:533–40.

Sewell HF, Jaffray B, Thompson WD. Reaction of monoclonal anti-Leu M1 – a myelomonocytic marker (CD15) – with normal and neoplastic epithelia. Journal of Pathology 1987;151:279–84.

Stein H, Hansmann ML, Lennert K, et al. Reed-Sternberg and Hodgkin's cells in lymphocyte-predominant Hodgkin's disease of nodular subtype containing J chain. American Journal of Clinical Pathology 1986;86:292–7.

Swerdlow SH, Wright SA. A spectrum of Leu M1 staining in lymphoid and hemopoietic proliferations. American Journal of Clinical Pathology 1986;85:283–8.

NOTES

CD 19

Sources/clones

Accurate (B19, CLB/B4/1, FMC63, polyclonal), Becton Dickinson (SJ25C1), Biodesign (BC3), Biogenex (B4), Biosource (BC3, SJ25C1), Caltag Laboratories (SJ25C1), Coulter (B4), Cymbus Bioscience (RFB9, SJ25-C1), Dako (HD37), Immunotech (386.12, J4.119), Novocastra (4G7/2E, FMC63), Pharmingen (B43, HIB19), Sanbio/Monosan (SJ25C1), Seralab, Sigma Chemical (SJ25C1), Zymed (SJ25-C1).

Fixation/preparation

The majority of these antibodies are only applicable to cryostat sections, although they may be used in acetone-fixed cryostat sections and smears. They are not suitable for formalin-fixed paraffin embedded sections.

Background

The CD19 gene (along with CD20 and CD22) encode transmembrane proteins with at least two extracellular immunoglobulin-like domains that are of vital importance to B-cell function. Similar to the immunoglobulin genes, they are expressed in a lineage-specific and developmentally regulated manner (Kehrl et al, 1994). In normal cells, CD19 antigen (90 kD polypeptide) (beta 2 integrin) is the most ubiquitously expressed protein in the B lymphocyte lineage (Scheuermann & Racila, 1995). CD19 expression is induced at the point of B lineage commitment during the differentiation of the hemopoietic stem cell. Its expression continues through pre-B and mature B cell differentiation, being down-regulated during terminal differentiation into plasma cells. Furthermore, CD19 expression is maintained in neoplastic B-cells enhancing its diagnostic usefulness. Since CD19 is not expressed in pluripotent stem cells, it has become the target for a variety of immunotherapeutic agents (Scheuermann & Racila, 1995).

Applications

B43 monoclonal antibody recognizes the same surface epitope as several other anti-CD19 monoclonal antibodies. Using clone B43 to test for CD19 expression on 340 leukemias and 151 malignant lymphomas, Uckun et al (1988) showed CD19 to be the most reliable B lineage surface marker. The advantage of immunodetection of CD19 expression is that B lineage leukemias and lymphomas rarely lose the epitope (Scheuermann & Racila, 1995). Furthermore, CD19 is not expressed on myeloid, erythroid, megakaryocytic or multilineage bone marrow progenitor cells (Uckun et al, 1988).

Comments

Although most B cells carry the CD19 antigen, the use of anti-CD19 is restricted to cryostat sections and therefore not useful to routine diagnostic histopathology practice.

CD19 is the first antigen to be expressed on B cells after HLA-DR. Positive staining seen in Pre B, B cells and follicular dendritic cells. Plasma cells are negative.

References

Kehrl JH, Riva A, Wilson GL, Thevenin C. Molecular mechanisms regulating CD19, CD29 and CD22 gene expression. Immunology Today 1994;15:432–6.

McMichael AJ (ed): Leucocyte Typing III, White Cell Differentiation Antigens. Oxford, England: Oxford University Press, 1987;305.

Scheuermann RH, Racila E. CD19 antigen in leukaemia and lymphoma diagnosis and immunotherapy. Leukemia and Lymphoma 1995;18:385–97.

Uckun FM, Jaszcz W, Ambrus JL, et al. Detailed studies on expression and function of CD19 surface determinant by using B43 monoclonal antibody and the clinical potential of anti-CD19 immunotoxins. Blood 1988;71:13–29.

CD 20

Sources/clones

Becton-Dickinson (Leu 16), Biodesign (BB6), Biogenesis (MEM97), Biogenex (L260), Coulter (B1), Cymbus Bioscience (MEM97, BC1), Dako (L26), Immunotech (L26, HRC20-B9E9), Monosan (MEM-97), Sanbio (MEM97), Sera-Lab (BC1), Serotec (B>B6, BC1), Signet, Novocastra, Pharmingen (2H7) and Zymed (L26).

Fixation/preparation

All the available antibodies to CD20 react in paraffin and frozen sections and can be used to label cells in suspension. Immunoreactivity is enhanced by heat-induced antigen retrieval but not proteolytic digestion.

Background

The CD20 molecule is one of the best markers of B cell lineage. It is a membrane-embedded, nonglycosylated phosphoprotein which appears in early pre-B cells and throughout its maturation into late pre-B cells. It is expressed on the surface of all mature B-lymphocytes but not in secreting plasma cells. The CD20 gene is a single copy gene located on chromosome 11q12-q13, near the site of the t(11;14)(q13; q32) translocation which is commonly noted in mantle zone lymphoma. The complete gene is 16 kbp long and comprises eight exons, with six exons encoding the protein. (Dorken et al, 1989; Tedder et al, 1989)

The exact function of the CD20 molecule is unknown but it is involved in the regulation of B cell activation, proliferation and differentiation. Certain anti-CD20 antibodies trigger resting B cells to enter the cell cycle and induce IgM production, while other antibodies to CD20 can inhibit B cell activation. (Ishii et al, 1984)

The CD20 antigen appears on the cell surface after light chain gene rearrangement and before the expression of intact surface Ig, remaining throughout the course of B cell development and is lost only prior to plasma cell differentiation. While it is expressed on both resting and activated B cell, its expression is about fourfold greater in the latter.

Virtually all lymphoid cells in the germinal center express CD20 besides CD19, CD22 and other pan-B cell antigens, and CD20 and CD19 are also expressed by cells of the mantle zone, but in lesser intensity. In the thymus, CD20 stains medullary B cells and cells within the epithelial meshwork of the thymic parenchyma. Cortical cells are negative for this antigen. (Norton & Isaacson, 1989)

Weak expression of CD20 may be seen in a subpopulation of T cells but the antigen is not expressed in normal myeloid, erythroid, monocytic or mesenchymal cells. Antigen-presenting dendritic cells in the blood do not stain for CD20 and the antigen is not expressed in cells of the normal skin or adnexal structures (Chang et al, 1996).

Applications

CD20 is the most useful marker for neoplasms of B cell derivation and is almost always expressed in B cell lymphomas of small cell type, prolymphocytic leukemia, follicular centre cell lymphomas, large or small cell types of both diffuse and follicular patterns, monocytoid lymphomas, mantle cell lymphomas, hairy cell leukemias/lymphomas and immunoblastic lymphomas. Originally, it was thought that neoplastic plasma cells mirrored the lack of expression in benign plasma cells but it has been shown that up to 20% of cases of myeloma may immunoexpress CD20 (Ruiz-Arguelles et al, 1994). The staining of CD20 in chronic lymphocytic leukemia/small cell lymphoma may be weak and often not in all cells. It has not been shown to stain the neoplastic cells T lymphomas. While CD20 has great diagnostic utility, it is of no prognostic relevance. Homogenous staining for CD20 in bone marrow lymphoid aggregates is more common in neoplastic aggregates than in benign ones and may be a useful discriminator in such settings.

About 10–20% of lymphoblastic lymphoma are non-T cell lineage and express B cell antigens, about half the latter group expressing CD20.

In Hodgkin's disease, 60–100% of cases of the nodular lymphocyte predominant subtype show CD20 staining of the L&H malignant cells. Up to 22 % of Reed Sternberg cells of classic Hodgkin's disease may stain for CD20 but this finding is not associated with different clinical outcomes after treatment with equivalent regimens (Rassidakis et al, 2002).

Occasional cases of acute myeloid leukemia and extramedullary myeloid tumors may show aberrant expression of CD20 but this is estimated to involve only 3% of cases, with no correlation between any lymphoid antigen expression and morphology. In the case of chronic myelogenous leukemia, about 25–30% of the cases that show blastic transformation display lymphoid differentiation by morphology, cytochemistry and immunophenotyping. The lymphoid cells usually display the immunophenotype of precursor

B cells, including the expression of CD20 as well as other B cell antigens such as CD10, CD19, increased TdT and rearranged immunoglobulin genes. Follicular dendritic cells, 40% of pure B ALL/LBL, 80% of lymphocyte predorminant Hodgkin's disease may show reactivity for CD20, which may also be dimly expressed in benign and neoplastic T cells in immunofluorescence labeling. As 90% of B cell lymphomas express CD20 in vivo ablation of malignant B cells may be achieved using antibodies directed to the CD20 antigen (Polyak & Deans, 2002). Immunoreactivity for CD20 has been observed in the epithelial cells of a subset of thymomas and seems to correlate with spindling of the neoplastic cells.

Comments

Antibodies to CD20 are mostly reactive in formalin-fixed paraffin-embedded tissues and is by far the most superior marker for B lymphocytes (Appendix 2.1), with a sensitivity and specificity of 95 and 100% respectively. (Bluth et al, 1993) The pattern of staining is membranous and continuous. It may be accompanied by nuclear, paranuclear and diffuse cytoplasmic staining but this should be generally weak. Heat-induced epitope retrieval has been reported to produce nucleolar staining. Very rare cases of low-grade B cell lymphomas may not stain for CD20 and may express CD43 in paraffin sections suggesting an erroneous interpretation of T cell lineage (Norton & Isaacson, 1989). However, an awareness of this

and the proper use of antibody panels will avoid such pitfalls. Clone L26 is the most commonly used of the CD20 antibodies.

CD20 is immunoexpressed on most B cells (after CD19 and CD10 expression) and before CD21/22 and surface immunoglobulin expression), retained on mature B cells until plasma cell development; also follicular dendritic cells, 90% of B cell lymphomas, 40% of pre B ALL/LBL; 80% of lymphocyte predominant Hodgkin's disease and weakly expressed on benign and neoplastic T cells. As many as 20% of cases of myeloma may express CD20. CD20 is generally not expressed on non-hematopoietic cells, most T cells and non-neoplastic plasma cells. Aberrant focal expression of CD20 on thymoma cells has been described. The staining is membranous and dendritic in outline and together with the presence of lymphoid cells with immature phenotype CD1a+, CD2+, CD99+ and TdT+ has been employed for the identification of thymoma (Attanoos et al, 2002).

Immunoexpression may be reduced in tissues fixed in Zenker's solution and following decalcification. Trypsinisation may similarly reduce immunoreactivity but heat induced antigen retrieval is useful.

References

Attanoos RL, Galateau-Salle F, Gibbs AR, et al. Primary thymic epithelial tumors of the pleura mimicking malignant mesothelioma. Histopathology 2002;41:42–9.
Bluth RF, Casey TT, McCurley TL. Differentiation of reactive from neoplastic small cell lymphoid

aggregates in paraffin-embedded marrow particle preparations using L26 (CD20) and UCHL1 (CD45RO) monoclonal antibodies. American Journal of Clinical Pathology 1993;99:150–6.

Chang KL, Arber DA, Weiss LM. CD20: A review. Applied Immunohistochemistry 1996;4:1–15.

Dorken B, Moller P, Pezzutto A, et al. B cell antigens: section report. In: Knapp W, Dorken B, Gilks WR, et al. Eds. Leukocyte typing IV. White cell differentiation antigens. Oxford: Oxford University Press, 1989, p22.

Ishii Y, Takami T, Yuasa H, et ai. Two distinct antigen systems in human B lymphocytes: identification of cell surface and intracellular antigens using monoclonal antibodies. Clinical and Experimental Immunology 1984;58:183–92.

Norton AJ, Isaacson PG. Lymphoma phenotyping in formalin-fixed and paraffin wax-embedded tissues. II. Profiles of reactivity in various tumor types. Histopathology 1989;14:557–79.

Polyak MJ, Deans JP. Alanine-170 and proline-172 are critical determinants for extracellular CD20 epitopes; heterogeneity in the fine specificity of CD20 monoclonal antibodies is defined by additional requirements imposed by both amino acid sequence and quanternary structure. Blood 2002;99:3256–62.

Rassidakis GZ, Medeiros LJ, Vivani S, et al. CD20 expression in Hodgkin and Reed Sternberg cells of classical Hodgkin's disease: associations with presenting features and clinical outcome. Journal of Clinical Oncology 2002;20:1278–87.

Ruiz-Arguelles GJ, San Miguel JF. Cell surface markers in multiple myeloma. Mayo Clinic Proceedings 1994;69:684–90.

Tedder TF, Klejman F, Schlossman SF, Saito H. Structure of the gene encoding the human B lymphocyte differentiation antigen CD20 (B1). Journal of Immunology 1989;142:2560–8.

NOTES

CD 21

Sources/clones

Dako (1F8), Coulter (B2),
Immunotech (BL13).

Fixation/preparation

CD21 is applicable to formalin-
fixed paraffin-embedded tissue
sections. Enzymatic digestion
with proteolytic enzyme trypsin
is essential for positive
immunoreaction but HIER
produces significant enhancement
of immunoreactivity. CD21 may
also be used for labeling acetone-
fixed cryostat sections or fixed
cell smears.

Background

CD21 antigen (CR2) (Isotype:
IgG1 kappa) represents the
purified receptor of the C3d
fragment of the third
complement component from
human tonsils (Weiss et al, 1984).
This membrane molecule is a
glycoprotein of MW 145 kD and
is involved in the transmission of
growth promoting signals to the
interior of the B cell. CD21 also
functions as a receptor for
Epstein-Barr virus (Nemerow et
al, 1985). IF8 reacts with an
epitope localized on trypsin
fragments of CR2 of molecular
weights 95,72,50,32 and 28 kD

(Mason et al, 1986). The 28kD
and 72 kD MW fragments of
CR2 contains the binding site for
the C3d receptor.

The CD21 antigen is a
restricted B cell antigen expressed
on mature B cells. The antigen is
also present on follicular
dendritic cells (FDCs), the
accessory cells of the B zones
(Appendix 2.8). IF8 labels B cells
moderately and demonstrates
FDCs strongly on cryostat
sections. However, on paraffin
sections, B cell immunoreaction
is abolished whilst the FDCs
remain highlighted similar to the
cryostat sections. Hence, in
normal and reactive lymph
nodes, tonsils and extra-nodal
lymphoid tissue, the antibody
demonstrates the FDC meshwork
remarkably clearly defined in the
germinal centers (Mason et al,
1986).

Applications

On paraffin sections, antibodies
to the CD21 antigen are useful
to demonstrate FDC meshwork
in lymphoid proliferations where
the germinal centres may be ill-
defined and difficult to delineate
morphologically, eg. HIV
lymphadenopathy. In the early
stages of progressive generalised
lymphadenopathy (PGL, stage I),

the large geographic reactive
germinal centers may occupy
large areas of the lymph node,
giving an appearance of
effacement of the architecture.
Similarly, in the late stage of PGL
(stage III), the atrophic germinal
centers are not easily definable.

The demonstration of the
nodular dense FDC meshwork of
follicular lymphomas is also a
potential application of the CD21
antibody. Similarly, the
follicular/nodular architecture of
nodular lymphocyte predominant
Hodgkin's disease may be
highlighted. Residual germinal
centers that have been colonized
in low-grade B-cell MALT
lymphomas may also be
demonstrated with antibody to
CD21, which reveals an
expanded and dense FDC
meshwork (Bagdi et al, 2001).
Nodal mantle cell lymphoma and
multiple lymphomatous polyposis
are characterized by the presence
of a monotonous small lymphoid
B-cell population, and
interspersed cells with "naked"
nuclei (FDCs), which is helpful
in distinguishing this lymphoma
from other low-grade B-cell
lymphomas (Chan, 1996).

The demonstration of a FDC
meshwork is also characteristic of
peripheral T-cell lymphomas of
angioimmunoblastic

lymphadenopathy (AILD) type. The FDC meshwork in AILD is typically around hyperplastic venules (Bagdi et al, 2001).

The diagnosis of angiofollicular lymph node hyperplasia or Castleman's disease (hyaline-vascular type) may also benefit from highlighting the follicles with anti-CD21. Dysplastic FDCs have been demonstrated in association with Castleman's disease of the hyaline vascular type and thought to be the precursor to FDC tumors (Chan et al, 2001). Again the characteristic dendritic processes in FDC tumors are well demonstrated with CD21 antibodies (Chan et al, 1997). Recent findings of chromosomal aberrations involving 12q13–15 targeting the gene HMGIC, a member of the high mobility group protein family suggests that FDC proliferation in the hyaline vascular type of Castleman's disease is clonal (Cokelaere et al, 2002).

Comments

Although sometimes patchy and focal, positivity with the paraffin section-reactive CD21 is essential for the diagnosis of FDC tumors, which are probably under diagnosed through under-recognition. CD35 generally produces stronger staining of FDC sarcomas compared to antibodies to CD21 (Biddle et al, 2002; Shimazaki et al, 2002). Both antibodies benefit from heat-induced antigen retrieval.

References

Bagdi E, Krenacs L, Krenacs T, et al. Follicular dendritic cells in reactive and neoplastic lymphoid tissues: a reevaluation of staining patterns of CD21, CD23, and CD35 antibodies in paraffin sections after wet heat-induced epitope retrieval. Applied Immunohistochemistry and Molecular Morphology 2001;9:117–24.

Biddle DA, Ro JY, Yoon GS, et al. Extranodal follicular dendritic cell sarcoma of the head and neck region: three new cases, with a review of the literature. Modern Pathology 2002;15:50–8.

Chan JKC. Gastrointestinal lymphomas: an overview with emphasis on new findings and diagnostic problems. Seminars in Diagnostic Pathology 1996;13:260–96.

Chan JKC, Fletcher CDM, Nayler SJ, Cooper K. Follicular dendritic cell sarcoma. Clinicopathologic analysis of 17 cases suggesting a malignant potential higher than currently recognized. Cancer 1997;79:294–313.

Chan AC, Chan KW, Chan JK, et al. Development of follicular dendritic cells sarcoma in hyaline vascular Castleman's disease of the nasopharynx: tracing its evolution by sequential biopsies. Histopathology 2001;32:745–9.

Cokelaere K, Debiec-Rychter M, De Wolf-Peerers C, et al. Hyaline vascular Castleman's disease with HMGIC rearrangement in follicular dendritic cells: molecular evidence of mesenchymal tumorigenesis. American Journal of Surgical Pathology 2002;26:662–9.

Mason DY, Ladyman H, Gatter KC. Immunohistochemical analysis of monoclonal anti-B cell antibodies. In: Reinherz EL, Haynes BF, Nadler LM, Bernstein ID, eds. Leukocyte Typing II, Volume 2. Human B lymphocytes. New York – Berlin – Heidelberg – Tokyo: Springer-Verlag, 1986;245–55.

Nemerow GR, Wolfert R, McNaughton ME, Cooper NR. Identification and characterization of the Epstein-Barr virus receptor on human B lymphocytes and its relationship to the C3D complement receptor (CR2). Journal of Virology 1985;55:347–51.

Shimazaki K, Ohshima K, Haraoka S, et al. Accessory cell tumor: a clinicopathological study of 16 aggressive tumors containing EBV-positive Hodgkin's and Reed-Sternberg-like giant cells. Histopathology 2002;40:12–21.

Weiss JJ, Tedder TF, Fearon DT. Identification of 145,000 Mr membrane protein as the C3d receptor (CR2) of human B lymphocytes. Proceedings of the National Academy of Science USA 1984;81:881–5.

CD 23

Sources/clones

Accurate, Biodesign (BB-10, 9P.25), Biotest (TU1), Cymbus Bioscience, Dako (MHM6), GenTrak, Immunotech (9P25), Novocastra (IB12, Tu1), Pharmingen (B3B4), RDI (TU1), Sanbio (BL-C/B8), Serotec (B-G6, BSL-23) www.bindingsite.co.uk (BU38).

Fixation/preparation

With exception of clones MHM6, Tu1 and 1B12 other available antibodies are immunoreactive only in fresh frozen sections and fresh cytologic preparations. Immunoreactivity in fixed paraffin-embedded sections follows heat-induced antigen retrieval.

Background

The antigen is an integral membrane glycoprotein of molecular weight 45–60 kD. The CD23 antigen has been identified as a low affinity receptor for IgE and may be involved in the regulation of IgE production as well as also being a receptor for lymphocyte growth factor. Following cross-linkage of antigen and Ig, CD23 becomes expressed and serves as an autocrine stimulus driving B cell proliferation. CD23 appears on B cells within 24hrs following a variety of stimuli. Surface CD23 has a half-life of only 1–2 hours and is shed in the form of soluble fragments of varying molecular weight that display the autocrine promoting activity. Two species of CD23 have been described. FcεRIIa and FcεRIIb, differing in the N-terminal cytoplasmic region and sharing the same C-terminal extracellular region. FcεRIIa is strongly expressed on IL-4-activated B cells and weakly on mature B cells; it also stains some dendritic reticulum cells, which probably acquire the antigen from neighboring B cells (Kikutani et al, 1986). FcεRIIa is not found on circulating B cells and its expression can only be induced on surface IgMD positive cells and not on those B cells that have lost IgD, undergone isotype switch, and express IgG, IgA, or IgE. FcεRIIb is expressed weakly on a range of cell types including monocytes, eosinophils, platelets, some T cells and NK cells. IL-4 treated monocytes show stronger staining (Armitage & Goff, 1988; Zola, 1987). CD23 is strongly expressed on EBV-transformed lymphoblastoid B cell lines. The aberrant expression of CD23 in B CLL appears to be the result of deregulation of Notch2 signaling, members of the Notch family encode transmembrane receptors that modulate differentiation, proliferation and apoptotic programs of many precursor cells including hematopoietic progenitors (Hubmann et al, 2002).

Applications

CD23 is found in most low-grade B cell lymphomas and in Reed-Sternberg cells in Hodgkin's disease (Rowlands et al, 1990). Activated B cells within germinal centers express CD23 in high density but mantle zone (resting) B cells are negative or only stain weakly. The majority of B cell CLLs and a variable proportion B cell non-Hodgkin's lymphoma are CD23 positive, whereas mantle cell lymphomas are generally negative, so that this marker is useful when applied with other markers to separate the small cell lymphomas (DiRaimondo et al, 2002) (Appendix 2.9). Precursor B cell and T cell ALL/LBL, acute myeloid leukemia, chronic myeloid leukemia and post-thymic T cell neoplasms are CD23 negative (Raghoebnier et al, 1991). The marker is upregulated by EBV infection.

Comments

CD23 negativity is rare in typical B cell CLL/SLL so that it is an important marker for the distinction of small cell lymphomas (Appendix 2.9). CD23 is positive on activated mature B cells expressing IgM or IgD, monocytes/macrophages, T cell subsets, eosinophils, Langerhans cells, follicular dendritic cells and B cell CLL/SLL. Mantle cells do not stain for CD23.

References

Armitage RJ, Goff LK. Functional interaction between B cell subpopulation defined by CD23 expression. European Journal of Immunology 1988;18:1753–60.

DiRaimondo F, Albitar M, Huh Y, et al. The clinical and diagnostic relevance of CD23 expression in the chronic lymphoproliferative disease. Cancer 2002;94:1721–30.

Hubmann R, Schwarzmeier JD, Shehata M, et al. Notch2 is involved in the overexpression of CD23 in B cell chronic lymphocytic leukemia. Blood 2002;99:3742–7.

Kikutani H, Suemura M, Owaki H, et al. Fcε receptor, a specific differentiation marker transiently expressed on mature B cells before isotype switching. Journal of Experimental Medicine 1986;164:1455–69.

Raghoebier S, Kramer MHH, Vankrieken JHJM, et al. Essential differences in oncogene involvement between primary nodal and extranodal large cell lymphoma. Blood 1991;78:2680–5.

Rowlands DC, Hansel TT, Crocker J. Immunohistochemical determination of CD23 expresssion in Hodgkin's disease using paraffin sections. Journal of Pathology 1990;160:239–43.

Thorley-Lawson DA, Nadler LM, Bhan AK, Schooley RT. BLAST-2 (EBVCS), an early cell surface marker of human B cell activation is superinduced by Epstein-Barr virus. Journal of Immunology 1985;134:3007–12.

Zola H. The surface antigens of human B lymphocytes. Immunology Today 1987;8:303–15.

CD 24

Sources/clones

Biodesign (ALB9), Cymbus
Bioscience (ALB9), Dako
(SN389), Immunotech (ALB9),
RDI (ALB9) and Serotec
(ALB9).

Fixation/preparation

Current antibodies are reactive in
fresh frozen sections and cell
preparations only.

Background

Antibodies to CD24 react with a
42 kD single chain cell surface
sialoglycoprotein which is
expressed throughout B cell
differentiation but, like other
pan-B cell antigens, is lost
following activation and before
the secretory (plasma cell) stage.
CD24 is not entirely restricted to
B cells and is expressed on
granulocytes, interdigitating cells,
renal epithelial cells, as well as
some benign and malignant
epithelial tumors (Abramson et
al, 1981; Melink & LeBien, 1983;
Kemshed et al, 1982; Hsu & Jaffe,
1984). CD24 can function as a
ligand for P-selectin and may
have a role in the lung
colonization of human tumors
(Friederichs et al, 2000) and
through glycolipid-enriched
membrane fractions may mediate
intracellular signaling and
apoptosis in human B
lymphocytes (Suzuki et al, 2001).
CD24 has adhesion molecule
functions and promotes invasion
of glioma cells in vivo (Senner et
al, 1999). In breast canrcinoma,
the binding of tumor cells to
platelets and the rolling of these
cells on endothelial P-selectin
facilitates metastasis (Fogel et al,
1999).

Applications

CD24 is expressed on the
majority of precursor B cell
ALL/LBLs and by virtually all
mature, TdT negative, SIg-
positive and SIg-negative B cell
non-Hodgkin's lymphoma
(Kersey et al, 1982). It is not
found in multiple myeloma nor
on benign and neoplastic T cells.
Anti-CD24 has been used for
purging bone marrow of B-ALL
cells in autologous bone marrow
transplantation.

CD24 is abundantly expressed
on breast cancer cell lines and
tumor tissues and has been
suggested as a possible marker for
breast carcinoma, with
cytoplasmic expression in
carcinoma cells compared to
apical expression in benign cell
(Fogel et al, 1999).

CD24 is positive on all B
cells, granulocytes, kidney cells,
epithelial cells, both benign and
malignant, most pre-B ALL/LBL
and virtually all B cell
lymphomas. It is not expressed on
plasma cells, myeloma, T cells,
monocytes, red blood cells and
platelets.

References

Abramson CS, Kersey JH, LeBien
TW. A monoclonal antibody
(BA-1) reactive with cells of
human B lymphocyte lineage.
Journal of Immunology
1981;126:83–8.

Fogel M, Friederichs J, Zeller Y, et al.
CD24 is a marker for human
breast carcinoma. Cancer Letters
1999;143:87–94.

Friederichs J, Zeller Y, Hafezi-
Moghadam A, et al. The
CD24/P-selectin binding
pathway initiates lung arrest of
human A125 adenocarcinoma
cells. Cancer Research
2000;60:6714–22.

Hsu SM, Jaffe ES. Phenotypic
expression of B lymphocytes. I.
Identification with monoclonal
antibodies in normal lymphoid
tissues. American Journal of
Pathology 1984;144:387–95.

Kemshed JT, Fritschy J, Asser U, et al.
Monoclonal antibodies defining
markers with apparent selectivity
for particular hematopoietic cell
types may also detect antigens on
cells of neural crest origin.
Hybridoma 1982;1:109–23.

Kersey JH, Abramson C, Perry G, et al. Clinical usefulness of monoclonal antibody phenotyping in childhood lymphoblastic leukemia. Lancet 1982;2:1419–23.

Melink GB, LeBien TW. Construction of an antigenic map for human B cell precursors. Journal of Clinical Immunology 1983;3:260–7.

Senner V, Sturm A, Baur I, et al. CD24 promotes invasion of glioma cells in vivo. Journal of Neuropathology and Experimental Neurology 1999;58:795–802.

Suzuki T, Kiyokawa N, Taguchi T, et al. CD24 induces apoptosis in human B cells via the glycolipid-enriched membrane domains/rafts-mediated signaling system. Journal of Immunology 2001;166:5567–77.

CD 30 (Ki-1)

Sources/clones

Accurate (Ki-1, Ber-H2),
Biodesign (HRS4), Bioprobe
(IC)-88), Cymbus Bioscience
(Ki-1), Dako (Ber-H2, Ki-1),
Diagnostic Biosystems (Ki-1,
Ber-H2), Immunotech (HRS4,
Ki-1), Serotec.

Fixation/preparation

The Ki-1 antibody produces
membrane staining only in frozen
sections and does not stain
paraffin-embedded tissues. BER–
H2 labels an epitope that survives
routine fixation and processing.

Background

The first CD30 antibody
generated was called Ki-1 and
was thought to be specific for
Reed-Sternberg cells. The Ki-1
antibody recognizes an
intracellular protein and a
membrane bound glycoprotein
that are apparently not related.
The membrane bound
glycoprotein is often referred to
as the true CD30 antigen. It has a
molecular mass of 105–120 kD
and is phosphorylated at serine
residues and contains a N- and
O-glycosidyl bound carbohydrate
portion. The extracellular domain
of CD30 shows significant

homology with members of the
tumor necrosis factor/nerve
growth factor receptor
superfamily (Stein et al, 1985).
The human CD30 gene has been
localized to the short arm of
chromosome 1 at 1p36, a band
frequently involved in neoplastic
disorders (Fonatsch et al, 1992).
Deletions, duplications,
translocations, and inversions of
this band have been observed in
non-Hodgkin's lymphomas and
abnormalities of the short arm of
chromosome 1 have been
described in Hodgkin's disease.
1p36 is also the location for the
TNF receptor-2 gene and
appears to be a preferential site
for integration of viruses such as
the Epstein-Barr virus.

CD30 appears to be a
lymphoid activation antigen and
its expression can be induced on
B- and T-lymphocytes in vitro by
a number of stimuli, which
include viruses and lectins. CD30
may act as a receptor whose
ligand is a cytokine. Recombinant
CD30L exhibits pleiotropic
cytokine activities, with CD30L
inducing proliferation of activated
T-cells in the presence of an anti-
CD3 co-stimulus and enhancing
the proliferation of a Hodgkin's
cell line HDLM2. CD30L
mRNA expression can be
induced on T-cells and

macrophages suggesting that a
variety of autocrine and paracrine
mechanisms may be operative.
Immunoelectron microscopic
studies have localized the antigen
in the cytoplasm and in
association with the nuclear
envelope, chromatin structures
and nucleoli.

Applications

CD30 antibodies do not react
against any resting peripheral
blood cells. Staphylococcus-
stimulated B-lymphocytes and
phytohaemagglutinin-stimulated
T-lymphocytes become CD30
positive, and expression of the
antigen can be induced by
activating T-helper lymphocytes
with autologous and allogeneic
stimulator cells. The antigen is
also expressed in Epstein-Barr
virus transformed B-cells and
human T-lymphotrophic virus-
transfected T-cell lines. Activated
T-cells express CD38, CD71,
CD25, epithelial membrane
antigen, HLA-DR and CD15
together with α-1-antitrypsin
and CD11C prior to the
expression of CD30. Scattered
large B- and T-cells localized
around lymphoid follicles and at
the margin of germinal centres
show CD30 positivity in normal
and reactive lymph nodes. These

cells may also co-express Ki-67 nuclear antigen indicating their proliferating state. Similarly, macrophages which are generally negative for CD30, may become CD30-positive in conditions such as miliary tuberculosis, sarcoidosis and other granulomatous reactions such as cat scratch disease and toxoplasmosis. BER–H2 may also label a subpopulation of plasma cells. Among non-haemopoietic tissues, exocrine pancreatic cells, some cerebral cortical neurons and Purkinje cells may be positive for CD30.

In initial studies, Hodgkin's disease was the only neoplasm that was CD30 positive. About 89% of cases of non-lymphocyte predominant Hodgkin's disease are positive for CD30 and the staining pattern is membranous, often with a strong paranuclear globule in the region of the Golgi and weaker cytoplasmic staining (Appendix 2.3). In frozen sections, BER–H2 produces stronger staining than Ki-1 and staining is also stronger in frozen sections than in paraffin sections. A variable degree of positivity was reported in the L & H cells of lymphocyte-predominant Hodgkin's disease (LPHD). About 25% of cases were said to show positivity in paraffin sections; the staining being generally weaker and limited usually to the cell membrane (Swerdlow & Wright, 1986) (Appendix 2.10). A more recent extensive study of 16 cases of nodular LPHD showed that CD30 remains negative in L&H cells even after enhanced antigen retrieval methods and advocates the use of the marker to distinguish nodular LPHD from classic Hodgkin's disease (Roberts et al, 2002).

CD30 expression is a characteristic of anaplastic large cell lymphoma (ALCL) that is defined in part by its nearly constant CD30 positivity. The pattern of staining is similar to that seen in Reed-Sternberg cells and may be expressed by ALCLs of both T and B-cell lineage as well as "null" cell types. The small cell variant of ALCL is prone to leukemic presentation and a discordant expression of CD30 and ALK protein has been found in such cases. Peripheral blood cells were negative for CD30 and ALK protein which were expressed on bone marrow tumor cells (Awaya et al, 2002). CD30 expression, however, is not limited to ALCL and may be found in other types of non-Hodgkin's lymphoma. In one study of about 500 cases of non-Hodgkin's lymphomas, 36 cases of lymphomas other than ALCL were CD30 positive. The expression of CD30 is highest in immunoblastic lymphomas, and among the T-cell lymphomas, both mycosis fungoides as well as other types of peripheral T-cell lymphomas including AILD-like T-cell lymphoma, Lennert's lymphoma and HTLV-I-positive T-cell leukemia/lymphoma may show a relatively high incidence of CD30 positivity. It has been suggested that primary CD30 positive lymphomas, particularly primary cutaneous lymphomas, have a better prognosis than their CD30-negative counterparts (Stein et al, 1985; Piris et al, 1990). However, the expression of CD30 in cutaneous lymphomas which arise in patients with a preceding history of another lymphoma may have a particularly poor prognosis. The expression of CD30 in

lymphomatoid papulosis and regressing atypical histiocytosis has suggested a close relationship between these disorders and cutaneous CD30+ ALCL. These three lesions may represent a spectrum with their histologic and clinical characteristics determined by the degree of biological aggressiveness of the neoplasm and the host immune defenses. Prognosis in primary cutaneous T cell lymphomas is determined by the expression of CD30, those expressing the antigen having excellent prognosis with 5 year survival of 96% compared to 15–21% in CD30- cases (Grange & Bagot, 2002).

Occasional cases of plasmacytomas and myelomas may show CD30 positivity. Hairy cell leukemia is consistently negative for CD30 and Langerhans' cell histiocytosis is also CD30 negative. Staining has also been reported to be negative in three cases of dendritic reticulum cell sarcoma and the expression in true histiocytic tumors is not known. CD30 positivity has not been reported in cases of leukemia (Piris et al, 1990).

CD30 positivity has been reported in embryonal carcinomas and in the embryonal elements of mixed germ cell tumours, and less commonly, has been observed in pancreatic and salivary gland carcinomas (Pallesen & Hamilton-Dutoit, 1988). CD30 expression in metastatic deposits of embryonal carcinoma may lost following chemotherapy (Berney et al, 2001). The combination of CD30 and CD117 (c-kit) staining has been advocated for the distinction of embryonal carcinoma from seminoma, these tumors staining CD30+CD117- and CD30-CD117+ respectively (Leroy et al, 2002). Occasionally, other paraffin-embedded carcinomas and malignant lymphomas may show weak, diffuse cytoplasmic staining and CD30 positivity has more uncommonly been observed in mesenchymal tumors including leiomyoma, leiomyosarcoma, rhabdomyosarcoma, synovial sarcoma, giant cell tumor of tendon sheath, malignant fibrous histiocytoma, osteogenic sarcoma, Ewing's sarcoma, malignant schwannoma, ganglioneuromas and aggressive fibromatosis. Occasional lipoblasts in liposarcoma may show positivity (Mechterscheimer & Moller, 1990; Chang, 1993).

Comments

We have found that BER-H2 staining is enhanced by MW epitope retrieval in citrate buffer with or without enzyme pre-treatment. Because it is expressed in stimulated B and T-lymphoid cells, BER-H2 should not be employed as a primary marker of Reed-Sternberg cells. However, it should be used in a panel for the identification of ALCL, bearing in mind that such tumors may be CD45-negative and EMA-positive, an immunophenotype, which may be mistaken for carcinoma (Appendix 2.10). From a practical standpoint, ALCLs do not express cytokeratin.

Staining is membranous, frequently accompanied by staining of the Golgi. Cytoplasmic staining per se should not be considered as positive. CD30 expression is seen in granulocytes, plasma cells, activated B, T and NK cells, lymphocytes infected with HIV, HTLV-1, EBV, HHV8 and hepatitis B, Reed Sternberg cells, 90% of anaplastic large cell lymphomas, lymphomatoid papulosis, peripheral T cell lymphomas and embryonal carcinoma. The available antibodies may not be immunoreactive in B5 fixed tissue.

References

Awaya N, Mori S, Takeuchi H, et al. CD30 and the NPM-ALK fusion protein (p80) are differentially expressed between peripheral blood and bone marrow in primary small cell variant of anaplastic large cell lymphoma. American Journal of Hematology 2002;69:200–4.

Berney DM, Shamash J, Pieroni K, Oliver RT. Loss of CD30 expression in metastatic embryonal carcinoma: the effect of therapy? Histopathology 2001;39:382–5.

Chang KL, Arber DA, Weiss LM. CD30: a review. Applied Immunohistochemistry 1993;1:244–55.

Fonatsch C, Latza U, Durkop H, et al. Assignment of the human CD30 (Ki-1) gene to 1p36. Genomics 1992;14: 825–6.

Grange F, Bagot M. Prognosis of primary cutaneous lymphomas. Annals of Dermatology and Venereology 2002;129: 30–40.

Leroy X, Augusto D, Leteurtre E, Gosselin B. CD30 and CD117 (c-kit) used in combination are useful for distinguishing embryonal carcinoma from seminoma. Journal of Histochemistry and Cytochemistry 2002;50:283–5.

Mechterscheimer G, Moller P. Expression of Ki-1 antigen (CD30) in mesenchymal tumours. Cancer 1990;66:1732–7.

Pallesen G, Hamilton-Dutoit SJ. Ki-1 (CD30) antigen is regularly expressed by tumour cells of embryonal carcinoma. American Journal of Pathology 1988;133:446–50.

Piris M, Brown DC, Gatter KC, Mason DY. CD30 expression in non-Hodgkin's lymphoma. Histopathology 1990;17:211–8.

Roberts C, Jack F,, angus B, et al. Immunohistochemical detection of CD30 remains negative in nodular lymphocyte-predominant Hodgkin's disease using enhanced antigen retrieval. Histopathology 2002;40:166–70.

Stein H, Mason DY, Gerdes J, et al. The expression of the Hodgkin's disease-associated antigen Ki-1 in reactive and neoplastic lymphoid tissues. Evidence that Reed-Sternberg cells and histiocytic malignancies are derived from activated lymphoid cells. Blood 1985;66:848–58.

Swerdlow SH, Wright SA. A spectrum of LeuM1 staining in lymphoid and haemopoietic proliferations. American Journal of Clinical Pathology 1986;85:283–8.

NOTES

CD 31

Sources/clones

Accurate (JC70A, CLB-HEC75), Becton Dickinson (L133.1), Biogenex (9G11), Coulter (56E), Dako (JC/70A), Monosan (CLB-58, VM64), Novocastra (HC1.6), Pharmingen (2ET, M290, WM59), Research Diagnostics, Sanbio (VM64).

Fixation/preparation

Antibodies to CD31 are generally immunoreactive in fixed, paraffin-embedded tissue sections as well as fresh cell preparations and cryostat sections. HIER enhances immunoreactivity and if employed, enzyme predigestion is not necessary.

Background

CD 31 is a 130 kD glycoprotein, also designated platelet endothelial cell adhesion molecule-1 (PECAM-1), that is normally expressed on endothelial cells and circulating and tissue-phase hematopoietic cells, including platelets, monocytes/macrophages, granulocytes and B-cells. This antigen is also expressed in sinusoidal endothelial cells in the liver, lymph node and spleen (Parums et al, 1990). The same endothelial cells display variable staining with *Ulex europeaus* agglutinin-I (UEA-1) and for von Willebrand factor (Factor VIII related protein), indicating that the sinusoidal endothelium differs from other vascular endothelium. CD 31 does not label connective tissue, basement membrane, squamous epithelium or adnexal structures of the skin (Suthipintawong et al, 1995). The exact function of CD 31 has not been fully elucidated but CD 31 appears to mediate platelet adhesion to endothelial cells and may promote vascular adhesion of leukocytes (Stokinger et al, 1990; Albelda et al, 1991).

Applications

The main application of CD 31 is as a marker of both benign and malignant endothelial cells (Leong et al, 1997). CD 31 is an apparently more sensitive marker than CD 34, von Willebrand factor or UEA-1 as a marker of malignant vascular endothelium (DeYoung et al, 1993) (Appendix 1.22 and 1.23). Despite earlier the suggestion that CD 31 is specific for vascular endothelium (Parums et al, 1990) with no expression by lymphangiomas, we clearly showed that there was distinct staining for CD 31 in all 19 cases of lymphangioma studied, albeit of lesser intensity than that observed in vascular endothelium (Suthipintawong et al, 1995). Indeed, the endothelium of blood and lymphatic vessels share many common antigens such as CD 34, von Willebrand factor and UEA-1 and none provides absolute distinction between the two types of vessels. In the light of these findings, claims that Kaposi's sarcoma shows vascular endothelial differentiation or derivation (Scully et al, 1988; Hoerl & Goldblum, 1997) will need to be reassessed. CD31 is thus employed as a marker of endothelial cells in the evaluation of tumor angiogenesis (Massi et al, 2002; Teo et al, 2002).

While CD31 is only occasionally found on Ewing's sarcoma/Peripheral Neuroendocrine Tumors (4/85 cases), it was consistently found in small lymphocytic lymphoma and lymphoblastic lymphoma and less often in mantle cell and follicular center cell lymphomas. Rhabdomyosarcomas and desmoplastic small round cell tumors did not express the antigen (Siobhan et al, 2000).

Comments

Some form of HIER should be used with anti-CD 31 to produce

optimal immunoreactivity in fixed tissue sections (we employ microwave stimulated HIER in citrate buffer). CD31 is useful as part of the panel for the identification of epithelioid and spindled tumors in the skin and soft tissue (Appendix 1.23, 1.24, 1.25). The antigen is localized to the cell membrane with some weaker staining of the cytoplasm. CD31 is expressed on macrophages, granulocytes, T/NK cells, endothelium and in epithelioid hemangioendothelioma. CD31 is also expressed on megakaryocytes (Hoda et al, 2002).

References

Albelda SM, Muller WA, Buck CA, Newman PJ. Molecular and cellular properties of PECAM-1 (endoCAM/CD31): a novel vascular cell-cell adhesion molecule. Journal of Cell Biology 1991;114:1059–61.

DeYoung BR, Wick MR, Fitzgibbon JF, et al. CD 31: An immunospecific marker for endothelial differentiation in human neoplasms. Applied Immunohistochemistry 1993;1:97–100.

Hoda SA, Resetkova E, Yusuf Y, et al. Megakaryocytes mimicking metastatic breast carcinoma. Archives of Pathology and Laboratory Medicine 2002;126:618–20.

Hoerl HD, Goldblum JR. Immunoreactivity patterns of CD 31 and CD 68 in 28 cases of Kaposi's sarcoma. Evidence supporting endothelial differentiation in the spindle cell component. Applied Immunohistochemistry 1997;5:173–8.

Leong AS-Y, Wick MR, Swanson PE. Immunohistology and electron microscopy of anaplastic and pleomorphic tumors. Cambridge: Cambridge University Press, 1997: pp 79–81 and 160–1.

Massi D, Franchi A, Borgognoni L, et al. tumor angiogenesis as a prognostic factor in thick cutaneous malignant melanoma. A quantitative morphologic analysis. Virchows Archives 2002;440:22–8.

Nicholson SA, McDermott MB, DeYoung BR, Swanson PE. CD31 immunoreactivity in small round cell tumors. Applied Immunohistochemistry and Molecular Morphology 2000;8:19–24.

Parums DV, Cordell JL, Micklem K, et al. JC70: a new monoclonal antibody that detects vascular endothelium associated antigen on routinely processed tissue sections. Journal of Clinical Pathology 1990;43:572–7.

Scully PA, Steinmann HK, Kennedy C, et al. AIDS-related Kaposi's sarcoma displays differential expression of endothelial cell surface antigens. American Journal of Pathology 1998;130:244–51.

Stokinger H, Gadd SJ, Eher R, et al. Molecular characterization and functional analysis of the leukocyte surface protein CD31. Journal of Immunology 1990;145:3889–97.

Suthipintawong C, Leong AS-Y, Vinyuvat S. A comparative study of immunomarkers for lymphangiomas and hemangiomas. Applied Immunohistochemistry 1995;3:239–44.

Teo NB, Shoker BS, Jarvis C, et al. Vascular density and phenotype around ductal carcinoma in situ (DCIS) of the breast. British Journal of Cancer 2002;86:905–11.

CD 34

Sources/clones

Becton-Dickinson (MY10), Biodesign (QBEND/10), Biogenex QBEND/10), Cymbus Bioscience, Dako (BIRMA-K3), GenTrak, Immunotech (QBEND/10, IMMU133.3), Oncogene, PerSeptive, RDI (9BI-3c5, ICH3), Sera-Lab (BI-3C5), Serotec (QBEND/10), and Selinus (BI-3C5)

Fixation/preparation

Antibodies are immunoreactive in fixed tissue and staining is significantly enhanced by HIER.

Background

The CD34 antigen is a 110 kD heavily glycosylated transmembrane protein of generally unknown function. Some evidence suggests that CD34 might play a role in cell adhesion with the highly glycosylated molecule allowing it to act as a ligand for lectins. In this way, CD34+ hematopoietic precursors might bind to lectin-expressing cells of the bone marrow stroma. The CD34 antigen was originally defined by monoclonal antibody MY10 raised against the human myeloid leukemia cell line KG1a. The gene for CD34 has been localized to chromosome 1 in the region of 1q32 and the DNA sequence demonstrates no homology with any previously known human genes (Baum et al, 1992; Greaves et al, 1992).

The CD34 antigen is present on ~1% of normal bone marrow mononuclear cells including hematopoietic precursors/stem cells. Thus, antibodies to CD34 can be used to purify the CD34+ stem cell population from CD34-malignant cells. The CD34+ bone marrow population contains not only hematopoietic stem cells but also more mature lineage-committed precursor cells for the erythroid, myeloid and lymphoid lineages. Included among these CD34+ cells are stromal cells necessary for the appropriate bone marrow environment for hematopoiesis (Baum et al, 1992).

The demonstration of CD34 on immature leukemias and vascular neoplasms has been the main contributions to its diagnostic utility. Besides bone marrow stem cells and normal endothelial cells, the antigen is found on cells in the splenic marginal zone, dendritic interstitial cells around vessels, nerves, hair follicles, muscle bundles and sweat glands in a variety of tissues and organs.

CD34+ cells appear in the peripheral blood after treatment with chemotherapy or cytokines. In blood vessel endothelium the antigen may be absent from large veins and arteries and from sinuses in the placenta and spleen. It is expressed on the luminal surface and membrane processes that interdigitate between endothelial cells. In new vessels such as in tumors, the location of the antigen is altered and it is found on the abluminal microprocesses of such vessels (van de Rijn & Rouse, 1994).

Among the hematopoietic neoplasms, CD34 is seen in the immature leukemias such as acute lymphoblastic leukemia of both T- and B-cell lineage, and acute myeloblastic leukemia. In myelodysplastic syndromes the expression of CD34 was predictive of transformation and poor survival outcome. There is some confusion over the value of CD34 as a prognostic parameter in the leukemias. Some studies have suggested that its expression is a poor prognosticator in AML; whereas, it is a marker of good prognosis in childhood ALL, probably those restricted to B cell lineage – all these studies being performed with flow cytometry analysis (van de Rijn & Rouse, 1994).

Applications

The expression of CD34 is retained in malignant endothelial cells so that it is a good marker for vascular tumors (Appendix 1.16, 1.23, 1.24 and 1.26). The endothelial cells of both vascular and lymphatic vessels express the antigen (Ramani et al, 1990; Suthipintawong et al, 1995). There is variable staining for CD34 in smooth muscle cells and their tumors. Antibodies to CD34 label gastrointestinal stromal tumors (GIST) very strongly (Appendix 1.29). Epithelioid smooth muscle tumors stain less frequently but the marker may serve as a useful discriminator from epithelial tumors which are generally negative for CD34 (Sergi et al, 1993). The antigen is displayed by nerve sheath tumors although in some series both neurofibromas and schwannomas failed to stain. In the latter, staining may be mainly in the Antoni B areas. While the staining in malignant nerve sheath tumors is largely negative, some series report a high frequency of reactivity, suggesting that CD34 may be a useful inclusion in the diagnostic panel for such tumors as S100 and CD57 are negative in such tumors (Weiss & Nickoloff, 1993). Epithelioid sarcoma and hemangiopericytoma show staining for CD34 and the marker is invariably found in solitary fibrous tumors and dermatofibrosarcoma protuberans, two tumors which are generally recognized from their histologic mimics by the absence of specific markers (Kutzner, 1993; Westra et al, 1994). Recently, CD34 was also demonstrated in four of 12 cases of angiomyofibroblastomas (Neilsen et al, 1996). Interestingly, reactivity for CD34 was found in giant cell fibroblastomas and one Bednar tumor, supporting the relationship of such tumors to dermatofibrosarcoma protuberans. CD34 stains a stroma fibrocyte which functions as a matrix-producing cells and possibly as an antigen-presenting cell capable of priming naïve T cells in situ and may have an important role in host response to tissue damage (Barth et al, 2002). Loss of this stromal CD34+ fibrocyte has been observed in invasive breast cancer and in ductal carcinoma in situ with the appearance of smooth muscle actin positive myofibroblasts, whereas, benign lesions of the breast and normal breast stroma contined CD34+ fibrocytes but no smooth muscle positive myofibroblasts (Barth et al, 2002). The expression of a common vimentin+/CD34+/Bcl-2+/CD99+ phenotype in spindle cell lipoma-like tumor, solitary fibrous tumor and myofibroblastoma of the breast suggested a common histogenesis (Margo et al, 2002).

CD34 is also a useful marker for early myeloid cells and hence stains granulocytic sarcoma.

Comments

Much of the earlier controversy concerning the staining of CD34 in spindle cell tumors was due to the sensitivity of the staining technique. CD34 staining is greatly enhanced by heat-induced epitope retrieval especially microwave-induced techniques. While widely employed for labeling vascular endothelial cells for the enumeration of vessels in neoplasms, the staining of stromal fibrocytes makes the use of other endothelial markers such as CD31 a preferable marker. Nonetheless, CD34 can be employed as a useful substitute for CD31 in antibody panels for the identification of epithelioid and spindled tumors in the skin and soft tissue (Appendix 1.23, 1.24, 1.25).

CD34 is expressed on hematopoietic progenitor cells, leukemic blasts, vascular and lymphatic endothelial cells, 40% of acute myeloid leukemias, 75% of pre-B acute lymphocytic leukemia, vascular neoplasms, hemangiopericytomas (50%), epithelioid sarcomas, dermatofibrosarcoma protuberans, solitary fibrous tumors and peripheral nerve sheath tumors.

References

Barth PJ, Ebrahimsade S, Ramaswamy A, Moll R. CD34+ fibrocytes in invasive ductal carcinoma, ductal carcinoma in situ, and benign breast lesions. Virchows Archives 2002;440:298–303.

Barth PJ, Ebrahimsade S, Hellinger A, et al. CD34+ fibrocytes in neoplastic and inflammatory pancreatic lesions. Virchows Archives 2002;440:128–33.

Baum CM, Weissman IL, Tsukamoto AS, et al. Isolation of a candidate human hematopoietic stem-cell population. Proceedings of the National Academy of Science USA 1992;89:2804–8.

Greaves MF, Brown J, Molgaard HV, et al. Molecular features of CD34: a hematopoietic progenitor cell-associated molecule. Leukemia 1992;1:31–6.

Kutzner H. Expression of the human progenitor cell antigen CD34 (HPCA-1) distinguished dermatofibrosarcoma protuberans from fibrous histiocytoma in formalin-fixed, paraffin-embedded tissue. Journal of American Academy of Dermatology 1993;28:613–7.

Margo G, Bisceglia M, Michal M, Eusebi V. Spinel cell lipoma-like tumor, solitary fibrous tumor and myofibroblastoma of the breast: a clinicopathological analysis of 13 cases in favour of a unifying histogenetic concept. Virchows Archives2002;440:249–60.

Neilsen GP, Rosenberg AE, Young RH, et al. Angiomyofibroblastoma of the vulva and vagina. Modern Pathology 1996;9:284–91.

Ramani P, Bradley NJ, Fletcher CMD. QBEND/10, a new monoclonal antibody to endothelium: assessment of its diagnostic utility in paraffin sections. Histopathology 1990;17:237–42.

Sirgi KE, Wick MR, Swanson PE. B72.3 and CD34 immunoreactivity in malignant epithelioid soft tissue tumors: adjuncts in the recognition of endothelial neoplasms. American Journal of Surgical Pathology 1993;17:179–85.

van de Rijn M, Rouse RV. CD34. A review. Applied Immunohistochemistry 1994;2:71–80

Weiss SW, Nickoloff BJ. CD34 is expressed by a distinctive population in peripheral nerve, nerve sheath tumors and related lesions. American Journal of Surgical Pathology 1993;17:1039–45

Westra WH, Gerald WL, Rosai J. Solitary fibrous tumor. Consistent CD34 immunoreactivity and occurrence in the orbit. American Journal of Surgical Pathology 1994;18:992–8.

NOTES

CD 35

Sources/clones

Dako (Ber-MAC-DRC, To5), Immunotech (J3D3).

Fixation/preparation

This antibody can be used on formalin fixed, paraffin embedded tissue section. Enzymatic digestion with proteolytic enzymes (e.g. pronase) for antigen retrieval must be performed for optimum immunoreaction. HIER enhances immunoreactivity especially when Target Retrieval Solution is employed. The CD35 antibody may also be applied to acetone-fixed cryostat sections or fixed cell smears.

Background

DAKO-CD35 (isotype: IgG 1, kappa) reacts with a formalin-resistant epitope of the receptor for the C3b fragment of the third component of human complement (Gerdes et al, 1982). This receptor, which is often referred to as CR1, consists of a single glycoprotein chain with a MW of approximately 220 kD. The antigen has been designated CD35 in the system for classifying human leukocyte antigens and is therefore equivalent to To5 (Bettelheim, 1989).

In frozen sections of normal tissues, DAKO-CD35 shows immunostaining of B-cell follicles of lymphoid tissue. The most strongly labeled cells within B-cell follicles are follicular dendritic cells (FDCs), but mantle zone lymphoid cells also immunoreact to a lesser degree. The C3b receptor on epithelial cells of renal glomeruli may also be clearly demonstrated with this antibody. Further, enzyme-treated, routinely processed paraffin sections show strong immunoreaction of FDCs in lymphoid tissue (both nodal and extra-nodal). The well-defined dense meshworks of FDCs in germinal centers are well demonstrated with this antibody (Fearon, 1980).

Applications

Immunohistological analyses of FDCs in paraffin sections are confined to the demonstration of FDC meshworks in reactive and neoplastic lymphoid tissue. In this regard identical immunoreaction of the dendritic cell processes of FDC are demonstrated with antibodies to both CD21 and CD35. Hence, the application of antibody to CD35 in surgical pathology (being similar to CD21) remains largely for the demonstration of FDC meshworks in follicles of HIV lymphadenopathy, Castleman's disease, follicular lymphoma, follicular colonization by low grade B-cell MALT lymphoma, and nodular lymphocyte predominant Hodgkin's disease. Demonstration of FDCs with CD35 antibody is also useful in mantle cell lymphoma and peripheral T-cell lymphoma – AILD type (Chan, 1996). In contrast to follicular lymphomas in which the lymphomas cells are encased within a network of proliferating FDCs, the network of FDCs in mantle cell lymphoma is loosely arranged. In angioimmunoblastic T cell lymphoma, there is a pronounced proliferation of FDCs around postcapillary venules (Badghi et al, 2001). CD35 has its greatest utility in the diagnosis of follicular dendritic cell tumors (see section on CD21) (Shimazaki et al, 2002; Chan et al, 2001) (Appendix 2.8).

Recently, another antibody to FDC has been generated. The CNA.42 antibody is reactive in fixed paraffin embedded sections and stains FDCs but apparently identifying an antigen different from other known anti-FDC antibodies (Raymond et al, 1997). The antibody also labels some T cell lymphomas as well as a variety of soft tissue tumors and a proportion of carcinomas of the gastrointestinal tract and lung. Aberrant expression of CD35 is seen on mast cells in mastocytosis (Escribano et al, 2002). The antigen is conserved in a wide spectrum of animal tissues other than man.

Comments

In postchemotherapy excision specimens, immunostaining with a CD21/CD35 antibody cocktail is useful to highlight dispersed small islands of residual tumor among the negative foamy histiocytes (Chan et al, 1997). Reactive germinal centers highlighted by antibodies to FDCs are ideal for use as positive control tissue.

CD35 is expressed on granulocytes, macrophages, B cells, T cells (10%), NK cells, follicular dendritic cells, glomerular podocytes and some astrocytes.

References

Badgi E, Krenacs L, Krenacs T, et al. Follicular dendritic cells in reactive and neoplastic lymphoid tissues: a reevaluation of staining patterns of CD21, CD23, and CD35 antibodies in paraffin sections after wet heat-induced epitope retrieval. Applied Immunohistochemistry and Molecular Morphology 2001;9:117–24.

Bettelheim P. M8, cluster report: CD35. In: Knapp W et al, eds. Leucocyte typing IV. White Cell Differentiation Antigens. Oxford-New York-Tokyo: Oxford University Press, 1989;829–30.

Chan JKC. Gastrointestinal lymphomas: an overview with emphasis on new findings and diagnostic problems. Seminars in Diagnostic Pathology 1996;13:260–96.

Chan JKC, Fletcher CDM, Nayler SJ, Cooper K. Follicular dendritic cell sarcoma. Clinicopathologic analysis of 17 cases suggesting a malignant potential higher than currently recognized. Cancer 1997;79:294–313.

Chan AC, Chan KW, Chan JK, et al. Development of follicular dendritic cell sarcoma in hyaline-vascular Castleman's disease of the nasopharynx: tacing its evolution by sequential biopsies. Histopathology 2001;38:510–8.

Esrcibano L, Diaz-Agustin B, Nunez R, et al. Abnormal expression of CD antigens in mastocytosis. International Allergy and Immunology 2002;127:127–32.

Fearon DT. Identification of the membrane glycoprotein that is the C3b receptor of the human erythrocyte, polymorphonuclear leukocyte, B lymphocyte, and monocyte. Journal of Experimental Medicine 1980;152:20–30.

Gerdes J, Naiem M, Mason DY, Stein H. Human complement (C3b) receptors defined by a mouse monoclonal antibody. Immunology 1982;45:645–53.

Raymond I, Al Saati TA, Tkaczuk J, et al. CAN.42, a new monoclonal antibody directed against a fixative-resistant antigen of follicular dendritic reticulum cells. American Journal of Pathology 1997;151:1577–85.

CD 38

Sources/clones

Accurate (BCAP38), Advanced Immunochemical (24G3), Biodesign (MIG-P12, T16), Biosource (BA6), Caltag Laboratories (BL-AC38, HIT2), Coulter (CD38, T16), Cymbus Bioscience (BA6), Dako (AT13/5), Immunotech (T16), Pharmingen (HIT2), Sanbio/Monosan (BL-D2, MIG-P12), Sanbio/Monosan/Accurate (BLD2), Seralab, Serotec (B-A6, AT13/5, T16).

Fixation/preparation

Most antibodies are reactive in fixed paraffin-embedded sections and HIER in Target Retrieval solution enhances immunoreactivity (Leong et al, 1997).

Background

The CD38 molecule, initially described as T10, consists of a single chain of 46 kD, spanning the membrane with its carboxyl terminus located in the extracellular compartment. CD 38 has been one of the most elusive molecules within the family of leukocyte multilineage markers (Reinherz et al, 1980) that has emerged as a multifunctional protein (Mehta et al, 1996). It is expressed on different precursor cells, monocytes, activated T cells, and terminally differentiated B cells, including plasma cells (Malavsi et al, 1994). This transmembrane glycoprotein appears to mediate several diverse functions such as signal transduction, cell adhesion (including binding to endothelium), with an important role in lymphocyte homing (Dianzani et al, 1994), and cyclic adenosine diphosphate-ribose synthesis, but its activities remain elusive (Malavasi et al, 1994). Immunoreactivity for CD 38 has also been described in a subset of pyramidal neurons and astrocytes and was predominantly distributed in the perikarya and dendrites in association with rough endoplasmic reticulum, ribosomes, small vesicles, mitochondria and cell membranes (Yamada et al, 1997). CD 38 has also been demonstrated in normal prostate epithelium within both basal and secretory epithelial cells and appeared to be lost in some cases of prostatic carcinoma, hyperplasia and in nonmalignant glands surrounding tumor. It was speculated that the role of CD 38 in intracellular calcium mobilization may contribute to smooth muscle contraction and/or sperm motility (Kramer et al, 1995). The ligand to CD38 is the adhesion molecule CD31 (Vallario et al, 1999).

Insulin secretion is one of the functions mediated by CD38. The molecule is the target of an autoimmune response and serum auto antibodies to CD38 have been detected in diabetic patients. Anti-CD38 auto antibodies have been suggested to be a new diagnostic marker of beta-cell autoimmunity in diabetes (Mallone et al, 2001).

The source of the antigen for raising anti-CD38 specific monoclonal antibody had mainly been preparations obtained from MLC cells, normal thymocytes and the plasmacytoma cell line LP-1 (Alessio et al, 1990).

This was used in the context of endometrial biopsy specimens to allow the definitive diagnosis of chronic endometritis to be made (Leong et al, 1997).

Applications

The expression of CD38 is not restricted to a specific lineage nor to a discrete activation step. It is found on precursor cells in the bone marrow, activated cells (T and B blasts), terminally differentiated cells (such as plasma cells), monocytes and most peripheral blood NK cells (Malavasi et al, 1992, Allessio et al, 1990). CD4+CD45RA+ cells also preferentially express CD38, but the antigen is not expressed by CD4+CD45RO+ cells. From a practical standpoint, CD 38 has been useful in the immunophenotyping of acute leukemias and in research into the role of activated T cells in immunodeficiency diseases and in autoimmune diseases. It is a useful marker for plasma cells as poorly differentiated plasma cells may mimic other blastic lymphoid cells and suboptimal cytomorphologic preservation may impede the accurate recognition of plasma cells (Appendix 1.6). It has been employed to identify plasma cells in synovial biopsies aiding in the differential diagnosis of early arthritis Kraan et al, 1999). We have found CD 38 to be a better antibody compared to VS 38 when employed to identify plasma cells such as in the diagnosis of chronic endometritis (Leong et al, 1997) as the latter also stains stromal and endometrial cells, reducing its usefulness in this setting. CD38 shows strong labeling of plasma

cells, enhancing their distinctive cytologic characteristics.

References

Alessio M, Roggero S, Funaro et al. CD38 molecule: structural and biochemical analysis on human T lymphocytes, thymocytes, and plasma cells. Journal of Immunology 1990;145:878–84.

Dianzani U, Funaro A, DiFranco D, et al. Interaction between endothelium and CD4+ CD45RA+ lymphocytes: Role of the human CD 38 molecule. Journal of Immunology 1994;153:952–9.

Kraan MC, Haringman JJ, Post WJ, et al. Immunohistoclogical analysis of synovial tissue for differential diagnosis in early arthritis. Rheumatology 1999;38:1074–80.

Kramer G, Steiner C, Fodinger D, et al. High expression of a CD-38 like molecule in normal prostatic epithelium and its differential loss in benign and malignant disease. Journal of Urology 1995;154:1636–41.

Leong AS-Y, Vinyuvat S, Leong FJW-M, Suthipintawong C. Anti-CD 38 and VS 38 antibodies for the detection of plasma cells in the diagnosis of chronic endometritis. Applied Immunohistochemistry 1997;5:189–93.

Malavasi F, Funaro A, Roggero S, et al. Human CD 38: A glycoprotein in search of a function. Immunology Today 1994;15:95–7.

MalloneR, Ortolan E, Baj G, et al. Autoantibody response to CD38 in Caucasian patients with type 1 and type 2 diabetes: immunological and genetic characterization. Diabetes 2001;50:752–62.

Mehta K, Shahid U, Malavasi F. Human CD 38, a cell-surface protein with multiple functions. FASEB Journal 1996;10:1408–17.

Reinherz EL, Kung PC, Goldstein G, et al. Discrete stages of human intrathymic differentiation: analysis of normal thymocytes and leukemic lymphoblasts of T cell lineage. Proceedings of /the National Academy of Sciences, USA 1980;77:1588–92.

Vallario A, Chilosi M, Adami F, et al. Human myeloma cells express the CD38 ligand CD31. British Journal of Haematology 1999;105:441–4.

Yamada M, Mizuguchi M, Otsuka N, et al. Ultrastructural localization of CD 38 immunoreactivity in rat brain. Brain Research 1997;756:52–60.

CD 40

Sources/clones

Ancell (BE1), Biodesign (BL–C4), Caltag Laboratories (BLB40), Coulter/Immunotech (MAB89), Cymbus Bioscience (B–B20), Immunotec (MAB89), Pharmingen (5C3), Sanbio/Monosan (BL–C4), Sanbio/Monosan/Accurate (BLC4), Serotec (B–B20).

Fixation/preparation

The antigen is resistant to formalin fixation with enhanced staining following heat-induced antigen retrieval at pH 8.0.

Background

CD40 is a 48 kD integral membrane protein expressed by B lymphocytes, follicular dendritic cells, interdigitating reticulum cells, monocytes, epithelial cells, endothelial cells and tumor cells including carcinomas, B cell lymphomas/leukemia and Reed Sternberg cells of Hodgkin's disease. CD40 has been clustered as a member of the nerve growth factor (NGF) /tumor necrosis factor (TNF) receptor superfamily. Its corresponding counterstructure, the CD40 ligand (CD40L) being mainly expressed by activated CD4+ T cells and also some activated CD8+ T cells, basophils, eosinophils, mast cells and stromal cells. CD40L shares significant amino acid homology with TNF particularly in its extracellular domain and is therefore viewed as a member of the TNF ligand superfamily. The flurry of publications relating to CD40 suggest that this receptor may have a pivotal role in the function of B lymphocytes and their survival (Klaus et al, 1997; van Kooten & Banchereau, 1997; Liu Arpin, 1997; Lipsky et al, 1997; Gulbranson-Judge et al, 1997). Binding of CD40L+ T cells to CD40+ B cells is thought to play a major role in the T cell-dependent B cell activation, B cell proliferation, Ig isotype switching, memory B cell formation and rescue of B cells from apoptotic death in germinal centers (Gruss et al, 1997). Mutations of the CD40L gene have been associated with the X-linked hyper-IgM immunodeficiency syndrome, indicating the critical role of the CD40/CD40L interaction in the T cell-B cell interplay. Accordingly, expression of CD40 has been found in most of the B cell neoplasms, Reed Sternberg cells of Hodgkin's disease and some carcinomas. In contrast, functional CD40/CD40L interactions appear to be critical for cellular activation signals during immune responses and neoplastic tumor cell growth. Lack of this important interaction results in greatly reduced activation of CD4+ T cells, while successful interaction of these molecules results in full activation of T cell effector functions such as help for B-cell differentiation and class switch, activation of monocytes and macrophages to produce lymphokines and to kill intracellular pathogens, and activation of autoreactive T cells to mount an autoimmune response (Klaus et al, 1997; Grewal & Flavell, 1997a, 1997b). CD40 may also play a similar role in the transduction of regulatory signals for cell functions such as proliferation and differentiation in non-lymphoid cells and has a role in the binding of tumor cells to endothelium, cell migration and enhancement of cell motility so that it is of interest in tumor metastasis and prognostication (Sviatoha et al, 2002).

Applications

The intense research interest in CD40 and its ligand has yet to be translated into diagnostic applications. Current uses of CD40 have mostly been for the immunodetection and identification of tumor cells in all subtypes of Hodgkin's disease. As many as 100% of Hodgkin's disease have displayed positivity for CD40, irrespective of their antigenic phenotype (Carbone et al, 1995). In contrast, CD40 was immunodetected in only one third of anaplastic large cell lymphomas, whereas almost 83% of B cell non-Hodgkin's lymphomas were positive (Carbone et al, 1995). In vitro engagement of CD40 by its soluble ligand CD40L enhanced both clonogenic capacity and colony cell survival of Hodgkin's disease cell lines. Recombinant CD40L induced interleukin-8 secretion and enhanced IL-6, TNF, and lymphotoxin-alpha release from cultured Reed Sternberg cells. These cytokines play a significant role in the clinical presentation and pathology of Hodgkin's disease, a tumor of cytokine-producing cells. CD40L has pleiotropic biologic activities on Reed Sternberg cells and the CD40-CD40L interaction might be a critical element in the deregulated cytokine network and cell contact-dependent activation cascade typical for Hodgkin's disease (Gruss et al, 1994; Carbone et al, 1995).

Other applications of CD40 include the study of ulcerative colitis in which an upregulation of CD40 has been demonstrated in epithelial cells of the colon in both the active state as well as in remission (Polese et al, 2002). Similarly, increased CD40 expression was found in the B cell, macrophage and dendritic cell compartments in acute ileitis

following oral infection with Toxoplasma in mice, suggesting that CD40/CD154 interaction is an essential component for development of inflammation in the experimental model (Li et al, 2002). CD40 is also expressed in neuronal cells of the brain (Tan et al, 2002).

Comments

CD40 shows distinctive immunolocalization to the cell membrane and as a paranuclear dot similar to that of CD30 and CD15.

CD40 is expressed on B cells, macrophages, dendritic cells, endothelial clls, fibroblasts, keratinocytes, carcinomas, most B cell lymphomas, some B-ALL and is not expressed on plasma cells.

References

Carbone A, Gloghini A, Gruss HJ, Pinto A. CD40 ligand is constitutively expressed in a subset of T cell lymphomas and on the microenvironmental reactive T cells of follicular lymphomas and Hodgkin's disease. American Journal of Pathology 1995;147:912–22.

Gray D, Bergthorsdottir S, van Essen D. Observations on memory B-cell development. Seminars in Immunology 1997;9:249–54.

Grewal IS, Flavell RA. The role of CD40 ligand in co-stimulation and T-cell activation. Immunology Reviews 1997a;153:85–106.

Grewal IS, Flavell RA. The CD40 ligand. At the center of the immune universe? Immunology Reviews 1997b;16:59–70.

Gruss HJ, Hirschstein D, Wright B, et al. Expression and function of CD40 on Hodgkin and Reed-Sternberg cells and the possible relevance for Hodgkin's disease. Blood 1994 84:2305–14.

Gulbranson-Judge A, Casamayor-Palleja M, MacLennan IC. Mutually dependent T and B cell responses in germinal centers. Annals of New York Academy of Sciences 1997;815:199–210.

Klaus GG, Choi MS, Lam EW, et al. CD40: a pivotal receptor in the determination of life/death decisions in B lymphocytes. International Reviews in Immunology 1997;15:5–31.

Li W, Buzoni-Gatel D, Debbabi H, et al. CD40/CD154 ligation is required for the development of acute ileitis following oral infection with an intracellular pathogen in mice. Gastroenterology 2002;122:762–73.

Lipsky PE, Attrep JF, Grammer AC, et al. Analysis of CD40-CD40 ligand interactions in the regulation of human B cell function. Annals of New York Academy of Science 1997;815:372–83.

Liu YJ, Arpin C. Germinal center development. Immunology Reviews 1997;156:111–26.

Polese L, Angriman I, Cecchetto A, et al. The role of CD40 in ulcerative colitis: histochemical analysis and clinical correlation. European Journal of Gastroenterology and Hepatology 2002;14:237–41.

Sviatoha V, Rundgren A, Tani E, et al. Expression of CD40, CD44, bcl-2 antigens and rate of cell proliferation on fine needle aspirates from metastatic melanoma. Cytopathology 2002;13:11–21.

Tan J, Town T, Mori T, et al. CD40 is expressed and functional on neuronal cells. EMBO Journal 2002;21:643–52.

Van Kooten C, Banchereau J. Functional role of CD40 and its ligand. Archives of Allergy and Immunology 1997;113:393–9.

CD 43

Sources/clones

Becton Dickinson (Leu22), Biodesign (BL-E/G3), Biogenesis (MEM59), Biogenesis/Biosource (WR14), Biogenex (MT1), Caltag Laboratories (BL-TP43), Coulter (DFT1), Cymbus Bioscience (DFT1), Dako (DF-T1), Labvision Corp (BRA7G), Novocastra (polyclonal), Pharmingen (HIS17, S7, 1G10), Sanbio/Accurate (BLEG3), Sanbio/Monosan (MEM-59), Serotec (DFT-1, DR-14), Shandon Lipshaw (DFT1).

Fixation/preparation

Generally (especially MT1 and DFT-1) applicable to formalin-fixed paraffin-embedded sections, but requires enzyme (trypsin) pre-treatment before immunostaining. HIER enhances immunoreactivity.

Background

MT1 (Poppema et al, 1987) and the identical antibody DFT-1 (Flavell et al, 1988) recognize a sialoantigen present on normal T-cells, myeloid cells and macrophages. Megakaryocytes are variably positive. Both antibodies belong to the CD43 cluster. There is evidence that the antibody MT1, originally thought to belong to CD45 (Poppema et al, 1987), binds to an entirely unrelated molecule (Flavell et al, 1988). Both MT1 and DFT-1 recognize surface antigens (190, 110 and 100 kD).

Applications

In a review of several published series, CD43 (MT1) was shown to immunoreact with 30% low grade B-cell lymphomas, approximately 90% T-cell lymphomas, 69% B-cell and 97% T-cell lymphoblastic lymphomas and 44% anaplastic large cell lymphomas. However, it should be noted that CD43 also highlights myeloid cells and macrophages (Norton and Isaacson, 1989) (Appendix 2.4) and may be employed as a marker of granulocytic tumors (Appendix 2.5). Although normal small B-lymphocytes are CD43 negative, most low-grade B-cell lymphomas are CD43 positive. However, hairy cell leukemia, MALT lymphoma and follicle center cell lymphomas are notable exceptions. Therefore CD43 is not useful to distinguish between T- and B-cell lymphocytic lymphoma. Furthermore, although CD43 is a reliable marker of mantle cell lymphoma (MCL), it cannot immunophenotypically distinguish MCL from T- or B-cell lymphoblastic lymphomas (Norton and Isaacson, 1986b). CD43 marks plasmacytoma/myeloma (Appendix 2.9) and is more often positive than negative in peripheral T-cell lymphomas.

An investigation of 28 extramedullary myeloid cell tumors using paraffin section immunohistochemistry with a panel of myeloid markers, revealed CD43 to be the only antibody that was positive in 100% of cases irrespective of the differentiation of the myeloid cells (Traweek et al, 1993). Furthermore, staining was always intense and widespread.

Comments

CD43 remains behind CD3 and UCHL1 (CD45RO) as a marker of T-cell lymphomas. Nevertheless, in appropriate immunohistochemical panels CD43 does play a role in the identification of low grade B-cell lymphomas (Appendix 2.1, 2.9) and myeloid disorders. Normal tonsil is useful as a control since paracortical cells are CD43 positive, whilst follicle center cells are negative. The expression of CD 43 in a large B cell lymphoma may be an indicator of dedifferentiation from a small cell lymphoma. There is ample evidence that CD43 is not specific for T cells (Kennedy et al, 2002). Together with CD79a and Tdt this marker is useful to separate lymphoblastic lymphoma from Ewing's sarcoma, which is consistently negative for these antigens (Ozdemirli et al, 2001).

CD43 is positive on most T cells, activated B cells, NK cells, granulocytes, monocytes, megakaryocytes, 90% of T cell lymphomas, co-expressed with CD20 in small lymphocyte lymphoma but not in benign cells, granulocytic sarcomas, acute myeloid leukemia, most acute lymphocytic leukemia, plasmacytomas and mast cell disease.

References

Flavell DJ, Flavell SU, Jones DB, Wright DH. Two new monoclonal antibodies recognising T-cells (DF-T1) and B-cells (DF-B1) in formalin fixed paraffin embedded tissue sections. Journal of Pathology 1988;155:343A.

Kennedy GA, Cull G, Gill D, et al. Identification of tumours with the CD43 only phenotype during investigation of suspected lymphoma: a heterogenous group not necessarily of T cell origin. Pathology 2002;34:46–50.

Norton AJ, Isaacson PG. Lymphoma phenotyping in formalin-fixed and paraffin wax-embedded tissues. I. Range of antibodies and staining patterns. Histopathology 1989;14:437–46.

Norton AJ, Isaacson PG. Lymphomas phenotyping in formalin-fixed and paraffin wax-embedded tissues: II. Profiles of reactivity in the various tumour types. Histopathology 1989;14:557–79.

Ozdemirli M, Fanburg-Smith JC, Hartmann DP, et al. Differentiating lymphoblastic lymphoma and Ewing's sarcoma: lymphocyte markers and gene rearrangement. Modern Pathology 2001;14:1175–82.

Poppema S, Hollema H, Visser L, Vos H. Monoclonal antibodies (MT1, MT2, MB1, MB2, MB3) reactive with leukocyte subsets in paraffin-embedded tissue sections. American Journal of Pathology 1987;127:418–29.

Traweek ST, Arber DA, Rappaport H, Brynes RK. Extramedullary myeloid cell tumors. An immunohistochemical and morphologic study of 28 cases. American Journal of Surgical Pathology 1993;17:1011–9.

CD 44

Sources/clones

CD44

Available from Biodesign (T2.F4, BU52), Cymbus Bioscience (F10–44–2), Dako (DF1485, 2B11), Immunotech (J.173), Oncogene (A3D8, AIG3), Pharmingen (OX-49), RDI (F10–44–2), Sanbio (MEM-85), Sera Lab (A3D8, AIG3), Serotec (F10–44–2) and Sigma (A3D8).

CD44v6

Available from R & D Systems (2F10) and various isoforms including v4, v5, v6, v7 and v7-v8 are available from Bender MedS.

Fixation/preparation

The antibodies, particularly CA1G3, are effective in formalin-fixed, paraffin embedded tissues but staining is optimal only after microwave-induced epitope retrieval in 10 m M citrate buffer at pH 6.0. Enzyme digestion should not be performed as this has been shown to be alter the integrity of the antigen.

Background

The CD44 receptor (also known as phagocytic glycoprotein (Pgp-1), extracellular matrix receptor III (ECM-III), B cell p80 antigen, lymphocyte homing receptor (Hermes antigen), hyaluronate cellular adhesion molecule (H-CAM). CD44 shows considerable homology with the cartilage link proteins involved in adhesion between hyaluronate and other proteoglycans in the extracellular matrix including collagen, fibronectin, and ankyrin. Besides this function, CD44 has since been found to have a role in recognition between lymphocytes and endothelial cells and in lymphocyte homing to the reticuloendothelial tissues. This latter function has led to interest in its possible role in the regulation of tumor cell dissemination.

The CD 44 family of glycoproteins exists in a number of variant isoforms, the most common being the standard 85–95kD or hematopoietic variant (CD 44s) that is found in mesodermal cells such as hematopoietic, fibroblastic, and glial cells, and in some carcinoma cell lines. The receptor is coded in five distinct domains located on the short arm of chromosome 11. The heterogeneity in the CD44 molecule results from post-translational modification of the protein and/or alternative splicing of up to 10 exons results in variant isoforms of higher molecular mass (140–160 kD) which may be expressed individually or in various combinations, with potentially diverse functions. Higher molecular weight isoforms have been described in epithelial cells (CD 44v) and are thought to function in intercellular adhesion and stomal binding. While the other functions and distributions of the CD 44 family have not yet been completely elucidated they are also know to participate in embryonic development and angiogenesis as well as other molecular processes associated with specific adhesions, signal transduction, and cell migration. The recent demonstration of a concordance of the cell proliferation nuclear antigen Ki-67 and CD 44 expression in adenomatous polyps, colonic carcinomas and adjacent mucosa raises the possibility of involvement of CD 44 in stimulating cell growth (Abassi et al, 1993).

Following the discovery that the splice variants, especially exon v4–7, initiated the lymphatic spread of rat pancreatic carcinoma cells, the role of the highly inter-species conserved CD 44 in human tumor progression and metastasis has been examined. It appears that the CD 44-hyaluronate interaction is central to tumor invasiveness; the receptor allowing the uptake and subsequent degradation of matrical hyaluronate. While many human tumors express CD 44, a positive correlation between increased CD 44v expression and tumor progression and/or dedifferentiation has been demonstrated in only some (East & Hart, 1993). Such tumors include non-Hodgkin's lymphoma (Stauder et al, 1995), hepatocellular carcinoma (Matthew et al, 1996), breast carcinoma, renal cell carcinoma (Terpe et al, 1993), colonic carcinoma (Abassi et al, 1993; Wielenga et al, 1993; Herrlich et al, 1995) and some soft tissue tumors (Wang et al, 1996). More recent additions to the list include metastatic melanoma (Sviatoha et al, 2002), prostatic carcinoma (Ekici et al, 2002), and gastric cancer (Yamaguchi et al, 2002). Conversely, CD 44v expression is downgraded in other tumors including neuroblastoma (Shtivelman & Bishop, 1991), squamous cell and basal cell carcinomas of the skin (Herold-Mende et al, 1996).

Applications

The suggestion that there is a positive association between CD 44 isoform expression and progression in human tumors has important implications for diagnosis and prognosis. Unfortunately, the situation is not yet clear-cut. Confusion over the complicated exon boundaries together with the different nomenclature employed by researchers have added to problems of identifying the true

metastasis-associated isoform. Furthermore, stromal cells may contribute to the isoform pattern detected. For example, activated lymphocytes may express the so-called metastasis-associated variant of CD 44, emphasizing the importance of immunohistological assessment as a method that allows morphologic discrimination.

Comments

Currently, applications of CD 44 still lie in the research domain. While antibodies to specific isoforms are available, some reactive in fixed paraffin-embedded tissues, the antibody to pan-CD44 molecule has been the most widely used in paraffin sections. Microwave epitope retrieval is essential for the demonstration of the antigen. While CD44 is a plasmalemmal determinant, both cytoplasmic and cell membrane staining patterns have been demonstrated in non-neoplastic and neoplastic cells. It has been suggested that exclusive cytoplasmic staining may reflect the overproduction of the protein so that not all of it can be incorporated into the cell membrane. Alternatively, the production of aberrant forms or massive shedding of the CD44 molecule from the cell membrane could account for this pattern of staining.

References

Abassi AM, Chester KA, Talbot IC, et al. CD 44 is associated with proliferation in normal and neoplastic human colorectal epithelial cells. European Journal of Cancer 1993;29A:294.

East JE and Hart IR. CD 44 and its role in tumor progression and

metastasis. European Journal of Cancer 1993;29A:1921–22.

Ekici S, Ayhan A, Kendi S, Ozen H. Determination of prognosis in patients with prostate cancer treated with radical prostatectomy: prognostic value of CD44v6 score. Journal of Urology 2002;167:2037–41.

Herold-Mende C, Seiter S, Born AI, et al. Expression of CD 44 splice variants in squamous epithelia and squamous cell carcinomas of the head and neck. Journal of Pathology 1996;179:66–73.

Herrlich P, Pals S and Ponta H. CD 44 in colon cancer. European Journal of Cancer 1995;31:1110–12.

Mathew J, Hines JE, Obafunwa JO, et al. CD 44 is expressed in hepatocellular carcinomas showing vascular invasion. Journal of Pathology 1996;179:74–9.

Shtivelman E and Bishop JM. Expression of CD 44 is repressed in neuroblastoma cells. Molecular and Cell Biology 1991;11:5446–53.

Stauder R, Eisterer W, Thaler J and Gunther U. CD 44 variant isoforms in non-Hodgkin's lymphoma: a new independent prognostic variable. Blood 1995;85:2885–99.

Sviatoha V, Rundgren A, Tani E, et al. Expression of CD40, CD44, bcl-2 anntigens and rate of cell proliferation on fine needle aspirates from metastatic melanoma. Cytopathology 2002;13:11–21.

Terpe HJ, Tajrobehkar K, Gunthert U and Altmannsberger M. Expression of cell adhesion molecules alpha-2, alpha-5 and alpha-6 integrin, E-cadherin, N-CAM and CD 44 in renal cell carcinoma: an immunohistochemical study. Virchow's Archives 1993;422:219–24.

Wang HH, DeYoung BR, Swanson PE and Wick MR. CD 44 immunoreactivity in soft tissue sarcomas. Applied

Immunohistochemistry 1996;4:184–89.

Wielenga VJM, Heider K-H, Offerhaus GJA, et al. Expression of CD 44 variant proteins in human colorectal cancer is related to tumour progression Cancer Research 1993;53:4754–6.

Yamaguchi A, Goi T, Yu J, et al. Expression of CD44v6 in advanced gastric cancer and its relationship to hematogenous metastasis and long-term prognosis. Journal of Surgical Oncology 2002;79:230–5.

NOTES

CD 45 (Leucocyte Common Antigen)

Sources/clones

CD45

Available from a large number of sources including Biodesign (ALB12, J.33, MEM 28, T29/33), Biogenex, Bioprobe (bra 55, ICO-46, LT46), Cymbus Bioscience (MEM 28, RVS-1, F10–89–4), Dako (T29/33, 2B11, PD7/26), GenTrak, Immunotech (J.33, ALB12), Oncogene (MEM 28, T29/33, J.33), Pharmingen (H130, CT-1, 30F11.1), RDI (F-10–89–4, CLB-T200/1), Sanbio (BL-leuk-45), Sera-Lab (F10–89–4), Serotec (YTH54.12, YTH24.5), and Sigma.

CD45R

Available from Accurate/Ancell (351C5), Biodesign (DFB1, F8–11–13, MEM56), Biogenex, Bioprobe (LT45R), Cymbus Bioscience (DFB1), GenTrak, RDI (DFB1), Sera-Lab, Serotec and Pharmingen (HIS24, DNL-1.9, 16A, 23G2, RA3–6B2).

CD45RO

Available from Accurate/Ancell (UCHL1), Biodesign (UCHL1), Biotest (UCHL1), Cymbus Bioscience (UCHL1), Dako (UCHL1, OPD4), GenTrak, Immunotech (UCHL1), Sera Lab (UCHL1), Serotec (UCHL1).

CD45RA

Available from Accurate (YTH80.103), Biodesign (ALB11, F8–11–13), Cymbus Bioscience (F8–1–3, MEM 56), Dako (4KB5), GenTrak, Immunotech (ALB11), RDI (F8–11–13), Sanbio (MEM-56), Sera-Lab, Serotec (B-C15, F8–11–13), and Pharmingen (14.8).

CD45RB

Available from Axcel/Accurate, Cymbus Bioscience, Dako (PD7/26),

CD45RC

Available from Pharmingen (HIS25) and Serotec (YTH80.103).

Fixation/preparation

The CD45 antibodies that are commercially available are mostly effective in paraffin-embedded tissues as well as in frozen sections.

Background

The CD45 cluster of antibodies recognises a family of proteins known as the leukocyte common antigen (LCA) exclusively expressed on the surface of almost all haematolymphoid cells and their progenitors. The CD45 antibody is one of the most specific antibodies currently available for diagnostic use. Virtually all haematolymphoid cells, including T- and B-lymphocytes, granulocytes and monocytes, and macrophages, with the exception of maturing erythrocytes and megakaryocytes express CD 45. This family of proteins has been called the leukocyte common antigen and, to date, has not been conclusively shown on any non-hematolymphoid cells.

The CD 45 proteins are coded for by a single gene located on chromosome 1q31–32. The gene is composed of 33 exons that code for the cDNA sequence as well as both 5' and 3' non-translated regions. Differential usage of three exons termed A, B and C is known to generate eight different mRNAs and at least five proteins in the CD 45 protein family. The complete CD 45 protein consists of a large cytoplasmic domain of 707 amino acids, a transmembrane region of 22 amino acids and an external domain of 391–552 amino acids depending on the pattern of exon splicing. By electron microscopy, the CD 45 proteins consist of a globular structure of 12 nm, representing the cytoplasmic domain, and a rod-like structure of 18 nm, representing the external domain.

There is high conservation of the cytoplasmic domain among mammals and it shows homology with placental tyrosine phosphatases. Consistent with this homology, the CD 45 protein has intrinsic tyrosine phosphatase activity and belongs to a family of protein tyrosine phosphatases that includes 16 other members, at least seven of which are transmembrane proteins (Trowbridge et al, 1991).

The precise function of the CD 45 proteins is not known but they appear to play an important role in early lymphocyte activation. Protein tyrosine phosphatase can counter the actions of protein tyrosine kinases, enzymes known to be induced in early T-cell activation that may represent the primary signaling event initiated by the T-cell receptor. CD 45 expression is inversely related to spontaneous tyrosine phosphorylation of multiple proteins, which has a fundamental role in regulating T-cell calcium levels. CD 45 is required for both T-cell antigen receptor and CD 2-mediated activation of T-lymphocyte protein tyrosine kinase and CD 45 is physically linked to both CD 2 and the T-cell receptor on the surface of memory T-lymphocytes. The difference in structure among the external domains of the different CD 45 proteins probably determines the specific target stimuli for the different cell types expressing CD 45. Similarly, CD 45 may also be important for B-cell function. Antibodies to CD 45 inhibit an early phase in the activation of resting B-cells and are able to inhibit *c-myc* induction in B-cells.

As a result of post-translocational change of the mRNA of the A, B and C exons, several isoforms are produced. By strict definition, CD 45 antibodies are monoclonal antibodies, which react with all isoforms of CD 45 proteins, and there are several subclusters of antibodies that detect different species of CD 45 proteins. These have molecular weights of 220 kD representing the ABC isoform, 205 kD probably representing distinct AB and BC isoforms, 190 kD representing the B isoform, and 180 kD representing the O isoform. The restricted CD 45 antibody refers to those that recognize subsets of CD 45 proteins but not the entire class and these CD 45R antibodies can be further subdivided into CD45RA, CD45RB, and CD 45RO depending on the isoform recognized by the antibody. To date, there are no monoclonal antibodies that specifically recognize the C isoform. CD 45RA antibodies generally precipitate the 200 and 205 kD (ABC, and AB isoforms), CD45RB the 220, 205 and 190 kD (ABC, AB, BC and B isoform) and CD 45RO the 180 kD protein (O isoform).

Many of the CD 45 antibodies are sensitive to neuraminidase consistent with the suggestion that these antibodies recognize epitopes that are associated with carbohydrates and possibly, terminal sialic acids. PD 7 is a CD 45RB antibody and labels all known CD 45 proteins with the exception of the ones lacking exons A, B and C, whereas 2B11 reacts against AB protein but not others. The combination of PD 7

with 2B11 as a CD 45-CD 45RB cocktail (Dako) allows a reliable method of detecting LCA in hematolymphoid cells. CD45 proteins are major components of the membranes of lymphocytes and form about 10% of the lymphocyte surface accounting for much of the carbohydrate present on the membrane. The staining with CD45 antibodies is membranous although there may be some staining of the Golgi. Histiocytes exhibit minimal cell membrane staining and phagocytic cells show immuno-localization of the antigen to secondary lysosomes (Weiss et al, 1993).

Applications

The CD 45 proteins are the most specific of diagnostic antibodies currently available. A cocktail of PD7–2B11 (CD 45-CD 45RB) antibodies is a reliable marker of cells fixed in formalin as well as in cryostat sections and fresh cell preparations. It is, therefore, an essential component of the panel to distinguish anaplastic large cell tumors, which include the entities, malignant lymphoma, melanoma and carcinoma (Appendix 1.10). It is also an essential component of panels to separate small cell tumors of lymph nodes, skin, bone and other sites (Appendix 1.6, 1.11, 1.12), both in adults as well as in children. The reactivity of anti-LCA antibodies is between 93–99% for a cross-spectrum of different subtypes of B- and T-cell lymphomas.

In classic Hodgkin's disease, excluding the nodular L and H lymphocyte predominant subtype, membrane staining for leukocyte common antigen is rare, although cytoplasmic staining may be seen (Appendix 2.10). Cytoplasmic staining may be spurious as similar cytoplasmic staining can be found in non-hematolymphoid neoplasms. By contrast, the majority of nodular L and H lymphocyte predominant Hodgkin's disease shows positivity for PD 7 and/or 2B11 and this subtype is now thought to be distinctly different from classic Hodgkin's disease.

Anaplastic large cell lymphoma may show positivity for LCA in only 50–87% of cases only, although this figure may be higher in frozen section material. Furthermore, anaplastic large cell lymphoma may also show staining for epithelial membrane antigen, making its immunohistochemical differentiation from anaplastic carcinoma difficult. These tumors express CD30 and, in 60% of cases, are of activated T-cell phenotype showing staining for CD 45RO and/or CD 43 in paraffin sections (Chott et al, 1990).

Among other hematolymphoid neoplasms, plasmacytomas show a variable degree of positivity for LCA ranging from 0–20% of cases. Hairy cell leukemia has been found to be uniformly positive for PD 7–2B11 and CD 45 expression has been found in all cases of acute leukemias of T-cell lineage and in over 80% of cases of B-cell lineage. Failure of expression of CD 45 in acute childhood lymphoblastic leukemia appears to be associated with other favorable prognostic features such as lower leukocyte counts and serum lactic dehydrogenase levels and is associated with chromosomal hyperdiploidy. Mast cell disease appears to be positive

for PD 7–2B11 and polycythemia vera and extramedullary hematopoiesis were reported to be negative although only a few cases were studied. In keeping with the low expression in histiocytes, true histiocytic tumors were found to be negative for PD 7–2B11, whereas cases of Langerhans' histiocytosis were reported to be positive. The rare cases of interdigitating reticulum cell sarcoma, which have been studied, have been reported to be positive for PD 7 similar to non-neoplastic interdigitating reticulum cells. Cases of CD45-negative, keratin-positive large cell lymphomas have been reported but these are exceptionally rare (Donner et al, 2001).

While larger series have reported a total absence of staining for LCA in non-hematolymphoid neoplasms, there have been rare case reports of staining examples of primitive sarcoma, probably rhabdomyosarcoma.

CD45RA (4KB5, MB1, KiB3 and MT2)

The CD 45RA group of antibodies recognize the 220 kD and 205 kD variants of CD 45 encoded by exon A. These isoforms are expressed on the surface of most B-cells, as well as post-thymic, naive T-cells and some medullary thymocytes. MT 2 is thought to recognize a carbohydrate moiety and is negative in normal germinal centers unlike antibodies MB1 and KiB3 which appear to bind to the peptide backbone of CD 45RA, staining mantle zone and follicular center cells. In the paracortical areas of lymph nodes, there are approximately equal

numbers of CD 45RO-positive and CD 45 RA-positive cells. In paraffin-embedded sections, MB1 and 4KB5 stain over 80% of cases of B-cell lymphomas, while MT2 stains only 57% of such cases. Small lymphocytic lymphoma has the highest rate of positivity while small non-cleaved cell lymphoma has the lowest. Fifty-seven percent of cases of follicular center lymphoma are positive for MT2 and this pattern of staining has been exploited for diagnostic purposes as only weak or absent scattered positivity for MT2 is seen in reactive germinal center cells (Browne et al, 1991). Neoplastic follicles are labeled by MT2 whereas reactive follicles are not. This difference in staining patterns with MT2 has been postulated to be due to differences in the sialation of the CD 45 protein present on these B-cells. T-cell lymphoma has a much lower incidence of positivity with CD 45RA antibodies and is seen in about 10% of cases.

CD45RA+ mycosis fungoides is a rare form of the disease with T helper phenotype (CD3+, CD4+, CD8-, CD45RO+), often with loss of lineage markers (Fierro et al, 2001).

CD 45RO (UCHL1, A6, OPD4)

CD 45RO antibodies recognize the 180 kD (O isoform) variant of CD 45. UCHL1 antibody reacts with approximately 90% of cortical thymocytes, 50% of medullary thymocytes and approximately 50–70% of CD 2-negative and CD 3-positive peripheral blood and lymph node T-cells. It rarely, if ever, reacts with benign B-cells. While most mature T-cells are CD 45RO positive (Appendix 2.2), some normal T-cell subsets are constitutively CD 45RO-negative and CD45RA-positive and the CD 45RO-positive cells slowly increase in number to reach the adult level of about 50% by the age 10–20 years. CD 45RO-negative cells include naive CD 4-positive T-cells which predominate in neonates, and some CD 8-positive or CD 4-negative CD 8-negative subsets found in intestinal intraepithelial T-cells and enteropathy-associated T-cell lymphoma.

In the differentiation of low-grade B-cell from T-cell lymphomas, the approximated test analysis figures for UCHL1 are as follows: sensitivity 95%, specificity 95%, accuracy 95%. In contrast, in high grade lymphomas, the same parameters are 80%, 85% and 83% respectively. Stem cells giving rise to both erythroid and myeloid cells as well as primitive erythroid colony-forming cells express the 180 kD isoform of the CD 45 protein recognized by CD 45RO but more mature erythroid forms lack CD 45 expression. Most granulopoietic colony-forming cells are CD 45RO-negative while mature monocytes or macrophages and myeloid cells are generally CD 45RO-positive. These latter cells do not stain with the antibody OPD4, the difference in reactivity possibly due to a difference in the carbohydrate structure of the epitope presented on these cells. (Norton & Isaacson, 1989; Chittal et al, 1988).

Enumeration of CD45RO+ inflammatory cells together with CD8, neutrophil elastase, CD68 and mast cell tryptase have been employed in an attempt to distinguish ulcerative colitis and Crohn's disease but the results require confirmation (Sasaki et al, 2002).

The OPD4 antibody is not, as originally claimed, specific for CD 4-positive T-cells. It reacts very similarly to clone UCHL1 and differs only in having a low sensitivity for T-cell lymphoma and is not reactive with monocytic cells (Poppema et al, 1991).

CD45 is positive on all hematopoietic cells, strong expression is seen on lymphocytes. The antigen may not be found on non-hematopoietic cells, lymphoplasmacytic lymphoma, lymphoblastic lymphoma, anaplastic lymphoma, and multiple myeloma. CD45RA is expressed on naïve and activated T cells and medullary thymocytes. CD45RO is expressed on memory and activated T cells, thymocytes, some B cells, and weakly on granulocytes and macrophages. The antigen is expressed on about 75% of T cell lymphomas, with variable expression of T cell lymphoblastic lymphoma.

References

Browne G, Tobin B, Carney DN, Dervan PA. Aberrant MT2 positivity distinguishes follicular lymphoma from reactive follicular hyperplasia in B5 and formalin-fixed paraffin sections. American Journal of Clinical Pathology 1991;96:90–4.

Chittal SM, Caveriviere P, Schwarting R, et al. Monoclonal antibodies in the diagnosis of Hodgkin's disease. The search for a rational panel. American Journal of Surgical Pathology 1988;12:9–21.

Chott A, Kaserer K, Augustin I, et al. Ki-1 positive large cell lymphoma. A clinicopathologic study of 41 cases. American Journal of Surgical Pathology 1990;14:539–48.

Donner LR, Mott FE, Tafur I. Cytokeratin-positive, CD45-negative primary centroblastic lymphoma of the adrenal gland: a potential for a diagnostic pitfall. Archives of Pathology and Laboratory Medicine 2001;125:1104–6.

Fierro MT, Novelli M, Savoia P, et al. CD45RA+ immunophenotype in mycosis fungoides: clinical, histological and immunophenotypical features in 22 patients. Journal of Cutaneous Pathology 2001;28:356–62.

Norton AJ, Isaacson PG. Lymphoma phenotyping in formalin-fixed and paraffin wax embedded tissues. II. Profiles of reactivity in the various tumour types. Histopathology 1989;14:557–79.

Poppema S, Lai R, Visser L. Monoclonal antibody OPD4 is reactive with CD45RO but differs from UCHL1 by the absence of monocyte activity. American Journal of Pathology 1991;139:725–9.

Sasaki Y, Tanaka M, Kudo H. Differentiation between ulcerative colitis and Crohn's disease by a quantitative immunohistochemical evaluation of T lymphocytes, neutrophils, histiocytes and mast cells. Pathology International 2002;52:277–85.

Trowbridge IS, Ostergaard HL, Johnson P. CD45 – a leucocyte-specific member of the protein tyrosine phosphatase family. Biochemica et Biophysica Acta 1991;1095:46–56.

Weiss LM, Arber DA, Chang KL. CD45. A review. Applied Immunohistochemistry 1993;1:166–81.

CD 54 (ICAM-1)

Sources/clones

Accurate (1304.100.40), Biodesign (84H10, 15.2, MEM-111, MEM-112), Biogenesis (MEM-12), Biogenex (BBIG-1), Biosource (BC14, RR1-1), Caltag Laboratories (MEM111), Coulter (84H10), Dako (6.5B5), Exalpha Co. (D3.6), Immunotech (84H10), Novocastra (15.2), Pharmingen (3E2, HA58), Sanbio/Monosan (MEM-111), Serotec (84H10), Zymed (MY13).

Fixation/preparation

Apart from clone My13 which is applicable to both frozen and paraffin-embedded tissue sections, all the other antibodies are only applicable to frozen sections only. In certain instances acetone fixation is recommended.

Background

Cell-cell adhesion is critical in the generation of effective immune responses and is dependent upon the generation of a variety of cell surface receptors (Ohh & Takei, 1996). Intercellular adhesion molecule-1 (ICAM-1; CD54) is an inducible cell surface glycoprotein expressed at a low level on a subpopulation of haematopoietic cells, vascular endothelium, fibroblasts and certain epithelial cells. However, its expression is dramatically increased at sites of inflammation, providing important means of regulating cell-cell interactions and hence inflammatory responses. ICAM-1 is induced by proinflammatory cytokines such as interleukin-1, tumor necrosis factor-alpha or interferon-gamma (Stratowa & Audette, 1995).

The CD54 antigen (ICAM-1) is a 90 kD integral membrane glycoprotein with seven potential N-linked glycosylation sites.

Applications

The CD54 antigen is expressed on monocytes and endothelial cells. It is also a lymphokine-inducible molecule and has been shown to be a ligand for LFA-1 mediated adhesion. Expression of the antigen can be induced or upregulated on many cell types including B and T lymphocytes, thymocytes, fibroblasts, keratinocytes and epithelial cells. In its function of mediating immune and inflammatory responses, CD54 antigen mediates adhesion of T-cells with antigen presenting cells and is involved in T-cell to T-cell and T-cell to B-cell interactions. (for review see Fleming, 1990; 1991). Mice bearing a null mutation of CD54 have been found to display no inflammatory cell infiltrate in the lung following thoracic irradiation suggesting that agents that block CD54 function may prevent radiation-induced pulmonary fibrosis (Hallahan et al, 2002).

Increased expression of ICAM-1 has been associated with many types of atherosclerotic lesions (Poston et al, 1992). In rejecting kidneys the antibody highlights all infiltrating cells strongly as well as glomerulus epithelium, endothelium on capillaries, vessels and mesangium (Knapp et al, 1989).

Comments

CD54 is expressed on both B and T cells, monocytes, endothelial cells and a variety of epithelial cells and thus has low specificity. CD54 may be strongly positive on mantle cell lymphomas of the spleen (Angelopoulou et al, 2002).

References

Angelopoulou MK, Siakantariz MP, Vassilakopoulos TP, et al. The splenic form of mantle cell lymphoma. European Journal of Haematology 2002;68:12–21.

Fleming S. Cellular functions of adhesion molecules. (Editorial). Journal of Pathology 1990;161:189–90.

Fleming S. Cell adhesion and focusing of inflammatory responses. (Commentary) Histopathology 1991;19:571–3.

Hallahan DE, Geng L, Shyr Y. Effects of intercellular adhesion molecule 1 (ICAM-1) null mutation on radiation-induced pulmonary fibrosis and respiratory insufficiency in mice. Journal of National Cancer Institutes 2002;94:704–5.

Knapp W, Dorken B, Gilks WR, Rieber EP, Schmidt RE, Stein H et al, (eds). Leucocyte Typing IV White Cell Differentiation Antigens. Oxford-New York-Tokyo; Oxford University Press 1989.

Ohh M, Takei F. New insights into the regulation of ICAM-1 gene expression. Leukemia and Lymphoma 1996;20:223–8.

Poston RN, Haskard DO, Coucher JR, et al. Expression of intercellular adhesion molecule-1 atherosclerotic plaques. American Journal of Pathology 1992;140:665–73.

Stratowa C, Audette M. Transcriptional regulation of the human intercellular adhesion molecule-1 gene: a short overview. Immunobiology 1995;193:293–304.

CD 56 (Neural Cell Adhesion Molecule)

Sources/clones

Dako (MOC-1, T199), Monosan (123C3), Research Diagnostics (ERIC-1), Zymed (123C3).

Fixation/preparation

Applicable to formalin-fixed paraffin sections. Requires pretreatment with microwave or pressure cooker antigen/epitope retrieval in citrate buffer. Enzymatic pretreatment has been shown to markedly decrease reactivity. The antibody to CD56 may also be applied to frozen sections or cell smears.

Background

CD56, the neural cell adhesion molecule (NCAM), was discovered in a search for cell–surface molecules that contribute to cell-cell interactions during neural development (Rutishauer et al, 1988). Human peripheral cells capable of non-MHC-restricted cytotoxicity express the CD56 antigen. NCAM has at least three isoforms, generated by differential splicing of the RNA transcript from a single gene located on chromosome 11 (Cunningham et al, 1987). The core polypeptide of the CD56 appears to be the 140kD isoform

of NCAM, which is variably glycosylated and sialylated to produce mature species with molecular weights ranging from 175–220 kD. The CD56 antigen itself appears not to participate directly in the cytolytic activity of NK cells (Ritz et al, 1988). Subsequent immunohistochemical studies have shown that NCAM is widely expressed in neural and neuroendocrine tissues (Bourne et al, 1991). Antibody clone 123C3 recognizes a heterodimeric glycoprotein with the 145 and 185 kD isoforms of NCAM (Schol et al, 1988), whilst clone ERIC-1 has been reported with two human isoforms 145 and 180 kD of NCAM. T199 is a 135/220 kD single chain glycosylated and sialylated protein expressed on CD2+, CD3-, CD16+ natural killer cells (NK) and neuroectodermal cells (Feidkert et al, 1989). Autopsy tissue has been used to demonstrate strong CD56 immunoreaction in peripheral nerve, adrenal zona glomerulosa and medulla, and synapses in cerebral cortex. CD56 also marks thyroid follicular epithelium, proximal renal tubules, hepatocytes, gastric parietal cells and pancreatic islet cells (Shipley et al, 1997).

Applications

Merkel cell carcinoma, neuroblastoma, ganglioglioma, oligodendroglioma, glioblastoma multiforme, pheochromocytoma, retinoblastoma, laryngeal and pulmonary squamous cell carcinoma, pulmonary and intestinal carcinoid, pulmonary small cell undifferentiated carcinoma, pancreatic islet cell tumor, hepatocellular carcinoma, renal cell carcinoma and follicular and papillary thyroid carcinoma mark positively with CD56 antibodies. CD56 has been found to be negative in Ewing's sarcoma, nasopharyngeal carcinoma, colonic adenocarcinoma, melanoma, meningioma, follicular center cell lymphoma, hairy cell leukemia (1 case each respectively) and multiple myeloma (5 cases). However, the current major application of CD56 on paraffin sections is in the diagnosis of NK and NK-like T-cell lymphoma, i.e., CD56 being a marker for natural killer cells (Chan, 1997) (Appendix 2.6). CD56-positive lymphomas are heterogeneous, encompassing several entities: nasal/nasopharyngeal NK/T-cell lymphoma, nasal type (extranasal) NK/T cell lymphoma, aggressive NK-cell leukemia/lymphoma, and the newly described blastoid NK-cell lymphoma. The nasal form represents the prototype of this group and is referred to as angiocentric lymphoma in the REAL classification. Besides coexpression of CD3, such tumors are often labeled by EBER-1 (Altemani et al, 2002; Hahn et al, 2002) so that therapeutic measures directed against the EB virsue should be researched (Hahn et al, 2002). Since CD56-positive lymphomas do not always show angiocentricity, and angiocentricity may occur in other lymphoma types, the term NK/T cell lymphoma or T/NK cell lymphoma appears to be more appropriate. Two other types of T-cell lymphoma show a particularly high frequency of CD56 expression: hepatosplenic δγT-cell lymphoma (63% CD56+) and S-100 protein-positive T-cell lymphoma (Wong et al, 1995; Chan et al, 1987).

Microvillous lymphomas are a group of B cell lymphomas that frequently express CD56. These rare, poorly defined transformed cell lymphomas are characterized by a cohesive sinus growth pattern and ultrastructural cytoplasmic processes and have been compared to transformed follicle centre cells and follicular dendritic cells and show clonal heavy chain immunoglobulin rearrangement, mark with CD74, CDw75 and CD20 but not DBA.44, CD21 or CD35. About half of such tumors express CD56, suggesting a role for adhesion molecules in the distribution of these lymphomas (Hammer et al, 1998).

A recently recognized unusual cutaneous blastic tumor co expresses CD56 and terminal deoxynucleatidyl transferase (TdT) and has been termed blastic natural killer cell lymphoma. These tumors are likely to be of primitive/undifferentiated hematopoietic origin and may progressively develop bone marrow involvement by blast cells with myeloid immunophenotype that are negative for CD56 and TdT (Khoury et al, 2002).

CD56 expression may predict occurrence of CNS disease in acute lymphoblstic leukemia (Ravandi et al, 2002) and the expression of this antigen in multiple myeloma correlates with the presence of lytic bone lesions and distinguished myeloma from lymphomas with plasmacytoid differentiation and from monoclonal gammopathy of undetermined significance. CD56 is expressed by both myeloma cells as well as osteoblasts, the expression of CD56 perhaps contributing to bone lysis by causing a decrease in osteoid formation (Ely & Knowles, 2002).

Another rare malignancy with CD56+CD4+ immunophenotype was recently shown to correspond to the so-called type 2 dendritic cell or plasmacytoid dendritic cell. Such tumors typically present with cutaneous nodules associated with lymphadenopathy or spleenic enlargement or both and massive bone marrow infiltration. The disease is rapidly fatal but there is a purely cutaneous form that is indolent (Feuillard et al, 2002).

Comments

Clearly CD56 antibodies are essential for the diagnosis of NK/T-cell lymphomas, which show a predilection for the upper aerodigestive tract, skin, testes, skeletal muscle, gastrointestinal tract and other extranodal sites and pursue an aggressive clinical course. Furthermore, this antibody may be used to detect residual disease in CD56-positive NK-T-cell lymphoma in which the neoplastic lymphoid cells are small and show minimal atypia, especially in small biopsies.

CD56 is expressed on NK cells, activated T cells, cerebellum, brain, at neuromuscular junctions, normal and neoplastic neuroendocrine tissues, myeloma and myeloid leukemia.

References

Altemani A, Barbosa AC, Kulka M, et al. Characteristic of nasal T/NK-cell lymphoma among Brazilians. Neoplasma 2002;49:55–60.

Bourne SP, Patel K, Walsh F, et al. A monoclonal antibody (ERIC-1), raised against retinoblastoma, that recognizes the neural cell adhesion molecule (NCAM) expressed on brain and tumors arising from the neuroectoderm. Journal of Neurological Oncology 1991;10:111–9.

Chan JKC. CD56-positive putative natural killer (NK) cell lymphomas: nasal, nasal-type, blastoid, and leukemic forms. Advances in Anatomical Pathology 1997;4:163–72.

Chan JKC. Ng CS, Chu YC, Wong KF. S-100 protein positive sinusoidal large cell lymphoma. Human Pathology 1987;18:756–9.

Cunningham BA, Hemperly JJ, Murray BA, Prediger EA, Brackenbury R, Edelman GM. Neural cell adhesion molecule: structure, immunoglobulin-like domains, cell surface modulation, and alternative RNA splicing. Science 1987;236:799–806.

Ely SA, Knowles DM. Expression of CD56/neural cell adhesion

molecule correlates with the presence of lytic bone lesions in multiple myeloma and distinguishes myeloma from monoclonal gammopathy of undetermined significance and lymphomas with plasmacytoid differentiation. American Journal of Pathology 2002;160:1293–9.

Feidkert HJ, Pietsch T, Hadam MR, Mildenberger H, Riehm H. Monoclonal antibody T-199 directed against human medulloblastoma: characterization of a new antigenic system expressed on neuroectodermal tumors and natural killer cells. Cancer Research 1989;49:4338–43.

Feuillard J, Jacob MC, Valensi F, et al. Clinical and biologic features of CD4(+)CD56(+) malignancies. Blood 2002;99:1556–63.

Hahn JS, Lee ST, Min YH, et al. Therapeutic outcome of Epstein-Barr virus positive T/NK cell lymphoma in the upper aerodigestive tract. Yonsei Medical Journal 2002;43:175–82.

Hammer RD, Vnencak-Jones CL, Manning SS, et al. Microvillous lymphomas are B cell neoplasms that frequently express CD56. Modern Pathology 1998;11:239–46.

Khoury JD, Medeiros LJ, Manning JT, et al. CD56(+) TdT (+) blastic natural killer cell tumor of the skin: primitive systemic malignancy related to myelomonocytic leukemia. Cancer 2002;94:2401–8.

Ravandi F, Cortes J, Estrov Z, et al. CD56 expression predicts occurrence of CNS disease in acute lymphoblastic leukemia. Leukemia Research 2002;26:643–9.

Ritz J, Schmidt RE, Michon J, Hercend T, Schlossman SF. Characterization of functional structures on human natural killer cells. Advances in Immunology 1988;42:181–211.

Rutishauer U, Acheson A, Hall AK, Mann DM, Sunshine J. The neural cell adhesion molecule (NCAM) as a regulator of cell-cell interactions. Science 1988;240:53–7.

Schol DJ, Mooi WJ, Van Der Gugten AA, et al. Monoclonal antibody 123C3, identifying small cell carcinoma phenotype in lung tumors, recognizes mainly, but not exclusively, endocrine and neuron-supporting normal tissues. International Journal of Cancer 1988;2 (Suppl):34–40.

Shipley WR, Hammer RD, Lennington WJ, Macon WR. Paraffin immunohistochemical detection of CD56, a useful marker for neural cell adhesion molecule (NCAM), in normal and neoplastic fixed tissues. Applied Immunohistochemistry 1997;5:87–93.

Wong KF, Chan JKC, Matutes E, et al. Hepatosplenic Tτδ T-cell lymphoma: a distinctive aggressive lymphoma type. American Journal of Surgical Pathology 1995;19:718–26.

NOTES

CD 57

Sources/clones

Becton-Dickinson (Leu7), Biodesign (NC1), GenTrak, Immunotech (NC1), Sanbio (6–13–19–1), Serotec (NC-1).

Fixation/preparation

Most antibodies are reactive in fixed paraffin-embedded tissues and immunoreactivity is enhanced by heat-induced epitope retrieval.

Background

CD 57 antibodies detect a 110kd protein encoded by a gene on chromosome 11. The protein is present on some peripheral lymphocytes but not in monocytes, granulocytes, platelets or erythrocytes. CD 57+ lymphocytes increase with age and represent 10–20% of lymphocytes in most adults. They mostly include a subset of CD 8+ T lymphocytes as well as natural killer (NK) cells (Abo & Balch, 1982). A sub-population of peripheral lymphocytes that reacts with this marker includes large granular lymphocytes. This antibody also reacts with both CD 3+ and CD 3-, non-B lymphocytes. The CD 3- lymphocytes demonstrate NK cell activity and have large cytoplasmic granules that are not seen in the CD 3+ cells. CD 3+/CD 57+ T cells are primarily suppressor lymphocytes with CD 8 expression though CD 4+/CD 8-/CD 57+ T cells have been described and CD 8+/CD 57+/HLA-DR+ T cells have also been identified. CD 3+/CD 8+/CD 57+ lymphocytes are positive for CD45RA but not CD 45RO. While this phenotype is characteristic of naïve T lymphocytes, the CD 57+ cells differ from other naïve T cells by failing to lose the CD45RA antigen when stimulated with alloantigens. These cells also differ from other T lymphocytes by their increased ability to acquire the HLA-DR antigen in the absence of antigen-specific cytotoxic activity against allogeneic target cells.

The frequency of CD 57+ lymphocytes in solid tissues varies according to site. CD 57+ lymphocytes are increased in term placental tissue, but not in decidua of early pregnancy. CD 57+ lymphocytes are decreased in bronchoalveolar lavage specimens compared with peripheral blood in the same patient, and they represent less than 2% of all nasal mucosal lymphocytes. CD 57+ lymphocytes are rare in both in the endometrium and uterine cervix. They are also rare in the thymus and in the bone marrow; they constitute no more than 1% of all nucleated cells.

CD 57+ lymphocytes have a different distribution to that of CD 8+ cells in the tonsils and lymph nodes, with the CD 57+ cells located primarily within the germinal centers. These germinal center cells are CD 3+ T cells, which also express the CD 4 antigen. Similar to the CD 57+/CD 4+ T cells in cytomegalovirus (CMV) carriers, the CD 4+ germinal center cells do not display the usual helper activity of classic CD 4+ lymphocytes (Swerdlow & Murray, 1984).

CD 57+ cells in the spleen are seen mostly in the germinal centers of the white pulp, or as a rim of cells around the central white pulp (Griffiths et al, 1989).

The HNK-1/Leu 7 antibody also reacts with cells other than lymphocytes. CD 57 antibodies react with an antigen present in the central and peripheral nervous system myelin and oligodendroglia and Schwann cells. Some neural adhesion molecules also contain a carbohydrate epitope that is recognized by CD 57 antibodies.

The reactivity is due to part of the myelin-associated glycoprotein having a similar molecular mass (110 kD) to the CD 57 lymphocyte antigen.

Besides neural-associated cells, CD 57 antibodies immunoreact with prostatic epithelium, pancreatic islets, adrenal medulla, renal loops of Henle and proximal tubules, chromaffin cells of the gut, gastric chief cells, epithelial cells of the outer thymic cortex and some cells in the fetal bronchus. It is also detected in the prostatic seminal fluid (Arber & Weiss, 1995).

Applications

CD 57+ lymphocytes are increased in patients following bone marrow transplantation. This increase often persists for years after the procedure. The majority of these cells are CD 57-/CD 8+ T lymphocytes which form up to two-thirds of the peripheral blood T lymphocytes, with a small expansion in CD 57+/CD 4+ cells.

The relationship of this increase in CD 57+ cells and graft versus host disease is controversial, some workers finding a correlation between the increase in CD 57+ cells and the onset of disease while others have not. Some investigators have noted the expansion of CD 57+ population with reactivation of CMV after transplantation, similar to the increase in CD 57+ cells seen in healthy carriers of CMV.

CD 57+ cells are also elevated in the peripheral blood in some solid organ transplant patients. Up to 20% or renal allograft, 66% of cardiac allograft, and 44% of liver allograft recipients had

greater than 20% peripheral blood CD 57+/CD 3+ lymphocytes, the majority of these cells also being CD 8+. As with bone marrow transplantation, the elevation of CD 57+ correlated with a rise in CMV titers and may show poorer graft survival (Legendre et al, 1989).

CD 57+ cells are also elevated in human immunodeficiency virus infections. CD 57+/CD 8+ lymphocytes are increased through the clinical progression of the infection while CD 57+/NK and CD 57- NK cells remain normal.

Peripheral blood CD 57+ cells may be increased in patients with adult–onset cyclic neutropenia whereas no elevation was seen in childhood onset cases. The adult-onset variant of cyclic neutropenia was found to be steroid responsive.

Circulating CD 57- lymphocytes are elevated in patients with Crohn's disease with many of these cells being CD 8+, corresponding to the increase in suppressor cell function found in such patients, Elevations in peripheral blood CD 57+ cells may also be seen in rheumatoid arthritis.

Large granular lymphocytosis (LGL) is by far the most common CD 57-positive lymphoproliferative disorder. LGL are usually CD 2+ and may be divided into T cell and NK cell types based on CD 3 expression. CD 3+ cases are generally associated with clonal T cell gene rearrangement. The T cell cases are usually CD 57- and CD 8-positive, and may be further typed according to the presence (Type 1) or absence (Type 2) of the NK-associated antigen CD

16. Immunostaining of the spleen may be useful in the evaluation of resected spleens in LGL patients. CD 57+ lymphocytes are found in the splenic red pulp, while the expanded while pulp nodules are usually not involved.

Elevations of peripheral blood CD 57+ lymphocytes may be associated with non-neoplastic states such as in CMV carriers, possibly in chronic hepatitis, in ankylosing spondylitis, and more frequently in rheumatoid arthritis and Felty's syndrome. Synovial fluid CD 57+ cells may also be elevated in rheumatoid arthritis. Clonal T cell receptor gene rearrangement has been demonstrated in some cases of rheumatoid arthritis especially those with Felty's syndrome.

NK/T cell lymphomas frequently affect the nasal and extranodal sites and show similarities to LGL. The lymphoma cells display large cytoplasmic granules with either a T cell or NK cell phenotype. They are also mostly positive for the Epstein-Barr virus and display an angiocentric pattern of infiltration with necrosis and an aggressive clinical course. Unlike LGL, NK/T cell lymphomas are CD 57-positive in less than 10% of cases, with most cases being CD 56+ so that CD 57 antibodies alone are unreliable NK cell markers of such lymphomas. (Ng et al, 1987; Nakumara et al, 1995)

CD 57 expression is seen in just over 20% of T lymphoblastic lymphomas, but the expression of CD 57 does not correlate with NK activity in these cases and the significance expression of this antigen being unknown. Less than 2% of other types of T cell lymphoma are CD 57+ and the antigen does not appear to be expressed in B cell lymphomas, monocytic leukemia or Langerhans' histiocytosis. Increases in presumably non-neoplastic CD 57+ cells may be seen in the neoplastic follicles of follicular lymphomas especially of the small cleaved cell type and in cases of nodular L & H Hodgkin's disease where the + cells often rosette around CD20-positive L & H cells, providing a useful pointer to the diagnosis. The CD 57+ cells in the latter condition are also CD 4+ and can be seen in about 25–30% of cases of nodular lymphocyte predominant Hodgkin's disease (Appendix 2.10). Interestingly, a recently described variant of classic Hodgkin's disease that produces follicles with small, eccentric germinal centres and expanded mantle zones that contained classic Reed-Sternberg cells showed similar CD57+ resetting of the latter cells, mimicking nodular L & H Hodgkin's disease (Kansal et al, 2002) Similar distribution and increases in CD 57+ cells were not found in nodular sclerosing Hodgkin's disease, T-cell rich B-cell lymphoma or follicular lymphoma (Sun et al, 1992; Kamel et al, 1993).

CD 57 expression may be observed in a variety of solid tumors most common of which are lung tumors. Almost half of small cell lung carcinomas and about 85% of carcinoid tumors are CD 57+. In non-small cell lung carcinoma the identification of neuroendocrine-associated antigens such as CD 57, has been shown to be predictive of response to chemotherapy. The expression of CD 57 antigen in small cell carcinoma and carcinoid is generally widespread in the tumor but only focal in non-small cell lung carcinomas. Sampling errors show be taken into consideration in the assessment and because of the low sensitivity and specificity of CD 57 antibodies, other neuroendocrine-associated markers such as chromogranin, synaptophysin and neuron specific enolase should be employed.

Other non-hematopoietic neoplasms that express CD 57 include the majority of thyroid carcinomas especially papillary carcinoma, while being present in only 30% of benign thyroid proliferations. CD 57 may be used to separate medullary carcinomas from other thyroid carcinomas, although there have been some reported examples of positivity in medullary carcinomas. Strong CD 57-staining of the majority of the tumor cells is indicative of papillary or follicular carcinoma and uncommon in benign thyroid proliferations and medullary carcinoma (Ghali et al, 1992).

The CD 57 antigen is expressed in prostatic epithelium but the marker does not discriminate between benign and neoplastic cells. Metanephric adenomas were strongly and diffusely positive for CD57 and WT1, with focal staining for CK7 but no staining fro CD56 and desmin. While Wilm's tumor was also strongly positive for WT1 in the blastema and epithelial components, there was no staining for CD57 in these components, and some cases were diffusely for CD56 (Muir et al, 2001).

Epithelial cells of thymomas are usually CD 57 positive while only some thymic carcinomas express the antigen. Over half of malignant mesotheliomas are reported to express CD 57 although they generally do not react with other neuroendocrine markers. Among the soft tissue tumors, the majority of neural tumors, especially neuromas, schwannomas, and neurofibromas, react with CD 57 antibodies. Most malignant peripheral nerve sheath tumors are CD 57-positive but the antigen may also be expressed by other sarcomas such as synovial sarcoma and leiomyosarcoma. Therefore the marker on its own is not a useful diagnostic discriminant and should be used in an appropriate panel of antibodies in order to separate the various spindled and pleomorphic soft tissue tumors. Similarly, because CD 57 may be expressed by a variety of small round cell tumors including neuroblastomas, it is not a useful diagnostic discriminant for this group of poorly differentiated tumors (Bunn et al, 1985; Michels et al, 1987; Linnoila et al, 1994).

In the central nervous system, CD 57 expression may be seen in normal oligodendroglia and other nervous system cells as well as in their corresponding tumors (Motoi et al, 1985). Oligodendrogliomas perhaps show the most extensive degree of CD 57-positivity compared to astrocytomas and glioblastomas that demonstrate fewer positive cells. Among skin tumors, the expression of CD 57 closely paralleled that of S100 protein although the two were not identical. Neither was useful in the distinction of eccrine from apocrine tumors (Kanitakis et al, 1987). Melanocytic proliferations and melanomas may show variable positivity for CD 57, whereas reports of the expression of this antigen in Merkel cell carcinoma are conflicting, the antigen being absent in some series and positive half the tumors in another study. CD 57 positivity is also seen in other tumors including a large proportion of granular cell tumors, paragangliomas and pheochromocytomas. Embryonal carcinomas and dysgerminomas are also reported to be positive for CD 57 in most cases.

Comments

The CD 57 antigen is most useful in the identification of large granular lymphocyte disorders (Appendix 2.6) and assists in the identification of L & H cells of lymphocyte predominant Hodgkin's disease (Appendix 2.10). The CD 57+ cells that are CD 4+ T cells form rosettes around CD 20+ L & H cells. Elevation of peripheral blood CD 57+ lymphocytes may be seen following some viral infections such as CMV, in patients following bone marrow or solid organ transplantation. CD 57 should not be used alone as a marker of NK cells, neuroendocrine cells, or neural cells and must be employed in combination with other antibodies in a panel, particularly if used for diagnostic purposes. The antibody is immunoreactive in fixed paraffin embedded tissues especially following heat-induced epitope retrieval.

CD57 is expressed on a NK cell subset, T cell subset, brain, neuroectodermal tumors, small cell lung carcinoma, prostatic epithelium and tumors, nerve sheath tissues and tumors.

References

Abo T, Balch CM. A differentiation antigen of human NK and K cells identified by a monoclonal antibody (HNK-1). Journal of Immunology 1982;129:1758–61.

Arber DA, Weiss LM. CD57. A review. Applied Immunohistochemistry 1995;3:137–52.

Bunn PA, Linnoila I, Minna JD, Carney D, Gazdar AF. Small cell lung cancer, endocrine cells of the fetal bronchus, and other neuroendocrine cells express the Leu 7 antigenic determinant present on natural killer cells. Blood 1985;65:764–8.

Ghali VS, Jimenez JS, Garcia RL. Distribution of Leu 7 antigen (HNK-1) in thyroid tumors: its usefulness as a diagnostic marker for follicular and papillary carcinomas. Human Pathology 1992;23:21–5.

Griffiths DFR, Jasani B, Standen GR. Pathology of the spleen in large granular lymphocytic leukemia. Journal of Clinical Pathology 1989;42:885–90.

Kamel Ow, Gelb AS, Shibuya RB, Warnke RA. Leu 7 (CD 57) reactivity distinguishes nodular lymphocyte predominance Hodgkin's disease from nodular sclerosing Hodgkin's disease, T-cell rich B-cell lymphoma and follicular lymphoma. American Journal of Pathology 1993;142:541–6.

Kanitakis J, Zambruno G, Viac J, et al. Expression of neural-tissue markers (S100 protein and Leu7 antigen) by sweat gland tumors of the skin. Journal of American Academy of Dermatology 1987;17:187–91.

Kansal R, Singleton TP, Ross CW, et al. Follicular Hodgkin lymphoma: a histopathologic study. American Journal of Clinical Pathology 2002;117:29–35.

Legendre CM, Forbes RDC, Loertscher R, Guttmann RD. CD 4+/Leu 7+ large granular lymphocytes in long-term renal allograft recipients. A subset of atypical T cells,. Transplantation 1989;47:964–71.

Michels S, Swanson PE, Robb JA, Wick MR. Leu-7 in small cell neoplasms. An immunohistochemical study with ultrastructural correlations. Cancer 1987;60:2958–64.

Muir TE, Cheville JC, Lager DJ. Metanephric adenoma, nephrogenic rests, Wilm's tumor: a histologic and immunophenotypic comparison. American Journal of Surgical Pathology 2001;25:1290–6.

Linnoila RI, Piantadosi S, Ruckdeschel JC. Impact of neuroendocrine differentiation in non-small cell lung cancer. The LCSG experience. Chest 1994;106 (Suppl):367S-71S.

Motoi M, Yoshino T, Hayashi K, et al. Immunohistochemical studies on human brain tumors using anti-Leu 7 monoclonal antibody in paraffin-embedded specimens. Acta Neuropathologica 1985;66:75–7.

Nakumara S, Suchi T, Koshikawa T, et al. Clinicopathologic study of CD 56 (NCAM)-positive angiocentric lymphoma occurring in sites other than the upper and lower respiratory tract. American Journal of Surgical Pathology 1995;19:284–96.

Ng CS, Chan JKC, Lo STH. Expression of natural killer cell markers in non-Hodgkin's lymphomas. Human Pathology 1987;18:1257–62.

Sun T, Brody J, Koduru P, et al. Study of the major phenotype of large granular T cell lymphoproliferative disorder. American Journal of Clinical Pathology 1992;98:516–21.

Swerdlow SH, Murray LJ. Natural killer (Leu 7+) cells in reactive lymphoid tissues and malignant lymphomas. American Journal of Clinical Pathology 1984;81:459–63.

CD 68

Sources/clones

Accurate (EVM11), Biodesign (BL-M68), Caltag Laboratories (BLM68), Dako (KP1, PG-M1, EBM 11), Sanbio/Monosan/Accurate (BLAD8), Serotech (KiM6)

Fixation/preparation

Apart from EBM 11 which is only applicable to frozen sections, KP1 and PG-M1 monoclonal antibodies are applicable to formalin-fixed paraffin sections, acetone-fixed cryostat sections and fixed cell smears. Anti-macrophage reagents recognizing formalin-resistant epitopes require microwave or enzyme pretreatment with trypsin or pronase before immunostaining to reduce background staining.

Background

The best macrophage reagents produced to date are those recognizing the CD68 antigen (Knapp, 1989). This 110 kD antigen belongs to a family of acidic, highly glycosylated lysosomal glycoproteins that include the lamp-1 and lamp-2 molecules (Fukuda, 1991). CD68 is the human homologue of the murine macrosialin antigen (Holness et al, 1993) and is present in the cytoplasmic granules of monocytes, macrophages, neutrophils, basophils and large lymphocytes (Pulford et al, 1990). This antigen is also expressed to some degree in the cytoplasm of some non-haemopoietic tissue. However, the function of the molecule is to date unknown.

The monoclonal antibody KP1 (IgG1, Kappa) was raised against lysosomal granules prepared from lung macrophages (Pulford et al, 1989) and recognizes the 110 kD CD68 antigen. This antibody labels monocytes and macrophages in a wide range of tissues e.g. lung macrophages, germinal centre macrophages and Kupffer cells. Osteoclasts and myeloid precursors in bone marrow are also strongly labelled. In frozen sections, KP1 stains endothelium and hepatocytes weakly. Strong labelling of blood monocytes (granular/cytoplasmic), neutrophils and basophils is also demonstrated with KP1. KP1 antigen is expressed as an intracytoplasmic molecule, associated with lysosomal granules.

The murine PG-M1 monoclonal antibody (IgG3, Kappa) was raised against spleen cells of Gaucher's disease (Falini et al, 1993). Reactivity with cells transfected with a human cDNA encoding for the CD68 antigen confirms PG-M1 as a member of the CD68 cluster. In normal tissue, PG-M1 is comparable to KP-1; however, in bone marrow paraffin sections, PG-M1 strongly stains macrophages but not granulocytes and myeloid precursors. PG-M1 also shows immunopositivity with mast cells and synovial cells.

Applications

Malignant histiocytosis and true histiocytic lymphoma express the CD68 macrophage marker (Ralfkiaer et al, 1990). These tumors should be CD68-positive, but be unlabelled with antibodies to CD30, T- and B-cell antigens and cytokeratins. Acute myeloid leukemias (AML) are identified by the presence of CD68 antigen (Warnke et al, 1989; Thiele et al, 1992). Whilst KP1 recognises M1-M5 types, PG-M1 immunoreaction is confined to M4 (myelomonocytic) and M5 (monocytic) types of AML. The CD68 antibodies are also able to distinguish between monocyte/macrophage and lymphoid leukemias (Appendix 2.4). Whilst this is useful in identifying granulocytic sarcoma (Appendix 2.5), some B cell neoplasms (notably small lymphocytic lymphoma and hairy cell leukemia) show weak cytoplasmic staining in the form of a few scattered granules. Mast cell proliferations and "plasmacytoid monocytes" are usually stained by both the KP1 and PG-M1 antibodies. The CD68 antigen is also expressed to varying degrees in Langerhans' and interdigitating reticulum cell sarcomas, as well as Langerhans' cell histiocytosis (Ruco et al, 1989). Other accessory cell tumors such as follicular dendritic cell sarcomas may be positive for CD68 (Shimazaki et al, 2002).

Interestingly, a recent study of atopic dermatitis suggests that CD68, a classic macrophage marker and CD1a, the prototypic dendritic cell marker could bind to the same cell population suggesting that a heterogenous pool of marcophage/dendritic cell-like cells may exist from which dermal macrophages and dendritic cells are derived (Kiekens et al, 2001). Not unexpectedly, as one of the antibodies was raised to Gaucher's cells, it is a good marker in this disease, accentuation the striations in the characteristic cells (Bogoeva & Petrusevska, 2001).

Macrophages may be present either as rare scattered cells or large cellular infiltrates in some T- and B- cell lymphomas, leading to erroneous diagnoses of histiocytic malignancies. Dual immunocytochemical labelling with CD68 antigen and T/B-cell antigen is useful in delineating the two populations. The identification of macrophages is also crucial in the diagnosis of granulomatous diseases, storage diseases and certain types of lymphadenitis, eg. Kikuchi's lymphadenitis. In the latter condition macrophages phagocytosing apoptotic bodies and cells known as "plasmacytoid monocytes" and "crescentic histiocytes" are easily recognised with antibodies against CD68, avoiding a misdiagnosis of a high-grade lymphoma.

Comments

Caution is advised in the immunophenotypic interpretation of histiocytes, since the distinction between "uptake" and "synthetic" patterns should be borne in mind. KP1 would appear to be superior to PG-M1, particularly with respect to the wider recognition of AML. The latter antibody also carries the distinct disadvantage of being demonstrated in about 10% of melanomas. Tissue rich in macrophages is suitable as a positive control.

CD68 is expressed on macrophages/monocytes, basophils, neutrophils, mast cells, dendritic cells, myeloid and CD34+ progenitor cells, B and T cells, 50% of acute myeloid leukemias, some B cell lymphomas, hairy cell leukemia, Langerhans cell histiocytosis, mastocytosis and some melanomas.

References

Bogoeva B, Petrusevska G. Immunohistochemical nd ultrastructural features of Gaucher's cells − five case reports. Acta Medica Crotiaca 2001;55:131−4.

Falini B, Flenghi L, Pileri S, et al. PG-M1: a new monoclonal antibody directed against a fixative-resistant epitope on the macrophage-restricted form of the CD68 molecule. American Journal of Pathology 1993;142:1359−72.

Fukuda M. Lysosomal membrane glycoproteins. Structure, biosynthesis, and intracellular trafficking. Journal of Biology and Chemistry 1991;266:21327−30.

Holness CL, Da Silva RP, Fawcett J, et al. Macrosialin, a mouse macrophage-restricted glycoprotein, is a member of the lamp/lgp family. Journal of Biology and Chemistry 1993;268:9661−6.

Kiekens RC, Thepen T, Oosting AJ, et al. Heterogeneity within tissue-specific macrophage and dendritic cell populations during cutaneous inflammation in atopic dermatitis. British Journal of Dermatology 2001;145:957−65.

Knapp W. Myeloid section report: In: Knapp W et al., eds. Leucocyte Typing IV. White Cell Differentiation Antigens. Oxford-New York-Tokyo: Oxford University Press. 1989;747−80.

Pulford KAF, Rigney EM, Micklem KJ, et al. KP1: a new monoclonal antibody that detects a monocyte/macrophage associated antigen in routinely processed tissue sections. Journal of Clinical Pathology 1989;42:414−21.

Pulford KAF, Sipos A, Cordell JL, Stross WP, Mason DY. Distribution of the CD68 macrophage/myeloid associated antigen. Immunology 1990;2:973−80.

Ralfkiaer E, Delsol G, O'Connor NTJ, et al. Malignant lymphomas of true histiocytic origin. A clinical, histological, immunophenotypic and genotypic study. Journal of Pathology 1990;160:9−17.

Ruco LP, Pulford KAF, Mason DY, et al. Expression of macrophage-associated antigens in tissues involved by Langerhans' cell histiocytosis (histiocytosis X). American Journal of Clinical Pathology 1989,92:273−9.

Shimazaki K, Ohshima K, Haraoka S, et al. Acessory cell tumors: a clinicopathological study of 16 aggressive tumors containing EBV-positive Hodgkin and Reed-Sternberg-like giant cells. Histopathology 2002;40:12–21.

Thiele J, Braeckel C, Wagner S, et al. Macrophages in normal human bone marrow and in chronic myeloproliferative disorders: an immunohistochemical and morphometric study by a new monoclonal antibody (PG-M1) on trephine biopsies. Virchows Archives A Pathologic Anatomy 1992,421:33–9.

Warnke RA, Pulford KAF, Pallesen G, et al. Diagnosis of myelomonocytic and macrophage neoplasms in routinely processed tissue biopsies with monoclonal antibody KP1. American Journal of Pathology 1989;135:1089–95.

NOTES

CD 74 (LN2)

Sources/clones

Ancell/Pharmingen (MB741), American Research Products (MB3), Biodesign (BU43, BU45), Biogenex (LN-2), Cymbus Bioscience (BU45), Harlan Sera Lab/Accurate (2G5), ICN Biomedicals (LN-2), Dako (LN-2), Immunotech (LN2), Novocastra (LN-2), Pharmingen (LN2), RDI (BU45, LN2), Serotec (BU 45), Sigma Chemical (LN2), Zymed (LN2).

Fixation/preparation

This antibody is applicable to formalin-fixed paraffin-embedded tissue sections, frozen sections and cytological preparations. Immunoreaction may be improved with microwave antigen retrieval in citrate buffer.

Background

The CD 74 antigen represents a membrane-bound subunit of the MHC Class II associated invariant chain (Wilson et al, 1993) that is encoded by the gene located on chromosome 5 region q31-q33 (Moller, 1995). The monoclonal antibody LN2 recognizes nuclear and cytoplasmic antigens of molecular weights 35kD and 31kD respectively in routinely processed tissues. MB-3, another mononuclear antibody, is thought to be identical to LN2. LN2 reacts with about 50% and 75% of activated and resting L20-positive B cell in the peripheral blood and tonsils respectively. LN2 is positive in less than 3% of CD 3-positive T cells. Very weak staining may be seen on circulating monocytes and granulocytes are negative.

In lymph nodes, LN2 positivity is seen primarily in germinal center and mantle cells. Staining is strongest in small germinal center cells and in mantle cells. Plasma cells are not labeled. The vast majority of cells in the interfollicular areas are negative except for interdigitating dendritic reticular cells, which are often strongly positive. Besides distinct staining of the nuclear membrane there may be diffuse or paranuclear cytoplasmic staining, the pattern of staining being similar in both fixed and frozen tissue sections.

Thymocytes are negative for LN2 but thymic dendritic cells may often be positive. Other cells that may be positive for LN2 include sinusoidal histiocytes, epithelioid histiocytes, splenic red pulp histiocytes and Langhans' type giant cells. In addition, some epithelial cells and corresponding carcinomas may be positive but the staining of LN2 in these cells is often diffuse in the cytoplasm and the distinctive nuclear membrane staining is not observed (Epstein et al, 1984; Okon et al, 1985).

Applications

The LN2 antibody stains about 90% and 20% of low-grade B and T cell lymphomas respectively. In high-grade lymphomas, the corresponding figures are 85% and 75% respectively so that its value as a discriminator is less in large cell lymphomas. The pattern of labeling is also different. In small lymphocytic lymphoma, LN2 shows either nuclear membrane or dot-like cytoplasmic positivity, whereas, in small cleaved cells nuclear membrane staining is the predominant pattern. In the mixed cell lymphomas and large cell lymphomas, LN2 stains the nuclear membranes of the small cleaved cells but only some of the larger cells exhibit cytoplasmic staining, the minority displaying bright cytoplasmic globules.

Reed Sternberg cells also stain with LN2, exhibiting cytoplasmic, cytoplasmic membrane and nuclear membrane staining in about two-thirds if cases. The antigen is expressed in about 60% of precursor B cell ALLs/LBLs, about 50% of AMLs (excluding FAB M6 AML), most cases of CML, granulocytic sarcomas and true histiocytic sarcomas (Norton & Isaacson, 1989a; 1989b).

A recent study showed that LN-2 antigen is strongly expressed by cells of malignant fibrous histiocytoma (MFH) but not atypical fibroxanthoma (AFX). LN-2 immuno-reactivity appears to distinguish between these two histologically similar yet biologically distinct tumors with a high degree of statistical significance. The antigen was not expressed or only weakly expressed on dermatofibroma and dermatofibrosarcoma protuberans (Lazova et al, 1997). LN-2 has also been observed to label some epithelial tumors including adenocarcinoma of the uterus, squamous cell carcinoma of the lung and transitional cell carcinoma of the bladder (Epstein et al, 1984) and renal cell carcinoma (Young et al, 2001).

Comments

LN2 is immunoreactive in formalin-fixed paraffin-embedded tissue sections. It is only poorly reactive in ethanol-fixed tissues and B5 fixation produces reduced positivity and a high background staining. The staining in B5 fixed tissues tends to be of the nuclear membranes and the perinuclear cytoplasm of B cells, whereas, in formalin-fixed tissues, paranuclear dot-like globules are more common. Trypsinization destroys LN2 reactivity and neuraminidase treatment does not affect it (Yoshino et al, 1990). Given the contrasting immunoreactivity of LN-2, it is possible that other applications of LN-2 are yet to be discovered. Benign or neoplastic B-cell tissue is recommended for optimisation of this antibody.

CD74 is expressed on B cells, activated T cells, macrophages, endothelial cells and a variety of epithelial cells and corresponding tumors.

References

Epstein AL, Marder RJ, Winter JN, Fox RI. Two new monoclonal antibodies (LN1 and LN2) reactive in B5 formalin fixed, paraffin-embedded tissues with follicular center and mantle zone human B lymphocytes and derived tumors. Journal of Immunology 1984;133:1028–36.

Lazova R, Moynes R, May D, Scott G. LN-2 (CD74). A marker to distinguish atypical fibroxanthoma from malignant fibrous histiocytoma. Cancer 1997;79:2115–24.

Moller P. CD74 Workshop panel report. In: Schlossman SF (ed). Leucocyte Typing V White Cell Differentiation Antigens. Oxford University Press 1995; p 568.

Norton AJ, Isaacson PG. Lymphoma phenotyping in formalin-fixed and paraffin wax-embeded tissues. I. Range of antibodies and staining patterns. Histopathology 1989a;14:437–46.

Norton AJ, Isaacson PG. Lymphoma phenotyping in formalin-fixed and paraffin wax-embedded tissues. II. Profiles of reactivity in the various tumour types. Histopathology 1989b;14:557–79.

Okon E, Felder B, Epstein A, et al. Monoclonal antibodies reactive with B lymphocytes and histiocytes in paraffin sections. Cancer 1985;56:95–104.

Wilson KM, Labeta MO, Pawelec G, Fernandex N. Cell-surface expression of human histocompatibility leucocyte antigen (HLA) class II-associated invariant chain (CD74) does not always correlate with cell-surface expression of HLA class II molecules. Immunology 1993;79:331–5.

Yoshino T, Hoshida Y, Murakami I, et al. Comparison of monoclonal antibodies reactive with lymphocyte subsets in routinely fixed paraffin-embedded material: flow cytometric analyses, immunoperoxidase staining and influence of fixatives. Acta Medica Okayama 1990;44:243–50.

Young AN, Amin MB, Moreno CS, et al. Expression profiling of renal epithelial neoplasms: a method for tumor classification and discovery of diagnostic molecular markers. American Journal of Pathology 2001;158:1639–51.

CD w75 (LN1)

Sources/clones

Biogenex (LN1), Dako (LN1), Immunotech (LN1), Novocastra, Sigma Chemical (LN1), Zymed (LN1).

Fixation/preparation

HH2 is applicable to formalin-fixed paraffin-embedded tissue sections. Enzyme or heat pretreatment before immunostaining improves immunodetection.

Background

The CDw75 epitope is a sialylated carbohydrate determinant generated by the beta–galactosyl alpha 2,6 sialyltransferase and has a molecular weight of 53 kD. Sialyltransferase catalyzes the incorporation of sialic acid to the carbohydrate group of glycoconjugates. Alterations on the cell surface of the oligosaccharide portion of glycoproteins and glycolipids are thought to play a role in tumorigenesis (Reed et al, 1993). Sialyltransferase has been found elevated in different tumor tissues and in serum of cancer patients. Further, the amount of sialic acid correlates with the invasiveness and metastasizing potential of several human tumors. Therefore the CDw75 epitope can be viewed as a target for identifying biologically aggressive tumors (David et al, 1993).

LN-1 belongs to the CDw75 group of antibodies and recognizes a sialo antigen (45–85 kD). LN-1 stains B lymphocytes in the germinal center with no reaction with T cells. It also reacts with a variety of epithelial cells including distal renal tubules, mammary glands, bronchus and prostate.

Applications

CDw75 antigen expression has been examined in breast lesions (Reed et al, 1993). Duct carcinoma showed diffuse cytoplasmic staining in 21% of in situ and 35% of invasive carcinomas respectively. No correlation was demonstrated between immunoreactivity for CDw75 in breast carcinoma and their metastatic potential. However, CDw75 was more frequently expressed in high-grade carcinomas. A positive immunoreaction was demonstrated in benign proliferating lesions: intraductal papillomas (2/3) and epitheliosis in fibrocystic disease (10/14). This high frequency of immunoreactivity among the benign breast lesions was ascribed to activation of epithelial cells.

CDw75 epitope expression has also been examined in gastric carcinomas and their metastases (David et al, 1993). Forty-one cases (47%) were immunopositive for CDw75 antigen in the primary tumors or metastases. In contrast to breast carcinomas, a close relationship was found between antigen in primary tumors and their respective metastases. In addition antigen expression correlated with an infiltrative growth pattern, lymphatic invasiveness and aneuploidy; whilst no correlation was found with gastric carcinoma morphology, lymphoid infiltrate, vascular invasion and gastric wall penetration. Hence, CDw75 expression appears to be a good indicator of biologic aggressiveness of gastric carcinoma, a finding recently confirmed (Elpek et al, 2001). In view of the contrasting results between breast and gastric carcinoma, further studies examining CDw75 expression in these and other cancers is awaited.

LN-1 is an excellent marker for B cell lymphomas especially follicular-derived lymphomas

(Appendix 2.1). In B cells, the LN-1 antibody produces a typical membrane and cytoplasmic (paranuclear "dot-like" or golgi) staining pattern. No immunoreaction is present with small lymphocytic lymphomas and T-cell lymphomas. LN-1 also reacts with L& H cells in nodular lymphocyte predominant Hodgkin's disease. In a study of CD10, bcl-6 and CDw75 as markers of follicle centre cell lymphomas, it was found that CDw75 was the most sensitive (97%), closely followed by bcl-6 (90%), with CD10 being the least sensitive (79%). A combination of all three markers produced a sensitivity of 100% (Dunphy et al, 2001).

Comments

Follicular lymphomas or epitheliosis of the breast or gastric carcinoma is most suitable for use as positive control tissue.

References

David L, Nesland JM, Funderud S, Sobrinho-Simoes M. CDw75 antigen expression in human gastric carcinoma and adjacent mucosa. Cancer 1993;72:1522–7.

Dunphy CH, Polski JM, Lance Evans H, Gardner IJ. Paraffin immunoreactivity of CD10, CDw75 and bcl-6 in follicle center cell lymphoma. Leukemia and Lymphoma 2001;41:585–92.

Elpek GO, Gelen T, Karpuzoglu G, et al. Clinicopathologic evaluation of CDw75 antigen expression in patients with gastric carcinoma. Journal of Pathology 2001;193:169–74.

Reed W, Erikstein BK, Funderud S, et al. CDw75 antigen expression in breast lesions. Pathology Research and Practice 1993;189:394–8.

CD 79a

Sources/clones

Becton-Dickinson (HM47), Dako (JCB117, HM57), Immunotech (HM47), Novocastra (11E3, 11D10, HM47/A9)

Fixation/preparation

This antibody is applicable to paraffin-embedded tissue sections. Heat pretreatment in citrate buffer is necessary for antigen retrieval to improve staining pattern. CD79a may also be applied to acetone-fixed cryostat sections and fixed cell smears.

Background

Membrane-bound immunoglobulin (mIg) on human B-lymphocytes is non-covalently associated with a disulfide-linked heterodimer, which consists of two phosphoproteins of 47 kD and 37 kD, encoded by the *mb*-1 and *B29* genes respectively (Mason et al, 1991; van Noesel et al, 1991). Association of IgM with the *mb*-1 protein is necessary for membrane expression of the B-cell antigen receptor complex. When antigen is bound to this B-cell complex, a signal transduction is transmitted to the interior of the cell, accompanied by phosphorylation of several components following induction of tyrosine kinase activity. The mb-1/B29 dimer seems to be analogous to the association of the T-cell receptor with the CD3 components (Hornback et al, 1990).

Studies have shown that mb-1 is present throughout B-cell differentiation and is B-cell specific (Mason et al, 1991). Its high degree of specificity is probably a reflection of its crucial role in signal transduction after antigen binding to the B-cell antigen receptor complex. The mb-1 and B29 proteins have been designated CD79a and CD79b at the Fifth International Workshop on Human Leucocyte Differentiation Antigens (Boston 1993). JCB117 was raised against the recombinant protein containing part of the extracellular portion of the CD79a (mb-1) polypeptide (Mason et al, 1995). Clone HM57 was raised against a synthetic peptide sequence comprising amino acids 202–216 of mb-1 protein (Sakaguchi et al, 1988). This oligopeptide represents the intracytoplasmic C-terminal part of the mb-1 protein.

Applications

The mb-1 (CD79a) chain appears before the pre-B cell stage and is still present at the plasma cell stage. JCB117 reacts with human B cells in paraffin embedded tissue sections including decalcified bone marrow trephines. When applied to 454 paraffin embedded tissue biopsies, it reacted with the majority (97%) of B-cell neoplasms. This covered the full range of B-cell maturation including 10/20 cases of myeloma/plasmacytoma. This antibody also labeled precursor B-cell acute lymphoblastic leukemia, making it the most reliable B-cell marker detectable on paraffin-embedded specimens (Mason et al, 1995). T cell and nonlymphoid neoplasms were negative, indicating that JCB117 may be of value in identification of B-cell neoplasms.

The mb-1 protein has also been detected in nodular lymphocyte predominance Hodgkin's disease using monoclonal antibody JCB117; however only 20% of non-lymphocyte predominance cases expressed mb-1. A rare phenotypic characterisation has been demonstrated in mediastinal large B-cell lymphomas, with the

majority being mb-1+/ Ig-
(Kanavaros et al, 1995).

Comments

We have found JCB117 to be
superior to HM57, the latter
demonstrating cross reactivity
with smooth muscle in paraffin
sections.

CD79a is a marker of
precursor B cells, expressed early
in B cell differentiation and often
positive when other mature B
cell markers are negative
(Appendix 2.1). It is expressed on
megakaryocytes. CD79a has been
shown on pre-T-acute
lymphoblastic leukemia and
rarely in peripheral T cell
lymphomas, normal T cell being
negative for the antigen (Chu &
Arber, 2001). As CD79a is only
weakly positive in some B cell
lymphomas it is preferable to use
CD20 as the first-line marker of
mature B cell lymphomas.

References

Chu PG, Arber DA. CD79: A review.
Applied Immunohistochemistry
and Molecular Morphology
2001;9:97–106.

Homback J, Tsubata T, Leclercq L,
Stappert H, Reth M. Molecular
components of B cell antigen
receptor complex of IgM class.
Nature 1990;343:760–2.

Kanavaros P, Gaulard P, Charlotte F,
et al. Discordant expression of
immunoglobulin and its associated
molecule mb-1/CD79a is
frequently found in mediastinal
large B cell lymphomas. American
Journal of Pathology
1995;146:735–41.

Mason DY, Cordell JL, Tse AGD
et al. The IgM associated protein
mb-1 as a marker of normal and
neoplastic B cells. Journal of
Immunology 1991;147:2474–82.

Mason DY, Cordell JL, Brown MH
et al. CD79a: a novel marker for
B cell neoplasms in routinely
processed tissue samples. Blood
1995;86:1453–9.

Sakaguchi N, Kashiwamura S,
Kimoto M, Thalmann P, Melchers
F. B lymphocyte lineage restricted
expression of mb-1, a gene with
CD3-like structural properties.
EMBO Journal 1988;7:3457–64.

Van Noesel CJM, van Lier RAW,
Cordell JL et al. The membrane
IgM-associated heterodimer on
human B cells is a newly defined
B cell antigen that contains the
protein product of the mb-1
gene. Journal of Immunology
1991;146:3881–8.

CD 99 (p30/32^{MIC2})

Sources/clones

Dako (12E7), Pharmingen (MIC2), Signet (013).

Fixation/preparation

All three clones of antibodies show enhanced immunoreactivity following some method of heat-induced epitope retrieval.

Background

The p30/32^{MIC2} antigen, also referred to as CD 99 or the MIC2 gene product is a cell-surface glycoprotein of relative molecular mass of 30,000–32,000 that appears to be involved in cell adhesion processes. It is recognized by a number of monoclonal antibodies including RFB-1, 12E7, HBA71 and 013, although there is some demonstrable difference in sensitivity and perhaps specificity.

CD 99 was first described as a polypeptide expressed in T-cell acute lymphoblastic leukemia and T-ALL derived cell lines, as well as in a subset of cortical thymocytes. CD 99 was also found on a group of hematopoietic precursor cells in the human bone marrow including terminal deoxynucleotidyl transferase-positive cells and myelo-monocyte progenitors, the expression decreasing with maturation of cells in the latter series. The MIC2 gene has been mapped to the terminal region of the short arm of the X chromosome (Xp22.32-pter) and the euchromatin region of the Y chromosome (Yq11-pter). The gene is expressed in both sexes and escapes X inactivation, making it the first described pseudo-autosomal gene in humans (Dracopoli et al, 1985; Fellinger et al, 1991).

The main application of this antigen has been for the differentiation of the group of small round cell tumors in childhood as the marker is strongly expressed in Ewing's sarcoma and the closely related peripheral/primitive neuroectodermal tumors (PNETs). Both show strong membrane and cytoplasmic staining with clones 12E7, HBA71 and 013 (Stevenson et al, 1994; Weidner & Tjoe, 1994; Vartanian et al, 1996). Subsequent studies have also demonstrated positive staining in acute lymphoblastic lymphoma and related leukemias, and rhabdomyosarcoma, although to a much lesser degree (Ramani et al, 1993). More recently, immunoreactivity for this marker has been shown in a much wide spectrum of normal tissues and ependymal cells, pancreatic islet cells, urothelium, some squamous cells, columnar epithelial cells, fibroblasts, endothelial cells and granulosa/Sertoli cells. Among the spindle cell neoplastic tissues which show variable positivity for CD 99 are synovial sarcomas, hemangiopericytomas, meningiomas, solitary fibrous tumors and only very rarely in mesotheliomas. Epithelial tumors expressing CD 99 include neuroendocrine tumors such as islet cell tumors, carcinoid tumors and pulmonary oat cell carcinomas but apparently not Merkel cell carcinomas of the skin (Soslow et al, 1966). Granulocytic sarcomas have been shown to stain for CD 99 (Cooper & Haffajee, 1995).

Applications

CD 99 antibodies have proven usefulness for the separation of Ewing's sarcoma and PNETs from the other small round cell tumors in childhood (Pappo et al, 1993; Lumadue et al, 1994) (Appendix 1.3, 1.11). In addition, this marker can be employed as a diagnostic discriminator for the identification of thymic cortical T cells associated with thymic neoplasms (Chan et al, 1995;

Dorfman & Pinkus, 1996) (Appendix 1.12), and in the differential diagnosis of spindle cell tumors (Appendix 1.23, 1.25). The latter include synovial sarcoma, hemangiopericytoma, meningioma and solitary fibrous tumors, all of which show variable extents of positivity (Renshaw, 1995). The recent demonstration of CD 99 in mesenchymal chondrosarcoma emphasizes the need for caution if this marker is to be employed as a diagnostic discriminator for small round cell tumors. Furthermore, the immunoexpression of CD99, while most common in ES/PNET (100%) may also be seen in rhabdomyosarcoma, non-Hodgkin's lymphoma, and synovial sarcoma and needs to be used in combination with antibodies to FLI-1 and Tdt to increase the diagnostic yield (Llombart-Bosch & Navarro, 2001; Lucas et al, 2001, Folpe et al, 2000). CD99 expression in retinoblastoma is much less common compared to PNET (Schwimer & Prayson, 2001). Ependydomas express CD99 strongly in a membraneous pattern with intracytoplasmic or intercellular dots (Choi et al, 2001). B cell lymphoblastic lymphoma have also been shown to immunoexpress CD99 (Kahwash et al, 2002). Benign spindle stromal tumors of the breast, which encompass spindle cell lipoma-like tumor, solitary fibrous tumor and myofibroblastoma, share the common immunophenotype of vimentin+/CD34+/bcl-2+/CD99+ and may have a common histiogenesis (Magro et al, 2002). CD99 has also been described on a number of other

tumors including superficial acral fibromyxoma (Fetsch et al, 2001), proximal epithelioid sarcoma (Hasegawa et al, 2001), spindle cell epithelioma of the vagina (Skelton & Smith, 2001), neuroepithelial tumors of the kidney (Parham et al, 2001) and tumors of sex cord-stromal differentiation (Kommoss et al, 2000).

Comments

Initial enthusiasm for the specificity of CD99 has been tempered by the realization of the wide spectrum of tumors that may express the antigen. Immunoreactivity is enhanced following heat-induced epitope retrieval. Both 013 and 12E7 have been very effective in our hands but it should be noted that they show different sensitivities, perhaps reflecting different specificities. Positive staining for CD 99 occurs as strong membrane immunolocalization whereas, variable heterogeneous staining may be seen in some cases of non-Hodgkin's lymphoma and in occasional Reed-Sternberg cells and their variants.

CD99 is expressed on a variety of cells and tumors that include Ewing's sarcoma/PNET, T cell lymphoblastic lymphoma, synovial sarcoma, rhabdomyosarcoma, some cases of Wilm's tumor, ovarian granulosa cells, pancreatic islets, infant thymus.

References

Chan JKC, Tsang WYW, Seneviratne S, Pau MY. The MIC2 antibody 013. Practical application for the study of thymic epithelial tumors. American Journal of surgical Pathology 1995;19:1115–23.

Choi YL, Chi JG, Suh YL. CD99 immunoreactivity in ependymoma. Applied Immunohistochemistry and Molecular Morphology 2001;9:125–9.

Cooper K, Haffajee Z. Immunohistochemical assessment of MIC2 gene product in granulocytic sarcoma using six epitope retrieval systems. Applied Immunohistochemistry 1995;3:198–201

Dei Tos AP, Wadden C, Calonje E, et al. Immunohistochemical demonstration of glycoprotein p30/32^{MIC2} (CD99) in synovial carcinoma. Applied Immunohistochemistry 1995;3:168–73.

Dorfman DM, Pinkus GS. CD99 (p30/32^{MIC2}) immunoreactivity in the diagnosis of thymic neoplasms and mediastinal lymphoproliferative disorders. A study of paraffin sections using monoclonal antibody 013. Applied Immunohistochemistry 1996;4:34–42.

Dracopoli NC, Rettig WJ, Albino AP, et al. Genes controlling gp25/30 cell-surface molecules map to chromosome X and Y and escape X-inactivation. American Journal of Human Genetics 1985;37:199–207.

Fellinger EJ, Garin-Chesa P, Su SL, et al. Biochemical and genetic characterization of the HBA71 Ewing's sarcoma cell surface antigen. Cancer Research 1991;51:336–40.

Fetsh JF, Laskin WB, Miettinen M. Superficial acral fibromyxoma: a clinicopathologic and immunohistochemical analysis of 37 cases of a distinctive soft tissue tumor with predilection for the fingers and toes. Human Pathology 2001;32:704–14.

Folpe AL, Hill CE, Parham DM, et al. Immunohistochemical detection of FLI-1 protein expression: study of 132 round cell tumors with emphasis on

CD99 positive mimics of Ewing's sarcoma/primitive neuroectodermal tumor. American Journal of Surgical Pathology 2000;24:1657–62.

Granter SR, Renshaw AA, Cletcher CDM, et al. CD99 reactivity in mesenchymal chondrosarcoma. Human Pathology 1996;27:1273–6.

Hasegawa T, Matsuno Y, Shimoda T, et al. Proximal-type epithelioid sarcoma: a cl;inicopathologic study of 20 cases. Modern Pathology 2001;14:655–63.

Kahwash SB, Qualman SJ. Cutaneous lymphoblastic lymphoma in children: report of six cases with precursor B cell lineage. Pediatric Developmental Pathology 2002;5:45–53.

Kommoss F, Oliva E, Bittinger F, et al. Inhibin-alpha CD99, HEA125, PLAP, and chromogranin immunoreactivity in testicular neoplasms and the androgen insensitivity syndrome. Human Pathology 2000;31:1055–61.

Llombart-Bosch A, Navarro S. Immunohistochemical detection of EWS and FLI-1 proteins in Ewing sarcoma and primitive neuroectodermal tumors: comparative analysis with CD99 (MIC-2) expression. Applied Immunohistochemistry and Molecular Morphology 2001;9:255–60.

Lucas DR, Bentley G, Dan ME, et al. Ewing sarcoma vs lymphoblastic lymphoma. A comparative immunohistochemical study. American Journal of Clinical Pathology 2001;115:11–7.

Lumadue JA, Askin FB, Perlman EJ. MIC2 analysis of small cell carcinoma. American Journal of Clinical Pathology 1994;102:692–4.

Magro G, Bisceglia M, Michal M, Eusebi V. Spindle cell lipoma-like tumor, solitary fibrous tumor and myofibroblastoma of the breast: a clinicaopathological analysis of 13 cases in favor of a unifying histogenetic concept. Virchows Archives 2002;440:249–60.

Pappo AS, Douglass EC, Meyer WH, et al. Use of HBA71 and anti-β_2-microglobulin to distinguish peripheral neuroepithelioma from neuroblastoma. Human Pathology 1993;24:880–5.

Parham DM, Roloson GJ, Feely M, et al. Primary malignant neuroepithelial tumors of the kidneys: a clinicopathologic analysis of 146 adult and pediatric cases from the National Wilm's Tumor Study Group Pathology Center. American Journal of Surgical Pathology 2001;25:133–46.

Ramani P, Rampling D, Link M. Immunocytochemical study of 12E7 in small round-cell tumors of childhood: an assessment of its sensitivity and specificity. Histopathology 1993;23:557–61.

Renshaw AA. 013 (CD99) in spindle cell tumors. Reactivity with hemangiopericytoma, solitary fibrous tumor, synovial sarcoma, and meningioma, but rarely with sarcomatoid mesothelioma. Applied Immunohistochemistry 1995;3:250–6.

Schwimer CJ, Prayson RA. Clinicopathogic study of retinoblastoma including MIB-1, p53, and CD99 immunohistochemistry. Annals of Diagnostic Pathology 2001;5:148–54.

Skelton H, Smith KJ. Spindle cell epithelioma of the vagina shows immunohistochemical staining supporting its origin from a primitive/progenitor cell population. Archives of Pathology and Laboratory Medicine 2001;125:547–50.

Soslow RA, Wallace M, Goris J, et al. MIC2 gene expression in cutaneous neuroendocrine carcinoma (Merkel cell carcinoma. Applied Immunohistochemistry 1966;4:235–40.

Stevenson AJ, Chatten J, Bertoni F, Mittinen M. CD99 (p30/32^MIC2) neuroectodermal/Ewing's sarcoma antigen as an immunohistochemical marker. Review of more than 600 tumors and the literature experience. Applied Immunohistochemistry 1994;2:231–40.

Vartanian RK, Sudilovsky D, Weidner N. Immunostaining of monoclonal antibody 013 (anti MIC2 gene product) (CD99) in lymphomas. Impact of heat-induced epitope retrieval. Applied Immunohistochemistry 1996;4:43–55.

Weidner N, Tjoe J. Immunohistochemical profile of monoclonal antibody 013: antibody that recognizes glycoprotein p30/32^MIC2 and is useful in diagnosing Ewing's sarcoma and peripheral neuroepithelioma. American Journal of Surgical Pathology 1994;18:486–94.

NOTES

CD117 (KIT)

Sources/clones

Dako (C-KIT/CD117, polyclonal rabbit).

Fixation/preparation

The antibody can be used on formalin-fixed, paraffin-embedded tissue sections without antigen retrieval but heat pretreatment provides the best staining. Proteolytic enzyme treatment should be avoided.

Background

Tyrosine kinase growth factor receptors are a family of membrane bound proteins essential for the regulation of cell growth and maintenance of the cells. *C-kit* is a proto-oncogene, which encodes for one such growth factor receptor protein, KIT (CD117). *C-kit* maps to chromosome 4 (4q11–12). The gene product KIT is the receptor for stem cell factor (SCF), also known as mast cell growth factor (Zsebo et al, 1990; Williams et al, 1990). As a transmembrane type III tyrosine kinase receptor, KIT is phosphorylated as a result of binding with SCF and begins a cascade of intracytoplasmic signals, which are important to the regulation of cell

development and growth (Ashman, 1999; Taylor & Metcalfe, 2000). Many investigators have shown that *c-kit* expression is essential for the proper development of certain hematopoietic cells, mast cells, melanocytes and germ cells.

KIT (CD117) is a 145–160 kDa protein, which is structurally related to platelet-derived growth factor (Taylor & Metcalfe, 2000). It was originally described in the late eighties as a cellular homologue of the feline sarcoma retrovirus HZ4-FeSV transforming gene (Besmer et al, 1986; Yarden et al, 1987). Since that time, several authors have shown that the KIT protein is constitutively expressed in hematopoietic stem cells, tissue mast cells, basal cells of the skin, epithelial cells of the breast, melanocytes, germ cells, and interstitial cells of Cajal. KIT is not expressed in normal squamous epithelium (Lammie et al, 1994). The central nervous system shows distinct immunopositivity in certain regions, which is absent in peripheral nerves (Lammie et al, 1994).

Several publications have extensively demonstrated the utility of KIT staining in the identification and diagnosis of

gastrointestinal stromal tumors (GISTs). Moreover, the study of this property of GISTs has lead to the development of new treatment modalities targeting the KIT protein as a tyrosine kinase receptor, which is activated in the majority of GISTs. The KIT protein is selectively and competitively bound by a newly developed molecule, STI-571, resulting in inhibition of tyrosine phosphorylation. The effect thereof is to shut down the transcriptional activity in the cell resulting in growth arrest (Joensuu et al, 2001). Recent data suggests that this molecule is effective in the treatment of GISTs (Joensuu et al, 2001; Fletcher, 2001).

The currently accepted terminology for mesenchymal tumors of the gastrointestinal tract assigns true smooth muscle tumors and neural tumors into separate categories from these spindled or epithelioid GISTs with KIT immunostaining and/or staining for CD34. The interstitial cells of Cajal, the proposed pacemaker cells of the gastrointestinal (GI) tract are believed to represent the cell of origin for GISTs due to their similar immunohistochemical profile, electron microscopic features and location within the

GI tract (Kindblom et al, 1998; Sircar et al, 1999; Robinson et al, 2000). Gastrointestinal autonomic nerve tumors (GANT) have features that overlap with GISTs, including immunoreactivity with KIT, and are viewed by some as a variant of GISTs (Lee et al, 2001).

Depending on the study design, 72–100% of GIST tumors are immunopositive with the CD117 antibody (Tazawa et al, 1999; Miettinen et al, 1999; Sarlomo-Rikala et al, 1998). The staining pattern is typically a diffuse cytoplasmic, granular staining with membrane accentuation with occasional cases showing focal perinuclear staining (Miettinen et al, 2000). The panel including CD117, CD34, as well as S-100, desmin, and smooth muscle actin (SMA), can effectively differentiate between GISTs, true smooth muscle tumors and neural tumors (Appendix 1.29); since GISTs do not typically express desmin or S-100, but demonstrate immunopositivity for CD117 and/or CD34 and occasionally SMA (Miettinen et al, 2000; Schmid & Wegmann, 2000). Occasional tumors with S-100 and desmin positivity may also be classified as GISTs (Miettinen et al, 2000). Recent reviews of GISTs have reported similar findings (Chan, 1999). C-kit mutations appear to occur preferentially in the spindle rather than in the epithelioid variant of GIST (Wardelmann, et al. 2002).

Mast cells are well known to show distinctive membranous and cytoplasmic staining for KIT. Furthermore, similar staining is seen in mast cell disorders and can be used to identify neoplasms of mast cells in bone marrow,

skin, lymph nodes and solid organs (Natkunam & Rouse, 2000; Arber et al, 1998). Germ cells and germ cell neoplasms have been the subject of numerous studies looking at *c-kit* mutations and KIT protein expression. Studies have shown membranous staining of malignant germ cells in intratubular germ cell neoplasia (ITGCN) (Rajpert-De Meyts et al, 1996) and seminomas, in contrast to cytoplasmic staining in non-seminomatous germ cell neoplasms (Rajpert-De Meyts et al, 1996). The combination of CD30 and CD117 is useful for distinguishing seminomas from embryonal carcinomas (Appendix 1.5), seminomas being CD117+/CD30-, none being CD117-/CD30+; whereas, embryonal carcinomas were CD30+/CD117-, none being CD30-/CD117+ (Leroy et al, 2002).

Other tumors have been shown to have KIT immunoreactivity, predominantly with weak to moderate cytoplasmic staining intensity. These include small cell carcinomas of the lung, ovarian epithelial neoplasms, endometrial carcinomas, thyroid carcinomas, melanomas, certain salivary gland neoplasms, angiosarcomas, breast carcinomas and malignant phyllodes tumors and acute myelogenous leukemia (AML). The deep dermal or nodular components of melanomas tend to show loss of staining for KIT, while the in-situ component stains strongly (Monotone et al, 1997). Angiomyolipomas generally show strong immunostaining for CD117 in the epithelioid, spindle and intermediate small round cell

components in a frequency slightly higher than Melan A and HMB45 (Makhlouf et al, 2002). Other more recent additions to the CD117-positive list include pediatric solid tumors such as osteosarcomas, Ewing's sarcoma, and synovial sarcomas and, less frequently, neuroblastomas, Wilm's and rhabdomyosarcoma (Smithey et al, 2002). In addition, occasional immunoreactivity was encountered in extraskeletal myxoid chondrosarcoma, melanotic schwannoma, metastatic melanoma and angiosarcoma (Hornick & Fletcher, 2002).

Applications

The potential uses of the KIT (CD117) antibody include the diagnosis of GISTs, mast cell disorders and potential use in the diagnosis of seminomatous germ cell neoplasms (Appendix 1.5). As with most antibodies in immunohistochemistry, CD117 should be used in conjunction with others in a panel targeted towards the differential diagnosis. Within the spectrum of mesenchymal neoplasms of the GI tract, CD117, CD34, desmin, S-100 and SMA should be the primary panel of choice for most circumstances (Appendix 1.29). In the case of mast cell disorders, care must be taken to include antibodies to B-cells, T-cells, myeloid markers (since CD117 can stain AML), and histiocytic markers. Despite its expression in diverse tumors, selective application with attention to specific staining patterns makes it a useful marker for tumor diagnosis (Gibson & Cooper, 2002).

CD117 is expressed on hematopoietic progenitor cells,

melanocytes, embryonic/fetal brain, endothelium, gonads, gastrointestinal stromal tumors (GIST), gastrointestinal autonomic nerve tumors, omental mesenchymal tumors, acute myeloid leukemia, granulocytic sarcoma, small cell carcinoma of the lung, mast cell disease, some Reed-Sternberg cells and synovial sarcoma.

References

Arber DA, Tamayo R, Weiss LM. Paraffin section detection of *c-kit* gene product (CD117) in human tissues: value in the diagnosis of mast cell disorders. Human Pathology 1998;29:498–504.

Ashman LK. The biology of stem cell factor and its receptor *c-kit*. International Journal of Biochemistry and Cell Biology 1999;31:1037–51.

Besmer P, Murphy JE, George PC, et al. A new acute transforming feline retrovirus and relationship of its oncogene c-kit with the protein kinase gene family. Nature 1986;320:415–21.

Chan JKC. Mesenchymal tumors of the gastrointestinal tract. A paradise for acronyms (STUMP, GIST, GANT, and now GIPACT). Implications of *c-kit* in genesis, and yet another of many emerging roles of the interstitial cells of Cajal in the pathogenesis of gastrointestinal disease. Advances in Anatomical Pathology 1999;6:19–40.

Fletcher CDM. KIT (CD117) immunostaining and treatment with STI-571. Advances in Anatomical Pathology 2001;8:304.

Gibson PC, Cooper K. CD117 (KIT): a diverse protein with selective applications in surgical pathology. Advances in Anatomical Pathology 2002;9:65–9.

Hornick JL, Fletcher CD. Immunohistochemical staining for KIT (CD117) in soft tissue sarcomas is very limited in distribution. American Journal of Clinical Pathology 2002;117:188–93.

Joensuu H, Roberts PH, Sarlomo-Rikala M, et al. Effect of the tyrosine kinase inhibitor STI571 in a patient with metastatic gastrointestinal stromal tumor. New England Journal of Medicine 2001;344:1052–6.

Kindblom LG, Remotti HE, Aldenborg F, Meis-Kindblom J.: Gastrointestinal pacemaker cell tumor (GIPACT): gastrointestinal stromal tumors show phenotypic characteristics of the interstitial cells of Cajal. American Journal of Pathology 1998;152:1259–69.

Lammie A, Drobnjak M, Gerald W, et al. Expression of *c-kit* and kit ligand proteins in normal human tissues. Journal of Histochemistry and Cytochemistry 1994;42:1417–25.

Lee JR, Joshi V, Griffin JW, et al. Gastrointestinal autonomic nerve tumor: Immunohistochemical and molecular identity with gastrointestinal stromal tumor. American Journal of Surgical Pathology 2001;25:979–87.

Leroy X, Augusto D, Leteurtre E, Goselin B. CD30 and CD117 (c-kit) used in combination are useful for distinguishing embryonal carcinoma from seminomas. Journal of Histochemistry and Cytochemistry 2002;50:283–5.

Makhlouf HR, Remotti HE, Ishak KG. Expression of KIT (CD117) in angiolipoma. American Journal of Surgical Pathology 2002;26:493–7.

Miettinen M, Sarlomo-Rikala M, Lasota J. Gastrointestinal stromal tumors: Recent advances in understanding of their biology. Human Pathology 1999;30:1213–20.

Miettinen M, Sobin LH, Sarlomo-Rikala M: Immunohistochemical spectrum of GISTs at different sites and their differential diagnosis with a reference to CD117 (KIT). Modern Pathology 2000;13:1134–42.

Monotone KT, van Belle P, Elenitsas R, Elder DE. Proto-oncogene *c-kit* expression in malignant melanoma: Protein loss with tumor progression. Modern Pathology 1997;10:939–44.

Natkunam Y, Rouse RV. Utility of paraffin section immunohistochemistry for C-KIT (CD117) in the differential diagnosis of systemic mast cell disease involving the bone marrow. American Journal of Surgical Pathology 2000;24:81–91.

Rajpert-De Meyts E, Kvist M, Skakkebaek NE. Heterogeneity of expression of immunohistochemical tumour markers in testicular carcinoma in situ: pathogenic relevance. Virchows Archives 1996;428:133–9.

Robinson TL, Sicar K, Hewlett BR, et al. Gastrointestinal stromal tumors may originate from a subset of CD34-positive interstitial cells of Cajal. American Journal of Pathology 2000;156:1157–63.

Sarlomo-Rikala M, Kovatich A, Barusevicius A, et al. CD117: A more sensitive marker for gastrointestinal stromal tumors that is more specific than CD34. Modern Pathology 1998;11:728–34.

Schmid S, Wegmann W. Gastrointestinal pacemaker cell tumor: Clinicopathological, immunohistochemical, and ultrastructural study with special reference to *c-kit* receptor antibody. Virchows Archives 2000;436:234–42.

Sircar K, Hewlett BR, Huizinga JD, et al. Interstitial cells of Cajal as precursors of gastrointestinal stromal tumors. American Journal of Surgical Pathology 1999;23:377–89.

Smithey BE, Pappo AS, Hill DA. C-kit expressionj in pediatric solid tumors: a comparative immunohistochemical study. American Journal of Surgical Pathology 2002;26:486–92.

Taylor ML, Metcalfe DD. KIT signal transduction. Hematology-Oncology Clinics of North America 2000;14:517–35.

Tazawa K, Tsukada K, Makuuchi H, Tsutsumi Y. An immunohistochemical and clinicopathological study of gastrointestinal stromal tumors. Pathology International 1999;49:786–98.

Williams DE, Eisenman J, Baird A, et al. Identification of a ligand for *c-kit* proto-oncogene. Cell 1990;3:167–74.

Yarden Y, Kuang WJ, Yang-Feng L, et al. Human proto-oncogene *c-kit*: A new cell surface receptor kinase for an unidentified ligand. EMBO Journal 1987;6:3341–51.

Zsebo KM, Williams DA, Geissler EN, et al. Stem cell factor is encoded at the SI locus of mouse and is ligand for the *c-kit* tyrosine kinase receptor. Cell 1990;63:213–24.

Wardelmann E, Neidt I, Bierhoff E, et al. c-kit mutation in gastrointestinal stromal tumors occur preferentially in the spindle rather than in the epithelioid cell variant. Modern Pathology 2002;15:125–36.

c-erbB-2 (Her-2, neu)

Sources/clones

Accurate (CB11, CBE1, polyclonal), Becton Dickinson (3B5), Biogenesis (2G2–91, LY369), Biogenex (EGFR), Coulter (3B5), Dako (polyclonal A0485), Lab Vision (9G6.10, L87, N12, N24, N28.6), Novocastra (CB11, CBE1), Oncogene Science (CNeu), Pharmingen (9G6), Zymed (TAB250).

Fixation/preparation

Most antibodies are immunoreactive in fresh frozen tissue sections as well as in fixed paraffin-embedded sections. HIER enhances immunoreactivity. Enzyme treatment is not necessary.

Background

The c-erbB-2 oncogene was discovered in the 1980s by three different avenues of investigation. The neu oncogene was detected as a mutated transforming gene in neuroblastomas experimentally induced in fetal rats. The c-erbB-2 was a human gene discovered by its homology to the retroviral gene

v-erbB, and HER-2 was isolated by screening a human genomic DNA library for homology with v-erbB. When the DNA sequences were determined subsequently, c-erbB-2, HER-2 and neu were found to represent the same gene.

The c-erbB-2 gene is located on human chromosome 17q21 and codes for the c-erbB-2 mRNA (4.6 kb), which translates to the c-erbB-2 protein (p185). The c-erbB-2 oncogene is homologous with, but not identical to, c-erbB-1, which is located on chromosome 7 and encodes for the epidermal growth factor receptor. The c-erbB-2 protein, a member of the epidermal growth factor receptor family, is a normal cell membrane component of all epithelial cells with extracellular, transmembrane and intracellular tyrosine kinase activity (Lupu et al, 1992). Apart from a growth stimulatory function, the molecule plays an important role in the motility of tumor cell. Cell migration depends mainly on actin polymerization and intracellular organization, which is influenced by a vast variety of actin binding proteins. Second messengers such as phosphoinositides and calcium mediate the regulation of these proteins. Signaling via these second messengers is initiated and regulated by membrane receptors, e.g., receptor tyrosine

kinases, and by adhesion molecule interactions (e.g., integrins and selectins) and focal adhesion kinases. As c-erbB-2 is a receptor tyrosine kinase it has a major role in steering second-messenger signaling and thus in actin cytoskeleton reorganization and motility of the cell (Feldner & Brandt, 2002). The erbB-2 is unique among the erbB family in that no ligand has yet been identified. Due to this absence, alternative mechanisms are use for erbB-2 activation. With overexpression kinase activation occurs in the absence of ligand because of constitutive homodimerization. At normal expression levels erbB-2 acts as the shared co-receptor for the erbB family, and these heterodimeric complexes are activated in response to the partner ligand (Penuel et al, 2001).

c-erbB-2 gene alterations have been reported in diverse human neoplasms and almost exclusively involve amplification of the gene. Amplification involves the repeated duplication of a particular gene sequence, resulting in multiple gene copies within each cell. This results in overexpression of the gene product, as reflected in the levels of mRNA and gene oncoprotein.

There is generally good correlation of the c-erbB-2 gene amplification with overexpression (Smith et al, 1994).

Applications

c-erbB-2 has been shown to be amplified in about 20–30% of invasive breast carcinomas and various studies have correlated the gene amplification or overexpression with other prognostic variables in breast cancer patients. Almost all reported studies have shown a strong correlation with various established adverse factors including large tumor size, unfavorable histologic subtype, high histologic grade, high mitotic index and proliferative activity, positive nodal status, presence of hematogenous spread and aneuploidy (De Potter et al, 1990; 1994; Borg et al, 1991; Horiguchi et al, 1994). Recently, c-erbB-2 expression has also been shown to be an independent significant prognostic factor in both node-positive as well as node-negative breast cancer and the combination of c-erbB-2 positivity and estrogen receptor negativity made it possible to identify a subgroup of patients with the worst clinical outcome (Tsutsui et al, 2002).

c-erbB-2 overexpression is more common in invasive ductal and medullary carcinomas than in lobular, colloid and papillary carcinomas. In intraductal carcinomas, it is almost exclusively seen in large cell, high nuclear grade, estrogen receptor negative, and comedo type intraductal carcinoma (interestingly, a larger percentage of DCIS compared to infiltrating ductal carcinoma is positive for c-erbB-2). In situ lobular carcinoma seldom shows overexpression of the oncoprotein. Overexpression is more common in invasive tumors associated with an intraductal component than in those without, and there is usually concordance between the invasive and intraductal components of an individual tumor. The rates of overexpression and gene amplification did not appear to be different in ductal carcinoma in situ and invasive carcinoma but appeared to be significantly higher in invasive carcinoma with intraductal spread (Kobayashi et al, 2002).

Despite the universal observation of a strong correlation with various adverse prognostic factors, conflicting data regarding the prognostic value of c-erbB-2 suggest that overexpression of the oncoprotein may not be a powerful predictor by itself. In any individual patient it should be employed as part of a multivariate approach to guiding treatment and determining prognosis. Overexpression of c-erbB-2 may also serve as a predictor of response to adjuvant treatment, predicting a poor response to chemotherapy and a lack of response to endocrine therapy on relapse, and identifying those patients who are most likely to benefit from high dose regimens (Muss et al, 1994). Furthermore, as c-erbB-2 protein has an extracellular domain and tends to be expressed in more aggressive tumors, it is the target for immunotherapy with the humanized anti-HER 2/neu antibody, trastuzumab (Herception; Genentech, Inc, South San Francisco, CA, USA) that became available in 1998, particularly for patients with metastatic carcinoma.

Comments

Occasional reports have noted discrepancies between the demonstration of amplification of the c-erbB-2 gene and detection of protein overexpression by immunostaining. Despite this drawback, immunohistochemistry now appears to be the method of choice in most institutions for assessing c-erbB-2 overexpression (Bobrow et al, 1996). A number of factors account for variability of immunohistochemical results and these include fixation, storage, antigen retrieval, reagent optimization, antibody specificity and its domain, controls, scoring system employed, and interobserver variability. Numerous antibodies to c-erbB-2 are available, including both polyclonal and monoclonal antibodies. In general, monoclonal antibodies are considered more specific. The HercepTest uses a polyclonal antibody (A0485). In general, the Food and Drug Administration approved antibodies detect the internal domain of the c-erbB-2 receptor. Some antibodies such as Zymed TAB250 are against the external domain of the receptor. There is some concern that the external domain of c-erbB-2 may be cleaved so that antibodies to the external domain may not be as sensitive (Ceccarelli et al, 1999), although this concern has not been substantiated.

Only membrane staining should be accepted as positive staining and we have found the polyclonal antibody from Dako and monoclonal Cneu to be the most sensitive. HIER enhanced staining, although producing some increase in cytoplasmic staining was not a hindrance to interpretation. There is no standardized scoring system for Her 2/neu by immunostaining and disparate systems have been employed; some take into consideration the proportion of positive cells; some only regard the intensity of staining, while others combine the two parameters into one score. The heterogeneity of staining in any section is due to variability of fixation and embedding and probably not to intrinsic tumor properties. The majority of publications score immunostaining of c-erbB-2 in the following manner: 0 = no staining; 1+ occasional tumors cells show membranous staining that is fragmented and not circumferential; 2+ scattered tumors cells or small groups of tumor cells show circumferential staining; 3+ strong membrane staining throughout the tumor that may be associated with some cytoplasmic staining. The area of highest intensity of staining is assessed; the area occupying at least 10–20% of the tumor in the section. Successful antigen retrieval will result in normal expression in benign epithelial cells, as the c-erbB-2 is a normal gene. However, such internal controls of benign breast epithelium must not display >1+ staining. Data from clinical trials suggest that 3+ immunoexpression reflects gene amplification and 0 and 1+ are negative. Scores of 2+ should proceed to FISH analysis as a small portion of these cases represent true gene amplification.

Besides fixed, paraffin-embedded sections, we have shown that c-erbB-2 immunostaining can also be performed on formalin-fixed cytological preparations (Suthipintawong et al, 1997); however, scoring of staining in such preparations has not been correlated with gene amplification.

c-erbB-2 immunoexpression has been demonstrated in a number of epithelial tumors including carcinomas of the prostate (Fossa et al, 2002), bile duct (Aishima et al 2002), colon and rectum (McKay et al, 2002), lung (Bakir et al, 2002), stomach (Takehana et al 2002) and head and neck region (O-charoenrat et al, 2002) and other organs and may have a role in such tumors.

References

Aishima SI, Taguchi KI, Sugimachi K, et al. c-erbB-2 and c-Met expression relates to cholangiocarcinogenesis and progression of intrahepatic cholangiocarcinoma. Histopathology 2002;40:269–78.

Bakir K, Ucak R, Tuncozgur B, et al. Prognostic factors and c-erbB-2 expression in non-small cell lung carcinoma (c-erbB-2 in non small cell lung carcinoma). Thoracic and Cardiovascular Surgery 2002;50:55–8.

Bobrow LG, Happerfield LC, Millis RR. Comparison of immunohistological staining with different antibodies to the c-erbB-2 oncoprotein. Applied Immunohistochemistry 1996;4:128–34.

Borg A, Baldetorp B, Ferno M, et al. ErbB2 amplification in breast cancer with a high rate of proliferation. Oncogene 1991;6:137–43.

Ceccarelli C, Santini D, Gamberini M, et al. Immunohistochemical expression of internal and external ErbB-2 domains in invasive breast caner. Breast Cancer Research and Treatment 1999;58:107–14.

DePotter CR, Beghin C, Marak AP, et al. The neu oncogene protein as a predictive factor for hematogenous metastasis in breast cancer patients. International Journal of Cancer 1990;45:55–8.

DePotter CR. The neu-oncogene: More than a prognostic indicator? Human Pathology 1994;25:1264–8.

Feldner JC, Brandt BH. Cancer cell motility – on the road from c-erbB-2 receptor steered signaling to actin reorganization. Experimental Cell Research 2002;15:93–108.

Fossa A, Lilleby W, Fossa SD, et al. Independent prognostic significance of HER-2 oncoprotein expression in pN0 prostate cancer undergoing curative radiotherapy. International Journal of Cancer 2002;99:100–5.

Horiguchi J, Iino Y, Takei H, et al. Immunohistochemical study on the expression of c-erbB-2 oncoprotein in breast cancer. Oncology 1994;51:47–51.

Kobayashi M, Ooi A, Oda Y, Nakanishi I. Protein overexpression and gene amplification of c-erbB-2 in breast carcinomas: a comparative study of immunohistochemistry and fluorescence in situ hybridization of formalin-fixed, paraffin-embedded tissues. Human Pathology 2002;33:21–8.

Lupu R, Colomer R, Kannan B, Lippman ME. Characterization of a growth factor that binds exclusively to the erbB-2 receptor and induces cellular responses. Proceedings of the National Academy of Sciences USA 1992;89:2287–91.

McKay JA, Loane JF, Ross VG, et al. c-erbB-2 is not a major factor in the development of colorectal cancer. British Journal of Cancer 2002;86:568–73.

Muss HB, Thor AD, Berry DA, et al. *C-erb*B-2 expression and response to adjuvant therapy in women with node-positive early breast cancer. New England Journal of Medicine 1994;330:1260–6

O-charoenrat P, Rhys-Evans PH, Archer DJ, Eccles SA. C-erbB-2 receptors in squamous cell carcinomas of the head and neck: clinical significance and correlation with matrix metalloproteinases and vascular endothelial growth factors. Oral Oncology 2002;38:73–80.

Smith KL, Robbins PD, Dawkins HJS, et al. C-erbB-2 amplification in breast cancer: detection in formalin fixed, paraffin-embedded tissue by in situ hybridization. Human Pathology 1994;25:413–8.

Suthipintawong C, Leong AS-Y, Chan KW, Vinyuvat S. Immunostaining of estrogen receptor, progesterone receptor, MIB1 and c-erbB-2 in cytological preparations – a simplified method. Diagnostic Cytopathology 1997;17:127–33.

Takehana T, Kunitomo K, Kono K, et al. Status of c-erbB-2 in gastric adenocarcinoma: a comparative study of immunohistochemistry, fluorescence in situ hybridization and enzyme-linked immuno-sorbent assay. International Journal of Cancer 2002;98:833–7.

Tsutsui S, Ohno S, Murakami S, et al. Prognostic value of c-erbB-2 expression in breast cancer. Journal of Surgical Oncology 2002;79:216–23.

Chlamydia

Sources/clones

American Research Products (C512F), American Research Products/EY Labs (polyclonal), Biogenex (LM-9, 16-UB), Dako (RR402), Fitzgerald (polyclonal).

C. trachomatis

Accurate (115), Biogenesis (polyclonal), Biodesign (168, JDC1), Pharmingen (CHL888).

C. trachomatis 60kD

Biodesign (168), Biogenesis (polyclonal),

C. psittaci

Biogenesis (73–0200, 77–05), Kallestadt Diagnostics, Chaska, MN

C. pneumoniae

Fitzgerald (M73066)

Fixation/preparation

Most antibodies are applicable to routine formalin-fixed, paraffin-embedded tissue.

Background

Genital chlamydial infection is recognized as the world's most common sexually transmitted disease (WHO, 1990). In the majority of cases the condition is asymptomatic. *C. trachomatis* is associated with various complications of pregnancy (Lan et al, 1995) and with premature birth and neonatal difficulties (Gencay et al, 1995; Donders et al, 1991). A monoclonal antibody specific for the outer membrane proteins of *C.trachomatis* is available.

C. psittaci is the causative agent of psittacosis. It infects a diverse group of animals, including birds, humans, and other mammals. It is a cause of abortion in sheep, cattle and goats (Schlossberg, 1995). Transmission to humans is incidental, with a history of direct contact with contaminated products of conception. The disease is characterized as a mild-to-moderate flu-like illness (Gherman et al, 1985). However, in pregnancy the human host is especially vulnerable. Gestational psittacosis typically present as a progressive febrile illness with headaches, complicated by abnormal liver enzymes, low grade disseminated intravascular coagulapathy, atypical pneumonia and abnormal renal function. Management includes termination of pregnancy with aggressive antibiotic therapy (Khatib et al, 1995).

Applications

Diagnosis of gestational psittacosis is dependent on histopathological findings which consist of an intense acute intervillositis, perivillous fibrin deposition with villous necrosis, and large irregular basophilic intracytoplasmic inclusions within the syncytiotrophoblast (Wong et al, 1985). The application of genus-specific monoclonal anti-chlamydial antibody is useful for the rapid confirmation of the diagnosis.

C.trachomatis is a major cause of genital infection. The acquired infection tends to persist and is usually symptom free (Beatty et al, 1994). Consequently fetal exposure to chlamydial infection is high, with *C.trachomatis* being demonstrated in the placenta (Gencay et al, 1997). More often, basophilic intracytoplasmic inclusions are detected in cervical smears, where genus-specific antibody may be applied for diagnostic confirmation. In lymphogranuloma venereum, a small ulcerating primary lesion develops in the genitalia, following by involvement of draining lymph nodes with a suppurative granulomatous inflammation, necrosis and scarring.

Inclusion bodies may also be demonstrated in lung tissue and secretions in atypical pneumonias caused by *C.trachomatis*. Trachoma/Trachoma inclusion conjunctivitis or TRIC infection is common in the tropical zones being responsible for blindness. The organism initially infects the conjunctival epithelium and it can be demonstrated in smears of these cells by the presence of characteristic intracytoplasmic inclusion bodies.

Recent interest centres around the role of *C. pneumoniae* in cardiovascular disease. Chlamydia infection of the cardiovascular system is associated with pericarditis, endocarditis and myocarditis and chlamydia particles have also been observed in damaged heart valves and may be associated with lesions of arteriosclerosis and aortic aneurysm. In addition patients with myocardial infarction show seroconversion against Chlamydia lipopolysaccharide (Saikku, 1996). Young patients who died of sudden death showed immunohistochemically detectable *C. pneumoniae* in 53% (17/32) cases of advanced arteriosclerosis of left anterior descending coronary arteries and in 21% (8/37) cases of early lesions. *C. pneumoniae* was found most often in macrophages and less often in smooth muscle cells (Hortovanyi et al, 2002). The

organism has similarly been demonstrated in atherosclerotic plaques in a variety of other vascular sites (Rassu et al, 2001).

References

Beatty WL, Morison RP, Byrne GI. Immunoelectron microscopic quantitation of differential levels of chlamydial proteins in cell culture model of persistent Chlamydia trachomatis infection. Infection Immunology 1994;62:4059–62.

Donders GG, Moerman P, De-Wet GH, et al. The association between Chlamydia cervicitis and neonatal complications. Archives of Gynecology and Obstetrics 1991;249:79–85.

Gencay M, Koskiniemi M, Saikku P, et al. *C trachomatis* seropositivity during pregnancy is associated with perinatal complications. Clinical Infectious Disease 1995;21:424–6.

Gencay M, Puolakkainen M, Wahlström, et al. *Chlamydia trachomatis* detected in human placenta. Journal of Clinical Pathology 1997;50:852–5.

Gherman RB, Leventis LL, Miller RC. Chlamydial psittacosis during pregnancy: a case report. Obstetrics and Gynecology 1985;86:648–50.

Hortovanyi E, Illyes G, Glasz T, Kadar A. Chlamydia pneumoniae in different coronary artery segment in the young. Pathology Research and Practice 2002;198:19–23.

Hyde SR, Benirschke K. Gestational Psittacosis:Case report and literature review. Modern Pathology 1997;10:602–7.

Khatib R, Muthayipalayam C, Thirumoorthi MC, et al. Severe psittacosis during pregnancy and

suppression of antibody response with early therapy. Scandinavian Journal of Infectious Disease 1995;27:519–21.

Lan J, Van Der Brule AJ, Hemrika DJ et al. Chlamydia trachomatis and ectopic pregnancy: retrospective analysis of salpingectomy specimens, endometrial biopsies, and cervical smears. Journal of Clinical Pathology 1995;48:815–9.

Mahoney JB, Sellors J, Chernesky MA. Detection of Chlamydial inclusions in cell culture or biopsy tissue by alkaline phosphatase–anti-alkaline phosphatase staining. Journal of Clinical Microbiology 1987;25:1864–7.

Rassu M, Cazzavillan S, Scagnelli M, et al. Demonstration of Chlamydia pneumoniae in atherosclerotic arteries from various vascular regions. Atherosclerosis 2001;158:73–9.

Saikku P. Chlamydia pneumoniae and cardiovascular disease. Clinical Microbiology and Infection 1996;1 (Suppl 1):S19–22.

Schlossberg D. *Chlamydia psittaci* (psittacosis). IN: Mandell G, Bennet J, Dolin R. eds. Principals and practice of infectious diseases. 4th ed. New York, Churchill Livingstone, 1995, 1693–5.

WHO, Guidelines for the prevention of genital chlamydial infections. World Health Organisation, Regional Office for Europe, 1990.

Wong SY, Gray ES, Buston D, et al. Acute placentitis and spontaneous abortion caused by *Chlamydia psittaci* of sheep origin: a histological and ultrastructure study. Journal of Clinical Pathology 1985;38:707–11.

Chromogranin

Sources/clones

Antibodies to chromogranin A are available from Accurate (A3), Biogenesis (A11, LK2H10), Biogenex (A11, LK2H10), Camon (LK2H10), Cymbus Bioscience (LK2H10), Dako (DAK-A3, polyclonal), Enzo (PHE5), Immunotech (LK2H10, C3420), Milab (CH), RDI (LK2H10), Novocastra (LK2H10), Medac, Sanbio (LK2H10), Saxon, Serotec (LK2H10, C3420), Zymed.

Fixation/preparation

The antibodies are immunoreactive in fixed, paraffin-embedded sections and frozen sections. HIER does not result in significant enhancement. Fixation in Bouin's or B5 fixative may improve immunogenicity but background staining is correspondingly increased. Proteolytic digestion does not improve immunostaining.

Background

The chromogranins are a family of soluble acidic proteins of about 68 kD. They are the major proteins in the peptide-containing dense core (neurosecretory) granules of neuroendocrine cells and sympathetic nerves.

Ultrastructural examination has confirmed the localization of chromogranins to the matrix of neurosecretory granules of neuroendocrine cells. While having different molecular weights, the chromogranin subunits are neither identical nor entirely dissimilar and may differ in only two or three amino acid residues, with a minimum homology between any pair of polypeptides of about 33%. The chromogranins in neuroendocrine tissues displays both quantitative and qualitative variability. They occur in the highest concentration in the following rank order: the adrenal medulla; anterior, intermediate and posterior pituitary; pancreatic islets; small intestine; thyroid C cells; and hypothalamus.

The antibody clone LK2H10 to chromogranin of 68 kD labels most normal neuroendocrine cells and their corresponding neoplasms. The LK2H10 clone was derived from human pheochromocytoma exhibits cross-reactivity with monkey and pig chromogranins (Wilson & Lloyd, 1984).

Chromogranins are thought to stabilize the soluble portion of neurosecretory granules by interaction with adenosine tri-phosphate and catecholamines and are released into the serum after splanchnic stimulation. They have multiple roles in the secretory process of hormones. Intracellularly, they play role in targeting peptide hormones and neurotransmitters to granules of the regulated pathway by virtue of their ability to aggregate in the low-pH, high-calcium environment of the trans-Golgi network. Extra-cellular peptides formed as a result of proteolytic processing of chromogranins regulate hormone secretion. The synthesis of chromogranins is regulated by many different factors, including steroid hormones and agents that act through a variety of signaling pathways (Hendy et al, 1995).

Applications

The major applications of antibodies to the chromogranins are for the identification of neuroepithelial/neuroendocrine differentiation in normal and neoplastic tissues (Hirose et al, 1005; Blumenfeld et al, 1996), as well as the neural elements of the brain (Schiffer et al, 1995) and gut (Shen et al, 1994). Initial experience with clone LK2H10 to chromogranin A revealed less than 100% sensitivity for neuroendocrine cells, especially among those cells and tumors with low concentrations of neurosecretory granules and among tumors such as insulinomas, somatostatinomas, prolactinomas and corticotrophin- and growth hormone-producing adenomas. However, the rate of positivity has improved with the use of more sensitive immunolabelling procedures.

Chromogranin is the most specific marker for neuroendocrine differentiation and corresponds to the neurosecretory granule, the hallmark of the neuroendocrine cell (Appendix 1.3, 1.4, 1.9, 1.20, 1.29, 1.30, 1.35, 1.37). While it may be used with other neuroendocrine markers such as NSE and PGP9.5 to improve the diagnostic yield, chromogranin and synaptophysin are the most specific of all neuroendocrine markers.

Comments

As neurosecretory granules tend to be localized beneath the plasma membranes of neuroendocrine cells, their highest density is within the cytoplasmic processes characteristic of such cells. As such staining for chromogranin highlights the cytoplasmic processes often not visible in H & E stains; these processes when cut in cross section show dot-like staining. Aberrant immunoreactivity for chromogranin has been described in normal and neoplastic urothelium, particularly in the umbrella cells, attributed to reactivity with chromogranin-like proteins in the transitional cells (Mai et al, 1994).

Chromogranin immunostaining has been employed to resolve the problem of argyrophilia seen in some breast cancers. A subset of such carcinomas (10–18%) have been confirmed to show neuroendocrine differentiation by chromogranin immunolabelling but the phenomenon appears to have no relationship to established prognostic factors or patient outcome (Miremadi et al, 2002). Histologic grade appears to overcome the phenotype in determining prognosis of neuroendocrine differentiation in breast carcinomas (Sapino et al, 2001).

References

Blumenfeld W, Chandhoke DK, Sagerman P, Turi GK. Neuroendocrine differentiation in gastric adenocarcinomas. An immunohistochemical study. Archives of Pathology and Laboratory Medicine 1996;120:478–81.

Hirose T, Scheithauer BW, Lopes MB, et al. Olfactory neuroblastoma. An immunohistochemical, ultrastructural and flow cytometric study. Cancer 1995;76:4–19.

Hendy GN, Bevan S, Mattei MG, Mouland AJ. Chromogranin A. Clinical Investigative Medicine 1995;18:47–65.

Mai KT, Perkins DG, Parks W, et al. Unusual immunostaining pattern of chromogranin in normal urothelium and in transitional cell neoplasms. Acta Histochemia 1994;96:303–8.

Miremadi A, Pinder SE, Lee AH, et al. Neuroendocrine differentiation and prognosis in breast adenocarcinoma. Histopathology 2002;40:215–22.

Sapino A, Papotti M, Right L, et al. Clinical significance of neuroendocrine carcinoma of the breast. Annals of Oncology 2001;12 (S2):S115–7.

Schiffer D, Cordera S, Giordana MT, et al. Synaptic vesicle proteins, synaptophysin and chromogranin A in amyotropic lateral sclerosis. Journal of Neurological Science 1995;129:68–74.

Shen Z, Larsson LT, Malmfors G, et al. Chromogranin A and B in neuronal elements in Hirschsprung's disease: an immunocytochemical and radioimmunoassay study. Journal of Pediatric Surgery 1994;29:1293–301.

Wilson BS, Lloyd RV. Detection of chromogranin in neuroendocrine cells with a monoclonal antibody. American Journal of Pathology 1984;115:458–68.

c-Myc

Sources/clones

Biogenesis (9E11), Caltag Laboratories (polyclonal), Chemicon, Fitzgerald (polyclonal), Novocastra (polyclonal), Oncogene (9E10, 8, 33), Pharmingen (9E10), Serotec (CT14, polyclonal).

Fixation/preparation

Several clones including 9E10 are immunoreactive in acetone- or formalin-fixed, paraffin-embedded tissue sections.

Background

Myc is the product of the early-response gene *myc*. The *myc* family of oncogenes, *c-myc* and N-*myc*, on chromosome 8, encodes three highly related regulatory cycle cycle-specific nuclear phosphoproteins. Myc protein contains a transcriptional activation domain and a basic helix-loop-helix-leucine zipper DNA-binding and dimerisation domain. As a heterodimer with a structurally related protein, Max, Myc can bind DNA in a sequence-specific manner suggesting that the Myc/Max heterodimer functions as a transcriptional activator of genes that are critical for the regulation of cell growth (Prins et al, 1993; Vastrik et al, 1994). When overexpressed or hyperactivated as a result of mutation in certain types of cells, *myc* can cause uncontrolled proliferation. There is evidence that *myc* may have a critical role in the normal control of cell proliferation and cells in which *myc* expression is specifically prevented in vitro will not divide even in the presence of growth factors. Conversely, cells in which *myc* expression is specifically switched on independently of growth factors cannot enter G_0. If the cells are in G_0 when Myc protein is provided, they will leave G_0 and begin to divide even in the absence of growth factors, a behavior that ultimately causes them to undergo programmed cell death or apoptosis. The presence of a single oncogene is not usually sufficient to turn a normal cell into a cancer cell. In transgenic mice that are endowed with *myc* oncogene, some of the tissues that express the oncogene grow to an exaggerated size, and with the passage of time, some cells undergo further changes and give rise to cancers. However, the vast majority of cells in the transgenic mouse that express the *myc* oncogene do not give rise to cancers, showing that the presence of a single oncogene is not enough to cause neoplastic transformation. Nonetheless, *myc* expression produces an increased risk as the presence of another oncogene such as *ras* results in a synergistic effect known as oncogene collaboration. The synergism increases the incidence of cancers in the transgenic mouse to a much higher rate, although the cancers originate as scattered isolated tumors among non-cancerous cells. Even with the presence of two expressed oncogenes, the cells must undergo further, randomly generated changes to become cancerous.

In follicular B cell lymphomas, collaboration between *myc* and the *bcl-2* gene occurs. If *myc* alone is overexpressed, cells are driven round the cell cycle inappropriately but this does not result in lymphoma because the progeny of such forced divisions die by apoptosis. If *bcl-2* is overexpressed at the same time, the excess progeny survive and proliferate as *bcl-2* acts as an oncogene by inhibiting apoptosis.

Applications

The ability to stain for c-Myc in tissue sections has understandably been received with great interest and several attempts to use the oncoprotein as a prognostic marker have been made. For example, in squamous cell carcinoma of the head and neck significant negative correlation has been shown between c-myc levels and the number of metastatic nodes and clinical stage of disease but no correlation was found with tumor size or degree of differentiation (Gapany et al, 1994). Other applications have included c-myc protein expression in prostatic carcinoma (Fox et al, 1993), pituitary adenomas (Lloyd & Osamura, 19970, ovary (King et al, 1996), lung (Prins et al, 1993), and colon (Agnantis et al, 1991), among other tumors (Gilbertson et al, 2001; Nagashima et al, 2001;Channa et al, 2000; Jamec et al, 2000; Kee et al, 2001).

The examination of c-myc as a marker for persons at risk of various types of cancer including breast carcinoma is another potential useful application (Hehir et al, 1993) and a recent study claimed between c-myc immunostaining with proliferation index, differentiation, patient age and estrogen receptor status (Naidu et al, 2002).

Comments

Clone 9E10 is immunoreactive in formalin-fixed, paraffin-embedded tissue sections.

References

Agnantis NJ, Aapostolikas N, Sficas C, et al. Immunohistochemical detection of ras p21 and c-myc p62 in colonic adenomas and carcinomas. Hepatogastroenterology 1991;38:239–42.

Fox SB, Persad RA, Royds J, et al. P53 and c-myc expression in stage A1 prostatic adenocarcinoma: useful prognostic determinants? Journal of Urology 1993;150:490–4.

Gapany M, Pavelic ZP, Kelley DJ, et al. Immunohistochemical detection of c-myc protein in head and neck tumors. Archives of Otolaryngology and Head and Neck Surgery 1994;120:255–9.

Gilbertson R, Wickramasinghe C, Hernan R, et al. Clinical and molecular stratification of disease risk in medulloblastoma. British Journal of Cancer 2001;85:705–12.

Hehir DJ, McGreal G, Kirwan WO, et al. C-myc oncogene expression: a marker for females at risk of breast carcinoma. Journal of Surgical Oncology 1993;54:207–9.

Jamec B, Chana J, Grover R, Grobbelaar AO. The Merkel cell carcinoma: survival and oncogene markers. Journal of European Academy of Dermatology and Venereology 2000;14:400–4.

Kee KH, Lee MJ, Ro JY. Oncoprotein changes in the flat lesions with atypia and invasive neoplasms of the urinary bladder. Oncology Reports 2001;8:579–83.

King LA, Okagaki T, Gallup DG, et al. Mitotic count, nuclear atypia, and immunohistochemical determination of Ki-67, c-myc, p21-ras, c-erbB2, and p53 expression in granulosa cell tumors of the ovary: mitotic count and Ki-67 are indicators of poor prognosis. Gynecological Oncology 1996;61:227–32.

Lloyd RV, Osamura RY. Transcription factors in normal and neoplastic pituitary tissues. Miscroscopic Research and Technology 1997;39:168–81.

Naidu R, Wahab NA, Yadav M, Kutty MK. Protein expression and molecular analysis of c-myc gene in primary breast carcinomas using immunohistochemistry and differential polymerase chain reaction. International Journal of Molecular Medicine. 2002;9:189–96.

Nagashima G Aoyagi M, Yamamoto S, et al. Involvement of disregulated c-myc but not c-sis/PDGF in atypical and anaplastic meningiomas. Clinical Neurology and Neurosurgery 2001;103:13–8.

Prins J, De Vries EG, Mulder NH. The myc family of oncogenes and their presence and importance in small cell carcinoma and other tumor types. Anticancer Research 1993;13:1373–85.

Vastrik I, Makela TP, Koskinen PJ, et al. Myc protein: partners and antagonists. Critical Reviews in Oncology 1994;5:59–68.

Collagen Type IV

Sources/clones

Accurate (COL-4), Biodesign (1o42, MC4-HA), Biogenesis (2D8/29), Biogenex (CIV22), Biotec (XCD02), Dako (CIV22), ICN (polyclonal, 1042), Immunotech (CIV22), Milab, Sanbio (SB11), Serotec (PHM-12), Sera-Lab (1042), Serotec (CIV22, PHM-12).

Fixation/preparation

Most commercial clones of antibodies are immunoreactive in fixed paraffin-embedded sections but only following HIER and enzymatic predigestion with trypsin before the application of the primary antibody.

Background

Basal lamina is mostly formed by a dense 40–60 nm-thick layer called the lamina densa and an electron lucent layer adjacent to the cell membrane known as the lamina lucida. A loose layer of connective tissue known as the lamina reticularis may be present under the lamina densa. Type IV collagen localizes exclusively to the lamina densa and by immunoelectron microscopy is found in both lamina densa and lamina lucida. Laminin has the same distribution but appears to be more intensely localized to the lamina lucida. Other components of basal lamina include heparin sulfate proteoglycan, entactin, fibronectin and type V collagen, the latter probably a stromal rather than basal lamina component.

Applications

Diagnostic applications of collagen type IV immunostaining have mostly centered around the demonstration of basal lamina in invasive tumors, particularly epithelial tumors, and their changes with tumor invasion and metastasis (Birembaut et al, 1985). In particular, the demonstration of an intact basal lamina has been used to distinguish benign glandular proliferations such as microglandular adenosis and sclerosing adenosis from well-differentiated carcinoma like tubular carcinoma of the breast (Raymond & Leong, 1991; Tavassoli & Bratthauer, 1993). Immunostaining for collagen type IV has also been applied to discriminate between C-cell hyperplasia and microscopic medullary carcinoma of the thyroid. The former showed complete investment of the C-cells by a continuous rim of basal lamina, whereas, the latter was typified by deficiencies of the basal lamina so that the constituent C-cells were extrafollicular in location (McDermott et al, 1995). There was also focal reduplication of basal lamina, apparently tumor derived. Studies of collagen type IV in the matrix proteins and basal lamina of glomeruli and tubules have been reported (Schleucher & Olgemoller, 1992; Ziyadeh, 1993). Immunostaining for basal lamina has been shown to be a rapid and useful way to distinguish major variants of congenital epidermolysis bullosa, especially when electron microscopy is not available (Bolte & Gonzalez, 1995). Fragmentation of the basal lamina has been demonstrated with collagen type IV immunostaining in the mucosa of patients with celiac disease (Verbeke et al, 2002) and decreased or discontinuous staining for basal lamina has been employed to distinguish invasive foci of adenocarcinoma from misplaced submucosal epithelial deposits in adenomatous polyps (Yantiss et al, 2002).

Distinctive patterns of basal distribution were recently demonstrated in various types of soft tissue tumors, adding to the

163

diagnostic armamentarium for this group of neoplasms, which are often difficult to separate (Leong et al, 1997) (Appendix 1.25). While the presence of basal lamina cannot be used as an absolute discriminant for blood vessels and lymphatic spaces, the latter lack the reduplication of the basal lamina characteristic of blood vessels and generally show thin and discontinuous staining for collagen type IV and laminin (Suthipintawong et al, 1995). The distinctive staining observed around blood vessels has been employed as a marker when performing capillary density measurements (Madsen & Holmskov, 1995).

Glomus tumors of the stomach have been shown to be invested by net-like pericellular staining for both collagen IV and laminin (Miettinen et al, 2002) and cytological preparations of the same type of tumor were described to be strongly positive for collagen IV, smooth muscle actin and muscle specific actin (Gu et al, 2002).

Interestingly, besides being typically a major component of basal lamina, collagen type IV is also expressed in the interstitial stroma of extrahepatic bile duct carcinoma and schirrous gastric carcinoma where it may play a role in desmoplastic stroma formation (Chen et al, 2000).

Comments

Earlier work on basal lamina immunostaining was restricted to the use of immunofluoresence techniques in frozen sections because of the lack of sensitivity of the available antibodies and techniques. The application of HIER combined with proteolytic digestion makes it possible to produce consistent immunostaining of paraffin-embedded, routinely prepared tissue sections.

References:

Birembaut P, Caron Y, Adnet J-J. Usefulness of basement membrane markers in tumoral pathology. Journal of Pathology 1985;145: 283–96.

Bolte C, Gonzalez S. Rapid diagnosis of major variants of congenital epidermolysis bullosa using a monoclonal antibody against collagen type IV. American Journal of Dermatopathology 1995;17:580–3.

Chen Y, Sasatomi E, Satoh T, et al. Abnormal distribution of collagen type IV in extrahepatic bile duct carcinoma. Pathology International 2000;50:884–90.

Gu M, Nguyen PT, Cao S, Lin F. Diagnosis of gastric glomus tumor by endoscopic ultrasound-guided fine needle aspiration biopsy. A case report with cytologic, histologic and immunohistochemical studies. Acta Cytologica 2002;46:560–6.

Leong AS-Y, Vinyuvat S, Suthipintawong C, Leong FJ. Patterns of basal lamina immunostaining in soft-tissue and bony tumors. Applied Immunohistochemistry 1997;5:1–7.

Madsen K, Holmskov U. Capillary density measurements in skeletal muscle using immunohistochemical staining with anti-collagen type IV antibodies. European Journal of Applied Physiology 1995;71:472–4.

McDermott MB, Swanson PE, Wick MR. Immunostains for collagen type IV discriminate between C-cell hyperplasia and microscopic medullary carcinoma in multiple endocrine neoplasia, type 2a. Human Pathology 1995;26:1308–12.

Miettinen M, Paal E, Lasota J, Sobin LH. Gastrointestinal glomus tumors: a clinicopathologic, immunohistochemical, and molecular genetic study of 32 cases. American Journal of Surgical Pathology 2002;26:301–11.

Raymond WA, Leong AS-Y. Assessment of invasion in breast lesions using antibodies to basement membrane components and myoepithelial cells. Pathology 1991;23:291–7.

Schleicher ED, Olgemoller B. Glomerular changes in diabetes mellitus. European Journal of Clinical Chemistry and Clinical Biochemistry 1992;30:635–40.

Suthipintawong C, Leong, AS-Y, Vinyuvat S. A comparative study of immunomarkers for lymphangiomas and hemangiomas. Applied Immunohistochemistry 1995;3:239–44.

Tavassoli FA, Bratthauer GL. Immunohistochemical profile and differential diagnosis of microglandular adenosis. Modern Pathology 1993;6:318–22.

Verbeke S, Gottel M, Fernandez M, et al. Basement membrane and connective tissue proteins in interstinal mucosa of patients with celiac disease. Journal of Clinical Pathology 2002;55:440–5.

Yantiss RK, Bosenberg MW, Antonioli DA, Odze RD. Utility of MMP-1, p53, E-cadherin, and collagen IV immunohistochemical stains in the differential diagnosis of adenomas with misplaced epithelium versus adenomas with invasive adenocarcinomas. American Journal of Surgical Pathology 2002;26:206–15.

Ziyadeh FN. Renal tubular basement membrane and collagen type IV in diabetes mellitus. Kidney International 1993;43:114–20.

Cyclin D1 (bcl-1)

Sources/clones

Dako (DCS-6), Immunotech (5D4), Novocastra (P2D11F11, DCS-6).

Fixation/preparation

Clone DCS-6 is effective on paraffin wax embedded tissue. We have found that microwave antigen unmasking in Tris buffer produces an optimum immunoreaction. Alkaline pH of 8–10 produces the best results although tissue sections do not tolerate the higher pH. The combination of superheating to 120°C and Tris buffer at pH 8 produces optimal immunostaining (Leong et al, 2002).

Background

The G1 cyclin gene, cyclin D1 (PRAD-1, CCND-1), located on chromosome 11q13, exhibits characteristics of known cellular oncogenes (Schuuring et al, 1992). It plays an integral role in normal cell growth control and a complementary role in the in vitro transformation of cultured cells (Hinds et al, 1994; Hirama & Koeffler, 1995). Mechanisms of abnormal 11q13 regulation leading to cyclin D1 overexpression include genomic amplification in a variety of carcinomas (Foulkes et al, 1993; Proctor et al, 1991;

Karlseder et al, 1994), characteristic t(11; 14) (q13; q32) reciprocal chromosomal translocations in mantle cell lymphoma (Ott et al, 1996; Brynes et al, 1997; Williams et al, 1991) and chromosome 11 pericentric inversions in parathyroid adenomas. Together, cyclin D1 and cyclin-dependent kinase (Cdk) activities are required for completion of the G1/S transition in the normal mammalian cell cycle (Bartkova et al, 1994). Further, cyclin D1 inhibits the growth suppressive function of retinoblastoma tumor-suppressor protein (Ewen et al, 1993). Cyclin D1 is a 36 kD protein with a maximum expression of cyclin D1 occurring at a critical point in mid to late G1 phase of the cell cycle. Recombinant prokaryotic fusion protein is used as the antigen to raise antibody to cyclin D1 (Class IgG2a). In normal tissues, cyclin D1 expression is found restricted to the proliferative zone of epithelial tissues, and is absent from several other tissues such as lymph node, spleen and tonsil.

Applications

Many neoplasms, including mantle cell lymphoma, parathyroid adenomas and a spectrum of carcinomas including breast, supradiaphragmatic squamous cell, ovarian and bladder transitional cell carcinomas demonstrate overexpression of cyclin-D1 antibody on paraffin sections. Immunohistochemical demonstration of nuclear cyclin D1 protein was observed in 75 per cent of mantle cell lymphoma; and was not found in normal B-cells and other B-cell lymphomas (including follicle center cell lymphoma, diffuse large B-cell lymphoma, lymphocytic lymphoma and MALT lymphoma) (Ott et al, 1996). More recent interest in this marker involves its potential as a prognostic indicator in a variety of epithelial tumors. Cyclin D1 overexpression was demonstrated in metastasizing papillary microadenocarcinomas of the thyroid (Khoo et al, 2002). Overexpression of the protein predicted for poor prognosis in estrogen receptor-negative breast cancer patients (Umekita et al 2002), recurrence in nasopharyngeal carcinoma (Lai et al, 2002) and reduced disease-free survival in papillary bladder carcinoma (Sgambato et al, 2002).

Comments

Cyclin D1 is the main marker currently available to distinguish mantle cell lymphoma from the other small B-cell lymphomas (Appendix 2.9). Breast cancer tissue may be used as positive controls.

References

Bartkova J, Lukas J, Strauss M, Bartek J. Cell cycle-related variation and tissue-restricted expression of human cyclin D1 protein. Journal of Pathology 1994;172:237–45.

Brynes RK, McCourty A, Tamayo R, Jenkins K, Battifora H. Demonstration of Cyclin D1 (Bcl-1) in mantle cell lymphoma. Enhanced staining using heat and ultrasound epitope retrieval. Applied Immunohistochemistry 1997;5:45–8.

Ewen ME, Sluss HK, Sherr CJ, Matsushime H, Kato J, Livingston DM. Functional interactions of the retinoblastoma protein with mammalian D-type cyclins. Cell 1993;73:487–97.

Foulkes WD, Campbell IG, Stamp GWH, Trowsdale J. Loss of heterozygosity and amplification on chromosome 11q in human ovarian cancer. British Journal of Cancer 1993;67:268–73.

Hinds PW, Dowdy SF, Eaton EN, Arnold A, Weinberg RA. Function of a human cyclin gene as an oncogene. Proceedings of the National Academy of Science USA 1994;91:709–13.

Hirama T, Koeffler HP. Role of the cyclin-dependent kinase inhibitors in the development of cancer. Blood 1995;86:841–54.

Karlseder J, Zeillinger R, Schneeberger C, Czerwenka K, Speiser P, Kubista E, Birnbaum D, Gaudray P, Theillet C. Patterns of DNA amplification at band q13 of chromosome 11 in human breast cancer. Genes, Chromosomes and Cancer 1994;9:42–8.

Khoo ML, Ezzat S, Freeman JL, Asa SL. Cyclin D1 protein expression predicts metastatic behavior in thyroid papillary microcarcinomas but is not associated with gene amplification. Journal of Clinical Endocrinology and Metabolism 2002;87:1810–3.

Lai JP, tong CL, Hong C, et al. Association between high initial tissue levels of cyclin D1 and recurrence of nasopharyngeal carcinoma. Laryngoscope 2002;112:402–8.

Leong AS-Y, Lee ES, Yin H et al. Superheating antigen retrieval. Applied Immunohistochemistry and Molecular Morphology 2002;10:263–8.

Motokura T, Bloom T, Kim HG, Juppner H, Ruderman JV, Kronenberg HM, Arnold A. et al. A novel cyclin encoded by a bcl-1-linked candidate oncogene. Nature 1991;350:512–5.

Ott MM, Helbing A, Ott G, Bartek J, Fischer L, Dürr A, Kreipe H, Müller-Hermelink HK. bcl-1 rearrangement and cyclin D1 protein expression in mantle cell lymphoma. Journal of Pathology 1996;179:238–42.

Proctor AJ, Combs LM, Cairns JP, Knowles MA. Amplification at chromosome 11q13 in transitional cell tumors of the bladder. Oncogene 1991;6:789–95.

Sgambato A, Migaldi M, Faraglia B, et al. Cyclin D1 expression in papillary superficial bladder cancer: its association with other cell cycle-associated proteins, cell proliferation and clinical outcome. International Journal of Cancer 2002;97:671–8.

Schuuring E, Verhoeven E, Mooi WJ, Michalides RJ. Identification and cloning of two overexpressed genes, U21B31/PRADI and EMS1, within the amplified chromosome 11q13 region in human carcinomas. Oncogene 1992;7:355–61.

Umekita Y, Ohi Y, Sagara Y, Yoshida H. Overexpression of cyclin D1 predicts for poor prognosis in estrogen receptor-negative breast cancer patients. International Journal of Cancer 2002;98:415–8.

Williams ME, Meeker TC, Swerdlow SH. Rearrangement of the chromosome 11 bcl-1 locus in centrocytic lymphomas: analysis with multiple breakpoint probes. Blood 1991;78:493–8.

Cytokeratins

Cytokeratins (CKs) belong to a group of proteins known as intermediate filaments that constitute the cytoskeletal structure of virtually all epithelial cells. Being intermediate between microfilaments (6 nm) and microtubules (25 nm), the intermediate filaments comprise five characteristic groups based on cellular origin: CKs (epithelium), glial (astrocytes), neurofilaments (nerve cells), desmin (muscle) and vimentin (mesenchymal cells). More recently, these families of cytoskeletal proteins – the intermediate filaments, have been reclassified into six sub-types (Table 1) (Miettinen, 1993). Intermediate filament proteins are composed of a 310 amino acid residue central region known as the rod domain, which is flanked by end domains of varying length and sequence, known as the head and tail. It is these flanking sequences that are the most immunogenic, responsible for the different properties and functions of the intermediate filament proteins. Being exposed, these molecules are also sensitive to fixation artefact due to the formation of cross linkages. It is also important to note that due to the 30–50% sequence homology between the amino acid sequences of intermediate filaments of different types, monoclonal antibodies may cross react with different intermediate filament types (Battifora, 1988).

Table 1 Classification of intermediate filaments	
Type	**Intermediate filament protein**
I	acidic cytokeratin (CK9-CK20).
II	basic cytokeratin (CK1-CK8).
III	vimentin (mesenchymal cells), desmin (muscle), glial fibrillary acid protein (glial cells and astrocytes), peripherin (neuronal cells).
IV	neurofilaments protein triplet (neurones)
V	nuclear laminin proteins (nuclear lamina)
VI	nestin (CNS stem cells).

CKs are present in both benign and malignant epithelial cells, independent of cellular differentiation. However, CK immunohistochemistry utilizing subset selective antibodies has extended beyond the typing of epithelial tumors, with recent descriptions of non-epithelial cells and tumors expressing CK.

The CKs are a family of proteins coded by different genes and the expression in epithelial cells is dependent on the embryonic development and degree of cellular differentiation. Practically, the most important CKs have been classified and numbered, based on the catalogue of Moll et al (Table 2) (Moll et al, 1982). These CKs were identified by the biochemical properties in two-dimensional gel electrophoresis of tissue extracts with their identification based on their isoelectric points and molecular weight. Hence, two groups of CKs emerge: Type I/A (CK 9–20) with an acidic isoelectric point and type II/B (CK 1–8) with a basic-neutral isoelectric point. Apart from a few exceptions, CKs are numbered from the highest to the lowest molecular weight in each group (Table 3) (Miettinen, 1993).

An interesting phenomenon is the existence of the keratin intermediate filaments as pairs. With some exceptions, all other CKs form polymers with their corresponding member from each type (Table 3). Hence, it follows that all epithelial cells contain at least two CKs. For example, whilst hepatocytes harbor a single pair of CK 8 and 18, keratinocytes may contain as many as ten CKs.

Table 2 Cytokeratins according to Moll's classification

Moll's cytokeratin groups	Chromosome localisation	Molecular weight (x10^{-3})	Isoelectric point
K1	12	67	7.8
K2	12	65	6.1
K3	12	64	7.5
K4	12	59	7.3
K5	12	58	7.4
K6	12	56	7.8
K7	12	54	6.0
K8	12	52	6.1
K9	17	64	5.4
K10	17	56.5	5.3
K11	17	56	5.3
K12	17	55	4.9
K13	17	51	5.1
K14	17	50	5.3
K15	17	50	4.9
K16	17	48	5.1
K17	17	46	5.1
K18	17	45	5.7
K19	17	40	5.2
K20	17	46	5.7

Table 3 Keratins 1–20 with their molecular weight, and most important distribution (Modified from Mietten, 1993)

Type II	MW(kd)	Distribution	Type I	MW(kd)
		Epidermis – palms and soles	9	64
1	67	Epidermis, keratinizing squamous epithelia	10	56.5
2	65		11	56
3	63	Cornea	12	55
4	59	Non-keratinizing squamous epithelia (internal organs)	13	51
5	58	Basal cells – squamous and glandular epithelia, myoepithelium, mesothelium.	14	50
		Squamous epithelia	15	50
6	56	Squamous epithelia (hyperproliferative)	16	48
7	54	Simple epithelial. Basal cells – glandular epithelia, myoepithelium	17	46
8	52	Simple epithelia.	18	45
		Simple epithelia, most glandular, some squamous epithelia (basal).	19	40
		Simple epithelia – intestines and stomach, Merkel cells	20	46

Keratin pairs appear in the same line
MW = molecular weight; kD = Kilodalton.

Thus, these laws governing the expression of various CKs are observed in part by neoplastic cells, forming the basis for the application of antibodies to CKs within neoplastic cells (indicating epithelial differentiation) using immunohistochemical methods (Schaafsma et al, 1994). The emergence of selective monoclonal antibodies identifying individual CKs now offers the advantage of immunohistochemical detection with morphological correlation (Heatley, 1996). Monoclonal antibodies to CKs may be divided into two categories: (i) a broad group that recognizes many members of the keratin family (see later in chapter) and (ii) a selective group that reacts with isolated CKs; in this regard, only CKs 7 and 20 will be considered in detail. Nevertheless, Table 4 provides a list of the most important CK subtypes in some epithelial neoplasms (Miettinen, 1993). In addition, popular commercially available antibodies to broad groups of CKs (Table 5) will also be detailed individually. False-negativity due to masking of keratin epitopes and loss of antigenicity warrants antigen retrieval in most instances. Hence, the need for extensive and carefully controlled optimization of every new antibody before diagnostic application cannot be overemphasized.

References

Battifora H. Diagnostic uses of antibodies to keratins: a review and immunohistochemical comparison of seven monoclonal and three polyclonal antibodies. In: Fenoglio-Preiser CM, Wolff M, Rilke F. eds. Progress in Surgical Pathology, Vol. VIII. Springer-Verlag, 1988, pages 1–15.

Heatley, MK. Cytokeratins and cytokeratin staining in diagnostic histopathology (commentary). Histopatholpgy 1996;28:479–83.

Miettinen M. Keratin immunohistochemistry: update of applications and pitfalls. In: Rosen PP, Fechner RE. eds. Pathology Annual, Part 2/Vol 28. Appleton & Lange, 1993, pp 113–143.

Moll R, Franke WW, Schiller DL, Geiger B, Krepler R. The catalog of human cytokeratins: patterns of expression in normal epithelia, tumors and cultured cells. Cell 1982;31:11–24.

Schaafsma HE, Ramaekers FCS. Cytokeratin subtyping in normal and neoplastic epithelium: basic principles and diagnostic applications. In: Rosen PP, Fechner RE. eds. Pathology Annual, Part I/Vol 29. Appleton & Lange, 1994, pp 21–62.

Table 4 Summary of the most important keratin subtypes of some epithelial tumors (Modified from Miettinen, 1993)

Carcinoma Type	Keratin Composition (Moll's Catalog)									
	4	5	7	8	13	14	17	18	19	20
Squamous cell carcinoma, skin		+				+			+*	
Squamous cell Ca of oesophagus	+				+	+			+	
Ductal carcinoma of breast			+	+		+*	+*	+	+	
Malignant mesothelioma		+	+	+		+		+	+	
Adenocarcinoma, lung			+	+				+	+	
Adenocarcinoma, colon				+				+	+	+
Adenocarcinoma, pancreas			+	+				+	+	+*
Hepatocellular carcinoma				+				+	+*	
Carcinoid tumor/small cell carcinoma				+				+	+**	
Merkel cell carcinoma				+				+	+	+
Renal (cell) adenocarcinoma				+				+	+**	
Transitional cell carcinoma, low gr.	+		+	+	+			+	+	+*
Transitional cell carcinoma, high gr.			+	+	+*			+	+	
Thyroid carcinoma, papillary				+				+	+	
Thyroid carcinoma, follicular				+				+	+*	
Adenocarcinoma of prostate			+*	+				+	+	
Adenocarcinoma of ovary			+	+				+	+	+*

*Occasionally present/minor component
**often but inconsistently present

Cytokeratins

Table 5 †Specificities of Selected Cytokeratin Antibodies

Mol Wt (kD)	35βH11	34βE12	AE1	AE3	*Anti-Bovine keratin	*Anti-Callus keratin	Cam 5.2	KL1	MNF116
39							+		+
40			+					+	
45							+	+	+
48			+	+					
50		+	+					+	
51				+					
52			+	+					+
52.5							+	+	
54	+								
56				+		+		+	+
56.5		+	+	+					
57		+							
58		+		+	+		+	+	
60					+				
64						+			
65				+					
65.5								+	
66				+					
67				+					
68		+							

Antibody sources: 35βH11 and 34βE12 (Dakopatts, California, USA); Anti-Bovine keratin, Anti-Callus keratin (Dakopatts, California, USA); AE1, AE3 (available as AE1/3 cocktail) (Boehringer, Sydney, Australia; Dakopatts, California, USA); Cam 5.2 (Becton Dickinson, California, USA); KL1 (Immunotech, Marseille, France); MNF116 (Dakopatts, California, USA).
*polyclonal antisera
†specificities as supplied by manufacturers
Other cytokeratin cocktails not included above: Pankeratin cocktail (Bio Tek solution, Inc, Santa Barbara, Ca, USA – cocktail of AE1, AE3, Cam 5.2 and 35 BH11); LP34 (Dako Corp, Capinteria, Ca, USA – K5, K6, K17 and K19); Pancytokeratin antibodies (Novocastra, Burlingame, Ca, USA – K5, K6, K8 and K18); Anti-cytokeratin 5/6 (Chemicon International, Inc, Temecula, Ca, USA – K5 and K6).

Cytokeratin 20 (CK 20)

Sources/clones

American Research Products (IT-Ks 20.10, IT-Ks 20.3, IT-Ks 20.5), Biodesign, Cymbus Biosciences (Ks 20.8, Ks 20.3, Ks 20.5), Dako (K 20.8). Progen (IT-Ks 20.3, IT-Ks 20.5, IT-Ks 20.8).

Fixation/preparation

Formalin-fixed, paraffin-embedded tissue is ideally suited for this antibody. Immunoreactivity requires pre-treatment with a sodium citrate buffer with heated antigen retrieval. Enzyme pretreatment (trypsin or pronase) should not be used as it abolishes signal. The antibody is not recommended for cryostat sections or cell smears due to cross reactivity with cytokeratin 20- (CK 20) negative epithelia.

Background

CK 20 is a low-molecular weight cytokeratin, that was originally identified by Moll et al as protein IT in two-dimensional gel electrophoresis of cytoskeletal extracts of intestinal epithelia (Moll et al, 1990). The antibody reacts with the 46KD cytokeratin intermediate filament isolated from villi of duodenal mucosa.

CK 20 is less acidic than other type 1 cytokeratins and is particularly interesting because of its restricted range of expression.

In normal tissues it is expressed only in gastrointestinal epithelium, urothelium and Merkel cell. Other epithelial cells, including breast epithelia do not react with CD20, nor does it recognize other intermediate filament proteins.

Applications

Following extensive testing on both primary and metastatic carcinomas, it was concluded that tumors expressing CK 20 were derived from normal epithelia expressing CK 20 (Moll et al, 1992). Hence, colorectal carcinomas consistently express CK 20 while gastric adenocarcinomas and other carcinomas of the gastrointestinal tract express this cytokeratin isotype less frequently. In addition, adenocarcinomas of the biliary tree, pancreatic duct, mucinous ovarian tumors and transitional-cell carcinomas also demonstrate positive immunoreaction. Hence, the application of CK 20 antibody for determining the site of origin of carcinomas has been recently mooted largely due to absence of

CK 20 expression in adenocarcinomas of the breast, lung, endometrium and non-mucinous tumors of the ovary (Appendix 1.14, 1.15, 1.20, 1.32). In fact CK 20 has recently contributed to immunohistochemical evidence supporting the appendiceal origin of pseudomyxoma peritonei in women (Ronnett et al, 1997).

Immunostaining for CK 7 and CK 20 has been shown to be useful in the differentiation of ovarian metastases from colonic carcinoma and primary ovarian carcinoma (Loy et al, 1996). A CK 7-/CK 20+ immuno-phenotype was seen in 94% of metastatic colonic carcinomas to the ovary, 5% of primary ovarian mucinous carcinomas and none of the primary ovarian endometrioid or serous carcinomas.

The almost consistent staining of Merkel cell carcinoma for CK 20 and the very low frequency of CK 20 reactivity in other small cell carcinomas (except those salivary gland of origin) can help to resolve the diagnostic dilemma between Merkel cell carcinoma and metastatic small cell carcinoma presenting in the skin (Chan et al, 1997) (Appendix 1.20). In fact, it was recently shown that CK 20 positivity in a small cell carcinoma of uncertain origin is strongly predictive of Merkel cell carcinoma, especially when the majority of tumor cells are positive. In contrast, a negative CK 20 reaction practically rules out Merkel cell carcinoma, provided an effective antigen retrieval technique is used and appropriate immunoreaction obtained with other cytokeratin antibodies.

Finally, CK 20 positivity is often encountered in transitional cell carcinomas of the bladder but is rare in squamous carcinomas of that organ or adenocarcinoma of prostate (Moll et al, 1992).

Comments

The combined application of CK20 and CK7 allows the separation of a number of epithelial tumours as shown in Table 1.

CK 20 works extremely well in paraffin sections with microwave antigen retrieval in citrate buffer. It is extremely useful for the distinction between colonic and non-mucinous ovarian adenocarcinomas. Identifying Merkel cell carcinoma from metastatic small cell carcinoma to the skin is also easily accomplished with CK 20. Colonic carcinoma tissue sections should be used as positive control tissue.

Table 1 CK7 and CK20 Immunoexpression in Epithelial Tumors

	CK20+	CK20-
CK7+	Bladder	Cervical
	Breast	Endometrium
	Colon	Esophagus
	Bile duct	Breast
	Ovary	GIT carcinoid
	mucinous	Bile duct
	Pancreas	Pancreas
	Stomach	Kidney
		Liver
		Lung carcinoid
		Neuroendocrine
		Lung squamous
		Lung small cell
		Mesothelioma
		Ovary
		Salivary gland
		Thyroid
CK7-	Merkel	Adrenal cortex
	cell	Esophagus
	Stomach	GIT carcinoid
	Colon	Germ cell
		Kidney
		Liver
		Lung carcinoid
		Neuroendocrine carcinoma
		Lung squamous
		Lung small
		Mesothelioma
		Prostatic
		Soft tissue epithelioid sarcoma
		Thymus

References

Chan JKC, Suster S, Wenig BM, Tsang WYW, Chan JBK and Lau ALW. Cytokeratin 20 immunoreactivity distinguishes Merkel cell (primary cutaneous neuroendocrine) carcinomas and salivary gland small cell carcinomas from small cell carcinomas of various sites. American Journal of Surgical Pathology 1997;21:226–234.

Loy TS, Calaluce RD, Keeney GL. Cytokeratin immunostaining in differentiating primary ovarian carcinoma from metastatic colonic adenocarcinoma. Modern Pathology 1996;9:1040–1044.

Moll R, L''we A, Laufer J, Franke WW. Cytokeratin 20 in human carcinomas. A new histodiagnostic marker detected by monoclonal antibodies. American Journal of Pathology 1992;140:427–447.

Moll R, Schiller DL, Franke WW. Identification of protein IT of the intestinal cytokeratin as a novel type I cytokeratin with unusual properties and expression patterns. Journal of Cell Biology 1990;111:567–580.

Ronnett BM, Shmookler BM, Diener-West M, Sugarbaker PH, Kurman RJ. Immunohistochemical evidence supporting the appendiceal origin of pseudomyxoma peritonei in women. International Journal of Gynecologic Pathology 1997;16:1–9.

Cytokeratin 7 (CK 7)

Sources/clones

Accurate (LP5K), American Research Products (RCK105), Biodesign, Biogenesis (C35, C18), Biogenex (OV-TL 12/30), Bioprobe (C-35, C68), Boehringer Mannheim (KS7–18), Chemicon, Dako (OV-TL 12/30), Cymbus Bioscience (C46, LP5K), Dako (OV-TL 12/30), Intracell Corp (RCK105), Japan Tanner (C35, C68), Milab (RCK 105), Novocastra (LP5K), Sanbio (OV-TL 12/30, RCK105), Saxon (RCB105), Sera Lab (CK7), Sigma (LD5 68).

Fixation/preparation

Cytokeratin 7 (CK 7) can be used on formalin-fixed paraffin-embedded tissue sections. Enzymatic digestion with proteolytic enzymes such as trypsin should be performed before staining. Pronase digestion has been found to be harsh on CK 7. This antibody may also be used on acetone and/or methanol-fixed cryostat sections or fixed cell smears. It enjoys the additional advantage of being used on cytological preparations already stained by the Papanicolaou stain. For cell smears, the APAAP technique is recommended.

Background

CK 7 antibody reacts with the 54 kDa cytokeratin intermediate filament protein isolated from human OTN II ovarian carcinoma cells and other cell lines. Identified as CK 7 according to Moll's catalog, it is a basic cytokeratin found in most glandular and transitional epithelia (Moll et al, 1982).

In normal tissue CK 7 reacts with many ductal and glandular epithelia, but not stratified squamous epithelia. It is also reactive with transitional epithelium of urinary tract. Hepatocytes are negative whilst bile ducts are positive. In addition, lung and breast epithelia are positive with this antibody, whilst colon and prostate epithelial cells are negative (van Niekerk et al, 1991).

Applications

CK is expressed in specific subtypes of ovarian, breast and lung adenocarcinoma, whilst carcinomas of the colon are negative (Ramackers et al, 1990). Recent studies have indicated that a CK 7+CK 20-immunophenotype is helpful in distinguishing metastatic colonic adenocarcinoma from primary ovarian carcinomas, particularly the endometrioid type (with the exception of the mucinous type) (Loy et al, 1996) (Appendix 1.14, 1.15). Occasional ovarian mucinous carcinomas may show the same immunophenotype as metastatic colonic carcinomas (CK 7-CK 20+). Using the same immunophenotypic profile (together with CK 18), CK 7 was recently shown to assist in determining that most ovarian mucinous tumors in pseudomyxoma peritonei in woman are secondary to appendiceal adenoma (Ronnett et al, 1997).

CK 7 is also useful to distinguish transitional cell carcinomas (+ve) from prostate cancer (-ve). The failure of CK 7 to interact with squamous cell carcinomas presents the potential for specificity for adenocarcinoma and transitional cell carcinoma.

Comments

We have found the combined use of CK 7 and CK 20 to be extremely useful in distinguishing ovarian carcinomas (except mucinous) from colonic adenocarcinomas. Serous ovarian carcinoma tissue is recommended for positive control tissue.

References

Loy TS, Calaluce RD, Keeney GL. Cytokeratin immunostaining in differentiating primary ovarian carcinoma from metastatic colonic adenocarcinoma. Modern Pathology 1996;9:1040–44.

Moll R, Franke WW, Schiller DL, Geiger B, Krepler R. The catalog of human cytokeratins: patterns of expression in normal epithelia, tumors and cultured cells. Cell 1982;31:11–24.

Ronnett BM, Shmookler BM, Diener-West M, Sugarbaker PH, Kurman RJ. Immunohistochemical evidence supporting the appendiceal origin of pseudomyxoma peritonei in women. International Journal of Gynecologic Pathology 1997;16:1–9.

Ramackers F, van Niekerk C, Poels L, Schaafsma E, Huijsman A, Robben H, et al. Use of monoclonal antibodies to keratin 7 in differential diagnosis of adenocarcinomas. American Journal of Pathology 1990;136:641–55.

van Niekerk CC, Jap PHK, Raemaekers FCS, van de Molengraft F, Poels LG. Immunohistochemical demonstration of keratin 7 in routinely fixed paraffin embedded tissues. Journal of Pathology 1991;165:145–52.

Cytokeratins-MNF 116

Sources/clones

Dako (MNF 116), Immunotech (MNF 116).

Fixation/preparation

MNF 116 performs well on formalin-fixed, paraffin-embedded tissue sections. Enzymatic predigestion with proteolytic enzymes such as trypsin and pronase is essential prior to immunodetection, trypsin being superior for MNF116. This antibody may also be applied to acetone-fixed cryostat sections or fixed cell smears. Incubation of the primary antibody for 1 hr at 37°C yields better immuno-reaction.

Background

MNF 116 antibody detects an epitope that is present in a wide range of keratins. These comprise a number of discrete polypeptides, whose molecular weights range from 45–56.5 kD. These correspond to Moll's keratin numbers 5,6,8, 17 and probably 19 (Moll et al, 1982). The MNF 116 immunogen was derived from a crude extract of splenic cells in a nude mouse engrafted with MCF-7 cells.

In normal tissue, the MNF 116 antibody shows a broad pattern of reactivity with epithelial cells from simple glandular to stratified squamous epithelium. Epithelial cells are labeled irrespective of ectodermal, mesodermal or endodermal origin. However, due to the cross reactivity with the other members of the family of intermediate filaments, this antibody (not unlike other monoclonal anti-keratin antibodies) cross reacts with non-epithelial cells including smooth muscle, dendritic cells in lymph nodes, syncytiotrophoblasts, some cortical neurons and a minority of plasma cells.

Applications

MNF 116 demonstrates excellent immunopositivity with a wide range of benign and malignant epithelial neoplasms. A strong pattern of staining is observed in squamous cell carcinoma (including nasopharyngeal carcinoma), small cell carcinoma, sarcomatoid carcinoma, spindle cell carcinoma, adenocarcinoma and mesotheliomas. In small cell carcinomas, a characteristic juxtanuclear globular pattern of staining has been found to be extremely useful in identifying

these neoplasms. Both epithelioid and spindle cell components of mesotheliomas react with this antibody (Miettinen, 1993).

MNF 116 is also useful in confirming the diagnosis in a wide range of soft tissue neoplasms. Monophasic and biphasic synovial sarcomas demonstrate strong positivity (albeit focal in the spindle cells). Vascular neoplasms that react with this broad range cytokeratin antibody include epithelioid hemangioendothelioma (focal), epithelioid angiosarcoma and sinonasal hemangiopericytoma (Mentzel et al, 1997). Epithelioid sarcoma (and the recently described proximal variant) require cytokeratin positivity for diagnosis (Evans & Baer, 1993; Guillou et al, 1997). Other tumors in which cytokeratin positivity is essential for diagnosis include desmoplastic small round-cell tumors, chordomas and extra-renal rhabdoid tumors that are consistently positive. Mixed tumors and myoepitheliomas arising in soft tissue were recently described and shown to express pan-keratin (Kilpatrick et al, 1997).

Among germ cell tumors, embryonal carcinoma and yolk sac tumors are consistently positive with MNF 116.

The following neoplasms may demonstrate aberrant staining with MNF 116. The co-expression of cytokeratins in smooth muscle tumors is well-described (Ramackers et al, 1988). Cytokeratin-positive cells have been revealed in plasmacytoma (Wotherspoon et al, 1989). A few primitive neuroectodermal tumors may show focal cytokeratin expression. Rarely, myofibroblasts may demonstrate focal cytokeratin positivity (Hojo et al, 1995; Jones et al, 1993). Quite logically all of these potential diagnostic pitfalls may clearly be avoided if relevant panels of immunohistochemical antibodies are applied.

Comments

MNF 116 has developed into a first line antibody in the application of cytokeratins to surgical pathology. It is however necessary to be aware of the aberrant immunoreactions in order to avoid misdiagnosis. It is therefore unwise to arrive at a diagnosis based on the assessment of a single cytokeratin marker without the application of other relevant antibodies used in a diagnostic panel to exclude other possibilities. Any epithelial tissue – glandular or squamous – is suitable for use as positive control for MNF116.

References

Evans HL, Baer SC. Epithelioid sarcoma: a clinicopathologic and prognostic study of 26 cases. Seminars in Diagnostic Pathology 1993;10:286–91.

Guillou L, Wadden C, Coindre JM, Krausz T, Fletcher CDM. Proximal-type epithelioid sarcoma: a distinctive aggressive neoplasm showing rhabdoid features. American Journal of Surgical Pathology 1997;21:130–46.

Hojo H, Newton WA, Hamondi AB et al. Pseudosarcomatous myofibroblastic tumour of the urinary bladder in children: A study of 11 cases with review of the literature: An Intergroup Rhabdomyosarcoma Study. American Journal of Surgical Pathology 1995;19:1224–36.

Jones EC, Clement PB, Young RE. Inflammatory pseudotumour of the urinary bladder. A clinicopathological, immunohistochemical, ultrastructural and flow cytometric study of 13 cases. American Journal of Surgical Pathology 1993;17:264–74.

Kilpatrick SE, Hitchcock MG, Kraus MD, Calonje E, Fletcher CDM. Mixed tumours and myoepitheliomas of soft tissue: a clinicopathologic study of 19 cases with a unifying concept. American Journal of Surgical Pathology 1997;21:13–22.

Mentzel T, Beham A, Calonje E et al. Epithelioid haemangioendothelioma of skin and soft tissue: clinicopathologic and immunohistochemical study of 30 cases. American Journal of Surgical Pathology 1997;21:363–74.

Miettinen M. Keratin immunohistochemistry: update of applications and pitfalls. In: Rosen PP, Fechner RE. eds. Pathology Annual, Part 2/Vol 28. Appleton & Lange, 1993, pages 113–43.

Moll R, Franke WW, Schiller DL, Geiger B, Krepler R. The catalog of human cytokeratins: patterns of expression in normal epithelia, tumors and cultured cells. Cell 1982;31:11–24.

Ramackers FCS, Pruszczynski M, Smedts F. Cytokeratins in smooth muscle cells and smooth muscle tumors. Histopathology 1988;12:558–61.

Wotherspoon AC, Norton AJ, Isaacson PG. Immunoreactive cytokeratins in plasmacytomas. Histopathology 1989;14:141–50.

Cytokeratins-CAM 5.2

Sources/clones

Becton Dickinson (Cam 5.2).

Fixation/preparation

CAM 5.2 can be applied to both frozen and formalin-fixed paraffin embedded tissue. Trypsin enzyme pretreatment for antigen retrieval is essential for paraffin sections.

Background

CAM 5.2 was derived from hybridization of mouse P3/NS1/1-Ag4–1 cells with spleen cells from BALB/c mice immunized with a human colorectal carcinoma line, HT29 (Makin et al, 1984). It comprises mouse IgG_{2a} heavy chain and kappa light chains from spleen parent and myeloma cell lines. The antibody CAM 5.2 detects human cytokeratin epitopes with molecular weights 52kDa and 45kDa corresponding to Moll's catalog numbers 8 and 18 respectively (Moll et al, 1982). In normal tissue CAM 5.2 reacts with secretory epithelia but not stratified squamous epithelium.

Applications

Anti-cytokeratin antibody CAM 5.2 is useful for the detection of adenocarcinomas, mesotheliomas and certain carcinomas derived from squamous epithelia; the latter including spindle cell carcinomas (Battifora, 1988). It should, however, be noted that some squamous cell carcinomas do not stain with CAM 5.2, e.g., those in the cervix, vagina and esophagus. The ability of CAM 5.2 to detect epithelial neoplasms but not normal stratified squamous epithelium (e.g. skin) can be exploited to distinguish between Paget's disease (both mammary and extra-mammary) from superficial spreading melanoma. CAM 5.2 is especially useful in the demonstration of subtle metastatic deposits of breast carcinoma cells in lymph nodes (Raymond & Leong, 1987) and bone marrow. It also successfully reacts with renal cell carcinomas, hepatocellular carcinomas and cholangio-carcinomas (Johnson et al, 1987). CAM 5.2 also detects neuroendocrine carcinomas, (including small cell carcinoma and Merkel cell carcinomas) germ cell tumors (with the exception of seminoma), synovial and epithelioid sarcomas (Leader et al, 1986). This antibody is also useful for the detection of epithelial cells in thymomas, particularly when masked by lymphocytes. It is reputed not to detect melanomas (except in cryostat sections). (Leader et al, 1986).

Non-epithelial tissues which react with anti-cytokeratin CAM 5.2 include smooth muscle, rare sarcomas of breast (Pitts et al, 1987), meningiomas (hyaline bodies or malignant variants) (Theaker et al, 1986), and rosettes of neuroblastomas. B-cell anaplastic large cell lymphoma, confirmed by immunohistochemistry and immunoglobulin gene rearrangements, has been shown to be immunoreactive with CAM 5.2 (Frierson et al, 1994).

It should also be noted that large-cell lymphoma of B-cell lineage (verified with PCR) has been shown to be rarely reactive for cytokeratin 8 (Lasota et al, 1996)

Comments

Although CAM 5.2 has a narrow range of cytokeratin immunodetection in surgical pathology, it has been proven to be useful as a second line marker in specific circumstances. For example, in the identification of spindle cell carcinoma of the skin, subtle metastatic deposits of carcinoma in lymph nodes and to distinguish Paget's disease from superficial spreading melanoma. It also shows strong staining reaction with neuroendocrine carcinomas.

References

Battifora H. Diagnostic uses of antibodies to keratins: A review and immunohistochemical comparison of seven monoclonal and three polyclonal antibodies. In: Fenoglio-Preiser, CM., Wolff M, Rike F. Progress in Surgical Pathology (Vol VIII), Springer-Verlag 1988, pages 10–15.

Frierson HF Jr, Bellafiore FJ, Gaffey MJ, McCary WS, Innes DJ Jr, Williams ME. Cytokeratin in anaplastic large cell lymphoma. Modern Pathology 1994;7:317–21.

Gatter KC, Ralfkiaer E, Skinner J et al. An immunohistochemical study of metaplastic carcinomas and sarcomas of the breast. Journal of Clinical Pathology 1985;38:1353–7.

Johnson DE, Warnke R, Herndier B, Rouse R. An immunohistochemical study of the cytokeratin profiles of hepatocellular carcinomas and cholangiocarcinomas. Laboratory Investigation 1987;56:34A.

Lasota J, Hyjek E, Koo CH, Blonski J, Miettinen M. Cytokeratin-positive large-cell lymphomas of B-cell lineage. American Journal of Surgical Pathology 1996;20:346–54.

Leader M, Patel J, Makin C, Henry K. An analysis of the sensitivity and specificity of the cytokeratin (CAM 5.2) for epithelial tumours. Results of a study of 203 sarcomas, 50 carcinomas and 28 malignant melanomas. Histopathology 1986;10:1315–24.

Makin CA, Bobrow LG, Bodmer WF. Monoclonal Antibody to Cytokeratin for use in Routine Histopathology. Journal of Clinical Pathology 1984;37:975–83.

Moll R, Franke WW, Schiller DL, Geiger B, Krepler R. The catalog of human cytokeratins: Patterns of expression in normal epithelia, tumors and cultured cells. Cell 1982;31:11–24.

Pitts MD, Rojas BS, Rouse RV, Kempson RL. An immunohistochemical study of metaplastic carcinomas and sarcomas of the breast. Laboratory Investigation 1987;56:61A.

Theaker JM, Gatter KC, Esiri MM et al. Epithelial membrane antigen and cytokeratin expression by meningiomas: an immunohistological study. Journal of Clinical Pathology 1986;39:435–9.

Cytokeratins-AE1/AE3

Sources/clones

Dako (AE1/AE3), Zymed (AE1, AE3).

Fixation/preparation

This antibody is suitable for immunohistochemical staining of formalin-fixed paraffin-embedded or frozen tissue sections. Trypsin or pepsin digestion/antigen retrieval is necessary before staining of formalin-fixed paraffin-embedded tissue sections, although pepsin has been found to be superior to trypsin. The Zymed antibody is prediluted and ready to use. However, if DAB is used as a chromogen for immunodetection, then a further dilution of the primary antibody may be required.

Background

The antibody AE1/AE3 is a mixture of two monoclonal antibodies, raised against human epidermal keratins (Woodcock-Mitchell et al, 1982). AE1 recognizes most of the acidic (type 1) keratins with molecular weights 56.5, 50, 50[1],48, and 40 kD. AE3 recognizes all known basic (type II) cytokeratins (Moll et al, 1982) . This combination shows broad reactivity and is claimed to stain

almost all epithelia and their neoplasms. It is also reputed not to cross react with other members of the intermediate filaments.

Applications

The wide reactivity of AE1/AE3 expressed in simple epithelia and their tumors, including cytokeratins expressed in complex stratified squamous epithelia, permits identification of a wide range of epithelial-derived tumors. Hence, strong staining of AE1/AE3 has been demonstrated in adenocarcinomas (eg. colorectal, gastric, breast, prostate), renal cell carcinoma, hepatocellular carcinoma, transitional cell carcinoma, small cell carcinoma, carcinoid tumors, epithelial component of pleomorphic adenoma and squamous cell carcinoma of the skin (including the spindle cell variant), cervix and bronchus. Thymomas, mesotheliomas (including the sarcomatoid component) and chordomas consistently stain with AE1/AE3. Non-epithelial tumors that demonstrate AE1/AE3 positivity include germ cell tumors (except seminomas), synovial sarcoma and epithelioid sarcoma. Cross reactivity in some leiomyosarcomas has been

documented (Battifora, 1988; Goddard et al, 1991; Spagnolo et al, 1983; Tseng et al, 1982).

In a recent study of 290 cases of hepatocellular carcinoma, immunohistochemical evidence of biliary differentiation (reactivity with AE1/AE3 or cytokeratin 19) was found in 29.3% of cases. These hepatocellular carcinomas with biliary differentiation showed clinical features of greater aggressiveness with poorer cellular differentiation and higher expression of proliferation markers (Wu et al, 1996).

Comments

The pan-keratin marking potential of antibody AE1/AE3, places it in an ideal position to screen for neoplasms of epithelial origin, especially poorly differentiated carcinomas of diverse origin and to distinguish these from melanoma and lymphoma. Another useful role is the identification of micrometastases e.g., breast secondaries in lymph nodes and bone marrow.

References

Battifora H. Diagnostic uses of antibodies to keratins: a review and immunohistochemical comparison of seven monoclonal and three polyclonal antibodies. In: Fenoglio-Preiser CM, Wolff M, Rilke F. eds. Progress in Surgical Pathology, Vol. VIII. Springer-Verlag, 1988, pages 1–15.

Goddard MJ, Wilson B, Grant JW. Comparison of commercially available cytokeratin antibodies in normal and neoplastic adult epithelial and non-epithelial tissues. Journal of Clinical Pathology 1991;44:660–3.

Moll R, Franke WW, Schiller DL, Geiger B, Krepler R. The catalog of human cytokeratins: Patterns of expression in normal epithelia, tumors and cultured cells. Cell 1982;31:11–24.

Spagnolo DV, Michie SA, Crabtree GS, Warnke RA, Ronse RV. Monoclonal anti-keratin (AE1) reactivity in routinely processed tissue from 166 human neoplasms. American Journal of Clinical Pathology 1983;84:697–704.

Tseng SCG, Jarvinen M, Nelson WG, Twang J-W, Woodcock-Mitchell J, Sun T-T. Correlation of specific keratin with different types of epithelial differentiation: Monoclonal antibody studies. Cell 1982;30:361–72.

Woodcock-Mitchell J, Eichner R, Nelson WG, Sun T-T. Immunolocalisation of keratin polypeptides in human epidermis using monoclonal antibodies. Journal of Cell Biology 1982;95:580–8.

Wu PC, Fang JWS, Lau VKT et al. Classification of hepatocellular carcinoma according to hepatocellular and biliary differentiation markers, clinical and biological implications. American Journal of Pathology 1996;149:1167–75.

Cytokeratins-MAK-6®

Sources/clones

Triton Diagnostics, Zymed
(MAK-6® – clones KA4 and
UCD/PR10.11).

Fixation/preparation

MAK-6® works well in routinely
fixed, paraffin-embedded tissue
sections. Trypsin pretreatment is
necessary for antigen unmasking.
Incubation of the primary
antibody for 1 hr at 37°C or
overnight incubation at room
temperature yields superior
immunostaining. Pre-incubated
with blocking reagents to reduce
non-specific background staining
has been recommended, however,
we have found this to be
unnecessary.

Background

MAK-6® antibody cocktail
contains an optimized mixture of
two murine monoclonal
antibodies of IgG1 isotype.
Antibody kA 4 recognizes human
cytokeratin types, 14,15,16 and
19 while antibody UCD/PR-
10.11 recognizes human
cytokeratin 8 and 18.

Antibody UCD/PR 10.11
was produced using shed
extracellular antigen purified
from MCF-7 tissue culture media
and was selected for its specificity
to cytokeratin types 8 and 18
(Chan et al, 1986). Antibody KA4
was produced against human sole
epidermis and was selected for its
specificity to cytokeratin types
14,15,16 and 19.

Applications

MAK-6® is reputed to stain all
cases of squamous cell carcinomas
and the majority of
adenocarcinomas, carcinoid
tumors and undifferentiated
carcinomas. Lymphomas,
melanomas, gliomas/astrocytomas
and the majority of sarcomas do
not demonstrate MAK-6®
positivity. The latter is related to
the expected cytokeratin
expression in synovial sarcomas
and epithelioid sarcomas. It
should be noted that the majority
of ependymomas and basal cell
carcinomas of the skin also do
not express MAK-6®. Caution
should be observed in assessing
metastatic carcinomas to the
brain, since MAK-6® may rarely
show cross-reactivity with neural
tissue. In these instances
application of antibody to glial
fibrillary acidic protein (GRAP)
would be helpful (Cooper et al,
1985; McNutt et al, 1988).

Comments

We have found MAK-6® to be a
useful pan-keratin marker.
Strong immunoreaction is
demonstrated in tissue of
epithelial origin. Used in
conjunction with other pan-
keratin markers, the majority of
neoplasms showing cytokeratin
expression may be identified.

References

Chan R, Rossitto PV, Edwards BF,
Cardiff RD. Presence of
proteolytically processed keratins
in the culture medium of MCF-7
cells. Cancer Research 1986;46
(Pt 1): 6353–9.

Cooper D, Schermer A, Sun T-T.
Classification of human epithelia
and their neoplasms using
monoclonal antibodies to
keratins: strategies, applications
and limitations. Laboratory
Investigation 1985;52:243–56.

McNutt MA, Bolen JW, Vogel AM et
al. In: Wick MR & Siegel GP.
Eds. Monoclonal antibodies in
diagnostic immunohistochemistry.
Marcel Dekker Inc, New York
1988, pgs 51–70.

NOTES

Cytokeratins 34βE12

Sources/clones

Dako, Enzo diagnostics.

Fixation/preparation

34β12 may be used on formalin-fixed, paraffin-embedded tissue sections. Although reactivity on formalin-fixed tissue is obtainable, better consistency is observed on Carnoy's or methacarn-fixed material. Proteolytic treatment with pronase (for prostatic basal cells) and microwave antigen retrieval (for papillary carcinoma of thyroid) is essential for formaldehyde-fixed material. This antibody may also be used on acetone-fixed cryostat sections and fixed cell smears. Incubation of the primary antibody for 1 hr at room temperature is sufficient for prostatic basal cells. However, incubation of primary antibody at 4°C overnight is necessary for papillary carcinoma of the thyroid gland.

Background

34βE12 identifies keratins of approximately 66 kD and 57 kD in extracts of stratum corneum. The antibody reacts with keratins 1,5,10 and 14 in Moll's catalog (MW 68 kD, 58 kD, 56.5 kD, 50 kD) respectively (Moll et al, 1982). In normal tissue the antibody labels squamous, ductal and other complex epithelia.

Applications

Perhaps the most useful application for 34βE12 is in the detection of basal cells of the prostatic acini (O'Malley et al, 1990; Amin, 1995). Demonstration of this high molecular weight cytokeratin in the basal cells of prostatic acini is indicative of benignity. Further 34βE12 is negative in adenocarcinoma of the prostate. In this context 34βE12 is also useful to demonstrate the basal cells in basal cell hyperplasia (partial or atypical) and atypical adenomatous hyperplasia of the prostate; the latter being difficult to distinguish morphologically from prostatic adenocarcinoma.

More recently the role of 34βE12 in diagnostic thyroid pathology was highlighted (Appendix 1.30). It was shown that 34βE12 positivity was confined to papillary carcinoma of the thyroid, whereas follicular neoplasms and hyperplastic nodules were either negative or showed focal staining (Raphael et al, 1995).

34βE12 is also consistently positive in squamous cell carcinomas, ductal carcinoma of breast, pancreas, bile duct and salivary gland. It has also been demonstrated in transitional cell carcinomas of the bladder, nasopharyngeal carcinoma, thymomas and epithelioid mesotheliomas (Gown & Vogel, 1985).

Whilst this antibody has a variable positivity with adenocarcinomas, it is negative in hepatocellular carcinoma, renal cell carcinoma and endometrial carcinoma. Mesenchymal tumors, lymphomas, melanomas, neural tumors and neuroendocrine tumors are negative.

Comments

We have found 34βE12 to be extremely useful in both diagnostic prostatic and thyroid pathology. It should be noted that different incubation protocols need to be followed for these two applications of 34βE12.

References

Amin MB. Prostate mesonephric remnant hyperplasia. Advances in Anatomical Pathology 1995;2:110–2.

Gown AM, Vogel AM. Monoclonal antibodies to intermediate filament proteins . III. Analysis of

tumors. American Journal of
Clinical Pathology
1985;84:413–424

Moll R, Franke WW, Schiller DL,
Geiger B, Krepler R. The catalog
of human cytokeratins: Patterns of
expression in normal epithelia,
tumors and cultured cells. Cell
1982;31:11–24.

O'Malley FP, Grignon DJ, Shum DT.
Usefulness of immunoperoxidase
staining with high-molecular-
weight cytokeratin in the
differential diagnosis of small-
acinar lesions of the prostate
gland. Virchows Archives A
Pathologic Anatomy
1990;417:191–6.

Raphael SJ, Apel RL, Asa SL.
Detection of high-molecular-
weight cytokeratins in neoplastic
and non-neoplastic thyroid
tumors using microwave antigen
retrieval. Modern Pathology
1995;8:870–2.

Cytokeratin 5/6 (CK 5/6)

Sources/clones

Chemicon International;
Boehringer Mannheim, Zymed
Laboratories, Dako (Clone
D5/16B4).

Fixation/preparation

The antibody is immunoreactive
in formalin-fixed tissues and
reactivity is enhanced by heat-
stimulated antigen retrieval
combined with enzyme
digestion.

Background

Cytokeratins 5 and 6 correspond
to keratins of 58 and 56 kD
respectively. Clone D5/16B4 is a
monoclonal antibody raised
against cytokeratin 5 (CK5). The
CK5 (58kDa) is a high molecular
weight, basic type of cytokeratin
expressed in the basal,
intermediate and superficial layers
of stratified epithelia, transitional
epithelium and mesothelium.
CK6 (56kDa) is also a high
molecular weight, basic
cytokeratin expressed by
proliferating squamous
epithelium, palmoplantar cell,
mucosa and epidermal
appendages. Although this
combination of cytokeratins is
expressed by a number of

different epithelia its popularity
stems from its use in the
diagnosis of mesothelioma.
Morphologically, the
mesothelium is similar to simple
epithelium, and like,
adenocarcinomas, mesotheliomas
express simple epithelial keratins
such as CK7, CK8, and CK19.
Similar to squamous cell
carcinoma, mesothelioma also
express the stratified epithelial
keratins such as CK14, CK5/6
andCK17 (Chu et al, 2001;
2002).

Using the AE14 monoclonal
antibody that recognizes keratin
5, Moll et al (1989) reported
immunopositivity in 92% (12/13)
of epithelial and biphasic
mesotheliomas with negative
results in pulmonary
adenocarcinomas. Whilst
recommended as a useful marker
to distinguish epithelial
mesotheliomas from pulmonary
adenocarcinomas, these results
were not repeated, probably due
to the restricted use of keratin 5
on frozen tissue. More recently, a
study using CK5/6 on formalin-
fixed paraffin-embedded tissue
demonstrated positive
immunostaining in 100% pleural
epithelial mesothelioma with
81% pulmonary adenocarcinomas
being negative (Clover et al,
1997). The remaining

adenocarcinomas were weak,
equivocal or focally positive.
However, the majority of
sarcomatoid or desmoplastic
mesotheliomas in this study were
negative for CK5/6. Another
study produced a 100%
cytokeratin 5/6 immunopositivity
in epithelial mesotheliomas with
reciprocal negativity in
pulmonary adenocarcinomas
(Ordonez, 1998). The frequency
of CK5/6 positivity in
mesotheliomas varies because of
case selection, sarcomatoid
mesothelioma being less likely to
be positive than biphasic and
epithelioid mesothelioma. Chu et
al (2002) found two thirds of
biphasic mesothelioma and only
one third of sarcomatoid
mesothelioma to be positive for
CK5/6, the immunostaining
being focal and only restricted to
areas of squamous differentiation
(Chu et al, 2001; 2002).

Applications

CK5/6 is useful in
discriminating between epithelial
mesotheliomas and pulmonary
adenocarcinomas but does not
exclude metastatic carcinomas
from some sites as the latter may
be positive for CK5/6 (Chu &
Weiss, 2002). Furthermore, as it
is often negative in sarcomatoid

mesothelioma, CK5/6 is best utilized in a panel of antibodies for this differential diagnosis. CK5/6 also stains both reactive and neoplastic mesothelium. It has also been suggested for use in the differential diagnosis of squamous cell carcinoma and adenocarcinoma, being positive in basal cells and stratum spinosum cells of squamous epithelium so that the immunoexpression of CK5/6 in a poorly differentiated metastatic carcinoma is highly predictive of a primary tumor of squamous differentiation (Kaufman et al, 2001). It has been reported that intense CK5/6 positivity in ductal hyperplasia and negative staining of most cases of atypical ductal hyperplasia and DCIS may assist in the differential diagnosis of atypical proliferations of the breast (Otterbach et al, 2000) but this requires confirmation. It should be noted that this marker is of low specificity as adenocarcinoma of the salivary gland and lung, squamous cell carcinoma of the lung, anus, esophagus, cervix, upper aerodigestive tract and skin, and carcinomas of the urinary bladder, breast, and pancreas, as well as synovial sarcoma have been reported to immunoexpress CK5/6.

CK5/6 immunostaining has been employed successfully as a substitute for 34βE12 for the identification of basal cells in benign prostatic glands, allowing their distinction from neoplastic glands (Abrahams et al, 2002)

Comments

CK5/6 demonstrates a diffuse cytoplasm immunopositive reaction. Skin or prostate gland may be a useful source of positive control tissue.

References

Abrahams NA, Ormsby AH, Brainard J. Validation of cytokeratin 5/6 as an effective substitute for keratin 903 in the differentiation of benign from malignant glands in prostate needle biopsies. Histopathology 2002;41:35–41.

Clover J, Oates J, Edwards C: Anti-Cytokeratin 5/6: A positive marker for epithelioid mesothelioma. Histopathology 1997;31:140–3.

Chu PG, Weiss LM. Expression of cytokeratin 5/6 in epithelial neoplasms: an immunohistochemical study of 509 cases. Modern Pathology 2002;15:6–10.

Chu PG, Weiss LM. Cytokeratin 14 expression in epithelial neoplasms: a survey of 435 cases with emphasis on its value in differentiating squamous cell carcinomas from other epithelial neoplasms. Histopathology 2001;39:9–16.

Chu PG, Weiss LM. Keratin expression in human tissues and neoplasms. Histopathology 2002;40:403–39.

Kaufman O, Fietze E, Mengs J, et al. Value of p63 and CK5/6 as immunohistochemical markers for the differential diagnosis of poorly differentiated and undifferentiated carcinomas. American Journal of Clinical Pathology 2001;116:823–30.

Moll R, Dhouailly D, Sun T-T: Expression of cytokeratin 5 as a distinctive feature of epithelial and biphasic mesotheliomas. Virchows Archives. B Cellular Pathology 1989;58:129–45.

Ordonez NG: In search of a positive immunohistochemical marker for mesothelioma: An update. Advances in Anatomical Pathology 1998;5:53–60.

Otterbach F, Bankfalvi A, Bergner S, et al. Cytokeratin 5/6 immunohistochemistry assists the differential diagnosis of atypical proliferations of the breast. Histopathology 2000;37:232–40.

Other Pan-cytokeratin Cocktails

A number of other pan-cytokeratin cocktails are commercially available.

Pankeratin cocktail (Bio Tek Solution, Inc, Santa Barbara, Ca, USA) is a cocktail comprising monoclonal antibodies to AE1, AE3, Can 5.2 and 35βH11. This is a useful cocktail which reacts to virtually all epithelia and their corresponding tumors.

Pan-cytokeratin antibodies (Novocastra, Burlingame, Ca, USA) contains monoclonal antibodies to K5, K6, K8 and K18. This cocktail is said to recognise almost all epithelial tissues and their neoplasms.

Clone L34 Antibody (Dako Corp. Carpinteria, Ca. USA). A broad spectrum monoclonal antibody that detects K5, K6,

K17 and K19. It thus labels both simple glandular and stratified squamous epithelium.

Wide-spectrum Screening Antibody (Dako Corp., Carpinteria, Ca., USA). This is a useful polyclonal antibody raised to bovine skin that cross reacts with human keratins.

NOTES

Cytomegalovirus (CMV)

Sources/clones

Accurate (E13, CCH2), American Research Products (1692–18), Axcel (CCH2), Biodesign (084, BM204, BM219, polyclonal), Biogenesis (BM204, polyclonal), Biogenex (BM204, polyclonal), Chemicon, Dako (AAC10, CCH2), EY Labs, Fitzgerald (M2103126, M210312), Sera Lab (E13), Zymed (DDG9/CCH2).

Fixation/preparation

These antibodies are suitable for immunohistochemical staining of paraffin-embedded tissue sections. Enzymatic pre-digestion with trypsin or pepsin is required for clone CCH2. These antibodies may also be used to detect CMV early nuclear proteins in infected human embryonic fibroblasts 24 hours following inoculation of clinical specimens on cell culture.

Background

The CCH2 clone recognizes a 43kD protein, whilst the DDG9 clone recognizes a 76kD protein, both having been demonstrated in glycine extracted CMV antigen. These proteins are expressed in the immediate early and early stage of CMV replication in infected cells (Zweygberg et al, 1986). Early viral proteins are expressed in the nucleus of infected cells within 6–24 hours of infection and prior to viral DNA replication. Several late viral proteins may be demonstrated in the nucleus and the cytoplasm of infected cells. The different viral proteins can be demonstrated in infected cell cultures as well as in infected tissue (Senson & Kaplan, 1985). These antibodies do not cross react with adenoviruses or other herpes viruses.

Applications

These antibodies to CMV demonstrate the virus in infected cells producing a nuclear immunopositive reaction. However, at a later stage, both a nuclear and cytoplasmic immunoreaction with the early CMV antigen is produced, especially with the Zymed product. Antibodies to CMV have a wide application to diagnostic surgical pathology, especially when characteristic CMV inclusions are not clearly evident. CMV infection (latent or active) may be seen in salivary glands, lungs, kidneys, GIT and lymph nodes. Awareness of CMV as an opportunistic infection in the context of immunosuppression, invokes the use of CMV immunohistochemistry for definitive diagnosis (Schwartz & Wilcox, 1992). Recently CMV esophagitis has been observed as a florid aggregate of macrophages without typical inclusions (Greenson, 1997). Small biopsy specimens with such a morphological picture warrants further immunohistochemical study to identify CMV as has been shown in a case of a 6 week old infant with upper gastrointestinal hemorrhage from CMV esophagitis (Weinstein et al, 2001). Conversely, chemotherapy toxicity may mimic CMV gastritis, necessitating CMV immunohistochemistry to exclude false-positives (Canioni et al, 1995). Antibodies to CMV may also be applied for the identification of atypical CMV inclusions in gastrointestinal mucosal biopsy specimens, where classic inclusions are rarely found (Schwartz & Wilcox, 1992). The proper recognition of CMV-infected cells in the context of immunosuppression is critical, so that effective therapy is not delayed, preventing further viral dissemination. A study of colonoscopic biopsies from asymptomatic 82 patients with acquired immunodeficiency syndrome using immunostaining detected 34 patients with CMV colitis (Ornstein & Dieterich, 2001). Immunolabelling for CMV in transbronchial biopsies of transplanted lung revealed alveolar epithelial cells and capillary endothelial cells as the major targets of CMV, with rare involvement of ciliated and bronchiolar smooth muscle cells (Morbini & Arbustini, 2001).

Comments

It has been shown that immunohistochemistry with CCH2 detects a higher number of CMV infected cells than in situ hybridisation (Niedobitek et al, 1988). Hence, for routine diagnostic purposes at least, CMV immunohistochemistry would appear to be the method of choice for a rapid, sensitive and specific method of CMV detection.

References

Canioni D, Vassal G, Donadieu J, Hubert PH, Brousse N. Toxicity induced by chemotherapy mimicking cytomegalovirus gastritis. Histopathology 1995;26:473–5.

Greenson JK. Macrophage aggregates in cytomegalovirus esophagitis. Human Pathology 1997;28:375–8.

Morbini P, Arbustini E. In situ characterization of human cytomegalovirus infection in bronchiolar cells in human transplanted lung. Virchows Archives 2001;438:558–66.

Niedobitek G, Finn T, Herbst H et al. Detection of cytomegalovirus by in situ hybridisation and immunohistochemistry using new monoclonal antibody CCH2: a comparison of methods. Journal of Clinical Pathology 1988;41:1005–9.

Orenstein JM, Dieterich DT. The histopathology of 103 consecutive colonoscopy biopsies from 82 symptomatic patients with acquired immunodeficiency syndrome: original and look-back diagnoses. Archives of Pathology and Laboratory Medicine 2001;125:1042–6.

Schwartz DA, Wilcox CM. Atypical cytomegalovirus inclusions in gastrointestinal biopsy specimens from patients with the acquired immunodeficiency syndrome: diagnostic role of in situ nucleic acid hybridization. Human Pathology 1992;3:1019–26.

Swenson PD, Kaplan MH. Rapid detection of cytomegalovirus in cell culture by indirect immunoperoxidase staining with monoclonal antibody to an early nuclear antigen. Journal of Clinical Microbiology 1985;21:669–73.

Weinstein M, Ford-Jones E, Cutz E. Esophagitis and perinatal cytomegalovirus infection. Pediatric Infectious Disease Journal 2001;20:545–6.

Zweygberg WB, Wirgart B, Grillner L. Early detection of cytomegalovirus in cell culture by a monoclonal antibody. Journal of Virological Methods 1986;14:65–9.

Cytotoxic Molecules (TIA-1, Granzyme B, Perforin)

Sources/clones

TIA-1

Coulter (2G9).

Granzyme B

Coulter (GB7), Sanbio/Monosan (GrB7), clone GB9 (Dr Kummer, Amsterdam, The Netherlands).

Perforin

Kaimya (KM583), Sumitomo Denko, Osaka, Japan (1B4), T cell Diagnostics (polyclonal),

Fixation/preparation

All antibodies against cytotoxic molecules can be used in formalin-fixed paraffin embedded tissues. High temperature antigen retrieval in citrate buffer is essential for staining.

Background

Natural killer cells and cytotoxic T lymphocytes are characterized by the presence of cytoplasmic granules that are released in response to target cell recognition. Among the wealth of cytotoxic molecules found in cytotoxic cells, perforin and granzyme B are two well-characterized proteins involved in one major pathway leading to apoptosis in target cells (Smyth et al, 1995; Lou et al, 1995). Perforin allows for the entry of granzyme molecules into the target cells, which then activate the apoptotic protease CPP32 (Darmon et al, 1995). The genes for perforin (Lichtenheld and Podack, 1989) and granzyme B (Smyth et al, 1995) have been cloned and antibodies directed against these molecules have been generated (Kummer et al, 1993). T-cell-restricted intracellular antigen (TIA-1), another molecule found in cytotoxic cells, is recognized by the antibody 2G9 (Anderson et al, 1990). The exact function of TIA-1 has not been elucidated. Since it induces DNA fragmentation of digitonin-permeabilized thymocytes (Tian et al, 1991), it may be implicated in the killing induced by cytotoxic lymphocytes. TIA-1 has been demonstrated in many intestinal intraepithelial lymphocytes of normal proximal small intestine and a corresponding increase of TIA-1 positive cells in active celiac disease (Russel et al, 1993).

Applications

The expression of all the three cytotoxic molecules appear to be largely restricted to cytotoxic cells. In addition, *in vitro* findings have also suggested that with rare exceptions, expression of perforin and granzyme B is also restricted to cytotoxic cells, including natural killer cells and cytotoxic T-cells (Liu et al, 1995; Smyth et al, 1995). Analysis of these antigens in conjunction with other marker molecules can therefore further specify the cellular origin of lymphocytes and lymphoid malignancies (Daum et al, 1997). In this regard, granzyme B, TIA-1 and perforin have been demonstrated in the majority of intestinal T-cell lymphomas but not in intestinal B-cell lymphomas and CD8-negative peripheral nodal T-cell lymphomas (Daum et al, 1997). Antibody 2G9, which recognizes TIA-1, proved to be the most sensitive immunohistological marker, being demonstrated in the highest number of cases and also in high numbers of neoplastic cells in positive cases (Daum et al, 1997). Hence, the cytotoxic differentiation in intestinal T-cell lymphoma was clearly shown, supporting derivation from intraepithelial cytotoxic T-lymphocytes.

Anaplastic large-cell lymphomas of T-cell (T-ALCL) have also been shown to express cytotoxic molecules with antibody GB9 to granzyme B, whilst being absent in B-cell anaplastic large-cell lymphomas, proving that T-ALCL are derived from activated cytotoxic T cells (Foss et al, 1996). Granzyme B-positive T-cell lymphomas have also been mainly found in mucosa-associated lymphoid tissue, being more often associated with angioinvasion: nasal, gastrointestinal tract and lung (de Bruin et al, 1994). It has also been shown that immunohistochemical staining with anti-TIA-1 can be used to identify cytolytic T lymphocytes in epidermal lesions of human graft versus host disease (Sale et al, 1992). Recent work with antibodies to cytotoxic molecules has shown that the predominant mechanism of cellular destruction in Kikuchi's lymphadenitis was apoptosis mediated by cytolytic lymphocytes (Takakuwa et al, 1996; Felgar et al, 1997).

Cutaneous CD8+ and CD56+ lymphomas appear to show different expressions of cytotoxic molecules with the former expression only one or two of the cytotoxic proteins compared to the latter, which expresses the entire panel of cytotoxic antigens. Such differences may explain differences in their biological behavior (Kamarashev et al, 2001). Primary CD30+ cutaneous lymphomas and lymphomatoid papulosis frequently express at least one of the cytotoxic proteins (Boulland et al, 2000). Sinonasal lymphomas of CD3+ CD56+ phenotype invariably expressed all three cytotoxic antigens and Epstein Barr viral RNA but not CD57 (Gaal et al, 2000). In general the aggressive T cell lymphomas including gastrointestinal T cell lymphoma (Katoh et al, 2000), gastric T cell lymphoma (Barth et al, 2000), hepatosplenic gammadelta T cell lymphoma (Ohshima et al, 2000), and some nodal T cell lymphomas (Ohshima et al, 1999) express varying quantities of the cytotoxic proteins.

Comments

Until recently, it was impossible to differentiate most functional T-cell subsets, e.g. suppressor and cytotoxic T-cell by membrane characteristics on paraffin-embedded tissue. The production of monoclonal antibodies against cytotoxic molecules has enabled the identification of the major components of the cytotoxic granules found in the cytoplasm of activated cytotoxic and natural killer cells. Intestinal T-cell lymphomas provide an ideal positive control for antibodies to cytotoxic molecules.

References

Anderson P, Nagler-Anderson C, O'Brien C, et al. A monoclonal antibody reactive with a 15-kDa cytoplasmic granule associated protein defines a subpopulation of CD8+ T lymphocytes. Journal of Immunology, 1990;144:574–82.

Barth TF, Leithauser F, Dohner H, et al. Primary gastric apoptosis-rich T-cell lymphoma co-expressing CD4, CD8, and cytotoxic molecules. Virchows Archives 2000;436:357–64.

Boulland ML, Wechsler J, Bagot M, et al. Primary CD30-positive cutaneous T-cell lymphomas and lymphomatoid papulosis frequently express cytotoxic proteins. Histopathology 2000;36:136–44.

Darmon AJ, Nicholson DW, Bleackley RC. Activation of apoptotic protease CPP32 by cytotoxic T-cell derived granzyme B. Nature 1995;377:446–8.

Daums S, Foss H-D, Anagnostopoulos I, et al. Expression of cytotoxic molecules in intestinal T-cell lymphomas. Journal of Pathology 1997;182:311–7.

De Bruin PC, Kummer JA, van der Valk P, et al. Granzyme B-expressing peripheral T-cell lymphomas: neoplastic equivalents of activated cytotoxic T cells with preference for mucosa-associated lymphoid tissue localization. Blood 1994;84:3785–91.

Felgar RE, Furth EE, Wasik MA, Gluckman SJ, Salhany KE. Histiocytic necrotizing lymphadenitis (Kikuchi's Disease): in situ labeling, immunohistochemical, and serologic evidence supporting cytotoxic lymphocyte-mediated apoptotic cell death. Modern Pathology 1997;10:231–41.

Foss HD, Anagnostopoulos I, Araujo I, et al. Anaplastic large cell lymphoma of T-cell and null-cell phenotype express cytotoxic molecules. Blood 1996;88:4005–11.

Gaal K, Sun NC, Hernandez AM, Arber DA. Sinonasal NK/T-cell lymphomas in the United States. American Journal of Surgical Pathology 2000;24:1511–7.

Kamarashev J, Burg G, Mingari MC, et al. Differential expression of cytotoxic molecules and killer cell inhibitory receptors in CD8+ and CD56+ cutaneous lymphomas. American Journal of Pathology 2001;158:1593–8.

Katoh A, Ohshima K, Kanda M, et al. Gastrointestinal T cell lymphoma: predominant cytotoxic phenotypes, including alpha/beta, gamma/delta T cell and natural killer cells. Leukemia and Lymphoma 2000;39:91–111.

Kummer JA, Kamp A, van Katwijk M, et al. Production and characterization of monoclonal antibodies raised against recombinant human granzymes A and B and showing cross reactions with the natural proteins. Journal of Immunological Methods 1993;163:77–83.

Lichtenheld MG, Podack ER. Structure of the human perforin gene. A simple gene organization with interesting potential regulatory sequences. Journal of Immunology 1989;143:4267–74.

Liu C-C, Walsh CM, Young JD-E. Perforin: structure and function. Immunology Today 1995;16:194–201.

Ohshima K, Suzumiya J, Sugihara M, et al. Clinical, immunohistochemical and phenotypic features of aggressive nodal cytotoxic lymphomas, including alpha/beta, gamma/delta T-cell and natural killer cell types. Virchows Archives 1999;435:92–100.

Ohshima K, Haraoka S, Harada N, et al. Hepatosplenic gammadelta T-cell lymphoma: relation to Epstein-Barr virus and activated cytotoxic molecules. Histopathology 2000;36:127–35.

Russell GJ, Nagler-Anderson C, Anderson P, Bhan AK. Cytotoxic potential of intraepithelial lymphocytes (IELs): presence of TIA-1, the cytolytic granule associated protein in human IELs in normal and diseased intestine. American Journal of Pathology 1993;143:350–4.

Sale GE, Anderson P, Browne M, Myerson D. Evidence of cytotoxic T-cell destruction of epidermal cells in human graft-vs-host disease: immunohistology with monoclonal antibody TIA-1. Archives of Pathology and Laboratory Medicine 1992;116:622–5.

Smyth MJ, Trapani JA. Granzymes: exogenous proteinases that induce target cell apoptosis. Immunology Today 1995;16:202–6.

Takakuwa T, Ohnuma S, Koike J, Hoshikawa M, Koizumi H. Involvement of cell-mediated killing in apoptosis in histiocytic necrotizing lymphadenitis (Kikuchi-Fujimoto disease). Histopathology 1996;28:41–8.

Tian Q, Streuli M, Saito H, Schlossman SF, Anderson P. A polyadenylate binding protein localized to the granules of cytolytic lymphocytes induced DNA fragmentation in target cells. Cell 1991;67:629–39.

NOTES

DBA.44 (Hairy Cell Leukemia)

Sources/clones

Dako, Immunotech

Fixation/preparation

The antibody is immunoreactive in formalin-fixed, paraffin-embedded tissues with immunoreactivity enhanced by proteolytic digestion but not by HIER.

Background

DBA.44 recognizes an unknown fixation–resistant B-cell differentiation antigen expressed by mantle-zone lymphocytes, reactive immunoblasts, monocytoid B-cells and a small proportion of high and low-grade lymphomas (al Saati et al, 1989; Hounieu et al, 1992). The monoclonal antibody was one of four generated against a B-lymphoma cell line (DEAU-cell line) grafted in athymic nude mice. Within the group of low-grade B-cell lymphomas, DBA.44 reacted principally with hairy-cell leukemia. Among node-based lymphomas, the strongest membrane staining was observed in centroblastic, immunoblastic and monocytoid B-cell lymphomas.

Applications

In a study of bone-marrow specimens from 166 patients with hairy-cell leukemia, strong positive staining of the "hairy" surface membranes was observed in routinely fixed and decalcified bone marrow biopsies of nearly all cases (Hounieu et al, 1992). Subsequent studies have proven the usefulness of DBA.44 in the identification of hairy cell leukemia, particularly in the detection of minimal residual disease following treatment (Wheaton et al, 1996). DBA.44 has been successfully applied to peripheral blood cytospin preparations and for ultrastructural labeling (Cordone et al, 1995).

The antibody has also been successfully applied to methyl-methacrylate embedded bone marrow biopsies (Kreft et al, 1997). DBA.44 appears to be a more sensitive marker of hairy cells than the traditional tartrate-resistant acid phosphatase (TRAP) activity which has long been a cornerstone in the diagnosis of hairy cell leukemia (Hoyer et al, 1997). Mantle zone lymphocytes and their corresponding lymphoma were DBA.44 and CD44 positive, with a weaker reaction for CDw75 than marginal zone lymphocytes and monocytoid B-cells whereas monocytoid B-cell lymphoma showed positivity for CD74 and CDw75 with positivity for DBA.44 observed in only occasional cases. Hairy cell leukemia, in contrast, were all positive for DBA.44, with a weak reaction for CD74 and a stronger positivity for CDw75 than either mantle cell lymphoma or monocytoid B-cell lymphoma specimens (Ohsawa et al, 1994).

Comments

While useful as a diagnostic marker, DBA.44 is not specific for hairy cells and should be used in a panel of antibodies to separate other B-cell lymphomas such as large cell lymphoma, mantle cell lymphoma and paraimmunoblasts of small cell lymphoma that may express the antigen (Hoyer et al, 1997). In one study that included a variety of neoplastic and non-neoplastic hematological disorders, the combined positivity for DBA.44 and tartrate-resistant acid phosphatase (TRAP) was found only in hairy cell leukemia (Hoyer et al, 1997) when an antibody to TRAP was used (Janckila et al, 1998).

References

al Saati T, Caspar S, Brousset P, et al. Production of anti-B monoclonal antibodies (DBB.42, DBA.44, DNA.7, and DND.53) reactive on paraffin-embedded tissues with a new B-lymphoma cell line grafted into athymic nude mice. Blood 1989;74:2476–85.

Cordone I, Annino L, Masi S, et al. Diagnostic relevance of peripheral blood immunocytochemistry in hairy cell leukaemia. Journal of Clinical Pathology 1995;48:955–60.

Hounieu H, Chittal SM, al Saati T, et al. Hairy cell leukaemia. Diagnosis of bone marrow involvement in paraffin-embedded sections with monoclonal antibody DBA.44. American Journal of Clinical Pathology 1992;98:26–33.

Hoyer JD, Li CY, Yam LT, et al. American Journal of Clinical Pathology 1997;108:308–15.

Janckila AJ, Wlaton SP, Yam LT. Species specificity of monoclonal antibodies to human tartrate-resistant acid phosphatase. Biotechnology and Histochemistry 1998;73:316–24.

Kreft A, Busche G, Bernhards J, Georgii A. Immunophenotype of hairy-cell leukaemia after cold polymerization of methyl-methacrylate embeddings from 50 diagnostic bone marrow biopsies. Histopathology 1997;30:145–51.

Ohsawa M, Kanno H, Machii T, Aozasa K. Immunoreactivity of neoplastic and non-neoplastic monocytoid B lymphocytes for DBA.44 and other antibodies. Journal of Clinical Pathology 1994;47:928–32.

Wheaton S, Tallman MS, Hakimian D, Peterson L. Minimal residual disease may predict bone marrow relapse in patients with hairy cell leukaemia treated with 2-chlorodeoxyadenosine. Blood 1996;87:1556–60.

Desmin

Sources/clones

Accurate (DEU10, 4B4B2, 33), American Research Products/Research Diagnostics (DEU10), Biodesign (33), Biogenesis (BIO-41H), Boehringer (DEB5), Dako (DE-R-11, D33), Eurodiagnostica (D9), EY Labs, Immunotech (D33, HHF35), Shandon Lipshaw (D33), Sigma (DEU10), Zymed (ZSD1).

Fixation/preparation

Most of the available antibodies are immunoreactive in fixed tissues and are enhanced by HIER (Pollock et al, 1995). Enzyme digestion is not required if HIER is employed. Clone D33 can be used without enzyme predigestion.

Background

Desmin belongs to the class of "intermediate" (10nm) filaments and is a cytoplasmic protein, which is characteristically found in myogenic cells. It has a molecular weight of 53 kD and is composed of an N-terminal "headpiece" and a C-terminal "tailpiece", both of which are nonhelical in conformation. The two pieces bracket an α-helical middle domain of about 300 amino acid residues which is highly conserved from species to species, with striking interspecies homology. This homology is even more than that exhibited between intermediate filament proteins in the same species, with cytokeratin, vimentin, glial fibrillary acidic protein, neurofilaments and desmin exhibiting sequence homology of about 30% (Nagai et al, 1985; Li et al, 1993).

In smooth muscle cells, desmin is associated with cytoplasmic dense bodies and subplasmalemmal dense plaques and in striated muscle it is linked to sarcomeric Z disks. Muscle cells depleted of desmin (skeletin) are still able to contract in response to adenosine triphosphate and calcium suggesting that desmin played no role in contractility but rather serves to maintain the relationship and orientation of actin and myosin filaments and to anchor them to the plasmalemmal. More recent findings suggest that, like other intermediate filaments of nonepithelial cells, desmin also serves a nucleic acid-binding function, are susceptible to processing by calcium-activated proteases, and are substrates for cyclic adenosine monophosphate-dependent protein kinases. With its shared structural homology to lamins, the proteins of the nuclear envelope, desmin may also serve as a modulator between extracellular influences governing calcium flux into the cell and may have a role in nuclear transcription and translation. These newer roles of the intermediate filaments including desmin, relegate the supportive cytoskeletal function of intermediate filaments to a secondary role (Goldman et al, 1985).

Applications

The development of sensitive and specific antibodies to the intermediate filaments including desmin heralded a new era in diagnostic immunohistochemistry as they allow the subtyping of many seemingly undifferentiated and pleomorphic tumors through intermediate filament analysis. Through the application of judiciously selected panels of antibodies directed to the differential diagnoses derived from the histologic and clinical findings, it is possible to separate the different entities in the diagnostic categories of pleomorphic spindle cell tumors and round cell tumors in soft tissues and skin (Leong et al,

Desmin

1989) (Appendix 1.11, 1.23, 1.24, 1.25, 1.26 and 1.27). The former group includes rhabdomyosarcoma, leiomyosarcomas and tumors with focal myogenic differentiation such as Triton tumors and malignant mixed Müllerian tumors. The latter group includes embryonal rhabdomyosarcoma, epithelioid leiomyoma and leiomyosarcoma and focal myogenic differentiation in small round cell tumors such as desmoplastic small round cell tumors and primitive/peripheral neuroepithelial tumors. All of these tumors may express desmin (Azumi et al, 1988; Leong & Wannakrairot, 1992, Parham et al, 1992). In this context, it is important to remember that although myogenous cells often express desmin, it is also seen in myofibroblasts. Focal staining for desmin will be observed in tumors of myofibroblastic differentiation such as the fibromatosis, dermatofibrosarcoma protuberans (Leong et al, 1997) and in reactive conditions with abundant myofibroblasts such as inflammatory pseudotumor and post-operative spindle cell nodule (Hojo et al, 1995) (Appendix 1.31). Equally important is the observation that not all muscle cells contain desmin. For example, among mammalian vascular smooth muscle, three immunophenotypes have been observed. Those that display vimentin only, those coexpressing vimentin and desmin and a third group which expresses desmin only (Coindre et al, 1988).

Focal staining for desmin may also be seen in tumors with a background of reactive myofibroblasts or with focal myofibroblastic differentiation

such as malignant fibrous histiocytoma.

Desmin has been employed with h-caldesmon, calponin, CD10, CD34, CD99, inhibin and keratin to separate leiomyomas, leiomyosarcomas, endometrial stromal tumors and uterine tumors resembling ovarian sex cord tumors. Desmin was positive in all smooth muscle tumors with the exception of the epithelioid type, which were positive in only about half the cases. It also stained areas of smooth muscle differentiation in endometrial stromal tumors and uterine tumors resembling ovarian sex cord tumors (Oliva et al, 2002).

Reactive mesothelial cells were shown to be strongly positive for desmin in cell block preparations of serous fluids (22/24 cases) but was not expressed by malignant mesothelioma and adenocarcinoma suggesting that desmin may be a useful marker to separate these three entities. Other muscle markers including actin, myoglobin and myogenin were not expressed by the reactive mesothelial cells or any of the tumors (Afify et al, 2002).

Comments

While initial antibodies to desmin lacked sensitivity and specificity, current commercial antibodies are more reliable. Both monoclonal and polyclonal antibodies are useful but as desmin shares some common epitopes with actin and myosin, it should be ensured that the antibody employed does not show cross-reactivity. We employ clones DE-R-11 and D33, both antibodies being enhanced by HIER.

Afify AM, Al-Khafaji BM, Paulino AF, Davila RM. Diagnostic use of muscle markers in the cytologic evaluation of serous fluids. Applied Immunohistochemistry and Molecular Morphology 2002;10:178–82.

Azumi N, Ben-Ezra J, Battifora H. Immunophenotypic diagnosis of leiomyosarcomas and rhabdomyosarcomas with monoclonal antibodies to muscle-specific actin and desmin in formalin-fixed tissue. Modern Pathology 1988;1:469–74.

Coindre J-M, De Mascarel A, Trojani M, De Mascaral I. Immunohistochemical study of rhabdomyosarcoma. Unexpected staining with S-100 protein and cytokeratin. Journal of Pathology 1988;155:127–32.

Goldman R, Goldman AE, Green K, et al. Intermediate filaments: possible functions as cytoskeletal connecting links between the nucleus and the cell surface. Annals of New York Academy of Sciences 1985;455:1–17.

Hojo H, Newton WA, Hamoudi AB, et al. Pseudosarcomatous myofibroblastic tumor of the urinary bladder in children. American Journal of Surgical Pathology 1995;19:1224–36.

Leong AS-Y, Wick MR, Swanson PE. Immunohistology and electron microscopy of anaplastic and pleomorphic tumors. Cambridge: Cambridge University Press, 1997, pp59–93, 161–69.

Leong AS-Y, Wannatrairot P. A retrospective analysis of immunohistochemical staining in identification of poorly differentiated round cell and spindle cell tumors – results, reagents and costs. Pathology 1992;24:254–60.

Leong AS-Y, Kan A, Milios J. Immunohistochemical analysis of malignant round cell tumors in childhood. Surgical Pathology 1989;2:5–17.

Li Z, Colucci E, Babinet C, Paulin D. The human desmin gene: a specific regulatory program in skeletal muscle both in vitro and in transgenic mice. Neuromuscular Disorders 1993;3:423–7.

Nagai J, Capetanaki YG, Lazarides E. Expression of the genes coding for the intermediate filament proteins vimentin and desmin. Annals of New York Academy of Sciences 1985;455:144–55.

Oliva E, Young RH, Amin MB, Clement PB. An immunohistochemical analysis of endometrial stromal and smooth muscle tumors of the uterus: a study of 54 cases emphasizing the importance of using a panel because of overlap in immunoreactivity for individual antibodies. American Journal of Surgical Pathology 2002;26:403–12.

Parham DM, Dias P, Kelly DR, et al. Desmin positivity in primitive neuroectodermal tumors of childhood. American Journal of Surgical Pathology 1992;16:483–92.

Pollock L, Rampling D, Greenwald SE, Malone M. Desmin expression in rhabdomyosarcoma: influence of the desmin clone and immunohistochemical method. Journal of Clinical Pathology 1995;48:535–8.

NOTES

Desmoplakins

Sources/clones

American Research Products, Chemicon, Cymbus Bioscience (DP2.15), Biodesign (DP2.15), Boehringer Mannheim (2.15), ICI (DP2.17), Research Diagnostic Inc (DP2.15), Progen (DP2.15, Serotec (polyclonal)

Fixation/preparation

Avaliable antibodies are immunoreactive only in fresh frozen sections or cell preparations.

Background

Epithelial cells contain complexes of cytokeratin filaments (tonofilaments) associated with specific domains of the plasma membrane that appear as symmetrical junctions known as desmosomes, or as asymmetrical hemi-desmosomes. These regions of filament-membrane-attachment are characterized by 14–20 nm thick dense plaque; these desmosomal plaques comprise a dense mixture of intracellular attachment proteins including plakoglobin and desmoplakins (Mueller & Franke 1983). Transmembrane linker proteins, which belong to the cadherin family of cell-cell adhesion molecules, bind to the plaques and interact through their extracellular domains to hold the adjacent membranes together by a Ca^{2+}-dependent mechanism. Desmoplakins I and II (DPI and DPII) are two polypeptides which make up the desmoplakins and are of molecular masses 46 and 24 kD respectively, suggesting that DPI may be a dimer in solution and DPII a monomer (O'Keefe et al, 1989).

Applications

The widespread presence of desmosomes in epithelial cells and their corresponding tumors makes the presence of desmoplakins a specific marker of epithelial differentiation. Unfortunately, these proteins are fixative sensitive, restricting the use of antibodies to desmoplakins to fresh cellular preparations or frozen sections. Applications in diagnostic pathology have therefore been limited to some studies in bullous skin diseases (Burge & Garrod, 1991; Setoyama et al, 1991). In autoimmune acantholytic diseases such as pemphigus vulgaris and pemphigus erythematosus desmoplakins are intact even in acantholytic cells, whereas in Hailey-Hailey's disease and Darier's disease the normal plasma membrane localization of desmoplakins is lost and the protein is internalized and present diffusely in the cytoplasm (Setoyama et al, 1991).

Desmoplakins have been demonstrated in follicular dendritic cells and their corresponding tumors (Chan et al 1997). More recent studies employing anti-desmoplakins have included the progression of squamous intraepithelial lesions of the uterine cervix where the assembly of desmosomes have been shown to be affected during progression of atypia with a dramatically decreased expression of desmoplakins and desmogleins (de Boer et al, 1999)

Comments

Acetone fixation followed by plastic embedding allows the immunostaining of the desmoplakins in permanent sections. Trypsin digestion needs to be employed (Carmichael et al, 1991).

References

Burge SM, Garrod DR. An immunohistological study of desmosomes in Darier's disease and Hailey-Hailey disease. British Journal of Dermatology 1991;124:242–51.

Carmichael RP, McCulloch CA, Zarb GA. Immunohistochemical localization and quantification of desmoplakins I & II and keratins 1 and 19 in plastic-embedded sections of human gingiva. Journal of Histochemistry and Cytochemistry 1991;39:519–28.

Chan JK, Flketcher CD, Nayler SJ, Cooper K. Follicular dendritic cell sarcoma. Clinicopathologic analysis of 17 cases suggesting a malignant potential higher than currently recognized. Cancer 1997;79:294–313.

De Boer CJ, van Dorst E, van Krieken H, et al. Changing roles of cadherins and catenins during progression of squamous intraepithelial lesions in the uterine cervix. American Journal of Pathology 1999;155:505–15.

Mueller H, Fanke WW. Biochemical and immunological characterization of desmoplakins I and II, the major polypeptides of the desmosomal plaque. Journal of Molecular Biology 1983;163:647–71.

O'Keefe EJ, Erickson HP, Bennett V. Desmoplakin I and desmoplakin II. Purification and characterization. Journal of Biological Chemistry 1989;264:8310–8.

Steoyama M, Choi KC, Hashimoto K, et al. Desmoplakin I and II in acantholytic dermatoses: preservation in pemphigus vulgaris and pemphigus erythematosus and dissolution in Hailey-Hailey's disease and Darier's disease. Journal of Dermatological Science 1991;1:9–17.

Epidermal Growth Factors: TGF-α AND EGFR

Sources/clones

EGFR

Accurate (21–1, F4), Biodesign (EGFR1, 2E9, L-4451, F5, E5), Biogenesis (C11, EGFR1), Biogenex (E30), Caltag Laboratories (2E9), Chemicon (polyclonal), Cymbus Bioscience (EGFR1), Dako (EGFR1), Fitzgerald (polyclonal), Immunotech (F4), Novocastra (polyclonal), Oncogene (R.1, 225, 455), Pharmingen (c11), Sigma Chemical (29.1, F4), Zymed (Z025).

TGF-α

Biodesign, Biogenesis (2D7/44, 2D7/45, 8A5/7, Rt, TB21), Chemicon (polyclonal), Oncogene (134A-2B3, 213.4–4, 189–2130.1).

Fixation/preparation

Applicable to formalin-fixed, paraffin-embedded tissue, although an antigen retrieval technique should be used prior to immunostaining, e.g., citrate buffer and microwave oven unmasking. May also be applied to cryostat sections or cell smears.

Background

Transforming growth factors (TGF) were discovered due to their ability to transform fibroblasts to a malignant phenotype (DeLarco & Todaro, 1978). Two distinct polypeptides were subsequently isolated: TGF-α and TGF-β. TGF-α is a polypeptide of 50 amino acids and is acid and heat-stable (Prigent & Lemoine, 1992). TGF-α belongs to the epidermal growth factor family, members of which share a common amino acid sequence and biological activities. They also bind to a common receptor, epidermal growth factor receptor (EGFR) on target cells (Carpenter, 1984).

EGFR is a 170-kD protein comprising a cell surface ligand-binding transmembrane domain and a highly conserved cytoplasmic tyrosine kinase domain. When TGF-α binds to EGFR, tyrosine kinase of the receptor is activated. This is followed by phosphorylation and an increase in cytosolic calcium ions within target cells. The resultant effect is an increased DNA synthesis with proliferation and differentiation of the cell (Chen et al, 1989).

TGF-α is a potent growth stimulator and is distributed in both fetal and adult tissues, playing a role in the physiological regulation of normal growth and differentiation (Yasui et al, 1992).

Applications

There is sufficient evidence showing that TGF-α is an important growth factor for transformation of various cell types to a malignant phenotype (Pusztai et al, 1993). The co-expression of both the ligand (TGF-α) and its receptor (EGFR) has been documented in a variety of carcinomas – both gastrointestinal and non-gastrointestinal carcinomas. This bond is thought to confer autonomy to tumor cells by autocrine or paracrine mechanisms (Sporn & Roberts, 1985). Whilst coexistent expression of a growth factor and its receptor would be expected to confer increased growth advantage to tumor cells, the ability of certain tumors to express both growth factor and/or the respective receptor may be lost during the carcinogenic transformation.

The EGFR antibody reacts with the majority of squamous cell carcinomas arising from both squamous epithelium and metaplastic squamous epithelium (Ozanne & Richards, 1986). Studies on breast cancer have shown that the expression of the EGF receptor may also be of prognostic value (Nicholson et al,

1991) although other studies of the expression of EGFR family ligands including EGF and TGF-α showed no associated with cancer-specific survival, tumor size, lymph node status, histologic grade, c-erbB-2 and hormone status (Suo et al, 2002).

EGFR is universally expressed in gastrinomas and in the minority (15–20%) in which it is overexpressed, the overexpression correlates with aggressive growth and lower curability (Peghini et al, 2002). In invasive thymoma EGFR expression has also been found to be strongly expressed, suggesting a potential therapeutic target Henley et al, 2002).

Comments

Growth factors and their receptors participate in the process of tumorigenesis by promoting the growth of tumor cells. During this process, tumor cells acquire an increasingly aggressive phenotype with loss of the physiological control for growth and differentiation. At the present time the availability of antibodies to growth factors/receptors can only contribute to our understanding of the complex mechanisms involved in tumorigenesis.

References

Carpenter G. Properties of the receptor for epidermal growth factor. Cell 1984;37:357–8.

Chen WS, Lazar CS, Lund KA, et al. Functional independence of the epidermal growth factor receptor from a domain required for ligand-induced internalization and calcium regulation. Cell 1989;59:33–43.

DeLarco JE, Todaro GH. Growth factors from murine sarcoma virus transformed cells. Proceedings of the National Academy of Sciences USA 1978;75:4001–5.

Henley JD, Koukoulis GK, Loehrer PJSr. Epidermal growth factor receptor expression in invasive thymoma. Journal of Cancer Research and Clinical Oncology 2002;128:167–70.

Nicholson S, Richard J, Sainsburg C, et al. Epidermal growth factor receptor (EGFr); results of a 6 year follow-up study in operable breast cancer with emphasis on the node negative subgroup. British Journal of Cancer 1991;63:146–50.

Ozanne B, Richards CS. Over-expression of the EGF receptor is a hallmark of squamous cell carcinomas. Journal of Pathology 1986;149:9–14.

Peghini PL, Iwamoto M, Raffeld M, et al. Overexpression of epidermal growth factor and hepatocytes growth factor receptors in a proportion of gastrinomas correlates with aggressive growth and lower curability. Clinical Cancer Research 2002;8:2273–85.

Prigent SA, Lemoine NR. Type 1 (EGF-R related) family of growth factor receptors and their ligands. Progress in Growth Factor Research 1992;4:1–24.

Pusztai L, Lewis CE, Lorenzen J, McGee OD. Growth factors: regulation of normal and neoplastic growth. Journal of Pathology 1993;169:191–201.

Sporn MB, Roberts AB. Autocrine growth factors and cancer. Nature 1985;313:745–7.

Suo Z, Risberg B, Karlsson MG, et al. The expression of EGFR family ligands in breast carcinomas. International Journal of Pathology 2002;10:91–9.

Yasui W, Ji Z-O, Kuniyasu H et al. Expression of transforming growth factor alpha in human tissues. Immunohistochemical study and Northern blot analysis. Virchows Archives A Pathology Anatomy 1992;421:513–9.

Epithelial Membrane Antigen (EMA)

Sources/clones

Accurate (E29), Biodesign, Biogenesis (2D5/11), Biogenex (E29, Mc-5), Bioprobe (HMFGP1.4), Chemicon, Dako (E29), Diagnostic Biosystems (E29), Immunon (polyclonal, E29), Immunotech (E29, E348KP), Medac, Novocastra, Oncogene (MC5), Sera-Lab (HMFG/5/11IC, polyclonal), Serotec, Zymed (ZCE113).

Fixation/preparation

Most antibodies are immunoreactive in fixed paraffin-embedded sections. Immunostaining is enhanced by proteolytic digestion or HIER, the latter producing less background staining.

Background

Anti-epithelial membrane antigen (EMA) antibodies recognize a group of closely related high molecular weight transmembrane glycoproteins with high carbohydrate content. The MUC1 gene, located on chromosome 1 in 1q21–24 region encodes EMA. EMA is very similar to the human milk fat globule (HMFG). A heterogeneous population of HMFG proteins can be recovered from the aqueous phase of skimmed milk following extraction in chloroform and methanol. EMA is related to the high molecular weight glycoproteins of HMFG, especially to HMFG2 (Heyderman et al, 1985). Preparations of EMA reacted with polyclonal antibodies raised to delipidized HMFG with avid binding to wheat germ agglutinin and peanut agglutinin. A similar mucin-containing glycoprotein was solubilized from HMFG and labeled PAS-O because of reactivity for PAS (Shimuzu & Yamauchi, 1982). PAS-O and EMA represent closely allied glycoprotein moieties, with common antigenic determinants on both proteins. From a practical standpoint, patterns of immunoreactivity for EMA and HMFG are very similar (Strickler et al, 1987).

EMA reactivity is found in a wide variety of epithelial cells and their corresponding tumors. When present immunoreactivity is usually limited to apical cell membranes in benign secretory epithelium and well-differentiated carcinomas such as those of the breast, but in poorly differentiated carcinomas, cytoplasmic staining is seen and there is loss of staining polarity in the cell membranes. Secretory epithelia and their fetal anlage that show EMA include eccrine sweat glands, sebaceous, and apocrine glands and may be employed with the appropriate panel to separate cutaneous adnexal tumors (Appendix 1.20). It is also expressed in salivary gland, exocrine pancreas, gastric and endometrium, bronchial glands, alveolar cells and the epithelium of bile ducats, stomach, bronchi, fallopian tube and vas deferens. In additional to glandular epithelium, EMA has also been demonstrated in non-secretory epithelia such as urothelium, renal distal and collecting tubules, and syncytiotrophoblast.

Applications

Despite the ready availability of anti-cytokeratin as a marker of epithelial differentiation, there is still widespread use of EMA as a marker of epithelial cells. This is fraught with inconsistencies. While EMA is generally not expressed by germ cells, normal hemato-lymphoid, mesenchymal, neural and neuroectodermal, it may be expressed by certain non-epithelial tissues such as fetal notochord, arachnoid granulations, ependyma, choroid plexus, epineurial and perineural fibroblasts, histiocytes and plasma cells and their corresponding neoplasms. EMA is normally expressed by plasma cells and is conserved and even increased in plasma cell neoplasms and by ultrastructural examination has been located diffusely on the cell membranes and focally within rough endoplasmic reticulum. Neoplasms from earlier stage B cell differentiation do not usually express EMA and in lymph node-based B cell lymphomas, EMA is found mainly in diffuse large cell lymphomas and T-cell-rich B cell lymphomas. EMA is more frequently seen in T cell neoplasms, occurring in about 20% of all T cell lymphomas (Chittal et al, 1997). EMA expression in Reed Sternberg cells is unusual although it is frequently found in the L & H cells of nodular lymphocyte predominant Hodgkin's disease. EMA is also found in almost 50% of cases of anaplastic large cell lymphoma of CD30 phenotype.

In our practice, staining for EMA is not generally employed as a marker of epithelial cells but more often for the identification of certain mesenchymal tumors including synovial sarcoma (Leong et al, 1997), anaplastic large cell lymphoma (CD30+), and perineurioma (Li et al, 1996). Cytokeratin expression in monophasic (spindle) synovial sarcoma may be focal but EMA is often more extensively positive in such cases, even in the rare pleuropulmonary synovial sarcoma (Essary et al, 2002). The expression of EMA in chordoma serves to distinguish from chondroma and chondrosarcoma (Gown & Leong, 1993; Jeffrey et al, 1995); E-cadherin being

another marker expressed in most chordomas as opposed to chondrosarcoma (Mori et al, 2002). EMA is expressed in solitary fibrous tumors (Carneiro et al, 1996). EMA immunostaining may help identify ovarian granulosa cell tumors from tumors that mimic their various histological patterns. While keratin may be expressed in granulosa cell tumors, the absence of EMA and immunoreactivity for smooth muscle actin allows distinction from primary and metastatic carcinomas (Costa et al, 1994).

Immunostaining for EMA is a valuable adjunct to the examination of effusions and biopsies for malignant mesothelioma (Appendix 1.17). By ultrastructural examination EMA has been demonstrated exclusively on the long microvillous surfaces of the tumors cells with virtually no cytoplasmic labeling (Van der Kwast et al, 1987). These findings have been transposed to cytologic preparations and biopsies and careful staining for EMA employing clone E29 shows membranous labeling of malignant mesothelial cells and demonstrate the long microvilli characteristic of the tumor. In contrast, adenocarcinomas display diffuse cytoplasmic staining, with or without membranous enhancement but long microvilli are not seen (Leong et al, 1990).

EMA and vimentin immunostaining was employed to differentiate chromophobe renal cell carcinoma from renal oncocytoma and conventional renal cell carcinoma but the same phenotype was found in all three tumor. All 21 cases of chromophobe carcinomas

co-expressed both antigens, which was present in 75% of renal oncocytoma in 21% of conventional renal cell carcinoma. The absence of this phenotype, however, would preclude the diagnosis of chromophobe carcinoma (Khoury et al, 2002).

Comments

For diagnostic applications we prefer to use anti-EMA (clone E29) instead of HMFG, both antigens having very similar tissue distribution.

References

Carneiro SS, Scheithauer BW, Nascimento AG, et al. Solitary fibrous tumor of the meninges: a lesion distinct from fibrous meningioma. A clinicopathologic and immunohistological study. American Journal of Clinical Pathology 1996;106:217–24.

Chittal S, Saati TA, Delsol G. Epithelial membrane antigen in hematolymphoid neoplasms. A review. Applied Immunohistochemistry 1997;5:203–15.

Gown AM, Leong AS-Y. Immunohistochemistry of 'solid' tumors: poorly differentiated round cell and spindle cell tumors II. IN: Leong AS-Y (ed). Applied immunohistochemistry for the surgical pathologist. London: Edward Arnold, 1993: pp74–109.

Heyderman E, Strudley I, Powell G, et al. A New monoclonal antibody to epithelial membrane antigen (EMA) – E29. A comparison of its immunocytochemical reactivity with polyclonal anti-EMA antibodies and with another monoclonal antibody HMFG-2. British Journal of Cancer 1985;52:355–61.

Essary LR, Vargas SO, Fletcher CD. Primary pleuropulmonary

synovial sarcoma: reappraisal of a recently described anatomical subset. Cancer 2002;94:459–69.

Jeffrey PB, Biava CG, Davis RL. Chondroid chordoma. A hyalinized chordoma without cartilaginous differentiation. American Journal of Clinical Pathology 1995;103:271–9.

Khoury JD, Abrahams NA, Levin HS, MacLennan GT. The utility of epithelial membrane antigen and vimentin in the diagnosis of chromophobe renal cell carcinoma. Annals of Diagnostic Pathology 2002;6:154–8.

Leong AS-Y, Parkinson R, Milios J. "Thick" cell membranes revealed by immunocytochemical staining: A clue to the diagnosis of mesothelioma. Diagnostic Cytopathology 1990;6:9–13.

Leong AS-Y, Wick MR, Swanson PE. Immunohistology and electron microscopy of anaplastic and pleomorphic tumors. Cambridge: Cambridge University Press, 1997: pp 155–7.

Li D, Schauble, Moll C, Fisch U. Intratemporal facial nerve perineurioma. Laryngoscope 1996;106:328–33.

Mori K, Chano T, Kushima R, et al. Expression of E-cadherin in chordomas: diagnostic marker and possible role of tumor cell affinity. Virchows Archives 2002;440:123–7.

Shimizu M, Yamauchi K. Isolation and characterization of mucin-like glycoprotein in human milk fat globule membrane. Journal of Biochemistry 1982;91:515–24.

Van der Kwast TH, Versnel MA, Delahaye M, et al. Expression of epithelial membrane antigen on malignant mesothelial cells. An immunocytochemical and immunoelectron microscopic study. Acta Cytologica 1987;32:169–74.

NOTES

Epstein-Barr Virus, LMP

Sources/clones

Accurate (CS1–4), Biodesign (polyclonal), Dako (CS1–4), EY Labs, Novocastra (polyclonal).

Fixation/preparation

Applicable to formalin-fixed, paraffin-embedded tissue sections. Enzymatic digestion (e.g. trypsin) is essential to enhance immunopositivity. The application of microwave irradiation for antigen retrieval has also been used to good effect (Kaczorowski et al, 1994). This antibody may also be used for labeling acetone-fixed cryostat sections or fixed cell smears.

Background

The antibody (Isotype: IgG1, Kappa) has been raised against recombinant fusion protein containing sequences of bacterial β-galactosidase and the EBV-encoded latent membrane protein (LMP-1). LMP is one of the few viral proteins that are expressed in a latent infection. The antibody reacts with a 60 kD latent membrane protein encoded by BNLF gene of the Epstein-Barr virus. Being a cocktail of clones CS1, CS2, CS3 and CS4, all four anti-LMP antibodies recognize distinct epitopes on the hydrophilic carboxyl region of LMP (Rowe et al, 1987). These four epitopes are present on the internal aspect of the membrane-associated viral LMP. Therefore the antibody does not react with viable cells, but with fixed cells in paraffin sections, cytological preparations, and cryostat sections and in immunoblotting.

Applications

The antibody is characterized by its strong positivity with EBV-positive lymphoblastoid cell lines and EBV-infected B cell immunoblasts in infectious mononucleosis. Although EBV is consistently present in nasopharyngeal undifferentiated carcinoma among Oriental patients, LMP-1 antibody is only positive in about 60% of cases (Hording et al, 1993; Lopategui et al, 1994). LMP protein expression is especially useful in identifying these cancers in cervical lymph node metastases. This antibody may also be useful in the diagnosis of lymphoepithelioma-like carcinoma of the lung, mediastinum, stomach, and paranasal sinuses (Dimery et al, 1988; Shibata et al, 1991; Weiss et al, 1989).

Posttransplantation lymphoproliferative disorders arising in patients treated with a variety of immunosuppressive regimens after organ transplantation, usually show a type III latency pattern with LMP-1 expression (Delecluse et al, 1995). The EBV-positive AIDS-associated B cell lymphomas, usually demonstrate a latency type III in the large cell lymphomas permitting the use of antibody to LMP-1 (Hamilton-DuToit et al, 1993).

Nasal T/NK cell lymphoma is strongly associated with EBV (Kanavaros et al, 1993). However, LMP-1 protein expression has been inconsistent on paraffin sections, although one study consistently demonstrated LMP-1 protein in frozen sections, suggesting a low level of protein expression. LMP-1 immunohistochemistry is positive in 17% of adult T-cell leukemia/lymphoma (Tokunaga et al, 1993). LMP-1 expression has also been associated with an aggressive clinical course and hepatosplenomegaly in nodal T-cell lymphomas (Bruin, 1993). About 20–30% of CD30 (Ki-1)-positive anaplastic large cell lymphoma show LMP-1 immunoreaction (Herbst et al, 1991).

Approximately 50% of Hodgkin's disease are associated with EBV. In almost all of these positive cases, nearly all of the Reed-Sternberg cells are positive for EBV. Using modern epitope retrieval techniques, an almost 1:1 correlation between the results of LMP-1 paraffin-based immunohistochemistry studies and EBER in situ hybridisation studies has been demonstrated in Reed-Sternberg cells and Hodgkin's cells of EBV-associated Hodgkin's disease (Delsol et al, 1992; Oudejans et al 1997; Pinkus et al, 1994). A note of caution with respect to antibodies against LMP is advised: strong staining of normal early myeloid and erythroid precursors may be seen despite a total absence of evidence of EBV by PCR (Hammer et al, 1996).

Recent attempts to correlate LMP and p53 immunoexpression in adult and pediatric nasopharyngeal carcinoma have produced conflicting results (Solomides et al, 2002; Preciado et al, 2002; Shi et al, 2002).

Comments

As a research tool EBV immunohistochemical investigation is superior to PCR, in that it excludes background/resident lymphocytes harboring EBV. It has been suggested that the interpretation of LMP immunostaining is more accurate when combined with EBER as LMP staining while usually strong among all Reed-Sternberg cells in Hodgkin's disease in a given case, may alternatively be focal and weak (Gulley et al, 2002). LMP is localized to the cytoplasm and cell membrane.

References

Bruin PCD. Detection of Epstein-Barr virus nucleic acid sequences and protein in nodal T-cell lymphomas: relation between latent membrane protein-1 positivity and clinical course. Histopathology 1993;23:509–18.

Delecluse H-J, Kremmer E, Rouault J-P, et al. The expression of Epstein-Barr virus latent proteins is related to the pathological feature of post-transplant lymphoproliferative disorders. American Journal of Pathology 1995;146:1113–20.

Delsol G, Brousset P, Chittal S, Rigal HF. Correlation of the expression of Epstein-Barr virus latent membrane protein and in situ hybridization with biotinylated BamH1-W probes in Hodgkin's disease. American Journal of Pathology 1992;140:247–53.

Dimery IW, Lee JS, Blick M, et al. Association of the Epstein-Barr virus with lymphoepithelioma of the thymus. Cancer 1988;61:2475–80.

Gulley ML, Glaser SL, Craig FE, et al. Guidelines for interpreting EBER in situ hybridization and LMP1 immunohistochemical tests for detecting Epstein-Barr virus in Hodgkin lymphoma. American Journal of Clinical Pathology 2002;117:259–67.

Hamilton-Dutoit SJ, Rea D, Raphael M, et al. Epstein-Barr virus-latent gene expression and tumor cell phenotype in acquired immunodeficiency syndrome-related non-Hodgkin's lymphoma: correlation of lymphoma phenotype with three distinct patterns of viral latency. American Journal of Pathology 1993;143:1072–90.

Hammer RD, Scott M, Shahab I, et al. Latent membrane protein antibody reacts with normal haematopoietic precursor cells and leukaemic blasts in tissues lacking EBV by PCR. American Journal of Clinical Pathology 1996;106:469–74.

Herbst H, Dallenbach F, Hummel M, et al. Epstein-Barr virus DNA and latent gene products in Ki-1 (CD30)-positive anaplastic large cell lymphomas. Blood 1991;78:2663–73.

Hording U, Nielsen HW, Albeck H, Daugaard S. Nasopharyngeal carcinoma: histopathological types and association with Epstein-Barr virus. European Journal of Cancer Clinical Oncology 1993;29B:137–9.

Kaczorowski S, Kaczorowska M, Christennson B. Expression of EBV encoded latent membrane protein 1 and bcl-2 protein in childhood and adult Hodgkin's disease: application of microwave irradiation for antigen retrieval. Leukemia and Lymphoma 1994;13:273–83.

Kanavaros P, Lecsc M-C, Briere J, et al. Nasal T cell lymphoma: a clinicopathologic entity associated with peculiar phenotype and with Epstein-Barr virus. Blood 1993;81:2688–95.

Lopategui JR, Gaffey MJ, Frierson HF, et al. Detection of Epstein-Barr viral RNA in sinonasal undifferentiated carcinoma from Western and Asian patients. American Journal of Surgical Pathology 1994;18:391–8.

Oudejans JJ, Jiwa NM, Meijer CJLM. Epstein-Barr virus in Hodgkin's disease: more than just an innocent bystander. Journal of Pathology 1997;181:353–6.

Pinkus GS, Lones M, Shinataku IP, Said JW. Immunohistochemical detection of Epstein-Barr virus-encoded latent membrane protein in Reed-Sternberg cells and variants of Hodgkin's disease. Modern Pathology 1994;7:454–61.

Preciado MV, Chabay PA, De Matteo EN, et al. Epstein Barr virus associated pediatric nasopharyngeal carcinoma: Its correlation with p53 and bcl-2 expression. Medical Pediatric Oncology 2002;38:345–8.

Rowe M, Evans HS, Young LS, et al. Monoclonal antibodies to the latent membrane protein of Epstein-Barr virus reveal heterogeneity of the protein and inducible expression in virus transformed cells. Journal of General Virology 1987;68:1575–86.

Shi W, Pataki I, MacMillan C, et al. Molecular pathology parameters in human nasopharyngeal carcinoma. Cancer 2002;94:1997–2006.

Shibata D, Tokunaga M, Uemura Y, et al. Association of EBV with undifferentiated gastric carcinomas with intense lymphoid infiltration. Americal Journal of Pathology 1991;139:469–74.

Solomides CC, Miller AS, Christman RA, et al. Lymphomas of the oral cavity: Histology, immunologic type and incidence of Epstein-Barr virus infection. Human Pathology 2002;33:153–7.

Tokunaga M, Imai S, Utemura Y, Tokudome T, Osato T, Sato E. Epstein-Barr virus in adult T-cell leukaemia/lymphoma. American Journal of Pathology 1993;1993:1263–9.

Weiss LM, Movahed LA, Butler AE, et al. Analysis of lymphoepithelioma and lymphoepithelioma-like carcinoma for Epstein-Barr viral genomes by in situ hybridization. American Journal of Surgical Pathology 1989;13:625–31.

NOTES

Erythropoietin

Source/clone

Genzyme Diagnostics (EPO, monoclonal), Santa Cruz Biotechnology (EpoR (C-20): polyclonal SC-695).

Fixation/preparation

This antibody is applicable to formalin-fixed paraffin sections. Antigen retrieval achieved by gentle boiling in water at high power for 5 minutes in a microwave oven.

Background

Erythropoietin (EPO) is a glycoprotein hormone that stimulates erythropoiesis in mammals. Its synthesis is increased in the anemic and hypoxic state. Although the liver is the major source of EPO production in the fetus, the kidney is the major organ of EPO production in adults (Jacobson et al, 1957). The EPO antibody is an immunoglobulin G antibody that binds to an epitope within the first 26 amino acids at the NH_2 terminus of human urinary and recombinant EPO (Sytkowski & Fisher, 1985).

The production of EPO is responsible for stimulating polycythemia in various malignancies: renal cell carcinoma, nephroblastoma, hepatocellular carcinoma and cerebellar hemangioblastoma. Studies attempting to precisely localize the cells responsible for production of EPO have used immunohistochemistry and in-situ hybridization on frozen tissue sections to demonstrate that tumor cells of epithelial origin are the sites of EPO production in renal cell carcinomas associated with polycythemia (DaSilva, 1990). A recent study using monoclonal antibody EPO on paraffin sections achieved success with 16/19 renal cell carcinomas (comprising clear cell and tubulopapillary type) showing cytoplasmic immunopositivity (Clark et al, 1998), irrespective of the presence or absence of polycythemia. Similarly, 6/12 cerebellar hemangioblastomas stained positively with EPO antibody within the cells of the vascular walls (Hufnagel et al, 1989). Significantly, the latter study demonstrated EPO immunopositivity in metastatic renal cell carcinomas.

To date EPO has been reported to be synthesized in the normal brain, placenta, and capillary endothelium, glandular and surface epithelial cells of the normal cervix and endometrium, and oocytes, granulosa, theca interna and lutein cells of the ovary (Yasuda et al, 2001). A case of uterine myoma with erythropoietin synthesis by tumor tissue and erythrocytosis has been reported (Suzuki et al, 2001). High levels of EPO and EPO receptor expression have been reported in malignant cells and tumor vasculature in breast cancer but not in normal breast tissue (Acs et al, 2001).

Applications

EPO immunopositivity is useful in the identification of both primary and metastatic renal cell carcinoma. This is useful to distinguish from other carcinomas; but not from hemangioblastoma, which may also be EPO positive. EMA helps in this distinction, being positive in renal cell carcinoma, but not in hemangioblastoma.

References

Acs G, Acs P, Beckwith SM, et al. Erythropoietin and erythropoietin receptor expression in human cancer. Cancer Research 2001;61:3561–5.

Clark D, Kersting R, Rojiani AM. Erythropoietin immunolocalization in renal cell carcinoma. Modern Pathology 1998;11:24–8.

Da Silva J-L, Lacombe C, Bruneval P, et al. Tumor cells are the site of erythropoietin synthesis in human renal cancers associated with polycythemia. Blood 1990;75:577–82.

Hufnagel TJ, Kim JH, True LD, et al. Immunohistochemistry of capillary hemangioblastoma: immunoperoxidase-labeled antibody staining resolves the differential diagnosis with metastatic renal cell carcinoma, but does not explain the histogenesis of the capillary hemangioblastoma. The American Journal of Surgical Pathology 1989;3:207–16.

Jacobson LO, Goldwasser E, Fried W, et al. Role of the kidney in erythropoiesis. Nature 1957;79:633–4.

Suzuki M, Takamizawa S, Nomaguchi K, et al. Erythropoietin synthesis by tumour tissues in a patient with uterine myoma and erythrocytosis. British Journal of Hematology 2001;113:49–51.

Sytkowski AJ, Fisher JW. Isolation and characterization of an antipeptide monoclonal antibody to human erythropoietin. Journal of Biology and Chemistry 1985;260:14727–31.

Yasuda Y, Fujita Y, Musha T, et al. Expression of erythropoietin in human femal reproductive organs. Italian Journal of Anatomy and Embryology 2001;106 (2 Suppl 2):215–22.

Estrogen Receptor (ER)

Sources/clones

Abbott (H222), Accurate (CC4.5), Biogenesis (ERLH1), Dako (1D5), Eurodiagnostics/Accurate (polyclonal), Immunotech (1D5), Novocastra (CC4.5, LH1, 6F11), Vector (6F11), Zymed (1D5).

Fixation/preparation

The method of preparation is very much dependent on the antibody clone employed. The ERICA antibody (clone H222) is mostly only immunoreactive in fresh frozen tissues although some laboratories showed success with tissues that had only short exposure to formalin (Raymond & Leong, 1988; 1990) or following the careful use of specific antigen retrieval agents such as DNAse. The development of clone 1D5 and later 6F11 made it possible for the immunostaining of routinely fixed paraffin-embedded sections but only following heat-induced epitope retrieval (HIER) (Leong & Milios, 1993). The latter procedure has no effect with the H222 antibody.

Background

The first monoclonal antibodies to the estrogen receptor (ER)

protein (estrophilin) were produced from a human breast cancer cell line, MCF-7, subjected to affinity column processing and elution (Greene et al, 1980). The antibodies were produced by immunization of rats with this partially purified estradiol-estrophilin complex. Fusion of splenic lymphocytes from the immunized animals with myeloma cells yielded three hybridoma cells lines after cloning by limited dilution techniques, the antibodies thus produced recognized estrogen-occupied as well as unoccupied receptors (Pousen et al, 1985).

The human ER is a member of a family of nuclear receptors for small hydrophobic ligands such as thyroid hormone, vitamin D, retinoic acid and the steroid hormones. Each receptor has a ligand binding domain, a hinge region, a DNA binding domain and a variable or regulatory domain. The ER gene is located on the long arm of chromosome 6 (q24–27) and comprises eight exons and intervening introns spanning at least 140 kilobases. Binding of the ligand to the receptor is thought to result in an allosteric alteration that allows the hormone-receptor complex to bind to its DNA response element in the promoter region

of a target gene. In the absence of hormone binding, the domain appears to be inhibitory in function, preventing transcriptional activation. Besides establishing the allosteric association of the hormone binding and the regulatory domains, the sequences contained in the hinge region are critical in directing the ER and progesterone (PR) proteins to the nucleus after they are synthesized in the cytoplasm. The DNA binding domain has many basic amino acids, some of which are repeating units folded into a "fingered" structure coordinated by a zinc ion, known as the "zinc finger" (Schwabe et al, 1990). The ER and PR appear to enhance the transcriptional activity of selected genes. The actual mechanism is not known but probably involves interactions between receptors and other transcriptional factors with the promoter regions of the respective genes. In the current model of ER action, estradiol diffuses into the cell and binds to the receptor, leading to its dimerisation and tight binding to its specific DNA target. Following this binding to the estrogen response element in target genes, there is stimulation to increase the transcription of target genes, some directly or indirectly leading to the establishment of both autocrine and paracrine growth stimulatory loops (Leong & Lee, 1995).

Early studies employing monoclonal antibodies to estrophilin reported both cytoplasmic and nuclear staining, the former being stronger. However, subsequent studies have established an exclusive nuclear localisation for ER proteins in both human breast carcinomas as well as other steroid responsive tissues. This has been confirmed by autoradiographic studies and immunoelectron microscopy has shown the ER protein to be present in the euchromatin portion of the nucleus in breast, endometrial and ovarian cancers as well as in benign endometrium. The cytoplasm in all cases did not reveal presence of the receptor although there was some reaction product in the ribosome. This latter reactivity was considered to be non-specific although the possibility of synthesis of ER at the ribosomal level was not completely ruled out. Studies demonstrating cytoplasmic localization of ER protein in addition to nuclear localization have mostly employed fluorescein-tagged estrogen analogs, whereas modern immunoenzyme techniques utilizing monoclonal antibodies to ER protein have shown only nuclear reactivity.

Applications

Over a hundred years ago it was recognized that oophorectomy was associated with clinical remission in women with metastatic breast cancer. Despite the usefulness of hormonal

manipulation in some women, only approximately 30% of unselected women with metastatic breast cancer responded to such treatment. There was therefore a need to identify those women whose breast cancers are hormone dependent from those whose tumors are hormone independent. Employing cytosol based ligand-binding assays, it was shown that about 50–60% of women with ER-rich breast cancers responded to hormone treatment, while less than 10% with ER-poor tumors showed a similar response. The relevance of ER status and hormonal treatment in node negative tumors, however, is less clear. It is also clinically recognized that a small proportion of patients whose tumors are receptor negative by cytosol-based assays will show a positive response to hormone treatment, and as many as one third of those with ER-positive tumors may fail to respond to such treatment. On the basis of comparative immunohistologic studies, it is believed that some of these discrepancies are caused by inherent errors of the biochemical method which assays homogenized tissue samples with resultant errors introduced by the inclusion of benign epithelium, the dilutional effect of abundant stroma, and inadequate tumor sampling. Indeed, there is recent persuasive evidence, based on hormonal response as the ultimate yardstick, that immunostaining in frozen or paraffin sections is the more accurate measurement of ER status (Pertschuk et al, 1996) and this, and many other advantages makes immunostaining the "gold

standard" to replace cytosol assays (Taylor, 1997).

It has been suggested that ER may be used to identify metastatic breast carcinoma but a variety of other lesions with epithelioid features may also express ER. These include epithelioid smooth muscle tumors, malignant melanoma, meningioma, sclerosing hemangioma (Leong et al, 1997), desmoid tumors, thyroid neoplasms, and cervical, endometrial and ovarian cancers, rendering the marker less useful as a diagnostic discriminant. Recently, the demonstration of ER in 56% of primary pulmonary carcinoma of bronchiolar alveolar type and 80% of adenocarcinoma of no special type emphasizes further the dangers of using ER as a marker of breast carcinoma especially in the metastatic setting (Dabbs et al, 2002). Interestingly, nuclear staining was obtained in these cases with clone 6F11 and not 1D5 confirming that the clones may detect different epitopes of the ER antigen.

Comments

Since the development of clones 1D5 and 6F11, it has become possible to perform immunostaining for ER in routinely fixed and processed tissues inexpensively, accurately and consistently. Some form of HIER procedure is essential when using clone 1D5 and 6F11; in contrast, H222 fails to stain following HIER, indicating that only one epitope of the ER, and not the entire antigen, is retrieved by the heating process. For this reason, it has been suggested that the procedure be called heat-induced epitope retrieval rather than the original term "heat-induced antigen retrieval". It is possible to obtain consistent staining of ER in cytologic preparations by employing clone 1D5 with HIER on smears, which are initially completely air-dried before fixation in 10% buffered formalin (Suthipintawong et al, 1997; Leong, et al, 1999).

It is important, like with most other antibodies employed for immunohistology, that each laboratory determines its optimal time for epitope retrieval and should not purely rely on the procedures developed for other laboratories (Elias et al, 1996).

A concordance of 77 to 100% between immunostaining in paraffin and frozen sections with the dextran-coated charcoal assay (DCC), and we have adopted 10% staining of tumors cells as the cut-off value as it corresponded with 10 fmol/mg of proteins by DCC assay. There is strong correlation of the percentage of positive cells with the intensity of staining. We have expressed the results of immunostaining subjectively as positive or negative, as a percentage of positive tumor cells, or as a score derived by adding grades of staining (1, 2 and 3, corresponding to mild, intermediate and strong staining) and the percentage as scores of 0, 1, 2, 3 and 4 (corresponding to <10%, 11–25%, 26–50%, 51–75% and >75%). Others have developed other scoring systems, which are claimed to be more objective (Allred et al, 1998). Selected cutoff points for ER positivity have varied in different reported studies and a defined cutoff point is difficult to

establish. The question of what levels of ER immunostaining are associated with better prognosis and predictive of response to hormonal therapy cannot be presently answered.

Computerized image analysis has been claimed to produce an increasing specificity and sensitivity relative to biochemical assays; however, other studies have shown identical results by image analysis and visual examination, and significantly similar agreement between the two and biochemical values. It is clear, however, that there is significant interlaboratory variation in sensitivity to warrant caution when comparing results between laboratories (Rhodes et al, 2000) much of this may be due to differences in antibody clones, duration of fixation and importantly antigen retrieval techniques (Rhodes et al, 2001). A recent study suggested that tissue microarray may be an efficient method for use in quality assurance programs (Parker et al, 2002).

While the antigen is largely nuclear in location, one form of ER is localized to the cell membrane and it appears that Her2/neu interacts with the latter. Tamoxifen resistance was found to be associated with Her2/neu downregulation and ER upregulation in breast cancer cell lines. Tamoxiphen-induced apoptosis occurred immediately after dissociation of Her2/neu from cell membrane ER (Chung et al, 2002).

Our preference is for the 6F11 clone over 1D5.

References

Allred DC, Harvey JM, Berardo M, Clark GM. Prognostic and predictive factors in breast cancer by immunohistochemical analysis. Modern Pathology 1998;11:155–68.

Balaton AJ, Mathieu M-C, Le Doussal V. Optimization of heat-induced epitope retrieval for estrogen receptor determination by immunohistochemistry on paraffin sections. Results of a multicentric comparative study. Applied Immunohistochemistry 1996;4:259–63.

Chung YL, Sheu ML, Yang SC, et al. Resistance to tamoxifen-induced apoptosis is associated with direct interaction between Her2/neu and cell membrane estrogen receptor in breast cancer. International Journal of Cancer 2002;97:306–12.

Dabbs DJ, Landreneau RJ, Liu Y, et al. Detection of estrogen receptor by immunohistochemistry in pulmonary adenocarcinoma. Annals of Thoracic Surgery 2002;73:403–5.

El-Badawy N, Cohen C, De Rose PB, Sgoutas D. Immunohistochemical estrogen receptor assay: quantitation by image analysis. Modern Pathology 1991;4:305–9.

Elias JM, Cartun RA, Eilers S, Leong AS-Y, et al. Interlaboratory comparison of estrogen receptor analysis in paraffin sections by a monoclonal antibody to estrophilin (H222). Journal of Histotechnology 1993;16:57–63.

Greene GL, Fitch FW, Jensen EV. Monoclonal antibodies to estrophilin: Probe for the study of estrogen receptors. Proceedings of the National Academy of Sciences USA 1980;77:157–61.

Leong AS-Y, Lee AKC. Biological indices in the assessment of breast cancer. Molecular Pathology 1995;48:M221-M238.

Leong AS-Y, Milios J. Comparison of antibodies to estrogen and progesterone receptors and the influence of microwave-antigen retrieval. Applied Immunohistochemistry 1993;1:282–8.

Leong AS-Y, Chan KW, Leong FJ. Sclerosing hemangioma. In: Corrin B (ed), Pathology of Lung Tumors. London: Churchill Livingstone, 1997, pp 175–88.

Parker RL, Huntsman DG, Lesack DW, et al. Assessment of interlaboratory variation in the immunohistochemical determination of estrogen receptor status using a breast cancer tissue microarray. American Journal of Clinical Pathology 2002;117:723–8.

Pertschuk L, Feldman J, Kim Y-D et al. Estrogen receptor (ER) immunocytochemistry in paraffin with ER1D5 predicts breast cancer endocrine response more accurately that H222Sp in frozen sections or cytosol-based ligand binding assays. Cancer 1996;77:2541–9.

Pousen HS, Ozello L, King WJ, Greene GL. The use of monoclonal antibodies to estrogen receptors (ER) for immunoperoxidase detection of ER in paraffin sections of human breast cancer tissue. Journal of Histochemistry and Cytochemistry 1985;33:87–92.

Raymond WA, Leong AS-Y. An evaluation of potentially suitable fixatives for immunoperoxidase staining of estrogen receptors in imprints and frozen sections of breast carcinoma. Pathology 1988;20:320–5.

Raymond WA, Leong AS-Y. Estrogen receptor staining of paraffin-embedded breast carcinomas following short fixation in formalin: A comparison with cytosolic and frozen section receptor analyses. Journal of Pathology 1990;160:295–303.

Rhodes A, Jasani B, Barnes DM, et al. Reliability of immunohistochemical demonstration of oestrogen receptors in routine practice: interlaboratory variance in the sensitivity of detection and evaluation of scoring systems. Journal of Clinical Pathology 2000;53:125–30.

Rhodes A, Jasani B. Balaton AJ, et al. Study of interlaboratory reliability and reproducibility of estrogen and progesterone receptor assays in Europe. Documentation of poor reliability and identification of insufficient microwave antigen retrieval time as a major contributory element of unreliable assays. American Journal of Clinical Pathology 2001;115:44–58.

Suthipintawong C, Leong AS-Y, Chan KW, Vinyuvat S. Immunostaining of estrogen receptor, progesterone receptor, MIB1 and c-erbB-2 in cytological preparations – a simplified method. Diagnostic Cytopathology 1997;17:127–33.

Schwabe JWR, Newhause D, Rhodes D. Solution structure of the DNA-binding domain of estrogen receptor. Nature 1990;348:458–61.

Taylor CR. Paraffin section immunocytochemistry for estrogen receptor. The time has come. Journal of Histotechnology 1997;20:97–100.

Factor VIII RA (von Willebrand factor)

Sources/clones

Accurate (KG7/30), Axell/Accurate (F8/86, polyclonal), Biodesign (101, 102, 103), Biogenesis (37–56/3, 21–43, WF7, polyclonal), Biogenex (polyclonal), Dako (F8/86, polyclonal), Sanbio (KG7/30), Serotec (F8, F8/86), Zymed (Z002, polyclonal).

Fixation/preparation

The antigen is fixation resistant. Proteolytic digestion or HIER enhances immunoreactivity.

Background

Factor VIII related antigen is more appropriately known as the von Willebrand factor (Marder et al, 1985). Factor VIII is a glycoprotein and is complexed with Factor VIII related antigen in plasma. Factor VIII is also present in endothelial cells where it shows a granular pattern of reactivity. It is also present in the cytoplasm of megakaryocytes.

Applications

Factor VIII related antigen or von Willebrand factor was one of the first markers employed for endothelial cell differentiation in angiosarcomas (Sehested et al, 1981), but it soon became apparent that the von Willebrand factor is seldom expressed in poorly differentiated vascular tumors (Swanson & Wick, 1993). Other markers of endothelial cells provide a higher diagnostic yield and they include CD34, CD31 (Appendix 1.23) and Ulex europeus agglutinin I. There is also considerable overlap between the expression of von Willebrand factor in vascular and lymphatic endothelium (Suthipintawong et al, 1995).

Von Willebrand factor remains a sensitive marker of benign blood vessels and has been used for the study of angiogenesis in neoplasms such as breast cancer (Weidner et al, 1991).

Comments

von Willlebrand factor must be used in conjunction with other more sensitive markers of endothelial cells when identifying angiosarcomas. It should be noted that seepage of the antigen may occur from surrounding blood, particularly in hemorrhagic or vascular lesions and interpretation should be made with caution in such situations. Although von Willebrand factor continues to be used to delineate vessels in studies of tumor angiogenesis (Guidi et al, 2002; Vacca et al, 2001; Juric et al, 2001), other markers of endothelial cells including CD34 and CD31 serve this purpose better, particularly CD31 which is more sensitive and more specific (Suthipintawong et al, 1995).

References

Guidi AJ, Berry DA, Broadwater G, et al. Association of angiogenesis and disease outcome in node-positive breast cancer patients treated with adjuvant cyclophosphamide, doxorubicin, and fluorouracil: a Cancer and Leukemia Group B correlative science study from protocols 8541/8869. Journal of Clinical Oncology 2002;20:732–42.

Jiric G, Zarkovic N, Nola M, et al. The value of cell proliferation and agngiogenesis in the prognostic assessment of ovarian granulose cell tumors. Tumori 2001;87:47–53.

Marder VJ, Mannucci PM, Firkin BG, et al. Standard nomenclature for factor VIII and von Willebrand factor: a recommendation by the International Committee on Thrombosis and Haemostasis. Thrombosis and Hemostasis 1985;54:871–2.

Sehested M, Hou-Jensen K. Factor VIII-related antigen as an endothelial cell marker in benign and malignant diseases. Virchow's Archives (Pathology and Anatomy) 1981;391:217–25.

Suthipintawong C, Leong AS-Y, Vinyuvat S. A comparative study of immunomarkers for lymphangiomas and hemangiomas. Applied Immunohistochemistry 1995;3:239–44.

Swanson PE, Wick MR. Immunohistochemistry of cutaneous tumors. IN: Leong AS-Y (editor): Applied Immunohistochemistry for Surgical Pathologists. London: Edward Arnold, 1993, pp 270–302.

Vacca A, Ribatti D, Roccaro AM, et al. Bone marrow angiogenesis in patients with active multiple myeloma. Seminars in Oncology 2001;28:543–50.

Weidner N, Semple JP, Welch WR, et al. Tumor angiogenesis and metastasis – correlation in invasive breast carcinoma. New England Journal of Medicine 1991;324:1–8.

Factor XIIIa

Sources/clones

Biocare (polyclonal), Calbiochem (polyclonal), Cell Marque (polyclonal), Novocastra (polyclonal).

Fixation/preparation

The antibodies are immunoreactive in routinely fixed, paraffin-embedded sections. Staining is enhanced by HIER.

Background

Factor XIIIa is a blood pro-enzyme found in plasma and platelets. The reaction of Factor XIIIa with fibrin is the last enzyme-catalysed step on the coagulation cascade, leading to the formation of a normal blood clot stabilized as a result of fibrin cross-linkage. This transglutaminase exists in two forms, as an extracellular or plasma Factor XIIIa subunit attached to a dimer of the carrier protein or Factor XIIIb and an intracellular Factor XIII, which is exclusively the dimer of subunit "a" only. Intracellular Factor XIIIa has been identified in a variety of cells including human dendritic reticulum cells in reactive lymphoid follicles, fibroblast-like mesenchymal cells in connective tissue, and neoplastic fibroblastic and fibrohistiocytic lesions (Cerio et al, 1990). The dermal dendrocytes have been characterized as Factor XIIIa-positive dendritic cells of bone marrow origin that are typically found in the adventitia of dermal blood vessels and in the interstitial dermal connective tissues. In one study of dermal dendritic cells using CD34 and Factor XIIIa, it was found that antigenic profiles differed among the dendritic cell types (Nestle & Nickoloff, 1995a). At ultrastructural level, subepidermal dendritic cells (probably identical with lining macrophages) expressed Factor XIIIa only, perivascular dermal dendritic cells reacted with both Factor XIIIa and CD34, and reticular dermal dendritic cells were negative for Factor XIIIa but positive for CD34. However, at light microscopic level, perivascular dermal dendritic cells also expressed CD34.

Applications

The current diagnostic applications of Factor XIIIa pertain largely to the identification of dermal dendritic cells and their presence and role in various cutaneous and soft tissue tumors (Takata et al, 1994). Factor XIIIa has been described in various so-called fibrohistiocytic tumors including aneurysmal fibrous histiocytoma (Zeler et al, 1006), malignant fibrous histiocytoma (Nemes & Thomaszy, 1988), dermatofibroma (Nestle & Nickoloff, 1995b) and dermatofibrosarcoma protuberans (Leong & Lim, 1994). In the latter two conditions, Factor XIIIa expression appears to be associated with early lesions, with loss of expression in late or "mature" lesions. The marker also shows promise as a diagnostic discriminator for hepatocellular carcinoma from its morphologic mimics cholangiocarcinoma and metastatic carcinoma in the liver.

With increased used of this marker, a large number of tumors have been shown to be positive for Factor XIIIa. Among these are calcifying fibrous pseudotumor (Hill et al, 2001), dermatofibroma (Mentzel et al, 2001), solitary fibrous tumor (Alawi et al, 2001), and a number of so-called histiocytic lesions including xanthoma, xanthogranuloma (Kraus et al, 2001), pigmented villonodular synovitis, fibroblastic reticular cell tumor, malignant fibrous histiocytoma, atypical fibroxanthoma and epithelioid histiocytic proliferations (Busam et al, 2000). Interestingly, the antigen is also immunoexpressed in hemangiopericytomas, contributing to the morphologic and immunohistochemical similarities of this lesion to solitary fibrous tumors, both lesions staining for CD34, bcl2 and CD99 (Alawi et al, 2001). Glomus tumor, meningioma, neurothekoma, inflammatory pseudotumor and cerebellar hemangioblastoma also express this antigen, albeit, less frequently.

Comments

Reactivity in frozen sections is generally weak. We employ the polyclonal antibody from Calbiochem for paraffin section immunostaining.

References

Alawi F, Stratton D, Freedman PD. Solitary fibrous tumor of the oral soft tissues: a cl;inicopathologic and immunohistochemical study of 16 cases. American Journal of Surgical Pathology 2001;25:900–10.

Busam KJ, Granter SR, Iversen K, Jungbluth AA. Immunohistochemical distinction of epithelioid histiocytic proliferations from epithelioid melanocytic nevi. American Journal of Dermatopathology 2000;22:237–41.

Cerio R, Spaull J, Oliver GF, Wilson-Jones E. A study of Factor XIIIa and MAC387 immunolabelling in normal and pathological skin. American Journal of Dermatopathology 1990;12:221–33.

Fucich LF, Cheles MK, Thung SN, et al. Primary versus metastatic hepatic carcinoma. An immunohistochemical study of 34 cases. Archives of Pathology and Laboratory Medicine 1994;118:927–30.

Hill KA, Gonzalez-Crussi, Chou PM. Calcifying fibrous pseudotumor versus inflammatory myofibroblastic tumor: a histological and immunohistochemical comparison. Modern Pathology 2001;14:784–90.

Kraus MD, Haley JC, Ruiz R, et al. "Juvenile" xanthogranuloma: an immunophenotypic study with a reappraisal of histiogenesis. American Journal of Dermatopathology 2001;23:104–11.

Leong AS-Y, Lim MHT. Immunohistochemical characteristics of dermatofibrosarcoma protuberans.

Applied Immunohistochemistry 1994;2:42–47.

Mentzel T, Kutzner H, Rutten A, Hugel H. Benign fibrous histiocytoma (dermatofibroma) of the face: cliinicopathologic and immunohistochemical study of 34 cases associated with an aggressive clinical behaviour. American Journal of Dermatopathology 2001;23:419–26.

Nemes Z, Thomaszy V. Factor XIIIa and the classic histiocytic markers in malignant fibrous histiocytoma. Human Pathology 1988;9:822–9.

Nestle FO, Nickoloff BJ. A fresh morphological and functional look at dermal dendritic cells. Journal of Cutaneous Pathology 1995a;22:385–93.

Nestle FO, Nickloff BJ, Burg G. Dermatofibroma: an abortive immunoreactive process mediated by dermal dendritic cells? Dermatology 1995b;190:265–8.

Takata M, Imai T, Hirone T. Factor XIIIa-positive cells in normal peripheral nerves and cutaneous neurofibromas of type-1 neurofibromatosis. American Journal of Dermatopathology 1994;16:37–43.

Zelger BW, Zelger BG, Steiner H, Ofner D. Aneurysmal and hemangiopericytoma-like fibrous histiocytoma. Journal of Clinical Pathology 1996;49:313–8.

Fas (CD95) and Fas-ligand (CD95L)

Sources/clones

FAS (CD95)

Alexis Corp (SM1/17, SM1/1, SM1/23, APO1–3), Dako (APO-1, DX2), Pharmingen (DX2, G254–274),

FAS-ligand (CD95L, anti-FAS)

Immunotech (4A5, 4H9), Pharmingen (NOK-1, NOK-2, G247–4)

Fixation/preparation

Several of the antibodies (clones APO-1, DX2) are immunoreactive in fixed, paraffin-embedded tissue sections as well as frozen sections and cell preparations.

Background

Fas (CD95) is a cell surface protein that belongs to the tumor necrosis factor family. Cross-linking of Fas and Fas-ligand (FasL) tranduces signals, which cumulate in apoptosis in sensitive cells. These proteins therefore, have a role in the genesis of neoplasms and have been extensively studied in this context. Their expression in certain malignancies has been implicated as a possible key

mechanism in the immune privilege of such tumors. FasL is also expressed in immunologically privileged sites in the non-neoplastic state. The induction of apoptosis by FasL in invading lymphocytes acts as a mechanism of immune privilege and is important in preventing graft rejection. The placenta, another immune privileged site, has also been shown to express high levels of FasL. The induction of apoptosis in lymphocytes by invading trophoblasts may account for the immune tolerance of the fetal semi-allograft (Hunt et al, 1997; Bamberger et al, 1997; Uckan et al, 1997). Experimentally, FasL can be employed to induce apoptosis in Fas-bearing cells. In coeliac disease mucosal flattening is thought to result from an increased enterocyte apoptosis triggered by Fas/FasL system and perforin cytolytic granules. This is not the case in autoimmune enteropathy where enterocyte autoantibody-dependent cellular cytotoxicity is the prevalent mechanism of enterocyte death (Ciccocioppo et al, 2002).

Fas and FasL expression has been studied in a wide variety of tissues and in other diseases besides neoplasms (Nichans et al, 1997; Muller et al, 1997;

Hellquist et al, 1997; Nonomura et al, 1996; Tachibana et al, 1996). These include idiopathic pulmonary fibrosis (Kazufumi et al, 1997), human cancers following ionizing radiation (Sheard et al, 1997), Alzheimer's disease (de la Monte et al, 1997), chronic hepatitis (Lou et al, 1997), alveolar type II pneumocytes (Fine et al, 1997), colonic epithelial cells (Strater et al, 1997), inflammatory myopathies (Behrens et al, 1997), diabetes (Chervonsky et al, 1997) and germ cells of the testis (Lee et al, 1997).

Applications

Interest in immunostaining for Fas and FasL centers around their role in tumor destruction. Macrophages and lymphocytes express high levels of Fas and it has been thought that expression of FasL by tumor cells allows destruction of Fas-positive lymphocytes, allowing the survival of the tumor cells in vivo. With the discovery that tumors may express both FasL and Fas, it is realized that tumors like melanoma may induce their own apoptosis in an autocrine and/or paracrine fashion and that the decline of tumor apoptosis rather than the apoptosis of infiltrating lymphocytes may affect prognosis (Shukuwa et al, 2002).

Macrophages heavily infected by tuberculosis or leprosy bacteria have been shown to be induced to express high levels of FasL, which may protect them from destruction by Fas-expressing lymphocytes (Mustafa et al, 2001).

References

Bamberger AM, Schulte HM, Thuneke I, et al. Expression of the apoptosis-inducing Fas ligand (FasL) in human first and third trimester placenta and choriocarcinoma cells. Journal of Clinical Endocrinology and Metabolism 1997;82:3173–5.

Behrens L, Bender A, Johnson MA, Hohlfeld R. Cytotoxic mechanisms in inflammatory myopathies. Co-expression of Fas and protective Bcl-2 in muscle fibres and inflammatory cells. Brain 1997;120 (Part 6):929–38.

Ciccocioppo R, D'Alo S, Di Sabatino A, et al. Mechanisms of villous atrophy in autoimmune enteropathy and coeliac disease. Clinical and Experimental Immunology 2002;128:88–93.

De la Monte SM, Sohn YK, Wands JR. Correlates of p53- and Fas (CD95)-mediated apoptosis in Alzheimer's disease. Journal of Neurological Sciences 1997;152:73–83.

Fine A, Aanderson NL, Rothstein TL, et al. Fas expression in pulmonary alveolar type II cells. American Journal of Physiology 1997;273:(1 Part 1):L64-L71.

Hellquist HB, Olejnicka B, Jadner M, et al. Fas receptor is expressed in human lung squamous cell carcinomas, whereas bcl-2 and apoptosis are not pronounced: a preliminary report. British Journal of Cancer 1997;76:175–9.

Hunt JS, Vassmer D, Ferguson TA, Miller L. Fas ligand is positioned in mouse uterus and placenta to prevent trafficking of activated leukocytes between the mother and the conceptus. Journal of Immunology 1997;158:4122–8.

Kazufumi M, Sonoko N, Masanori K, et al. Expression of bcl-2 protein and APO-1 (Fas antigen) in the lung tissue from patients with idiopathic pulmonary fibrosis. Microscopy Research Technology 1997;38:480–7.

Lee J, Richburg JH, Younkin SC, Bockelheide K. The Fas system is a key regulator of germ cell apoptosis in the testis. Endocrinology 1997;138:2081–8.

Luo KX, Zhu YF, Zhang LX, et al. In situ investigation of Fas/FasL expression in chronic hepatitis B infection and related liver diseases. Journal of Viral Hepatitis 1997;4:303–7.

Muller M, Strand S, Hug H, et al. Drug-induced apoptosis in hepatoma cells is mediated by the CD95 (APO-1/Fas) receptor/ligand system and involves activation of wild-type p53. Journal of Clinical Investigation 1997;99:403–13.

Mustafa T, Bjune TG, Jonsson R, et al. Increased expression of fas ligand in human tuberculosis and leprosy lesions: a potential novel mechanism of immune evasion in mycobacterial infection. Scandinavian Journal of Immunology 2001;54:630–9.

Nichans GA, Brunner T, Frizelle SP, et al. Human lung carcinomas express Fas ligand. Cancer Research 1997;57:1007–12.

Nonomura N, Miki T, Yokoyama M, et al. Fas/APO-1-mediated apoptosis of human renal cell carcinoma. Biochemistry Biophysiology Research Communications 1996;229:945–51.

Sheard MA, Vojtesek B, Janakova L, et al. Up-regulation of Fas (CD95) in human p53 wild-type cancer cells treated with ionizing radiation. International Journal of Cancer 1997;73:757–62.

Shukuwa T, Katayama I, Koji T. Fas-mediated apoptosis of melanoma cells and infiltrating lymphocytes in human malignant melanomas. Modern Pathology 2002;15:387–96.

Strater J, Wellisch I, Riedl S, et al. CD95 (APO-1/Fas)-mediated apoptosis in colon epithelial cells: a possible role in ulcerative colitis. Gastroenterology 1997;113:160–7.

Uckan D, Steele A, Wang BY, et al. Trophoblasts express Fas ligand: a proposed mechanism for immune privilege in placenta and maternal invasion. Molecular Human Reproduction 1997;3:655–62.

Tachibana O, Lampe J< Kleihues P, Obgaki H. Preferential expression of Fas/APO1 (CD95) and apoptotic cell death in perinecrotic cells of glioblastoma multiforme. Acta Neuropathologica (Berlin) 1996;92:431–4.

Fascin

Source/clone

Dako (clone 55K-2).

Fixation/preparation

Anti-fascin is applicable to formalin-fixed, paraffin-embedded tissue sections. A heat-induced isotope retrieval system is essential prior to the immunohistochemical staining procedure.

Background

Human fascin is a highly conserved 55-kD actin-bundling protein. Fascin is encoded by the human homolog for *hsn* gene and is thought to be involved in the formation of microfilament bundles. The clone 55K-2 was raised against fascin purified and characterized from HeLa cells (Yamashiro-Matsumura & Matsumura, 1985; Duh et al, 1994).

Fascin immunoexpression has been demonstrated in interdigitating reticulum cells, follicular dendritic cells and interstitial dendritic cells in lymph nodes. In addition, strong immunoreactivity has also been observed in dendritic cells of the thymus and spleen (Mosialos et al, 1996; Pinkus et al, 1997).

Histiocytes, smooth muscle cells, endothelial cells and squamous mucosal cells may also express fascin. Fascin-expressing dendritic cells are decreased or absent in the neoplastic follicles of germinal centres compared with hyperplastic follicular centres (Said et al, 1998). In contrast, cases of Castleman's disease revealed tight syncytial networks of fascin-positive follicular dendritic cells.

Fascin has been demonstrated in the cytoplasm of most Reed-Sternberg cells and their variants in Hodgkin's disease; whilst only a minority of non-Hodgkin's lymphoma was immunoreactive (Pinkus et al, 1997). More recently, fascin immunopositivity has highlighted Reed-Sternberg cells in follicular Hodgkin's lymphoma (Kansal et al, 2002). Follicular dendritic cell tumors (Biddle et al, 2002) and juvenile xanthogranulomas (Kraus et al, 2001) have demonstrated uniform immunopositivity with fascin. However, only 75% of interdigitating dendritic cell sarcomas were fascin positive (Gaertner et al, 2001).

Application

Fascin immunoreactivity in Hodgkin's disease may serve to complement CD15 and CD30 to identify Reed-Sternberg cells (Appendix 2.3). Similarly, addition of fascin to CD21 and CD35 would be useful to identify follicular dendritic cell tumors (Appendix 2.8).

References

Biddle DA, Ro JY, Yoon GS, et al. Extranodal follicular dendritic cell sarcoma of the heard and neck region: three new cases, with a review of the literature. Modern Pathology 2002;15:50–8.

Dako Corporation. Anti-human fascin, 55K-2 (data sheet).

Duh FM, Latif F, Weng Y, et al. CDNA cloning and expression of the human homolog of the sea urchin fascin and Drosophila singed genes which encodes an actin-bundling protein. DNA & Cell Biology 1994;13:821–7.

Gaertner EM, Tsokos M, Derringer GA, et al. Interdigitating dendritic cell sarcoma. A report of four cases and review of the literature. The American Journal of Clinical Pathology 2001:115:589–97.

Kansal R, Singleton TP, Ross CW, et al. Follicular Hodgkin lymphoma: a histopathologic study. The American Journal of Clinical Pathology 2002;117:29–35.

Kraus MD, Haley JC, Ruiz R, et al. "Juvenile" xanthogranuloma: an immunophenotypic study with a reappraisal of histogenesis. American Journal of Dermatopathology 2001;23:104–11.

Mosialos G, Birkenbach M, Ayehunie S, et al. Circulating human dendritic cells differentially express high levels of 55-kd actin-bundling protein. American Journal of Pathology 1996;148:593–600.

Pinkus GS, Pinkus JL, Langhoff E, et al. Fascin, a sensitive new marker for Reed-Sternberg cells of Hodgkin's disease: evidence for a dendritic or B-cell derivation? American Journal of Pathology 1997;150:543–62.

Said JW, Pinkus JL, Shintaku IP, et al. Alterations in fascin-expressing germinal center dendritic cells in neoplastic follicles of B-cell lymphomas. Modern Pathology 1998;11:1–5.

Yamashiro-Matsumura S, Matsumura F. Purification and characterization of an F-actin-bundling 55-kilodalton protein from HeLa cells. Journal of Biological Chemistry 1985;260:5087–97.

Ferritin

Sources/clones

American Research Products (047A1703), Axcel/Accurate (polyclonal), Biodesign (ME.110, S1, S2, 501, 502, 503, 504, polyclonal), Biogenesis (05, 7D3/7, polyclonal), Biogenex (M-3.170, polyclonal), Chemicon (polyclonal), Dako (polyclonal), Fitzgerald (M94156, M94157, M94159, M94160, M94212, M94258, polyclonal), Serotec (polyclonal), Zymed (ZMFE1).

Fixation/preparation

Ferritin is resistant to formalin fixation and immunoreactivity is enhanced following HIER.

Background

Ferritin, the iron storage protein, plays a key role in iron metabolism and its ability to sequester iron gives ferritin the dual functions of iron detoxification and iron reserve. The distribution of ferritin is ubiquitous among living species and its three-dimensional structure is highly conserved. All ferritins have 24 protein subunits arranged in 432 symmetry to give a hollow shell with an 80 A diameter cavity capable of storing up to 45000 Fe (III) atoms as an inorganic complex. Subunits are folded as 4-helix bundles each having a fifth short helix at roughly 60 degrees to the bundle axis (Harrison & Arosio, 1996).

Applications

Ferritin was one of the first markers employed for the identification of hepatocytes and their neoplastic counterparts (Imoto et al, 1985; Johnson et al, 1992), but it proved to be of low sensitivity and low specificity, being found in a wide range of benign and neoplastic tissues (Fleming 1987; Pennys et al, 1990; Tuccari et al, 1992; Momotani et al, 1992). Ferritin is expressed in hepatoid tumors such as those in the ovary (Nogales et al, 1993) and hepatoblastomas (Abenoza et al, 1987). Ferritin is employed as a marker of hemorrhage in the brain (Ozawa et al, 1994; Carter et al, 1991) and is employed as a marker of microglia (Kaneko et al, 1989). In bone marrow biopsies, ferritin has been found to correlate with marrow hemosiderin as detected by the Perl's stain and is advocated as a more sensitive tool for the evaluation of body iron stores (Navone et al, 1988). In the skin, ferritin is localized to the outer layer of the eccrine duct and in sweat gland neoplasms, two distinct patterns were noted. In syringoma the antibody decorated the outermost layer of cells in the epithelial cords of the tumor so that a characteristic ring was produced in cross sections; whereas, only sparse staining was observed with other eccrine duct tumors such as dermal duct tumor and eccrine poroma. Syringoma showed diffuse staining as did acrospiroma and a number of other adnexal carcinomas (Penneys & Zlatkiss, 1990).

The presence of ferritin in epithelial cells often indicates increased cell permeability and this property has been exploited in the demonstration that hyaline globules associated with a variety of tumors are the product of apoptotic cell death; the name "thanotosomes" being recently proposed for such hyaline globules (Papadimitriou et al, 2000).

Comments

The diagnostic applications of this marker are limited, and except perhaps for the assessment of bone marrow iron stores, ferritin immunostaining is never employed alone.

F

Ferritin

References

Abenoza P, Manivel JC, Wick Mr, et al. Hepatoblastoma: an immunohistochemical and ultrastructural study. Human Pathology 1987;18:1025–35.

Carter RL, Hall JM, Corbett RP. Immunohistochemical staining for ferritin in neuroblastomas. Histopathology 1991;18:465–8.

Fleming S. Immunocytochemical localization of ferritin in the kidney and renal tumors. European Urology 1987;13:407–11.

Harrison PM, Arosio P. The ferritins: molecular properties, iron storage function and cellular regulation. Biochemia Biophysiologica Acta 1996;1275:161–203.

Imoto M, Nishimura D, Fukuda Y, et al. Immunohistochemical detection of alpha-fetoprotein, carcinoembryonic antigen, and ferritin in formalin-fixed sections from hepatocellular carcinoma. American Journal of Gastroenterology 1985;80:902–6.

Johnson DE, Powers CN, Rupp G, et al. Immunocytochemical staining of fine needle aspiration biopsies of the liver as a diagnostic tool for hepatocellular carcinoma. Modern Pathology 1992;5:117–23.

Kaneko Y, Kitamoto T, Tateishi J, Yamaguchi K. Ferritin immunohistochemistry as a marker for microglia. Acta Neuropathologica (Berlin) 1989;79:129–36.

Momotani E, Wuscger N, Ravisse P, Rastogi N. Immunohistochemical identification of ferritin, lactoferrin and transferrin in leprosy lesions of human skin biopsies. Journal of Comparative Pathology 1992;106:213–20.

Navone R, Azzoni L, Valente G. Immunohistochemical assessment of ferritin in bone marrow trephine biopsies: correlation with marrow hemosiderin. Acta Hematologica 1988;80:194–8.

Nogales FF, Concha A, Plata C, Ruiz-Avila I. Granulosa cell tumor of the ovary with diffuse true hepatic differentiation simulating stromal luteinization. American Journal of Surgical Pathology 1993;17:85–90.

Ozawa H, Nishida A, Mito T, Takashima S. Immunohistochemical study of ferritin-positive cells in the cerebellar cortex with subarachnoid hemorrhage in neonates. Brain Research 1994;65: 345–8.

Papadimitriou JC, Drachenberg CB, Brenner DS, et al. "Thanatosomes": a unifying morphogenetic concept for tumor hyaline globules related to apoptosis. Human Pathology 2000;31: 1455–65.

Penneys NS, Zlatkiss I. Immunohistochemical demonstration of ferritin in sweat gland and sweat gland neoplasms. Journal of Cutaneous Pathology 1990;17: 32–6.

Tuccari G, Rizzo A, Crisafulli C, Barresi G. Iron-binding proteins in human colorectal adenomas and carcinomas: an immunohistochemical investigation. Histology and Histopathology 1992;7: 543–7.

Fibrin

Sources/clones

Accurate (T2G1), Biodesign (polyclonal), Biogenesis (2F7), Serotec (E8).

Fixation/preparation

The antigen is resistant to formalin fixation and proteolytic digestion or HIER enhances immunoreactivity.

Background

Proteolytic conversion of fibrinogen to fibrin results in self-assembly to form a clot matrix that subsequently becomes cross-linked by factor XIIIa to form the main structural element of the thrombus in vivo. The roles of fibrin and its precursor have been extensively studied both in vitro and in vivo (Lorand 1965; Blomback, 1994, 1996; Gaffney 1997; Mosessan 1992, 1997).

Applications

Diagnostic applications of fibrin are mainly limited to the study of glomerulopathy (Dowling 1993) with sporadic use of anti-fibrin to identify fibrin deposits and thrombi in extra-renal sites (Bini & Kudruk, 1994; Takahashi et al,

1996; Imokawa et al, 1997; Kahng et al, 2002).

Comments

The diagnostic applications of anti-fibrin are limited to specific situations. Applications in nephropathology, particularly with immunofluoresence techniques are still extensive (Bonsib, 2002).

References

Bini A, Kudryk BJ. Fibrinogen and fibrin in the arterial wall. Thrombosis Research 1994;75:337–41.

Blomback B. fibrinogen structure, activation and polymerization and fibrin gel structure. Thrombosis Research 1994;75:327–8.

Blomback B. Fibrinogen and fibrin – proteins with complex roles in hemostasis and thrombosis. Thrombosis Research 1996;83:1–75.

Bonsib SM. Differential diagnosis in nephropathology: an immunofluorescence-driven approach. Advances in Anatomical Pathology 2002;9:101–14.

Dowling JP. Immunohistochemistry of renal diseases and tumours. IN: Leong AS-Y (editor). Applied Immunohistochemistry ofr Surgical Pathologists. London: Edward Arnold, 1993, pp 210–59.

Gaffney PJ. Structure of fibrinogen and degradation products of

fibrinogen and fibrin. British Medical Bulletin 1997;33:245–51.

Imokawa S, Sato A, Hayakawa H, et al. Tissue factor expression and fibrin deposition in the lungs of patients with idiopathic pulmonary fibrosis and systemic sclerosis. American Journal of Respiratory and Critical Care Medicine 1997;156 (2 Pt 1):631–6.

Kahng HC, Chin NW, Opitz LM, et al. Cellular angiolipoma of the breast: immunohistochemical study and review of the literature. Breast Journal 2002;8:47–9.

Lorand L. Physiological roles of fibrinogen and fibrin. Federation Proceedings 1965;24:784–93.

Mosessan MW., the roles of fibrinogen and fibrin in hemostasis and thrombosis. Seminars in Hematology 1992;29:177–88.

Mosessan MW. Fibrinogen and fibrin polymerization: appraisal of the binding events that accompany fibrin generation and fibrin clot assembly. Blood Coagulation and Fibrinolysis 1997;8:257–67.

Takahashi H, Shibata Y, Fujita S, Okabe H. Immunohistochemical findings of arterial fibrinoid necrosis in major and lingual minor salivary glands of primary Sjogren's syndrome. Anatomical and Cellular Pathology 1996;12:145–57.

NOTES

Fibrinogen

Sources/clones

Accurate (2C2G7, 85D4), Axcel/Accurate (polyclonal), American Qualex (polyclonal), Biodesign (PA), Biogenesis (2D1–2, polyclonal), Biogenex (2D1–2, polyclonal), Calbiochem (polyclonal), Caltag Laboratories, Chemicon, Coulter (D1G10VL2, E3F8E5), Dako (polyclonal), EY Labs, Immunotech (D1G10VL2, E3F8E5), Seralab (polyclonal), Sigma (85D4, FG21)

Fixation/preparation

Fibrinogen is fixative-resistant.

Background

Fibrinogen is a 340 kD multi-subunit glycoprotein present in plasma and tissue of all classes of vertebrates. Fibrinogen has a variety of physiologically important functions, most of which, if not all, are assigned to certain structures of fibrin including double-stranded fibrin protofibrils and highly cross-linked fibrin networks (Shafer & Higgins, 1988; Mosesson 1997). Its role in hemostasis and thrombosis has been extensively studied (Henschen 1983; Mosesson, 1992; Blomback 1996; Gaffney 1970).

Applications

Diagnostic applications of fibrinogen are largely limited to the identification of fibrinogen deposition and breakdown products in glomerular diseases (Dowling 1993).

Comments

Immunostaining for fibrin/fibrinogen deposits is employed for the detection of microthrombi (Stewart et al, 2001).

References

Blomback B. Fibrinogen and fibrin – proteins with complex roles in hemostasis and thrombosis. Thrombosis Research 1996;83:1–75.

Dowling JP. Immunohistochemistry of renal diseases and tumours. In: Leong AS-Y (editor). Applied Immunohistochemistry for the Surgical Pathologist. London: Edward Arnold, 1993, pp 210–59.

Gaffney PJ. Structure of fibrinogen and degradation products of fibrinogen and fibrin. British Medical Bulletin 1997;33:245–51.

Henschen A. On the structure of functional sites in fibrinogen. Thrombosis Research 1983;5 (Suppl):27–39.

Mosesson MW. The roles of fibrinogen and fibrin in hemostasis and thrombosis. Seminars in Hematology 1992;29:177–88.

Mosesson MW. Fibrinogen and fibrin polymerization: appraisal of the binding events that accompany fibrin generation and fibrin clot assembly. Blood coagulation and Fibrinolysis 1997;8:257–67.

Shafer JA, Higgins DL. Human fibrinogen. Critical Reviews in Clinical Laboratory Science 1988;26:1–41.

Stewart FA, Te Poele JA, Van der Wal AF, et al. Radiation nephropathy – the link between functional damage and vascular mediated inflammatory and thrombotic change. Acta Oncology 2001;40:952–7.

NOTES

Fibronectin

Sources/clones

Accurate (2B6F9, 568), Axcel/Accurate (polyclonal), Biodesign (1601, 1602, 120–5), Biogenesis (BIO-FIBTN-001, Bo, Rt, polyclonal), Biogenex (2755–8), Calbiochem (3E1, polyclonal), Caltag Laboratories, Cymbus Bioscience (FN4), Dako (polyclonal), EY Labs, Fitzgerald (polyclonal), Harlan Sera Lab/Accurate (2.3F9), Novocastra (polyclonal), Serotec (polyclonal), Sigma Chemical (FN-15, FN3-E2), Zymed (Z068, FN12–8).

Fixation/preparation

The antibody is well suited for both formalin-fixed paraffin embedded sections and cryostat sections. Proteolytic predigestion with protease or pepsin of formalin-fixed tissue is recommended (Kirkpatrick & d'Ardenne, 1984).

Background

Fibronectin is a non-collagenous connective tissue glycoprotein found in association with both basement membranes and interstitial connective tissue (Stenman & Vaheri, 1978). The exact ultrastructural localisation of fibronectin within the basement membrane is controversial (Laurie et al, 1982). Fibronectin is a β-glycoprotein with a molecular weight of 44 kD, comprising two nearly identical sub chains. It is widely distributed throughout many normal tissues including connective tissues, blood vessel walls and basement membranes. Some of the properties of fibronectin include forming crosslinks with fibrin in blood clots through factor XIII and binding to heparin and collagen. It is also thought to play a role in cellular adhesion, wound healing and tissue repair (Mosher & Fiocht, 1981). Antiserum to human fibronectin was produced from purified human material isolated from a pool of normal human plasma.

Applications

Fibronectin (and laminin) has been demonstrated to line cystic lumina and around tumor islands in adenoid cystic breast and salivary gland carcinomas (d'Ardenne et al, 1986). This pattern of distribution has been recommended as an aid to the diagnosis of these tumors, whilst the absence may have important prognostic implications with an aggressive outcome. Fibronectin immunoreactivity in breast adenoid cystic carcinomas is also useful to distinguish from cribriform carcinoma, the latter being negative.

In a comparative study of epithelial neoplasms of gastrointestinal and salivary gland origin, the difficulty in distinguishing between fibronectin of epithelial and fibroblastic origin was emphasized (d'Ardenne et al, 1983). In addition, carcinoma fibronectin was sometimes, but not invariably lost from epithelial cell surfaces, suggesting that loss of cell surface fibronectin was unlikely to serve as a useful diagnostic marker for malignancy. In soft tissue tumors, fibronectin was found to be most abundant in the stroma, both benign and malignant (d'Ardenne et al, 1984). Fibronectin failed to be useful in the identification of vitality of human skin injuries because of low sensitivity of immunohistochemical staining (Ortiz-Rey et al, 2002), although it was shown to be useful with immunofluoresence techniques as for the demonstration of decreased basement membrane in the intestinal mucosa of patients with celiac disease (Verbeke et al, 2002).

Comments

The major role of fibronectin is in the diagnosis of adenoid cystic carcinoma of the salivary gland and breast, with the latter being distinguished from cribriform carcinoma. Either adenoid cystic carcinoma or connective tissue stroma may be used as a positive control.

References

D' Ardenne AJ, Burns J, Skyes BC, Bennett MK. Fibronectin and type III collagen in epithelial neoplasms of gastrointestinal tract and salivary gland. Journal of Clinical Pathology 1983;36:756–63.

D'Ardenne AJ, Kirkpatrick P, Sykes BC. The distribution of laminin, fibronectin and interstitial collagen type III in soft tissue tumors. Journal of Clinical Pathology 1984;37:895–904.

D'Ardenne AJ, Kirkpatrick P, Wells CA, Davies JD. Laminin and fibronectin in adenoid cystic carcinoma. Journal of Clinical Pathology 1986;39:138–44.

Kirkpatrick P, D'ardenne AJ. Effects of fixation and enzymatic digestion on the immunohistochemical demonstration of laminin and fibronectin in paraffin embedded tissue. Journal of Clinical Pathology 1984;37:639–44.

Laurie GW, Leblond CP, Martin GR. Localisation of type IV collagen, laminin, heparan sulphate proteoglycan and fibronectin to the basal lamina of basement membranes. Journal of Cell Biology 1982;95:340–4.

Mosher DF, Fiocht L. Fibronectin: Review of its structure and possible functions. Journal of Investigative Dermatology 1981;77:175–80.

Ortiz-Rey JA, Suarez-Penaranda JM, da Silva EA, et al. Immunohistochemical detection of fibronectin and tenascin in incised human skin injuries. Forensic Science International 2002;126:118–22.

Stenman S, Vaheri A. Distribution of a major connective tissue protein, fibronectin in normal human tissues. Journal of Experimental Medicine 1978;147:1054–64.

Verbeke S, Gotteland M, Fernandez M, et al. Basement membrane and connective tissue proteins in intestinal mucosa of patients with celiac disease. Journal of Clinical Pathology 2002;55:440–5.

FLI-1 protein

Sources/clones

Santa Cruz (SC-356 polyclonal antibody)

Fixation/preparation

Heat induced retrieval is necessary for paraffin-embedded sections.

Background

Ewing's sarcoma/primitive neuroectodermal tumor (ES/PNET) are characterized in approximately 90% of cases by a reciprocal translocation t(11;22) (q24;q12) which results in the fusion of the *EWS* gene on chromosome 22 to the *FLI-1* gene on chromosome 11 (Turc-Carel et al, 1988; Zucman et al, 1992). The *FLI-1* (Friend leukemia virus integration site 1) gene encodes for a truncated transcription factor, belonging to the avian Erythroblastosis virus transforming sequence (ETS) family of DNA-binding transcription factors, is involved in cellular proliferation and tumorigenesis.

Using a polyclonal antibody raised against the carboxy-terminal of FLI-1 protein, workers have demonstrated FLI-1 immunopositivity in cytologic preparations of ES/PNET cell lines known to contain an EWS/FLI-1 fusion gene, and 5/7 formalin-fixed paraffin-embedded ES/PNET (Nilsson et al, 1999). Evaluating 132 well-characterized small, blue, round cell tumors, an independent study demonstrated the following immunopositivity using formalin-fixed, paraffin-embedded tissue: 29/41 (71%) ES/PNET, 7/8 (88%) lymphoblastic lymphomas, 0/8 poorly differentiated synovial sarcomas (PDSS), 0/32 rhabdomyosarcomas (RMS), 0/30 neuroblastomas, 0/8 esthesioneuroblastomas, 0/3 Wilm's tumor, 0/1 mesenchymal chondrosarcoma and 1/1 desmoplastic round cell tumor (Folpe et al, 2000). Another study from the same group demonstrated FLI-1 protein expression in 50/53 (94%) benign and malignant vascular tumors, including angiosarcomas, hemangioendotheliomas, hemangiomas and Kaposi's sarcomas (Folpe et al, 2001). In contrast, FLI-1 expression was absent in 68 non-vascular tumors including sarcomas, melanomas and carcinomas.

Applications

FLI-1 nuclear transcription factor appears to be a relatively sensitive and specific marker for ES/PNET. However, a note of caution in the differential diagnosis of small round blue cell tumors is that the great majority of lymphoblastic lymphomas are also positive with FLI-1 protein. Nevertheless, FLI-1 protein is useful to distinguish ES/PNET from other CD99-positive tumors such as PDSS and RMS (Appendix 1.3). The FLI-1 immunopositivity in vascular tumors appears to equal or exceed those of established vascular markers such as CD31, CD34 and FVIII.

Comments

Being a transcription factor, FLI-1 immunopositivity is nuclear in location.

References

Folpe AL, Chand EM, Goldblum JR, Weiss SW. Expression of Fli-1, a nuclear transcription factor, distinguishes vascular neoplasms from potential mimics. American Journal of Surgical Pathology 2001;25:1061–6.

Folpe AL, Hill CE, Parham DM, et al. Immunohistochemical detection of FLI-1 protein expression: A study of 132 round cell tumors with emphasis on CD99-positive mimics of Ewing's sarcoma/primitive neuroectodermal tumor. American Journal of Surgical Pathology 2000;24:1657–62.

Nilsson G, Wang M, Wejde J, et al. Detection of EWS/FLI-1 by immunostaining. An adjunctive tool in diagnosis of Ewing's sarcoma and primitive neuroectodermal tumor on cytological samples and paraffin-embedded archival material. Sarcoma 1999;3:25–32.

Turc-Carel C, Aurias A, Mugneret F, et al. Chromosomes in Ewing's sarcoma. I: an evaluation of 85 cases of remarkable consistency of t(11;22)(q24;q12). Cancer Genetics and Cytogenetics 1988;32:229–38.

Zucman J, Delattre O, Desmaze C, et al. Cloning and characterization of the Ewing's sarcoma and peripheral neuroepithelioma t(11;22) translocation breakpoints. Genes Chromosomes and Cancer 1992;5:271–7.

FMC-7

Source/clone

Monoclonal antibody FMC-7
(Immunotech, Beckman Coulter
Company)

Fixation/preparation

This antibody has been largely
utilized by flow cytometry with
FMC-7-FITC. Its role in
immunophenotyping of mature
B-cell lymphomas has been
utilized in the recent World
Health Organization classification
for lymphomas.

Background

The monoclonal antibody FMC-
7, developed at the Flinders
Medical Centre (Australia) by
somatic hybridization against the
human B-cell line HRIK, appears
to define a subset of normal
human B-lymphocytes. It is also
useful to distinguish mature B-
cell leukemias from immature
variants (Drexler et al, 1987; Zola
et al, 1984; Zola et al, 1983;
Catovsky et al, 1981). The
antibody FMC-7 detects an
antigen on certain subgroups of
neoplastic and normal B-cells
that have arisen from cells in later
stages of B-cell maturation (Huh
et al, 1994). However, some
studies indicate that the use of

FMC-7 antibody in
immunophenotypic studies of
lymphomas does not contribute
any additional information or
diagnostic reliability (Hubl et al,
1998 ; Menon et al, 1986).

A recent study evaluated
FMC-7 and CD23 expression
pattern in 201 cases of B-cell
lymphoma (Garcia et al, 2001).
These authors concluded that the
CD23 negative/FMC-7 positive
pattern was most common in
large cell, mantle and marginal
zone lymphomas. The
CD23/FMC-7/CD5
coexpression pattern permitted
accurate classification of all 71
cases of small lymphocytic,
mantle cell and marginal zone
lymphomas. The widest variation
of patterns was with follicular cell
lymphomas. The CD23 and
FMC-7 antigen expression
pattern was predictive of subtypes
in more than 95% of lymphoma
cases and could narrow the
differential diagnosis in the
remaining cases.

Applications

It would appear that FMC-7
expression in combination with
CD23 facilitates accurate and
reproducible classification of B-
cell lymphomas in flow
cytometric analysis.

References

Catovsky D, Brooks D, Bradley J et al
1981. Heterogeneity of B-cell
leukemias demonstrated by the
monoclonal antibody FMC-7.
Blood 58:406–8.

Drexler HG, Menon M, Gaedicke G,
Minowada J 1987. Expression of
FMC7 antigen and tartrate-
resistant acid phosphatase
isoenzyme in cases of B-
lymphoproliferative diseases.
European Journal of Cancer and
Clinical Oncology 23:61–8.

Garcia DP, Rooney MT, Ahmad E,
Davis BH 2001. Diagnostic
usefulness of CD23 and FMC-7
antigen expression patterns in B-
cell lymphoma classification.
American Journal of Clinical
Pathology 115:258–65.

Hubl W, Iturraspe J, Braylan RC
1998. FMC7 antigen expression
on normal and malignant B-cells
can be predicted by expression of
CD20. Cytometry 34:71–4.

Huh YO, Pugh WC, Kantarjian HM,
Stass SA, Cork A, Turjillo JM,
Keating MJ 1994. Detection of
subgroups of chronic B-cell
leukemias as FMC7 monoclonal
antibody. American Journal of
Clinical Pathology 101:283–9.

Menon M. Drexler HG, Minowada J
1986. Heterogeneity of marker
expression in B-cell leukemias
and its diagnostic significance.
Leukemia Research 10:25–8.

Zola H, Moore HA, Hohmann A,
Hunter IK 1984. The antigen of
mature human B cells detected by

the monoclonal antibody FMC7: Studies on the nature of the antigen and modulation of its expression. Journal of Immunology 133:321–6.

Zola H, McNamara PJ, Moore HA, Smart IJ, Brooks DA, Beckman IG, Bradley J 1983. Maturation of human B lymphocytes: studies with a panel of monoclonal antibodies against membrane antigens. Clinical and Experimental Immunology 52:655–64.

Glial Fibrillary Acidic Protein (GFAP)

Sources/clones

Accurate (GA-5, 6F2, polyclonal), Amersham, Biodesign (DP46.10, GF-01), Biogenesis (GF-01, polyclonal), Biogenex (GA-5, polyclonal), Chemicon (monoclonal, polyclonal), Cymbus Bioscience (polyclonal), Dako (6F2, polyclonal), Enzo, EY Labs, ICN (polyclonal), Immunotech (DP46.10), Milab (polyclonal), Novocastra, Sanbio (6F2, polyclonal), Saxo (polyclonal), Sera Lab (GA-5), Serotec (GA5, MIG-G2), Sigma (GA-5, polyclonal), Signet, Zymed (ZSGFAP2, ZCG29).

Fixation/preparation

Glial fibrillary acidic protein (GFAP) is relatively resilient to fixation and most antibodies are immunoreactive in routinely fixed and processed tissue sections. GFAP staining seems more consistent after fixation in Bouin's fixative. Monoclonal antibodies are more fixative-sensitive and polyclonal antibodies show more intense and more extensive staining. GFAP immunoreactivity is mildly enhanced by HIER.

Background

GFAP is an intermediate filament (IF) protein of astroglia and belongs to the type III subclass of IF proteins. Like other IF proteins, GFAP is composed of an amino-terminal head domain, a central rod domain and a carboxyterminal tail domain. GFAP with a molecular mass of 50 kD, has the smallest head domain among the class III IF proteins. Despite its insolubility, GFAP is in dynamic equilibrium between assembled filaments and unassembled subunits. As with other IF proteins, assembly of GFAP is regulated by phosphorylation-dephosphorylation of the head domain by alteration of its charge. The frequent co-polymerization of GFAP with vimentin IF in immature, reactive or radial glial indicates that vimentin has an important role in the build up of the glial architecture (Inagaki et al, 1994). The human GFAP gene is localized to chromosome 17.

Applications

In the central nervous system, astrocytes, rare ependymal cells and cerebellar radial glia express GFAP (Appendix 1.2). Mature oligodendrocytes do not express GFAP. GFAP or a GFAP-like protein is also found in Schwann cells, enteric glia, cells in all portions of the pituitary, cartilage, the iris and lens epithelium and the fat-storing cells of the liver. While monoclonal antibodies are said to recognize the GFAP epitope exclusively, there may be cross-reactivity with common epitopes shared by other IFs like neurofilaments and vimentin.

Immunohistochemical staining of GFAP has proven use in the identification of benign astrocytes and neoplastic cells of glial lineage (Sillevis-Smitt et al, 1993). Its application to the developing nervous system has contributed to our understanding of the histogenesis of neural tissue and its identification in various forms of injury and neoplasia has helped in the understanding of the role of astrocytes in these processes.

While it was initially thought that the GFAP expression in salivary gland tissues and pleomorphic adenomas was in myoepithelial cells (Lee et al, 1993), more recent evidence from developmental and cell culture studies indicate that GFAP is expressed in the epithelial cells, the myoepithelial cells being uniformly negative for the antigen (Okura et al, 1996). GFAP has been demonstrated in cartilage cells in culture (Benjamin et al, 1994) but do not appear to occur in chondrosarcomas and mesenchymal chondrosarcomas (Swanson et al, 1990) and *in vivo* and immunohistochemical detection of GFAP is used to identify chordomas. Choroid plexus tumors (Radotra et al, 1994) and ependymomas express GFAP in addition to S100 protein and occasionally, cytokeratin and epithelial membrane antigen. In the setting of vacuolated clear cell tumors occurring in the retroperitoneal space, GFAP positivity would serve to identify chordoma and ependymoma from other mimics, including renal cell carcinoma and colorectal carcinoma (Coffin et al, 1993).

Comments

Polyclonal antibodies to GFAP produce more intense and more extensive staining than monoclonal antibodies (Wittchow & Landas, 1991). GFAP together with S100 are sensitive markers of glial differentiation (Giannini et al, 2002). GFAP is useful in the identification intracranial and intraventricular tumors

(Appendix 1.7 and 1.35 respectively) and the differential diagnosis of small cell tumors in the brain (Appendix 1.36).

References

Benjamin M, Archer CW, Ralphs JR. Cytoskeleton of cartilage cells. Microscopic Research Technology 1994;28:372–7.

Coffin CM, Swanson PE, Wick MR, Dehner LP. An immunohistochemical comparison of chordoma with renal cell carcinoma, colorectal adenocarcinoma, and myxopapillary ependymoma: a potential diagnostic dilemma in the diminutive biopsy. Modern Pathology 1993;5;531–8.

Giannini C, Scheithauer BW, Lopes MB, et al. Immunophenotype of pleomorphic xanthoastrocytoma. American Journal of Surgical Pathology 2002;26:479–85.

Inagaki M, Nakamura Y, Takeda M, et al. Glial fibrillary acidic protein: dynamic property and regulation by phosphorylation. Brain Pathology 1994;4:239–43.

Lee SK, Kim EC, Chi JG, et al. Immunohistochemical detection of S-100 alpha, S-100 beta proteins, glial fibrillary acidic protein, and neuron specific enolase in the prenatal and adult human salivary gland. Pathology Research and Practice 1993;189:1036–43.

Okura M, Hiranuma T, Tominaga G, et al. Expression of S-100 protein and glial fibrillary acidic protein in cultured submandibular gland epithelial cells and salivary gland tissues. American Journal of Pathology 1996;148:1709–16.

Radotra BD, Joshi K, Kak VK, Banerjee AK. Choroid plexus tumors – an immunohistochemical analysis with review of literature. Indian Journal of Pathology and Microbiology 1994;37:9–19.

Sillevis-Smitt PA, van der Loos C, de Jong VJM, Troost D. Tissue fixation methods alter the immunohistochemical demonstrability of neurofilament proteins, synaptophysin, and glial fibrillary acidic protein in human cerebellum. Acta Histochemia 1993;95:13–21.

Swanson PE, Lillemoe TJ, Manivell C, Wick MR. Mesenchymal chondrosarcoma. An immunohistochemical study. Archives of Pathology and Laboratory Medicine 1990;114:943–8.

Wittchow R, Landas SK. Glial fibrillary acidic protein expression in pleomorphic adenoma, chordoma and astrocytoma. A comparison of three antibodies. Archives of Pathology and Laboratory Medicine 1991;115:1030–3.

Gross Cystic Disease Fluid Protein-15 (GCDFP-15, BRST-2)

Sources/clones

Biogenex (GCDFP-15), Signet (GCDFP-15).

Fixation/preparation

The antigen is fixation stable and can be detected in paraffin-embedded sections as well as fresh frozen sections and cell preparations. HIER enhances Immunostaining and proteolytic digestion is unnecessary. Cytologic preparations should be fixed in 10% formalin or Bouin's solution. Alcohol-fixed preparations are not immunoreactive.

Background

Gross cystic disease fluid protein-15 (GCDFP-15) is one of four major component proteins found in the cystic fluid obtained from patients with fibro-cystic changes of the breast. GCDFP15 is a marker of apocrine glandular differentiation in both benign and malignant mammary epithelium (Haagensen et al, 1990). This protein has widespread distribution in apocrine glands elsewhere in the axillary and perianal tissues, as well as in the sublingual and submaxillary salivary glands. The

GCDFP15 protein is a 15 kD glycoprotein shown to be prolactin-inducible, the GCDFP-15 gene having been recently cloned (Myal et al, 1991). Ultrastructurally, the GCDFP-15 protein has been localized in Golgi vesicles and cytoplasmic granules. The protein is released by exocytosis at the apices of the mammary epithelial cells (Mazoujian et al, 1984).

Applications

Carcinoma of the breast is a treatable disease with a variable prognostic outcome. Its recognition is therefore of great therapeutic importance but in metastatic sites identification of breast carcinoma can be often difficult. A marker of mammary epithelial differentiation would be of diagnostic importance. GCDFP-15 goes some way towards fulfilling this role and is currently the best marker yet to identify breast cancer metastases. GCDFP-15 was identified by immunostaining in 55–74% of cases of breast carcinoma (Mazoujian et al, 1989; Wick et al, 1989) and has a higher rate of sensitivity and specificity than alpha-lactalbumin as a marker of both primary and metastatic breast cancer. Besides mammary

carcinomas, the major tumor types that expressed GCDFP-15 were salivary glands, sweat glands and prostate (Wick et al, 1989), bronchial glands, prostate and seminal vesicle (Satoh et al, 2000). It is also a marker of apocrine differentiation in the skin (particularly in combination with lysozyme) and can be suitably applied for the separation of cutaneous adnexal tumors (Appendix 1.20). A case of signet ring carcinoma of the eyelid was shown to immunoexpress GCDFP-15 in addition to estrogen and progesterone receptors and was negative for CK20 and Her-2, supporting an apocrine differentiation (Langel et al, 2001). It is worth noting that the expression of GCDFP-15 varies among the histologic subtypes of breast carcinoma, with highest incidence in infiltrating lobular carcinoma with signet ring cell differentiation (90%), compared to 70% in ordinary infiltrating ductal carcinoma and 75% in those subtypes showing apocrine differentiation (Mazoujian et al, 1989). Expression of the GCDFP-15 gene was significantly associated with relapse-free survival and was suggested to represent a marker of prognostic relevance (Pagani et al, 1994). GCDFP-15 expression appears to be androgen receptor mediated and can be inhibited by anti-androgens (Loos et al, 1999) and androgen receptor, in turn, appear to be involved with apocrine differentiation in neuroendocrine carcinomas of the breast (Sapino et al, 2001).

Antibodies to GCDFP-15 have been used successfully to identify metastases from breast carcinoma in the brain (Perry et al, 1997), ovary (Monteagudo et al, 1991), lung (Nonami et al, 2001), and other sites (Chaubert & Hurlimann 1992). Immunodistinction of metastasis from breast cancer and eccrine and apocrine tumors in the skin can be difficult as the latter tumors also express this antigen (Tsubura et al, 1992; Wallace et al, 1995; Wallace & Smoller 1996). However, as with other metastatic sites, the highest diagnostic yield was obtained when anti-GCDFP-15 was employed together with other antibodies in a diagnostic panel. Similarly when used in conjunction with estrogen and progesterone receptors, CA125, CK7, CD20 and CEA, it provided discriminant analysis between primary adenocarcinomas of the ovary, ovarian metastases of colonic and breast origin (Lagendijk et al, 1999).

GCDFP-15 is also a suitable marker in cytological specimens and the best results are obtained following fixation in 10% formalin or Bouin's solution, alcohol-fixed samples showing no immunoreactivity for this antigen (Fiel et al, 1996).

Comments

The immunoreactivity of monoclonal antibodies and polyclonal antisera to GCDFP-15 appear to be the same (Mazoujian et al, 1988), HIER enhancing immunoreactivity of both antibodies.

References

Chaubert P, Hurlimann J. Mammary origin of metastases. Immunohistochemical determination. Archives of Pathology and Laboratory Medicine 1992;116:1181–8.

Fiel MI, Cernainu G, Burstein DE, Batheja N. Value of GCDFP-15 (BRST-2) as a specific immunocytochemical marker for breast carcinoma in cytologic specimens. Acta Cytologica 1996;40:637–41.

Haagensen DE Jr, Dilley WG, Mazoujian G, Wells SAJr. Review of GCDFP-15. An apocrine marker protein. Annals of New York Academy of Sciences 1990;586:161–73.

Langel DJ, Yeatts RP, White WL. Primary signet ring cell carcinoma of the eyelid: report of a case demonstrating further analogy to lobular carcinoma of the breast with a literature review. American Journal of Dermatology 2001;23:444–9.

Lagendijk JH, Mullink H, van Diest PJ et al. Immunohistochemical differentiation between primary adenocarcinomas of the ovary and ovarian metastases of colonic and breast origin. Comparison between a statistical and an intuitive approach. Journal of Clinical Pathology 1999;52:283–90.

Loos S, Schulz KD, Hakenberg R. Regulation of GCDFP-15 expression in human mammary cancer cells. International Journal of Molecular Medicine 1999;4:135–40.

Mazoujian G, Wahol MJ, Haagensen DEJr. The ultrastructural localization of gross cystic disease fluid protein-15 (GCDFP-15) in breast epithelium. American Journal of Pathology 1984;116:305–10.

Mazoujian G, Parish TH, Haagensen DEJr. Immunoperoxidase localization of GCDFP-15 with mouse monoclonal antibodies versus rabbit antiserum. Journal of Histochemistry and Cytochemistry 1988;36:377–82.

Mazoujian G, Bodian C, Haagensen DEJr, Haagensen CD. Expression of GCDFP-15 in breast carcinomas. Relationship to pathologic and clinical factors. Cancer 1989;63:2156–61.

Monteagudo C, Merino MJ, LaPorte N, Neumann RD. Value of gross cystic disease fluid protein-15 in distinguishing metastatic breast carcinomas among poorly differentiated neoplasms involving the ovary. Human Pathology 1991;22:368–72.

Myal Y, Robinson DB, Iwasiow B, et al. The prolactin-inducible protein (PIP/GCDFP-15) gene: cloning, structure and regulation. Molecular and Cellular Endocrinology 1991;80:165–75.

Nonami Y, Hisa S, Yamamoto A, et al. Immunohistochemical study with antibody to glycoprotein GCDFP-15 for metastatic lung cancer from breast cancer. Journal of Cardiovascular Surgery 2001;42:561–4.

Pagani A, Sapino A, Eusebi V, et al. PIP/GCDFP-15 gene expression and apocrine differentiation in carcinomas of the breast. Virchows Archives 1994;425:459–65.

Perry A, Parisi JE, Kurtin PJ. Metastatic adenocarcinoma to the brain: an immunohistochemical approach. Human Pathology 1997;28:938–43.

Sapino A, Righi L, Cassoni P, et al. Expression of apocrine differentiation markers in neuroendocrine breast carcinomas of aged women. Modern Pathology 2001;14:768–76.

Satoh F, Umemura S, Osamura RY. Immunohistochemical analysis of GCDFP-15 and GCDFP-24 in mammary and non-mammary tissue. Breast Cancer 2000;7:49–55.

Tsubura A, Senzaki H, Sasaki M et al. Immunohistochemical demonstration of breast-derived and/or carcinoma-associated glycoproteins in normal skin appendages and their tumors. Journal of Cutaneous Pathology 1992;19:73–9.

Wallace ML, Longacre TA, Smoller BR. Estrogen and progesterone receptors and anti-gross cytstic disease fluid protein-15 (BRST-2) fail to distinguish metastatic breast carcinoma from eccrine neoplasms. Modern Pathology 1995;8:897–901.

Wallace ML, Smoller BR. Differential sensitivity of estrogen/progesterone receptors and BRST-2 markers in metastatic ductal and lobular breast carcinoma to the skin. American Journal of Dermatopathology 1996;18:241–7.

Wick MR, Lillemoe TJ, Copland GT, et al. Cross cystic disease fluid protein-15 as a marker for breast cancer: immunohistochemical analysis of 690 human neoplasms and comparison with alpha-lactalbumin. Human Pathology 1989;20:281–7.

NOTES

HAM56 (Macrophage marker)

Sources/clones

Dako (HAM56)

Fixation/preparation

This antibody is applicable to both formalin-fixed paraffin sections and frozen sections. Either enzyme or microwave pretreatment is beneficial to the immunoreactivity with the HAM 56 antibody.

Background

Human alveolar macrophage-56 (IgM, Kappa) is a monoclonal antibody developed against human alveolar macrophages (Gown et al, 1986). The antigen being recognized by Ham 56 has not yet been identified. This antibody was developed specifically for the study of human atherosclerotic plaques, to identify tissue macrophages and monocyte-derived cells. (Gown et al, 1986).

Applications

HAM56 has wide immunoreactivity including tissue macrophages, germinal center macrophages, interdigitating reticulum cells, subset of monocytes, a small population of lymphocytes and endothelial cells. Variable reactivity with a small number of B cell lymphomas has also been reported. Inflammatory pseudotumors of lymph node have been shown to contain spindle-shaped macrophages resembling fibroblasts or myofibroblasts that have immunoreactivity for HAM56, CD68, HLA=DR and CD45 (Menke et al, 1996). Recent attempts using HAM56 to distinguish between ovarian and gastrointestinal carcinomas have proved inconclusive (Cheung et al, 1997; Fowler et al, 1994).

Comments

HAM56 can be added to the list of conventional markers of macrophages, which include CD68, Mac387 and lysozyme (Silver & Sherman, 1998). Tissue rich in macrophages is the recommended positive control.

References

Cheung ANY, Chiu P-M, Khoo U-S. Is immunostaining with HAM56 antibody useful in identifying ovarian origin of metastatic adenocarcinomas? Human Pathology 1997;28:91–4.

Fowler LJ, Maygarden SJ, Novotny DB. Human Alveolar Macrophage-56 and carcinoembryonic antigen monoclonal antibodies in the differential diagnosis between primary ovarian and metastatic gastrointestinal carcinomas. Human Pathology 1994;25:666–70.

Gown AM, Tsukadat, Ross R. Human atherosclerosis. II. Immunocytochemical analysis of the cellular composition of human atherosclerotic lesions. American Journal of Pathology 1986;125:191–207.

Menke DM, Griesser H, Araujo I, et al. Inflammatory pseudotumors of lymph node origin show macrophage-derived spindle cells and lymphocyte-derived cytokine transcripts without evidence of T cell receptor gene rearrangements. Implications for pathogenesis and classification as an idiopathic retroperitoneal fibrosis-like sclerosing immune reaction. American Journal of Clinical Pathology 1996;105:430–9.

Silver SA, Sherman ME. Morphologic and immunophenotypic characterization of foam cells in endometrial lesions. International Journal of Gynecological Pathology 1998;17:140–5.

NOTES

HBME-1 (Mesothelial Cell)

Sources/clones

Dako (HBME-1).

Fixation/preparation

The antibody is immunoreactive in formalin fixed, paraffin-embedded tissue sections and in frozen sections and cell preparations.

Background

The antibody reacts with an antigen present in the membrane of mesothelial cells and their neoplastic counterparts, particularly epithelioid mesotheliomas. In initial testing the antibody failed to decorate epithelial cells of the kidney, lung, liver, ovary and pancreas. The antibody was derived from human epithelioid mesothelioma cells.

Applications

The antibody was designed primarily for the identification of normal and neoplastic mesothelial cells from metastatic carcinoma and is useful in this context. However, like many previous attempts to produce a mesothelial cell specific antibody, HBME-1 has met with limited

success. In one study, HBME-1 labeled all 17 cases of mesothelioma but also adenocarcinoma cells in 10 of 14 cases (Bateman et al, 1997). Among other markers employed in the same study, the authors found that CA125 labeled 15 of 17 mesotheliomas and seven of 14 adenocarcinomas. They concluded that both HBME-1 and CA125 were not sufficiently specific to be employed on their own as mesothelial markers but made a contribution when used in an appropriate panel. Similar results have been previously reported (Attanoos et al, 1996). Negative staining for HBME-1 makes the diagnosis of mesothelioma unlikely. A study of serous effusions revealed HBME-1 reactivity on the membranes of all reactive and malignant mesothelial cells but also in 24% of metastatic carcinomas and as many as 83% of ovarian carcinomas (Ascoli et al, 1997). HBME-1 does not label sarcomatous malignant mesothelioma (Donna et al, 1997).

HBME-1 produces a "thick pattern of immunoreactivity of the cell surfaces, often including the intracytoplasmic lumina" and is said to show excellent correlation with the presence of

abundant long microvilli with electron microscopy (Battifora & McCaughey, 1995). There is usually no cytoplasmic labeling and although adenocarcinoma cells may show membrane staining, they do not display the characteristic "thick" membranes and may show cytoplasmic staining. A similar pattern of immunoreactivity with anti-epithelial membrane antigen (anti-EMA) was described earlier by Leong et al (1990) and corresponds to labeling of the cell membranes and long microvilli characteristic of mesothelioma cells (van der Kwast et al, 1987). It was emphasized that the microvillous processes that are visible with EMA immunostaining are not only abnormally long but the circumferential distribution around the cell is aberrant in nature and signifies malignancy (Leong & Vermin-Roberts, 1994). A comparison of EMA and HMFG-2 immunostaining in mesothelioma and adenocarcinoma concluded that membranous staining by EMA had a sensitivity of 65% and a specificity of 86% for the identification of malignant mesothelioma but HMFG-2 membranous staining was not a useful discriminator (King & Tucker, 1998).

A recent study with HBME-1 compared staining in mesothelioma to adenocarcinoma and confirmed the presence of distinctive microvillus brush border staining with the antibody in mesothelioma (negative in sarcomatoid and poorly differentiated mesotheliomas). Ultrastructural examination with immunogold revealed labeling of the membranes of the long microvilli (Dahlstrom et al, 2001). These ultrastructural findings were very similar to those described by van der Kwast et al (1987) with EMA. HBME-1 has been recognized to stain adenocarcinoma. Sixteen of 20 mesotheliomas and 14 of 22 lung adenocarcinomas reacted with HBME-1 compared, whereas 16 of 22 mesotheliomas and only 3 of 27 adenocarcinomas reacted were positive for thrombomodulin, suggesting that the latter may be of greater discrimatory value for these two entities (Ordonez, 1997). In another study MOC-31 was positive or equivocal in 5% of mesotheliomas and in 90% of adenocarcinomas (reactive pleural being negative) suggesting that it may be a useful addition to the panel for the diagnosis of mesothelioma versus carcinoma (Oates & Edwards, 2000).

Comments

As with EMA, immunostaining with HBME-1 is aimed at highlighting the cell membranes and the long microvilli characteristic of mesothelioma. We have not identified any difference in the staining patterns

or sensitivity of these two antibodies. Optimal dilutions of the antibody have to be determined before use in diagnostic panels, as high concentrations will result in cytoplasmic staining of both mesothelioma and adenocarcinoma cells, reducing the usefulness of HBME-1 as a diagnostic discriminator between the two entities. HBME-1 may be used as a substitute for EMA in the panel to distinguish mesothelioma from carcinoma (Appendix 1.17)

References

Attanoos RL, Goddard H, Gibbs AR. Mesothelioma-binding antibodies: thrombomodulin, OV 632 and HBME-1 and their use in the diagnosis of malignant mesothelioma. Histopathology 1996;29:209–15.

Ascoli V, Carnovale-Scalzo C, Taccogna S, Nardi F. Utility of HBME-1 immunostaining in serous effusions. Cytopathology 1997;8:328–35.

Bateman AC, al-Talib RK, Newman T, Williams, Herbert A. Histopathology 1997;30:49–56.

Battifora H, McCaughey WTE. Tumors of the serosal membranes. Atlas of tumor pathology, 3rd series, fascicle 15. Washington DC: Armed Forces Institute of Pathology, 1955, p 73.

Dahlstrom JE, Maxwell LE, Brodie N, et al. Distinctive microvillous brush border staining with HBME-1 distinguishes pleural mesotheliomas from pulmonary adenocarcinomas. Pathology 2001;33:287–91.

Donna A, Betta PG, Chiodera P, et al. Newly market tissue markers for malignant mesothelioma: immunoreactivity of rabbit AMAD-2 antiserum compared

with monoclonal antibody HBME-1 and a review of the literature on so-called mesothelioma antibodies. Human Pathology 1997;28:929–37.

King JA, Tucker JA. Evaluation of membranous staining of mesothelioma. Cell Vision 1998;5:24–7.

Leong AS-Y, Parkinson R, Milios J. "Thick" cell membranes revealed by immunocytochemical staining: A clue to the diagnosis of mesothelioma. Diagnostic Cytopathology 1990;6:9–13.

Leong AS-Y, Vermin-Roberts E. The immunohistochemistry of malignant mesothelioma. Pathology Annual 1994;29:157–9.

Oates J, Edwards C. HBME-1, MOC-31, WT1 and calretinin: an assessment of recently described markers for mesothelioma and adenocarcinoma. Histopathology 2000;36:341–7.

Ordonez NG. The value of antibodies 44-3A6, SM3, HBME-1, and thrombomodulin in differentiating epithelial pleural mesothelioma from lung adenocarcinoma: a comparative study with other commonly used antibodies. American Journal of Surgical Pathology 1997;21:1399–408.

Van der Kwast TH, Versnel MA, Delahaye M, et al. Expression of epithelial membrane antigen on malignant mesothelial cells. An immunocytochemical and immunoelectron microscopic study. Acta Cytologica 1987;32:169–74.

h-Caldesmon

Sources/clones

Dako (clone h-CD)

Fixation/preparation

h-CD requires microwave heat-induced epitope retrieval in citrate buffer. Some workers have combined this with pepsin pretreatment.

Background

Caldesmon is a protein that binds to calmodulin, tropomyosin and actin and is thought to play an important role in the regulation of smooth muscle contraction (Sobue et al, 1985). It exists in two isoforms: l-CD (molecular weight 70–80 kDa) and h-CD (120–150 kDa); the latter representing high molecular weight caldesmon (h-CD). Although l-CD is present in many cells, h-CD is exclusively expressed in vascular and visceral smooth muscle cells, and myoepithelial cells.

h-CD is expressed intensely and extensively in tumors with smooth muscle differentiation: leiomyomas, leiomyosarcomas, angiomyomas, and glomus tumors (Watanabe et al, 1999); whereas rhabdomyosarcomas, malignant fibrous histiocytomas,

desmoids and inflammatory myofibroblastic tumors were negative for h-CD. In addition, h-CD was not present in vascular pericytes and myofibroblasts (around ulcers and granulomas). Although non-neoplastic myoepithelial cells were immunopositive for h-CD, tumors with a myoepithelial cell participation (pleomorphic adenomas, chondroid syringoma, myoepithelioma and epimyoepithelial carcinoma) were completely negative for h-CD. A recent study noted that all 12 endometrial stromal sarcomas were negative with h-CD, whilst 8/11 uterine cellular leiomyomas showed heterogeneous but intense pattern of immunoreactivity with h-CD (Rush et al, 2001). An independent study confirmed these findings, showing all uterine leiomyomas (including usual and cellular types) to be positive with h-CD (albeit somewhat heterogeneous) and negative in all endometrial stromal neoplasms (Nucci et al, 2001). As the converse is generally true for CD10, the combined use of these two markers may serve to distinguish leiomyosarcoma from endometrial stromal neoplasms (McCluggage, 2002). This

specificity of h-CD for smooth muscle tumors has also been demonstrated in soft tissue tumors (Miettinen et al, 1999); however, it should be noted that another study, while confirming the specificity of this marker has shown significant variability in expression. H-CD was immunoexpressed in only 36% of leiomyosarcomas, which consistently expressed smooth muscle actin and muscle specific actin, expressed calponin in 86% and desmin in 76% of cases (n=30). Leiomyosarcomas confined to peripheral soft tissue were all negative for h-CD (Hisaoka et al, 2001).

Applications

h-CD appears to be useful in distinguishing smooth muscle tumors (h-CD+) from tumors with myofibroblastic and myoepithelial differentiation (h-CD-); however, its expression is not consistent and peripheral soft tissue leiomyosarcomas appear to show low immunoexpression. The other major application pertains to the differential diagnosis between cellular leiomyoma (positive) and endometrial stromal tumors, although the later may show focal muscle differentiation.

References

Hisaoka M, Wei-Qi S, Jian W, et al. specific but variable expression of h-Caldesmon in leiomyosarcomas. An immunohistochemical reassessment of a novel myogenic marker. Applied Immunohistochemistry and Molecular Morphology 2001;9:302–8.

McCluggage WG.Recent advances in immunohistochemistry in gynaecological pathology. Histopathology 2002;40:309–26.

Miettinen MM, Sarlomo-Rikala M, Kovatich AJ, Lasota J. Calponin and h-Caldesmon in soft tissue tumors: consistent h-Caldesmon immunoreactivity in gastrointestinal stromal tumors indicates traits of smooth muscle differentiation. Modern Pathology 1999;12:756–62.

Nucci MR, O'Connell JT, Huettner PC, et al. h-Caldesmon expression effectively distinguishes endometrial stromal tumors from uterine smooth muscle tumors. American Journal of Surgical Pathology 2001;25:455–63.

Rush DS, Tan J-Y, Baergen RN, Soslow RA. h-Caldesmon, a novel smooth muscle-specific antibody, distinguishes between cellular leiomyoma and endometrial stromal sarcoma. American Journal of Surgical Pathology 2001;25:253–8.

Sobue K, Tanaka T, Kanda K, et al. Purification and characterization of caldesmon 77: a calmodulin-binding protein that interacts with actin filament from bovine adrenal medulla. Proceedings of the National Academy of Science USA 1985;82:5025–9.

Watanabe K, Kusakabe T, Hoshi N, et al. h-Caldesmon in leiomyosarcoma and tumors with smooth muscle cell-like differentiation: its specific expression in the smooth muscle cell tumor. Human Pathology 1999;30:392–6.

Heat shock proteins (Hsps)

Sources/clones

Only clones of Hsp 27, Hsp 60 and Hsp 70 are listed.

Hsp 27

Biogenex (G3.1), Immunotech (G3.1), Stress Gen (G3.1)

Hsp 60

Accurate (LK1, LK2), Affinity Bio (4B9/89, 2E1/53), Sanbio (LK1, LK2), Sigma (LK2), Stress Gen (LK1, LK2, polyclonal)

Hsp 70

Affinity Bio (3a3, 5A5, 4G4, 7.10), Amersham, Biogenex (BRM22), Dako (polyclonal), Diagnostics Biosystems (polyclonal), Pharmingen (5G10), Sigma (BRM11), Stress Gen (N27F3–4, 1B5, C92F3A-5).

Fixation/preparation

Some of the antibodies are immunoreactive in fixed paraffin-embedded tissue sections, others are immunoreactive only in cryostat sections and fresh cell preparations. HIER produces enhancement of immunoreactivity.

Background

When prokaryotic or eukaryotic cells are submitted to a transient rise in temperature or to other proteolytic treatments, the synthesis of a set of proteins called heat shock proteins (Hsps) is induced. The structure of these proteins has been highly conserved during evolution. The signal leading to the transcriptional activation of the corresponding genes is the accumulation of denatured and/or aggregated proteins inside the cells after being subjected to stress. The expression of a subset of Hsp is also induced during early embryogenesis and many differentiation processes. Two different functions have been ascribed to Hsps: a molecular chaperone function whereby they mediate the folding, assembly or translocation across the intracellular membranes of other polypeptides, and a role in protein degradation. Some of the essential components of the cytoplasmic ubiquitin–dependent degradative pathway are Hsps (Mayer et al, 1991). These functions of Hsps are essential in every living cell and are required for repairing the damage that results from stress. In addition, the Hsps may also have a number of biological functions apparently distinct from their role during stress such as in tyrosine kinase and steroid hormone function (Welch 1987; Pratt & Welch 1994).

Current interest in Hsps lies in their role as prognostic markers in various tumors and in tumor resistance to chemotherapy, overexpression of Hsps allowing tumors cells to resist stressful situations and agents including cytotoxic drugs. In endometrial cancers, expression of Hsp27 has been correlated with the degree of tumor differentiation as well as with the presence of estrogen and progesterone receptors. In patients with cervical cancer, Hsp27 is predominantly expressed in well-differentiate and moderately-differentiated squamous cell carcinomas but the expression of this protein seems to be a negative prognostic factor for gastric cancer (Ciocca et al, 1993). In the case of malignant fibrous histiocytoma, the expression of Hsp27 was found to be the strongest prognostic factor, correlating with longer disease free intervals and overall survival, independent of tumor size, necrosis and histological subtype (Tetu et al, 1992). Different isoforms of Hsp27 have been found in lymphoid tissue of patients with acute lymphoblastic leukemia and the protein has been associated with viral infections.

The presence of Hsp70 appears to be associated with breast cancers of high histological grades (Lazaris et al, 1997) and it has been suggested that high levels of the protein identifies a subset of patients with node-negative breast cancer who show a high risk for disease recurrence (Ciocca et al, 1993). Increased Hsp70 expression has also been correlated with low levels of differentiation in colorectal cancer.

Immunostaining for Hsp27 and Hsp90 has been studied in a variety of central nervous system tumors (Kato et al, 1992; 1995) and it has been suggested that the presence of HSP and oxygen regulated protein demonstrated by immunostaining in the parieto-occipital lobe and hippocampus was indicative of prolonged survival from hypoxic attacks, whereas, a weak staining for excitatory amino acid transporter 2 was observed in almost all asphyxia deaths (Nakasono 2001). HSP27 immunoexpression has been reported to correlate inversely with survival in patients with oral squamous cell carcinoma (Mese et al, 2002).

Comments

The Hsps show immunolocalization in the cytoplasm as diffuse or finely granular staining. HSP70 appears to be selectively overexpressed in the blast cells of reactive germinal centers and paracortex of lymph nodes, the significance of which remains unknown (Leopardi et al, 2001).

References

Ciocca DR, Clark GM, Tandon AK, et al. Heat shock protein hsp70 in patients with axillary lymph node-negative breast cancer: prognostic implications. Journal of the National Cancer Institutes 1993;85:570–574.

Ciocca DR, Oesterreich S, Chamness GC, et al. Biological and clinical implications of heat shock protein 27,000 (Hsp27): a review. Journal of the National Cancer Institutes 1993;85:1558–1570.

Kato M, Herz F, Kato S, Hirano A. Expression of stress-response (heat-shock) protein 27 in human brain tumors: an immunohistochemical study. Acta Neuropathology (Berlin) 1992;83:420–422.

Kato S, Morita T, Takenaka T, et al. Stress-response (heat-shock) protein 90 expression in tumors of the central nervous system: an immunohistochemical study. Actsa neuropathology (Berlin) 1995;89:184–188.

Lazaris AC, Theodoropoulos GE, Davaris PS, et al. Heat shock protein 70 and HLA-DR molecules tissue expression. Prognostic implications in colorectal carcinoma. Diseases of Colon and Rectum 1995;38:739–745.

Lazaris AC, Chatzigianni EB, Panoussopoulos D, et al. Proliferating cell nuclear antigen and heat shock protein 70 immunolocalization in invasive ductal breast cancer not otherwise specified. Breast Cancer Research and Treatment 1997;43:43–51.

Leopardi O, Naughten W, Giannulis I, et al. HSP70 is selectively overexpressed in the blast cells of the germinal centers and paracortex in reactive lymph nodes. Histopathology 2001;39:566–71.

Mayer RJ, Lowe J, Landon M, et al. Ubiquitin and the lysosome system: molecular immunopathology reveals the connection. Biomedicine Biochemia Acta 1991;50:333–341.

Mese H, Sasaki A, Nakayama S, et al. Prognostic significance of heat shock protein 27 (HSP27) in patients with oral squamous cell carcinoma. Oncology Reports 2002;9:341–4.

Nakasono I. Application of immunohistochemistry for forensic pathological diagnosis: Finding of human brain in forensic autopsy (in Japanese). Nippon Hoigaku Zasshi 2001;55:299–309.

Pratt WB, Welsh MJ. Chaperone functions of the heat shock proteins associated with steroid receptors. Seminars in Cell Biology 1994;5:83–93.

Tetu B, Lacasse B, Bouchard HL, et al. Prognostic influence of HSP-27 expression in malignant fibrous histiocytoma: a clinicopathological and immunohistochemical study. Cancer Research 1992;52:2325–2328.

Welch WJ. The mammalian heat shock (or stress) response: a cellular defense mechanism. Advances in Experimental Medicine and Biology 1987;225:287–304.

Helicobacter pylori

Sources/clones

Biodesign (51–13), Biogenesis (1G6, CP15), Biogenex (UM01), Dako (polyclonal), Sanbio/Monosan (51–13).

Fixation/preparation

Applicable to 10% neutral buffered formalin or Bouin's fixed tissue.

Background

Helicobacter pylori (HP), is a spiral bacillus that can colonize the human gastric mucosa and induce a specific humoral immunologic reaction in the host. Colonization of the gastric mucosa by HP is a very common finding in gastric ulcers and active chronic gastritis. HP is increasingly recognized as one of the most prevalent human pathogens worldwide, and possibly plays a pathogenetic role in gastric carcinogenesis and primary gastric lymphogenesis. The details of the interaction between bacteria, epithelial cells and inflammatory cells are currently being explored. As effective specific treatment for HP associated gastroduodenal disorders emerges, surgical pathologists are requested to identify the organism in endoscopic biopsies. Histologic identification of HP (with special staining methods) has been shown to be as accurate as microbiologic culture techniques (Hui et al, 1992; Genta et al, 1994).

The Signet rabbit anti-HP polyclonal antisera was raised against *H.pylori* strain CH-20429 and detects antigens of the whole organism in formalin-fixed, paraffin-embedded, frozen and cytologic specimens.

Applications

Bacteria lying within the mucus and on the epithelial surface can be seen on sections stained with hematoxylin-eosin (H&E). However, organisms closely adherent to cells, insinuated in intercellular spaces or intimately associated with and perhaps phagocytosed by inflammatory cells are frequently difficult to identify.

There are several published special stains that demonstrate HP efficiently in the histologic sections (Genta et al, 1994). However, the use of immunohistochemical methods is highly specific and has an important role in selected situations (Cartun et al, 1991). For example, small gastric biopsies with a very low density of *H.pylori*, post-treatment biopsy specimens to assess therapeutic success or when abundant debris or mucus is present on gastric surface and pits, may benefit from identification of *H.pylori* with immunohistochemistry. A recent study demonstrated a concordance of 94.2% between touch smear cytology and immunohistochemical identification of *H pylori* (Yamamoto 2001) and fixation in Carnoy's fixative allowed immunohistochemical identification of the organism in both the surface mucus gel layer as well as surface mucus cells in patients with peptic ulceration (Ishihara et al, 2001).

Comments

Immunohistochemical methods for the detection of *H.pylori* are highly specific and play an important role in selected situations, but cannot be advocated for the routine diagnosis of *H.pylori* gastritis. HP-infected gastric tissue is recommended as positive control tissue.

References

Cartun RW, Kryzmowski GA, Pedersen CA, et al. Immunocytochemical identification of *H.pylori* in formalin-fixed gastric biopsies.

Modern Pathology
1991;4:498–502.

Genta RM, Robason GO, Graham DY. Simultaneous visualization of Helicobacter pylori and gastric morphology: A new stain. Human Pathology 1994;25:221–6.

Hui PK, Chan WY, Cheung PS, Chan JKC, Ng CS. Pathologic changes of gastric mucosa colonized by H.pylori. Human Pathology 1992;23:548–56.

Isihara S, Okuyama T, Ishimura N, et al. Intragastric distribution of Helicobacter pylori during short-term omeprazole therapy: study using Carnoy's fixation and immunohistochemistry for detection of bacteria. Alimentary Pharmacology and Therapeutics 2001;15:1485–91.

Yamamoto T. Evaluation of usefulness of touch smear cytology for the diagnosis of Helicobacter pylori infection (in Japanese). Kansenshogaku Zasshi 2001;75:856–62.

Hep Par 1 (Hepatocyte marker)

Sources/clones

Dako (OCH 1E5)

Fixation/preparation

The antibody is immunoreactive in fixed paraffin-embedded sections and immunoreactivity is slightly enhanced following HIER.

Background

Hep Par 1 (hepatocyte paraffin 1) is an IgGκ antibody to both normal and neoplastic hepatocytes raised at the Pittsburgh Cancer Institute. Hep Par 1 detects an antigen that is localized to the hepatocyte cytoplasm and produces no staining of bile ducts or other non-parenchymal cells. The staining is granular, occasionally ring-like and is seen diffusely throughout the hepatocyte cytoplasm, without canalicular accentuation. There is no apparent zonal preference in normal liver. In the first paper documenting its specificity in human tissue sections, the antibody labeled 37 of 38 cases of hepatocellular carcinoma (HCC), although four tumors had only rare positivity. The negative case was an example of the sclerosing variant of hepatocellular carcinoma. Five examples of fibrolamellar variant were positive. Two of 31 cases of cholangiocarcinoma (CC) were positive for Hep Par 1 and the antibody also decorated three of 10 cases of gastric carcinoma (Wennerberg et al, 1993). In our own recent study, Hep Par 1 labeled 31 of 32 HCCs as well as four of 27 cases of CC (Leong et al 1998), but was not found in metastatic adenocarcinomas. One other study has employed Hep Par 1 and showed staining in 289 of 290 HCCs (Wu et al, 1996). Hepatoblastomas were demonstrated to uniformly immunoexpress the antigen (Fasano et al, 1998). A recent study of cell blocks prepared from fine needle aspiration samples revealed Hep Par 1 staining in all 50 cases of hepatocellular carcinoma and in none of 5 cases of cholangiocarcinoma. However, 3 of 20 cases of metastatic carcinoma were reported to be positive (Siddiqui et al, 2002).

Applications

The highest diagnostic yield is obtained with Hep Par 1 when it is employed in a panel of antibodies in the context of the differential diagnosis (Appendix 1.8). Its main diagnostic application would be for the distinction of HCC from CC and metastatic adenocarcinoma in the liver. When employed with CK 19 and CK 20, it is able to provide useful diagnostic information to allow the separation of these three entities Leong et al 1998). CK 19 is largely limited to bile duct epithelium and their corresponding neoplasms including CC (Balaton et al, 1988; Terada et al, 1995), whereas CK 20 is a marker of gastrointestinal carcinomas, particularly those from the colon and less consistently the upper gastrointestinal tract and pancreas (Mittinen 1995).

Comments

As the staining of Hep Par 1 is heterogeneous and may be focal within HCCs, caution should be exercised in interpretation as small biopsies such as needle cores may produce false negative results. Despite its limitations, Hep Par 1 is still the best antibody yet for use in the context of the differential diagnosis of liver carcinomas. The OCH 1E5 antibody cross reacts with canine hepatocytes (Ramos-Vara et al, 2001).

References

Balaton AJ, Nehama-Sibony M, Gotheil C, et al. Distinction between hepatocellular carcinoma, cholangiocarcinoma, and metastatic carcinoma based on immunohistochemical staining for carcinoembryonic antigen and for cytokeratin 19 on paraffin sections. Journal of Pathology 1988;156:305–10.

Fasano M, Theise ND, Nalesnik M, et al. Immunohistochemical evaluation of hepatoblastomas with use of the hepatocyte-specific marker, hepatocyte paraffin 1, and the polyclonal anti-carcinoembryonic antigen. Modern Pathology 1998;11:934–8.

Leong AS-Y, Sormunen RT, Tsui WM-S, Liew CT. Immunostaining for liver cancers. Histopathology 1998;33:318–24

Miettinen M. Keratin 20: Immunohistochemical marker for gastrointestinal, urothelial, and Merkel cell carcinomas. Modern Pathology 1995;8:384–8.

Ramos-Vara JA, Miller MA, Johnson GC. Immunohistochemical characterization of canine hyperplastic hepatic lesions and hepatocellular carcinoma and biliary neoplasms with monoclonal antibody hepatocyte paraffin 1 and a monoclonal antibody to cytokeratin 7. Veterinary Pathology 2001;38:636–43.

Siddiqui MT, Saboorian MH, Gokasian ST, Ashfaq R. Diagnostic utility of HepPar1 antibody to differentiate hepatocellular carcinoma from metastatic carcinoma in fine needle aspiration samples. Cancer 2002,96.49–52.

Terada T, Hoso M, Nakanuma Y. Distribution of cytokeratin 19-positive biliary cells in cirrhotic nodules, hepatic borderline nodules (atypical adenomatous hyperplasia), and small hepatocellular carcinomas. Modern Pathology 1995;8:371–9.

Wennerberg AE, Nalesnik MA, Coleman WB. Hepatocyte paraffin 1: A monoclonal antibody that reacts with hepatocytes and can be used for differential diagnosis of hepatic tumors. American Journal of Pathology 1993;143:1050–4.

Wu P-c, Fand JW-S, Lau VK-T, et al. Classification of hepatocellular carcinoma according to hepatocellular and biliary differentiation markers. Clinical and biological implications. American Journal of Pathology 1996;149·1167–75.

Hepatitis B Core Antigen (HBcAg)

Sources/clones

Accurate/Axcel (polyclonal), American Research Products (1734–17), Biodesign (1841), Biogenesis (polyclonal), Biogenex (ESP512, polyclonal), Boegringer Mannheim (BW35A/312), Dako (polyclonal, B586), Fitzgerald (M29091, M22131), Immunon (polyclonal), Novocastra (polyclonal), Zymed (polyclonal).

Fixation/preparation

These antibodies are applicable to formalin fixed paraffin embedded tissue. No antigen unmasking is required. However, caution is advised when using the ABC immunodetection as hepatocytes contain biotin that may cross-react with the ABC system.

Background

The complete HB virus (Dane particle) is a 42 nm double stranded DNA virus (Hepadna virus), composed of a 27 nm core particle and envelope, 7 nm in thickness and is immunolocalized within endoplasmic reticulum of liver cells. The HB core protein of 183 amino acids is encoded by the gene C. It is self-assembling and has binding sites for HBV-RNA, which is encapsulated together with viral polymerase. Immuno-localization of HBcAg is cytoplasmic, cytoplasmic membranous and nuclear (Kakumu et al, 1989). Antibodies are raised against HBcAg obtained from recombinant core DNA of HB virus, purified from lysates of E.coli clones. HBcAg is expressed predominantly in the nuclei of liver cells, although variable immunoreaction may also be seen in the perinuclear cytoplasm (Burns, 1975; Chu & Liaw, 1990).

Applications

Antibody to HBcAg detects the replicative form of the virus found in the nucleus of HB infected cells. Perinuclear cytoplasmic immuno-localization is sometimes observed. In very actively replicating infections, cells with cytoplasmic reactivity may outnumber those with nuclear labeling. The presence of HBcAg on immunohistochemistry is usually correlated with complete viral synthesis as proved by positivity for viral DNA in both liver and blood, as well as circulating Dane particles in blood (Ballare et al, 1989). Demonstration of HBc in liver cells therefore reflects failure to eliminate cells with active viral replication. This is often associated with signs of active disease (piecemeal necrosis or chronic lobular hepatitis) with a membranous pattern of HBsAg. HBcAg is seen with the greatest frequency in immunosuppressed patients with chronic hepatitis (Tapp & Jones, 1977). Excess accumulation of core particles can be recognized in an H & E stain in rare cases as 'sanded' nuclei (Bianchi & Gudat, 1976).

HBcAg expression in liver biopsies of children with chronic hepatitis B showed a significant decrease after treatment with interferon-alpha, whereas HBsAg expression either increased or remained unchanged. Periportal piecemeal necrosis and intralobular confluent and spotty necrosis decreased but the extent of fibrosis and scoring of portal inflammation remained unchanged after treatment (Ozer et al, 1999).

Comments

It is assumed that viral DNA active in HBcAg production is episomal and not integrated into the host genome.

References

Ballare M, Lavarini C, Brunetto MR, et al. Relationship between the intrahepatic expression of e and c epitopes of the nucleocapsid protein of hepatitis B virus and viraemia. Clinical Experimental Immunology 1989;75:64–9.

Bianchi L, Gudat F. Sanded nuclei in hepatitis B. Laboratory Investigation 1976 35:1–5.

Bianchi L, Gudat F. Chronic hepatitis. In: MacSween RNM, Anthony PP, Scheuer PJ, Burt AD, Portmann BHC. eds. Pathology of the Liver. Churchill Livingstone, Edinburgh 1994; pp 363–73.

Burns J. Immunoperoxidase localization of hepatitis B antigen (HB) in formalin-paraffin processed liver tissue. Histochemistry 1975;44:133–5.

Chu CM, Liaw YF. Intrahepatic expression of HBcAg in chronic HBV hepatitis: lessons from molecular biology. Hepatology 1990;12:1443–5.

Kakumu S, Arao M, Yoshioka K, et al. Distribution of HBcAg in hepatitis B detected by immunoperoxidase staining with three different preparations of anti-HBc antibodies. Journal of Clinical Pathology 1989;42:284–8.

Ozer E, Ozer E, Helvaci M, et al. Hepatic expression of viral antigens, hepatocytic proliferative activity and histologic changes in liver biopsies of children with chronic hepatitis B after interferon–alpha therapy. Liver 1999;19:369–74.

Tapp E, Jones DM. HBsAg and HBcAg in the livers of asymptomatic hepatitis B antigen carriers. Journal of Clinical Pathology 1977;30:671–7.

Hepatitis B Surface Antigen (HBsAG)

Sources/clones

Accurate (BM51), American Research Products/EY Labs, Axcel/Accurate (polyclonal), Becton Dickinson, Biogenesis (1044–329, polyclonal), Biogenex (SI201), Calbiochem, Dako (polyclonal, 3E7), Fitzgerald (M94172, M94173, M94253, M94254, polyclonal), Harlan Sera Lab/Accurate (V2.5G4, V2.6E4), Novocastra (1044/341), Pharmingen (S1–210), Zymed (ZCH16, ZMHB5).

Fixation/preparation

These antibodies are applicable to formalin fixed paraffin embedded tissues. No antigen unmasking is required. However, caution is advised when using the ABC immunodetection method, as liver cells contain biotin and may cross-react with the ABC system.

Background

The complete hepatitis B virus (Dane particle) is a 42 nm double stranded DNA virus (Hepadna virus), composed of a 27 nm core particle and envelope, 7 nm in thickness and is immunolocalized within endoplasmic reticulum of liver cells. The glycosylated surface protein of hepatitis B (HB) virus is composed of 3 gene products: the small, middle and large HBs-protein, governed by the S-, pre S2- and pre S1 domain respectively (Gudat & Bianchi, 1977).

Applications

These antibodies react with antigen-positive cells in patients with type B viral hepatitis, cirrhosis and hepatocellular carcinoma. Immunoreaction may occur in seropositive as well as seronegative patients. HBsAg in human liver biopsies has two expression patterns with apparently different biological implications:

(i) Membranous HBsAg is strongly associated with HBcAg expression and is an indirect indication of replicative HBV infection.

Intracytoplasmic HBsAg in excess is visible by H & E staining as a homogeneous ground-glass appearance of the cytoplasm (Hadziyannis et al, 1973), and is an indicator of chronic elimination insufficiency for this antigen but is an unreliable marker of active replication. In contrast membrane-associated HBsAg should always raise suspicion of active viral replication.

The livers of children with chronic hepatitis B showed a significant decrease in HBcAg immunoexpression after treatment with interferon-alpha, whereas HBsAg expression either increased or remained unchanged (Ozer et al, 1999).

In patients with IgA nephropathy and HBV antigenemia polyclonal antibodies have demonstrated HBcAg and HBsAg in the nuclei of glomerular mesangial cells suggesting immune complex deposition as a possible mechanism of the nephropathy (Lai et al, 1987). In situ hybridization studies of HBV DNA in such patients showed coexpression of HBV DNA and HBsAg and (or) HBcAg suggesting the expression of HBsAg in situ in infected renal cells (Ma et al, 1999).

Comments

Liver tissue from known patients with hepatitis may be used as control tissue for both HBcAg and HBsAg.

References

Gudat F, Bianchi L. HGsAg: A target antigen on the liver cell? In: Popper H, Bianchi L, Reutter W, eds. Membrane alterations as basis of liver injury. Lancaster: MTP Press, 1977: pp 171–8.

Hadziyannis S, Gerber MA, Vissoulis C, Popper H. Cytoplasmic hepatitis B antigen in "ground glass" hepatocytes of carriers. Archives of Pathology 1973;96:327–30.

Lai KN, Lai FM, Lo S, et al. IgA nephropathy associated with hepatitis B virus antigenemia. Nephron 1987;47:141–3.

Ma X, Zhang Y, Du W. The relationship between IgA nephropathy and HBV infection (in Chinese). Zonghua Yi Xue Za Zhi 1999;79:417–21.

Ozer E, Ozer E, Helvaci M, Yaprak I. Hepatic expression of viarl antigens, hepatocytes proliferative activity and histologic changes in liver biopsies of children with chronic hepatitis B after interferon-alpha therapy. Liver 1999;19:369–74.

Herpes Simplex Virus I & II (HSV I & II)

Sources/clones

Polyclonal HSV I & HSV II

Biodesign, Biogenesis, Biogenex, Chemicon, Dako (polyclonal), Fitzgerald, Immunon, Pharmingen.

Monoclonal antibody

Accurate (A321, M22253A, HP2M222M53A), American Research Products (1697–151, 1589–136, 1645–18), Biodesign (203, 206, 016, 017), Biogenesis (CHA437, 10527, H62), Biogenex (G16, E10, 023A1909, 045A1930B), EY Labs, Fitzgerald (M22254, M22255, M2110155, M2110156), Sera Lab (CHA437).

Fixation/preparation

Both antibodies 302M and 303M are applicable to frozen-cryostat sections as well as fixed paraffin-embedded tissue sections. The latter requires microwave pretreatment to eliminate non-specific background staining.

Background

The antigens used in the production of these antibodies comprise detergent solubilized HSV I and HSV II infected whole rabbit cornea cell. The 302M antibody reacts with HSV I specific antigens whilst the 303M antibody reacts with HSV II specific antigens. Both antibodies react with antigens common for HSV I and II, all major glycoproteins present in the viral envelope and at least one core protein. There is no demonstrable cross-reactivity with Varicella zoster virus, cytomegalovirus or Epstein-Barr virus.

Applications

Both antibodies 302M and 303M detect the presence of HSV I and HSV II respectively, in tissue sections, e.g., skin and brain. A diffuse intranuclear signal is produced, often coinciding with the ground glass intranuclear inclusions of HSV. Similar intranuclear inclusions associated with biotin accumulation, have been observed in glandular epithelia of gestational endometrium (Sickel & di Sant'Agnese, 1944; Shigeo et al, 1993). Hence, to the unwary, any attempt to demonstrate HSV in these biotin inclusions may produce a false-positive immunoreaction, especially when the avidin-biotin immunodetection system is utilized. The application of pre-washing with 0.05% free avidin and 0.05% free biotin does *not* eliminate this cross immunoreactivity. It is therefore recommended that the PAP or APAAP immunodetection system be used for any HSV immunohistochemical investigation of gestational endometrium (Cooper et al, 1997).

Localized herpes simplex lymphadenitis which resulted in rapid lymph node enlargement clinically indistinguishable from Richter's transformation has been described in a patient with chronic lymphocytic leukemia (Joseph et al, 2001), emphasizing the need to make the correct diagnosis. Such infected nodes show marked germinal centre and paracortical hyperplasia with foci of necrosis. Viral inclusions may be present and HSV antigen may be demonstrated immunohistologically (Miliauskas & Leong, 1991).

Comments

Biotin-like activity has been observed in thyroid lesions as well (Kashima et al, 1997). Hence, awareness of this interference is crucial to avoid misinterpretation of immunohistochemical investigations, especially with the

ABC immunodetection system. Genital lesions with typical multinucleated giant cells with "ground glass" intranuclear inclusions should be used as positive control tissue.

References

Cooper K, Haffajee Z, Taylor L. Comparative analysis of biotin intranuclear inclusions of gestational endometrium using the APAAP, ABC and the PAP immunodetection systems. Journal of Clinical Pathology 1997;50:153–6.

Joseph L, Scott MA, Schichman SA, Zent CS. Localized herpes simplex lymphadenitis mimicking large cell (Richter's) transformation of chronic lymphocytic leukemia/small cell lymphoma. American Journal of Hematology 2001;68:287–91.

Kashima K, Yokoyama S, Tsutomu D, et al. Cytoplasmic biotin-like activity interferes with immunohistochemical analysis of thyroid lesions: a comparison of antigen retrieval methods. Modern Pathology 1997;10:515–9.

Miliauskas J, Leong AS-Y. Localized herpes simplex lymphadenitis: Report of three cases and review of the literature. Histopathology 1991;19:355–60.

Shigeo Y, Kenji K, Souichi I, et al. Biotin-containing intranuclear inclusions in endometrial glands during gestation and puerperium. American Journal of Clinical Pathology 1993;99:13017.

Sickel JZ, di Sant'Agnese A. Anomalous immunostaining of 'optically clear' nuclei in gestational endometrium. Archives of Pathology and Laboratory Medicine 1994;118:831–3.

HLA-DR

Sources/clones

Accurate (917D7, CLBHLADR, DR), Axcel/Accurate (DK22), Biogenesis (HL-12, polyclonal), Biogenex (Q513), Biosource (BF1), Boehringer Mannheim (CR3–43), Coulter (I2, I3), Cymbus Bioscience (DDII, IQU9 TAL1B), Dako (DK22, TAL.1B5), Harlan/Seralab/Accurate (MID3, YD1–63.4.10), Immunotech (B8.12.2), Novocastra (polyclonal), Pharmingen (TU36), Research Diagnostics (CLB-HLA-DR), Sanbio/Monosan (HL39), Sanbio/Monosan/Accurate (HL39), Sigma chemical (HA14), Zymed (LN3).

Fixation/preparation

These antibodies are applicable to B5 or formalin-fixed paraffin-embedded tissue section. In addition, cryostat sections and cell smears may also be used with the antibodies.

Background

HLA molecules are highly polymorphic glycoproteins with a single binding site for immunogenic peptides. The complex formed by HLA-DR molecules and peptides is the entity specifically recognized by the antigen receptor of CD4+ helper T lymphocytes. This biological function has been linked to the constitutive cell surface expression of HLA molecules on antigen-presenting cells, which provide immunogenic peptides through denaturation, or fragmentation of antigen (Jendro et al, 1991).

The HLA-DR is a member of the 11β subclass of HLA (the other members is HLA-DQ). B cells of the germinal centers and mantle zones express the HLA-DR antigen. It is also expressed by macrophages, monocytes and antigen-presenting cells like interdigitating reticulum cells and Langerhans cells of the skin. Activated T cells may express the HLA-DR antigen, but not inactive T cells. Some endothelial and epithelial tissues may also express HLA-DR.

Applications

Anti-HLA-DR may be useful in distinguishing B-cell follicle center lymphomas from T-cell lymphomas. The antibody also detects Class II antigens which may be expressed 'de novo' or increased in certain pathological states e.g., autoimmune diseases. Similarly, it will demonstrate aberrant expression of Class II antigen in various malignant cell types (Crumpton et al, 1984). Expression of HLA-DR was demonstrated in bladder carcinoma and may have a role in the treatment of such tumors with intravesicle Bacillus Calmette-Guerin (Leong et al, 1990) The expression of HLA-DR molecules on crypt epithelial cells of jejunal biopsies of patients with Hashimoto's thyroiditis together with other signs of mucosal T cell activation was interpreted to suggest the potential of developing coeliac disease (Valentino et al, 2002)

Comments

Tonsil or skin may be used as positive control tissue.

References

Crumpton MJ, Bodmer JC, Bodmer WF et al. Biochemistry of Class II Antigens: Workshop Report. In: Albert ED, Mayr WR, eds. Histocompatibility Testing. Berlin-Springer-Verlag, 1984;29–37.

Jendro M, Goronzy JJ, Weyand CM. Structural and functional characterization of HLA-DR molecules circulating in the serum. Autoimmunity 1991;8:289–96.

Leong AS-Y, Wannakrairot P, Jose J, Milios J. Bacillus Calmette-Guérin-treated superficial bladder cancer. Correlation of morphology with immunotyping.

Journal of Pathology 1990;162:35–42.

Valentino R, Savastano S, Maglio M, et al. Markers of potential celiac disease in patients with Hashimoto's thyroiditis. European Journal of Endocrinology 2002;146:479–83.

HMB-45 (Melanoma marker)

Sources/clones

Axcel/Accurate, Biodesign, Biogenesis, Biogenex, Dako, Enzo and Immunotech.

Fixation/preparation

The antibody is immunoreactive in paraffin-embedded tissue as well as frozen sections. Immunoreactivity is stronger in ethanol-fixed tissues than following formalin fixation with immunoreactivity diminishing significantly following prolonged fixation in the latter. Sensitivity is enhanced following heat-induced antigen retrieval. Mercury-based fixatives result in a high degree of non-specific staining.

Background

The HMB-45 monoclonal antibody was generated to a whole-cell extract of a heavily pigmented lymph node deposit of human melanoma and has been shown to be a highly specific and sensitive reagent for the identification of melanoma. The designation *HMB* is derived from the immunogen employed, i.e., *H*uman *M*elanoma, *B*lack. The antigen is intracytoplasmic and ultrastructural studies suggest that the antibody reacts with

melanosomes before melanin deposition with HMB-45 binding to stage 1 and 2 melanosomes and to the non-melanised portion of stage 3; whereas stage 4 melanosomes and melanosome complexes found in macrophages and keratinocytes have been negative. The antibody appears to label premature and immature melanosomes in retinal pigment epithelium from fetuses and neonates but not from adults, leading to the suggestion that this "oncofetal" pattern of expression may indicate a role in melanocytic cell proliferation. This thesis has not been confirmed and the sequential expression of the HMB-45 antigen in melanocytes may relate to the activation by specific growth factors, resulting in alterations in protein glycosylation during various ontogenic and pathologic states of melanocytes. The epitope recognized by HMB-45 appears to be, in part, the oligosaccharide side chain of a sialated glycoconjugate as the immunoreactivity can be abolished with neuraminidase treatment.

The gene corresponding to the HMB-45 defined proteins has recently been cloned and designated gp100-cl. This gene encodes the melanocyte lineage-specific antigens recognized by

HMB-45 and HMB-50 (one of two other monoclonal antibodies to melanocytes initially obtained with HMB-45) as well as another monoclonal antibody NKI-beteb. These three antibodies appear to recognize different epitopes of the same antigen; the melanosomal matrix protein or pmel 17 gene product defined by them being apparently related by differential splicing.

Applications

Immunoreactivity for HMB-45 is seen in normal fetal and neonatal melanocytes but not in adult resting melanocytes. Reactive or proliferating melanocytes in inflamed adult skin, wound healing, increased vascularity and in skin overlying certain dermal neoplasms may label for HMB-45 as a result of activation and stimulation by growth factors and "re-expression" of the antigen. HMB-45-positive melanocytes have been demonstrated in the anal squamous zone and transitional zone but not in the colorectal zone. Increased numbers of such melanocytes can be present adjacent to primary anal melanomas.

The staining for HMB-45 in melanocytic nevi depends on their location within the skin.

Junctional nevi and the junctional components of compound nevi are HMB-45-positive. In contrast, intradermal nevi and the dermal components of compound nevi are consistently negative. Thus, HMB-45 does not provide distinction between benign and malignant melanocytic proliferations and the difference in reactivity supports the concept, based on differences in morphology, enzyme activity and other immunological reactivity, that junctional and dermal cells are not identical. Junctional nevus cells are in an activated or proliferative state compared to their quiescent dermal counterparts and their immunoreactivity with HMB-45 is analogous to the proliferating fetal melanocytes that are positive for the antigen whilst quiescent, adult melanocytes are non-reactive.

Dysplastic nevi, in contrast, usually express HMB-45 in both the junctional nevus cells as well as in the dysplastic cells in the superficial dermis. Nevus cells within the deeper dermis do not usually react with HMB-45. In one study, minimally dysplastic nevi displayed intense immunolabelling of the junctional melanocytes but no staining of dermal nevus cells; whereas, with the moderately and severely dysplastic nevi, the dermal melanocytes showed focal cytoplasmic immunoreactivity. The likelihood of expression of HMB-45 paralleled the degree of dysplasia of the nevi. Common blue nevi and cellular blue nevi are generally HMB-45-positive, as are malignant blue nevi. Other nevi such as spindle and epithelioid cell nevi, congenital nevi and other nevi occurring in hormonally reactive sites show immunostaining in nevus cells in the deep dermis as well as those near the dermal-epidermal junction. Less common benign melanocytic proliferations such as plexiform spindle cell nevi, Spitz nevi and atypical melanocytic hyperplasias are also HMB-45-positive.

Malignant melanoma shows strong cytoplasmic positivity for HMB-45 in the majority of cases (65–95%), with the proportion of positive tumor cells ranging from a few to 100%. When the expression of the antigen is weak, staining may appear as a fine granularity similar to that seen in cytologic preparations. The positivity for HMB-45 is seen in almost all types of primary and metastatic melanoma including amelanotic melanoma, spindle cell melanoma and acral lentiginous melanoma (Appendix 1.10). One important exception is desmoplastic malignant melanoma, which consistently displays a much lower rate of positivity and may be completely negative. When positive, reactivity is usually seen in the superficial epithelioid cell rather than the dermal spindle cells, which only rarely stain for HMB-45. The newer markers of melanoma including tyrosinase, MiTF and Melan A do not appear to stain HMB45- desmoplastic melanomas (Xu et al, 2002). However, of 14 HMB45-negative non-desmoplastic tumors, tyrosinase was positive in 6, MiTF in 9 and Melan A in 9. S100 was positive in all cases of desmoplastic and non-desmoplastic tumors that were HMB45- proving to be the most sensitive marker, albeit, of lowest specificity. Other studies have confirmed the greater sensitivity of tyrosinase, MiTF and Melan A over HMB45 (Miettinen et al, 2001; Clarkson et al, 2001).

Attesting to the specificity of the antigen, HMB-45 reactivity has been demonstrated in malignant melanomas of diverse morphology such as signet ring melanoma, myxoid melanoma, small cell melanoma, balloon cell melanoma and in melanomas of different anatomic sites such as the gallbladder, urinary bladder, anorectal region, vulva, sinonasal region, uterine cervix, other mucosal sites and bone. Melanomas and melanocytic proliferations occurring in complex tumors such as pulmonary blastoma have also been HMB-45 positive.

HMB-45 staining has also application in the separation of melanin-containing macrophages from melanoma cells, allowing the accurate determination of tumor thickness and depth of invasion. Similarly, labeling for the antigen helps the identification of recurrence or residual spindle melanoma cells from desmoplastic fibroblasts at resection sites.

As HMB-45 immunoreactivity is melanocyte-specific, positivity can be encountered in lesions with melanin production such as adrenal pheochromocytoma, melanotic neuroectodermal tumor of infancy (progonoma), melanin-containing hepatoblastoma, malignant epithelioid schwannoma of the skin, pigmented carcinoid tumor and esthesioneuroblastoma.

More recently, HMB-45 positivity has been reported in a variety of lesions, which may have implications on their differentiation or histogenesis. These include angiomyolipoma, lymphangiomyomatosis and sugar tumor of the lung. While these tumors consistently manifest HMB-45 immunoreactivity, they do not display obvious pigmentation. However, recent ultrastructural studies confirm the presence of premelanosomes and all three lesions also manifest evidence of smooth muscle differentiation. The reactivity for HMB-45 can be a useful diagnostic discriminator especially in the case of clear cell or sugar tumor, which resembles metastatic renal cell carcinoma and clear cell carcinoma of the lung (Appendix 1.9). Similarly, immunoreactivity for HMB-45 can be helpful in the identification of lymphangiomyomatosis in transbronchial biopsies, obviating the need for an open biopsy for definitive diagnosis.

The expression of this antigen in angiomyolipoma and lymphangioleiomyomatosis, both manifestations of the tuberous sclerosis complex, has been linked by the recent demonstration of HMB-45 immunoreactivity in cardiac rhabdomyoma, brain lesions and other mesenchymal as well as neural lesions found in the tuberous sclerosis complex. These lesions have also shown ultrastructural granules suggestive of melanosome formation and are in agreement with previous suggestions that a smooth muscle cell with unusual features links the various lesions of tuberous sclerosis. HMB-45 immunoreactivity in these lesions now provides another common denominator. This group of tumors has been expanded to comprise angiomyolipoma,

lymphangiomyoma, lymphangioleiomyomaosis, renal capsuloma, clear cell myomelanocytic tumor of the falciform ligament, and clear cell "sugar" tumor and are known as PEComas because of their differentiation towards a putative perivascular epithelioid cells (Govender et al, 2002). The PEComas are characterized by strong immunoreactivity for HMB45 and variable expression of muscle markers. A recently described monotypic epithelioid angiomyolipoma has been described which showed HMB45 immunoreactivity (Insabato et al, 2002).

Comments

Immunoreactivity of formalin-fixed tissue is enhanced following heat-induced antigen retrieval. Enzyme pre-treatment does not significantly improve immunostaining for HMB-45. As in other diagnostic situations, heavily pigmented melanocytic lesions may pose a problem in differentiating melanin in other cells, such as macrophages, from tumor cells with true brown immunoreactivity when 3,3'-diaminobenzidine (DAB) is used as the chromogen. This problem can be simply eliminated by employing azure B as a substitute for hematoxylin as the counterstain. Azure B renders melanin granules blue-green, contrasting against the brown granules resulting from positive immunoreactivity.

The HMB-45 antibody has been reported to rarely show false-positive staining in non-melanomatous tumors and some normal tissues. These include breast carcinoma and normal

breast epithelium, sweat gland tumors and normal counterparts, pheochromocytomas, hepatocellular carcinoma, chordoma, adenocarcinomas, lymphoma, plasmacytoma and plasma cells. This spurious staining is usually apical or perinuclear in location and granular in nature. This false positivity has been attributed to contamination of commercial ascites fluid preparations with nonspecific antibodies and the culture supernatant fluid of the hybridoma cell line, now available from Dako, has been shown to eliminate this false-positivity with HMB-45.

Mercury-based fixatives such as B5 should be avoided as it results in extensive false-positive staining of mesenchymal cells including vessels, fibroblasts and inflammatory cells,

References

Bacchi CE, Bonetti, Pea M, Martignoni G, Gown AM. HMB-45. A review. Applied Immunohistochemistry 1996;4:73–85.

Bonetti F, Pea M, Martignoni G, et al. False-positive immunostaining of normal epithelia and carcinomas with ascites fluid preparations of antimelanoma monoclonal antibody HMB-45. American Journal of Clinical Pathology 1991;95:454–9.

Clarkson KS, Sturdgess IC, Molyneux AJ. The usefulness of tyrosinase in the immunohistochemical assessment of melanocytic lesions: a comparison of the novel T311 antibody (anti-tyrosinase) with S100, HMB45 and A10 (anti-Melan A). Journal of Clinical Pathology 2001;54:196–200.

Govender D, Sabaratnam RM, Essa AS. Clear cell "sugar" tumor of the breast: another extrapulmonary site and review of the literature. American Journal of Surgical Pathology 2002;26:670–5.

Insabato L, De Rosa G, Terracciano LM, et al. Primary monotypic epithelioid angiomyolipoma of bone. Histopathology 2002;40:286–90.

Leong AS-Y, Milios J. An assessment of a melanoma-specific antibody (HMB-45) and other immunohistochemical markers of malignant melanoma in paraffin-embedded tissues. Surgical Pathology 1989;2:137–45.

Miettinen M, Fernandez M, Franssila K, et al. Microphthalmia transcription factor in the immunohistochemical diagnosis of metastatic melanoma: comparison with four other melanoma markers. American Journal of Surgical Pathology 2001;25:205–11.

Ordonez NG, Sneige N, Hickey RC, Brooks TE. Use of monoclonal antibody HMB-45 in the cytologic diagnosis of melanoma. Acta Cytologica 1988;32:684–8.

Weeks DA, Chase DR, Malott RL, et al. HMB-45 staining in angiomyolipoma, cardiac rhabdomyoma, other mesenchymal processes and tuberous sclerosis-associated brain lesions. Journal of Surgical Pathology 1994;1:191–8.

Xu X, Chu AY, Pasha TL, et al. Immunoprofile of MiTF, tyrosinase, melan A and MAGE 1 in HMB45-negative melanomas. American Journal of Surgical Pathology 2002;26:82–7.

hMLH1 and hMSH2 – Mismatch repair proteins

Sources/clones

Anti-hMLH1 – Becton-Dickenson/PharMingen (monoclonal G168–15), anti-hMSH2 – Becton-Dickenson/PharMingen (monoclonal G219–1129), Oncogene Research Products (monoclonal FE11),

Fixation/preparation

Both antibodies are applicable to formalin-fixed, paraffin-embedded tissues. Microwave antigen retrieval in a citrate buffer is necessary pretreatment.

Background

The deoxyribonucleic acid (DNA) mismatch repair system comprises six genes and is required for the correction of DNA mismatches that occur during replication. Inactivation of DNA mismatch repair (MMR) genes most commonly involve *hMLH1* (human *mutL* homologue 1) and *hMSH2* (human *mutS* homologue 2) (Jiricny, 1998). The understanding of the role of mismatch repair in human neoplasia resulted from the study of colorectal carcinomas arising in patients with hereditary nonpolyposis colorectal cancer (HNPCC) (Kinzler and Vogelstein, 1996). This disorder is responsible for 1–5% of all colorectal carcinoma. These patients have a lifetime risk of 80–90% for developing colorectal carcinoma in the fourth and fifth decade (Dunlop et al, 1997). Patients with HNPCC are also at an increased risk for developing other types of tumors: endometrium, ovary, small intestine, stomach, pancreas, biliary tract, bladder and ureter.

Germline mutations of *hMLH1* or *hMSH2* result in loss of protein function, accounting for 80–90% of observed mutations in HNPCC patients with mismatch repair-deficient cancers (Papadopoulos and Lindblom, 1997). *hMLH2* is localized to chromosome 3p21 and encodes a 756 amino acid protein; whilst *hMSH2* is localized to chromosome 2p21–22 and encodes a 935 amino acid protein (Leach et al, 1993; Papadopoulos et al, 1994). With development of tumor, the second (wild-type) allele of these genes is also inactivated, resulting in mismatch repair deficiency. This leads to an increased rate of mutations in microsatellite regions, so called microsatellite instability (MSI) (Stahl, 2000). Such mutations also affect crucial genes that regulate growth, differentiation and apoptosis. The present definition of replication error (RER)-positive tumors is that 30–40% of MSI markers tested need to show rearrangements in order to justify the designation RER-positive tumor.

Colon cancers in HNPCC patients typically occur in right colon (in the absence of multiple polyps), show poor differentiation with a cribiform pattern and a lymphoid inflammatory infiltrate, but carry a better prognosis than "conventional tumors" (Stahl, 2000). DNA mismatch repair genes also play a role in approximately 10–15% of sporadic colon cancers. However, these genes are inactivated by somatic hypermethylation (Herman et al, 1998) rather than germline mutations, with the latter only identified occasionally in tumor DNA (Liu et al, 1996). Hence, it is not only the HNPCC cases, but also a significant number of sporadic colorectal carcinomas that share the molecular mechanisms with the familial counterparts as well as pathologic, clinical and, more importantly, prognostic features; these being "early onset" (<50 years), right sided cancers with an improved survival rate (Stahl,

2000). Further, similar to HNPCC patients, the sporadic colorectal carcinomas with MMR defects have an increased incidence of synchronous and metachronous tumors.

MSI testing requires the services of a molecular diagnostic laboratory but these tumors may alternatively be recognized with immunohistochemical staining. The absence of *hMLH1* or *hMSH2* nuclear expression may identify tumors with a MMR deficiency (Thibodeau et al, 1996). More recently, a larger study showed that 37/38 MSI colorectal carcinomas were predicted to have a MMR gene defect, as demonstrated by the absence of *hMLH1* and/or *hMSH2* immunoexpression (Marcus et al, 1999). This included concordance of 16 cases with germline mutations. An additional 34 microsatellite-stable cancers had intact staining with both antibodies. These findings clearly demonstrate that immunohistology can discriminate accurately between MSI and microsatellite-stable tumors. Subsequent studies confirmed the usefulness of immunostaining for these proteins. Loss of MLH1 or MSH2 was detected in 90.9% of MSI-high carcinomas, whereas all MSI-low and MS-stable tumors showed normal expression of both proteins. Lack of MLH1 nuclear staining was observed more frequently than absence of MSH2 (106 and 14 cases respectively of 132 cases) (Lanza et al, 2002). Another study, which identified a group of carcinomas on the left side of the colon with absence of staining for one mismatch repair protein (these patients also later developed a second colorectal carcinoma), recommended that all colorectal carcinomas be screened for loss of immunoexpression for *hMLH1* and *hMSH2* irrespective of the HNPCC status (Cawkwell et al, 1999).

Applications

It is important to identify patients with HNPCC for genetic counseling, screening and prevention. It is equally important to stratify sporadic MSI tumors for future chemotherapeutic protocols. This would also identify patients who may be at a higher risk of developing a second carcinoma including those of the endometrium, ovary and urinary bladder. The immunohistochemical detection of MMR gene proteins (*hMLH1* and *hMSH2*) places the pathologist at the center of this decision making process.

Comments

The ability to identify HNPCC with immunostaining has allowed the correlation of clinico-pathological features of such tumors. MSI-high MLH1/MSH2-positive carcinomas are more often located in the distal colon, are more frequently typed as ordinary adenocarcinoma, and are more likely to be well- or moderately-differentiated, p53+, and <7cm in diameter than MLH1-negative and MSH2-negative carcinomas (Lanza et al, 2002). Antibodies to other mismatch repair gene proteins that immunoreactive in fixed, paraffin-embedded tissues include anti-PMS2 and anti-MSH6 but abnormalities of these proteins are less common in HNPCC

References

Cawkwell L, Gray S, Murgatroyd H, Sutherland F, Haine L, Longfellows M, O'Loughlin D, Kronberg O, Fenger C, Mapstone N, Dixon M, Quirke P. Gut 1999;45:409–15.

Dunlop MG, Garrinton SM, Carothers AD, et al: Cancer risk associated with germline DNA mismatch repair gene mutations. Human Molecular Genetics 1997;6:105–10.

Herman JG, Umar A, Polyak K, et al: Incidence and functional consequences of hMLH1 promoter hypermethylation in colorectal carcinoma. Proceedings of National Academy of Science USA 1998;95:6870–5.

Jiricny J: Eukaryotic mismatch repair: An update. Mutation Research 1998;409:107–21.

Kinzler KW, Vogelstein B: Lessons from hereditary colorectal cancer. Cell 1996;87:159–70.

Lanza G, Gafa R, Maestri I, et al. Immunohistochemical pattern of MLH1/MSH2 expression is related to clinical and pathological features in colorectal adenocarcinomas with microsatellite instability. Modern Pathology 2002;15:741–9.

Leach FS, Nicolaides NC, Papadopoulos N, et al: Mutations of a mutS homolog in hereditary nonpolyposis colorectal cancer. Cell 1993;75:1215–25.

Liu B, Parsons R, Papadopoulos N, et al: Analysis of mismatch repair genes in hereditary non-polyposis colorectal cancer patients. Nature Medicine 1996;2:169–74.

Marcus VA, Madlensky L, Gryfe R, et al. Immunohistochemistry of hMLH1 and hMSH2: a practical test for DNA mismatch repair-deficient tumors. American Journal of Surgical Pathology 1999;23:1248–55.

Papadopoulos N, Lindblom A: Molecular basis of HNPCC: mutations of MMR genes. Human Mutation 1997;10:89–99.

Papadopoulos N, Nicolaides NC, Wei YF, et al: Mutation of a mutL homolog in hereditary colon cancer. Science 1994;263:1625–9.

Stahl J: Mismatch repair proteins and microsatellites hit clinical practice. Advances in Anatomical Pathology 2000;7:85–93.

Thibodeau SN, French AJ, Roche PC, et al: Altered expression of hMSH2 and hMLH1 in tumors with microsatellite instability and genetic alterations in mismatch repair genes. Cancer Research 1996;56:4836–40.

NOTES

Human Immunodeficiency Virus (HIV)

Sources/clones

American Research Products (HIV1–1, HIV1–2), Biosource (LOHIV1–1), Dako (Kal-1), Harlan Sera Lab/Accurate (1HIVp24).

Preparation/fixation

Applicable to formalin-fixed, paraffin embedded tissue sections. Pretreatment with proteolytic enzymes such as pronase improves immunoreactivity. May also be used for labeling cryostat sections and fixed cell smears. Although the manufacturers provide working dilutions, optimization in individual laboratories is necessary. We have found that sections require a dual pretreatment with 0,5% trypsin (37°C, 15 minutes) followed by microwave treatment in citrate buffer.

Background

Kal-1 reacts with the HIV type 1 capsid protein p24 and its precursor p55 as demonstrated by immunohistochemistry, immunoprecipitation, ELISA, and immunoblotting using lysates of purified virus and lysates of HIV type 1 infected cells (Daugharty et al, 1990). The antibody detects an epitope of the p24 protein, which is resistant to fixation and paraffin embedding (Kaluza et al, 1992). It does not cross-react with HIV type 2 or simian immunodeficiency virus (SIV) as shown by immunoblotting. During the phase of persistent generalized lymphadenopathy and subsequent stages of disease leading to development of AIDS, follicular dendritic cells forming the framework of lymphoid follicles degenerate (Tenner-Racz et al, 1986). The expression of HIV-1 proteins by follicular dendritic cells (FDC) in germinal centers in situ, and the presence of HIV-1 mRNA-positive cells in germinal follicles suggests that FDC are infected and able to produce HIV-1(Parmentier et al, 1990). Such infection may contribute significantly to the destruction of the FDC network during the lymphadenopathy phase after HIV-1 infection. Kal-1 reacts with the p24 protein in cells infected with HIV type 1, i.e., lymphocytes, monocytes and macrophages, Langerhans cells of the skin, follicular dendritic cells, and brain cells of monocyte/macrophage or microglia lineage. One study employing HIV p24 immunohistochemistry following microwave antigen retrieval, showed positivity in 89% of sections of HIV-related brain lesions in 18 patients with AIDS and a positive correlation with beta-amyloid precursor protein (Nebuloni et al, 2001).

In formalin-fixed, paraffin-embedded tissue, Kal-1 antibody produces a positive immunoreaction of HIV-infected dendritic reticulum cells in the germinal centers of lymph nodes. The dendritic processes are highlighted producing the typical network pattern within germinal centers. Occasional positive mononuclear cells and lymphocytes may be observed in the interfollicular areas of the lymph node. However, only immunopositivity confined to the follicular dendritic cells in lymph nodes should be considered as specific.

Comments

Interpretation of a positive lymph node biopsy with this antibody should always be confirmed with a serological assay or western blot. In some countries an informed consent is required from the patient before testing for HIV status. Hence, histopathologists should be cautious in the reporting of p24 positive lymph node biopsies.

References

Daugharty H, Long EG, Swisher BC, et al. Comparative study with in situ hybridization and immunocytochemistry in detection of HIV-1 in formalin-fixed paraffin-embedded cell cultures. Journal of Clinical Laboratory Analysis 1990;4:283–8.

Kaluza G, Willems WR, Lohmeyer J, et al. A monoclonal antibody that recognizes a formalin-resistant epitope on the p24 core protein of HIV-1. Pathology Research and Practice 1992;188:91–6.

Nebuloni M, Pellegrinelli A, Ferri A, et al. Beta amyloid precursor protein and patterns of HIV p24 immunohistochemistry in different brain areas of AIDS patients. AIDS 2001;15:571–5.

Parmentier HK, van Wicken D, Sie-Go DM, et al. HIV-1 infection and virus production in follicular dendritic cells in lymph nodes. A case report with analysis of isolated follicular dendritic cells. American Journal of Pathology 1990;137:247–51.

Tenner-Racz K, Racz P, Bofill M, et al. HTLV-III/LAV viral antigens in lymph nodes of homosexual men with persistent generalized lymphadenopathy and AIDS. Journal of Pathology 1986;123:9–15.

Human Milk Fat Globule (HMFG)

Sources/clones

Biodesign, Biogenesis (3.14.A3), Biogenex (115D8), Immunotech (KC4,1.10.F3, 3.14.A3), Novocastra (1.10.F3, 3.14.A3), Unipath (1.10.F3, 3.14.A3).

Fixation/preparation

Both antibody clones available are immunoreactive in fixed, paraffin-embedded section. HIER enhances staining.

Background

The human milk fat globule (HMFG) is a complex secretory product of mammary epithelium. HMFG is a relatively pure cell membrane product and is partially covered by a typical unit membrane that is extruded from the luminal surface of breast epithelial cells by reverse pinocytosis (Freudenstein et al, 1979). Besides the covering unit membrane, filamentous membrane structures, including cytoplasm-associated glycoproteins, can be detected on the inner coat of the HMFG. Similar to the plasma membrane, HMFG expresses considerable enzymatic activity, including that of glucose-6-phosphate dehydrogenase, acid and alkaline phosphatases, magnesium-dependent ATPase, aldolase, galactosyl transferase, and xanthine oxidase.

A heterogeneous population of HMFG proteins can be recovered from the aqueous phase of skimmed milk following extraction in chloroform and methanol. This pool of solubilized glycoproteins is derived from a human epithelial membrane and referred to as epithelial membrane antigen (EMA). HMFG is thus very similar to EMA and from a practical standpoint antibodies to these proteins have very similar patterns of immunoreactivity. A polyclonal antibody was initially shown to react with EMA and related HMFG protein determinants in formalin-fixed, paraffin-embedded sections and has been extensively used in normal and neoplastic tissues (Heyderman et al, 1979; Sloane et al, 1983).

Applications

The expression of HMFG is heterogeneous in both normal and neoplastic epithelium and its distribution bears no relationship to cellular morphology. The heterogeneity appears to be the result of normal cellular glycosylation patterns and appears to be reproducible in clonal proliferations of all epithelial cells (Edwards 1985). HMFG proteins are widely distributed in secretory epithelia and their corresponding tumors and fetal anlage. These include sweat glands, sebaceous, apocrine and salivary glands, epithelium of the intestines, bile ducts, endometrium and endosalpinx; pulmonary alveolar cells and exocrine pancreas. HMFG is also expressed by some non-secretory epithelia such as the distal and collecting tubules of the kidney, and urothelium. Syncytiotrophoblasts, glandular cells of the endocervix, prostate, epidydimis, rete testes and thyroid may also be reactive for HMFG. Generally, hepatocytes and proximal tubular epithelia are negative (see section on EMA for further descriptions).

HMFG-1 reacts with apocrine sweat glands but not with eccrine sweat glands (Saga, 2001) and may be used with other markers to distinguish skin adnexal tumors (see Appendix 1.20). It is also immunoexpressed in extra mammary Paget's disease, a tumor of apocrine differentiation (Ohnishi & Watanabe, 2001). The antibody has been applied with limited success for the detection of aspirated milk in lung sections in infant death cases, anti-human alpha lactalbumin producing showing the greatest sensitivity and clearest reaction (Iwadate et al, 2000).

Comments

We employ anti-EMA in preference to anti-HMFG but do not use it as a generic marker of epithelial differentiation as some mesenchymal cells such as mesothelial cells, plasma cells, and their corresponding tumors may express HMFG/EMA. In addition soft tissue tumors such as synovial sarcoma, epithelioid sarcoma, peripheral nerve sheath tumor, smooth muscle tumor, rhabdomyosarcoma, chordoma, ependymoma and choroid plexus tumors may express HMFG/EMA.

References

Edwards PAW. Heterogeneous expression of cell-surface antigens in normal epithelia and their tumours, revealed by monoclonal antibodies. British Journal of Cancer 1985;51:149–60.

Freudenstein C, Keenan TW, Eigel WN, et al. Preparation and characterization of the inner coat meterial associated with fat globule membranes from bovine and human milk. Experimental Cell Research 1979;118:277–94.

Heyderman E, Steele K, Omerod MG. A new antigen on the epithelial membrane: Its immunoperoxidase localisation in normal and neoplastic tissue. Journal of Clinical Pathology 1979;32:35–9.

Iwadate K, Doty M, Nishimaki Y, et al. Immunohistochemical examination of the lungs in infant death cases using antibodies against milk components. Forensic Science International 2000;110:19–28.

Ohnishi T, Watanabe S. Immunohistochemical analysis of human milk fat globulin expression in extramammary Paget's disease. Clinical and Experimental Dermatology 2001;26:192–5.

Saga K. Histochemical and immunohistochemical markers for human eccrine and apocrine sweat glands: an aid for histopathologic differentiation of sweat gland tumors. Journal of Investigative Dermatology symposium Proceedings 2001;6:49–53.

Sloane JP, Hughes F, Ormerod MG. An assessment of the value of epithelial membrane antigen and other epithelial markers in solving diagnostic problems in tumour histology. Histochemistry Journal 1983;15:645–54.

Human Papilloma Virus (HPV)

Sources/clones

Accurate (polyclonal), American Research Products (1535–18, 1501–17, 1502–17, 1505–17), Biodesign, Biogenesis (H11B, 16L1, C1P5), Biogenex (CHO613), Cymbus Bioscience (BF7), Cymbus Bioscience/Pharmingen (CAM-VIR1), Dako (polyclonal to HPV 1), Novocastra (4C4/F10/H7/83, 5A3/C8), Pharmingen (7H7, TVG401, TVG402, p16INK4 clone G175–405), Santa Cruz (16-E7 clone TVG710Y, 180E6 C-20).

Fixation/preparation

Antibodies to HPV are applicable to formalin-fixed paraffin embedded tissues and frozen/cryostat sections.

Background

The most extensively studied area of HPV infection has been in epithelia of the anogenital tract, particularly the uterine cervix. Over 25 HPV genotypes have been isolated to date from the female genital tract. HPV genotypes have enabled specific types to be correlated with morphological lesions, e.g. HPV 6/11 being commonly associated with condylomata, whilst HPV 16/18 is frequently associated with high grade cervical intraepithelial neoplasia (CIN) and invasive squamous cell carcinoma (for review see Cooper & McGee, 1996). It has recently been demonstrated that over 90% of cervical squamous cell carcinomas harbor a high risk HPV (Bosch et al, 1995), the genome of which is usually integrated into the host DNA. Hence, in conjunction with epidemiological data showing that HPV infection and cervical squamous cell carcinoma share several risk factors, the association between high risk HPV and cervical cancer is now firmly established. Although only a small proportion of high grade CIN progress to invasive carcinoma, it is thought that HPV detection may assist in predicting the invasive potential of high grade CIN.

Applications

The detection of HPV in clinical samples depends on the demonstration of viral components within cells and tissues. This entails the detection of either protein or nuclei acid. Viral proteins may be visualized with immunohistochemical techniques using either polyclonal or monoclonal antibodies (Graham et al, 1991). Antibodies directed to viral proteins are dependent on the expression/synthesis of the latter by the virus, which is dependent on transcription/translation of the viral genome within the nucleus. Polyclonal antibodies raised to bovine papillomavirus capsid protein are applicable to HPV types in human biopsy specimens as they cross-react with several human subtypes (Jenkins et al, 1986). The synthesis of bacterial fusion proteins and used as immunogens in mice has led to the generation of monoclonal antibodies to specific viral proteins to achieve viral specificity (Patel et al, 1989). The use of the HPV 16 L1 (capsid) protein has led to the production of several antibodies of varying specificity. The immunoreactivity of antibodies to HPV capsid protein is dependent on active viral replication, which is closely correlated with keratin production. This therefore produces an intranuclear signal in the upper third of the squamous epithelia harboring the virus. Apart from the cervix, the use of antibodies to HPV is applicable to the vulva, penis, anus, oral cavity, larynx and esophagus.

Clone E6H4 (MTM Laboratories, Heildelberg, Germany) has been applied to ThinPreps and overexpression of P16INK4A has been employed as a specific marker for dysplastic and neoplastic cervical epithelial cells (Bibbo et al, 2002) and P16INK4 in combination with cyclin E and Ki67 have been proposed as surrogate biomarkers for HPV-related preinvasive squamous cervical disease (Keating et al, 2001).

Comments

With the advent of advanced in situ hybridization technology for the detection of HPV DNA, the demand for HPV immunohistochemistry has fallen. Non-isotope in situ hybridization techniques are easily accessible and readily applicable to the routine diagnostic histopathology laboratory. Squamous epithelium showing the typical

morphological features of HPV infection is recommended for use as positive controls. Staining should be mainly intranuclear, with some perinuclear staining of koilocytes.

References

Bibbo M, Klump WJ, DeCecco J, Kovatich AJ. Procedure for immunocytochemical detection of P16INK4A antigen in thin-layer, liquid-based specimens. Acta Cytology 2002;46:25–9.

Bosch FX, Manos MM, Munoz N, et al. Prevalence of HPV in cervical cancer: a worldwide perspective. Journal of the National Cancer Institute 1995;87:796–802.

Cooper K McGee J O'D. Human papillomavirus, integration and cervical carcinogenesis: a clinicopathological perspective. Journal of Clinical Pathology: Molecular Pathology 1997;50:1–3.

Graham AK, Herrington CS, J O'D McGee. Simultaneous in situ genotyping and phenotyping of

human papillomavirus cervical lesions: Comparative sensitivity and specificity. Journal of Clinical Pathology 1991;44:96–101.

Jenkins D, Tay SK, McCance DJ, et al. Histological and immunocytochemical study of cervical intraepithelial neoplasia (CIN) with associated HPV 6 and HPV 16 infections. Journal of Clinical Pathology 1986;39:1177–80.

Keating JT, Cviko A, Riethdorf S, et al. Ki-67, cyclin E and p16INK4 are complementary surrogate biomarkers for human papilloma virus–related cervical neoplasia. American Journal of Surgical Pathology 2001;25:884–91.

Patel D, Shepherd PS, Naylor JA, McCance DJ. Reactivities of polyclonal and monoclonal antibodies raised to the major capsid protein of human papillomavirus type 16. Journal of Virology 1989;70:69–77.

Human Parvovirus B19

Sources/clones

Chemicon, Dako (polyclonal), Novocastra (R92F6), Vector Laboratories (R92F6).

Fixation/preparation

Applicable to archival formalin-fixed paraffin-embedded tissue sections. Before immunostaining, sections should be subjected to heat-induced epitope retrieval at 100°C for 20 minutes (Liu et al, 1997).

Background

Human parvovirus B19 was accidentally discovered in 1975 in human serum being screened for hepatitis B surface antigen (Cossart et al, 1975). Since discovery, this virus has been found to be the causative agent in erythema infectiosum, chronic anemia in immunosuppressed patients, fetal death associated with hydrops, and acute arthralgia/arthritis in adults (Liu et al, 1997).

Parvovirus B19, which is cytotoxic to erythroid progenitor cells in vivo and in vitro, enters the erythroid precursor cell via the blood group P antigen (Mortimer et al, 1983; Brown et al, 1993). Human parvovirus B19 has been reported as a cause of severe and persistent anaemia in patients immunocompromised from organ transplantation, autoimmune disease, hematologic malignancies, chemotherapy and congenital or acquired immunodeficiency states including HIV infection (Liu et al, 1997).

The R92F6 monoclonal antibody is directed against the VP1 and VP2 capsid protein of parvovirus B19.

Applications

On bone marrow smears and trephine biopsies the presence of giant erythroblasts and small erythroid precursors with nuclear inclusions (Lantern cells) establishes the diagnosis. However, the inexperienced observer may easily overlook these cells and the use of antibody to parvovirus B19 may be useful in establishing the diagnosis. A high index of suspicion when assessing bone marrow smear/biopsies in immunocompromised patients with chronic severe anemia is required. Although Liu et al (1977) found anti-parvovirus B19 antibody to be less sensitive than in situ hybridization (ISH), others have not had the same experience. Good correlation between R92F6 antibody staining and B19 DNA was found in 19 cases of fatal non-immune hydrops fetalis (Morey et al, 1992). Further, the same study demonstrated the virus with immunohistochemistry (and ISH) in two cases that lacked parvovirus B19 inclusions on H&E stains, indicating that low grade or resolving infections may be missed on simple morphological examination alone. Recent studies employing immunostaining and PCR have confirmed that the presence of parvovirus B19 is common in cases of late second-trimester and third-trimester fetal death, mostly of non-hydropic type intra uterine deaths (Skjoldebrand-Sparre et al, 2000; Tolfvenstam et al, 2001). Immune complex-type glomerulonephritis may also be caused by parvovirus B19 antigen-antibody complexes (Komatsuda et al, 2000).

Comments

Parvovirus B19 infection should be considered in any unexplained chronic persistent anemia in an immunocompromised patient.

References

Brown KE, Anderson SM, Young NS. Erythrocyte P antigen: Cellular receptor of B19 parvovirus. Science 1993;262:114–7.

Cossart YE, Fiedl AM, Cant B, et al. Parvovirus-like particles in human sera. Lancet 1975;1:72–3.

Komatsuda A, Ohtani H, Nimura T, et al. Endocapillary proliferative glomerulonephritis in a patient with parvovirus B19 infection. American Journal of Kidney Diseases 2000;36:851–4.

Liu W, Ittmann MD, Liu J, et al. Human parvovirus B19 in bone marrows from adults with acquired immunodeficiency syndrome: A comparative study using in situ hybridization and immunohistochemistry. Human Pathology 1997;28:760–6.

Morey AL, O'Neill HJ, Coyle PV, et al. Immunohistological detection of human parvovirus B19 in formalin fixed paraffin embedded tissues. Journal of Pathology 1992;166:105–8.

Mortimer PP, Humphries RK, Moore JG, et al. A human parvovirus-like virus inhibits hematopoietic colony formation in vitro. Nature 1983;302:426–9.

Skjoldebrand-Sparre L, Tolfvenstam T, Papadogiannakis N, et al. Parvovirus B19 infection: association with third-trimester intrauterine fetal death. British Journal of Obstetrics and Gynaecology 2000;107:476–80.

Tolfvenstam T, Papadogiannakis N, Norbeck O, et al. Frequency of human parvovirus B19 infection in intrauterine fetal death. Lancet 2001;357:1494–7.

Human Placental Lactogen (hPL)

Sources/clones

Accurate (KIHPL3–489D5F3, polyclonal), American Research Products (polyclonal), Biogenesis (LIP603), Chemicon (polyclonal), Dako (polyclonal), Fitzgerald (M310198, M310199, polyclonal), Seralab (polyclonal), Zymed (polyclonal).

Fixation/preparation

The antigen is resistant to formalin fixation and immunoreactivity is enhanced by proteolytic digestion.

Background

Human placental lactogen (hPL) is a member of an evolutionarily related gene family that includes human growth hormone (hGH) and human prolactin. hPL together with human chorionic gonadotropin and pregnancy specific beta 1 glycoprotein (SP1) are the three major proteins produced by the placenta. Although its expression is limited to the placenta, its physiological actions are far reaching. hPL has a direct somatotropic effect on fetal tissues. It alters maternal carbohydrate and lipid metabolism to provide for fetal nutrient requirements, and aids in the stimulation of mammary cell proliferation. Two hPL genes (hPL3 and hPL4) encoding identical proteins are responsible for the production of up to 1–3 g hPL hormone/day (Walker et al, 1991).

Applications

Several studies have employed hPL and other placental markers for the distinction of intrauterine from extra-uterine pregnancies. The presence of cytokeratin and hPL was found to be useful in identifying trophoblastic elements in endometrial curettings (Sorensen et al, 1991; Khong et al, 1994), with a sensitivity of 73d% in one study (Kaspar et al, 1991). hPL can also be employed in a panel for the distinction of trophoblastic proliferations (Appendix I.5, 1.33,1.34,1.37). Complete hydatidiform mole showed strong expression of human chorionic gonadotropin (hCG) and weak expression of placental alkaline phosphatase (PLAP), whereas, partial mole showed weak hCG and strong PLAP. Choriocarcinoma, on the other hand, showed strong hCG and weak hPL and PLAP. All tissues were positive for cytokeratin but negative for vimentin (Losch & Kainz, 1996).

Focal expression of hCG and diffuse expressions of hPL and PLAP was a profile not observed in complete moles (Brescia et al, 1987; Cheah & Looi, 1994).

hPL has also been employed as a marker of intermediate trophoblasts (IT) together with pregnancy specific glycoprotein, cytokeratin and vimentin are more reliable markers (Yeh et al, 1990; Shibata & Rutgers JL, 1994). Extra villous trophoblasts are diffusely and strongly positive for hPL in contrast to the focal staining in villous trophoblasts (Tarrade et al, 2001). There appears to be three subpopulations of IT with distinct morphologic and immunohistochemical features, this accounting perhaps for the differences in immunophenotype report for placental site tumors. Chorionic-type IT was found to comprise two populations – one with eosinophilic and the other with clear (glycogen-rich) cytoplasm. The former tended to be larger with more pleomorphic nuclei compared to the smaller more uniform nuclei of the clear cell type. Both cell types were diffusely positive for placental alkaline phosphatase but only focally positive for hPL, Mel-Cam (CD146) and oncofetal fibronectin. These cells corresponded to those found in chorion leave and placental site nodule and its neoplastic counterpart, epithelioid trophoblastic tumor, the latter also stain for alpha-inhibin (Ohira et al, 2000; Coulson et al, 2000; Kamoi et al, 2002;). In contrast, implantation site IT cells were strongly positive for hPL, Mel-Cam and oncofetal firbonectin, corresponding to cells in an exaggerated placental site and its neoplastic counterpart, placental site trophoblastic tumor (Shih et al, 1999; Arato et al, 2001).

Comments

Various tumors that show trophoblastic differentiation may express hPL (Boucher & Yoneda, 1995; Ulbright et al, 1997; Dirnhofer et al, 1998; Erhan et al, 2002).

References

Arato G, Fulop V, Degrell P, Szigetvari I. Placental site trophoblastic tumor. Clinical and pathological report of two cases. Pathology Oncology Research 2000;6:292–4.

Boucher LD, Yoneda K. The expression of trophoblastic cell markers by lung carcinomas. Human Pathology 1995;26:1201–6.

Brescia RJ, Kurman RJ, Main CS, et al. Immunocytochemical localization of chorionic gonadotropin, placental lactogen, and placental alkaline phosphatase in the diagnosis of complete and partial hydatidiform moles. International Journal of Gynecological Pathology 1987;6:213–29.

Cheah PL, Looi LM. Expression of placental proteins in complete and partial hydatidiform moles. Pathology 1994;26:115–8.

Coulson LE, Kong CS, Zaloudek C. Epithelioid trophoblastic tumor of the uterus in a postmenopausal woman: a case report and review of the literature. American Journal of Surgical Pathology 2000;24:1558–62.

Dirnhofer S, Koessler P, Ensinger C, et al. Production of trophoblastic hormones by transitional cell carcinoma of the bladder: association to tumor stage and grade. Human Pathology 1998;29:377–82.

Erhan Y, Ozdemir N, Zekioglu O, et al. Breast carcinomas with choriocarcinomatous features: case reports and review of the literature. Breast Journal 2002;8:244–8.

Kamoi S, Ohaki Y, Mori O, et al. Epithelioid trophoblastic tumor of the utrus: cytological and immunohistochemical observation of a case. Pathology Intenational 2002;52:75–81.

Kaspar HG, To T, Dinh TV. Clinical use of immunoperoxidase markers in excluding ectopic gestation. Obstetrics and Gynecology 1991;78:433–7.

Khong TY, Stewart CJ, Mott C, et al. The usefulness of human placental lactogen and keratin immunohistochemistry in the assessment of tissue from purported intrauterine pregnancies. American Journal of Clinical Pathology 1994;102:72–5.

Losch A, Kainz C. Immunohistochemistry in the diagnosis of the gestational trophoblastic disease. Acta Obstetrics Gynecology Scandinavia 1996;75:753–6.

Ohira S, Yamazaki T, Hatano H, et al. Epithelioid trophoblastic metastatic to the vagina: an immunohistochemical and ultrastructural study. International Journal of Gynecological Pathology 2000;19:381–6.

Shibata PK, Rutgers JL. The placental site nodule: an immunohistochemical study. Human Pathology 1994;25:1295–301.

Shih IM, Seidman JD, Kurman RJ. Placental site nodule and characterization of distinctive types of intermediate trophoblast. Human Pathology 1999;30:687–94.

Sorensen FH, Marcussen N, Daugaard HO, et al. Immunohistological demonstration of intermediate trophoblast in the diagnosis of uterine versus ectopic pregnancy: a retrospective survey and results of a prospective trial. British Journal of Obstetrics and Gynecology 1991;98:463–9.

Tarrade A, Lai KR, Malassine A, et al. characterization of human villous and extravillous trophoblasts isolated from first trimester placenta. Laboratory Investigation 2001;81:1199–211.

Ulbright TM, Young RH, Scully RE. Trophoblastic tumors of the testis other than classic choriocarcinoma: "monophasic" choriocarcinoma and placental site trophoblastic tumor: a report of two cases. American Journal of Surgical Pathology 1997;21:282–8.

Wright WH, Fitzpatrick SL, Barrera-Saldana HA, et al. The human placental lactogen genes: structure, function, evolution and transcriptional regulation. Endocrine Reviews 1991;12:316–28.

Yeh IT, O'Connor DM, Kurman RJ. Intermediate trophoblast: further immunocytochemical characterization. Modern Pathology 1990;3:282–7.

Immunoglobulins: Igκ, Igλ, IgA, IgD, IgE, IgG, IgM

Sources/clones

Both monoclonal and polyclonal antibodies to immunoglobulins of the various types are available from a wide variety of sources. Affinity-isolated F (ab')$_2$ fragments to Igκ and Igλ are also available.

Igκ

Accurate (EA2–38), Becton Dickinson (TB28–2), Biodesign/Pharmingen (polyclonal), Biogenesis (HK3, polyclonal), Biosource (LOHK3), Calbiochem (HP6062, polyclonal), Cymbus Bioscience (24K6), Dako (R10–21-F3, A8B5, polyclonal), Immunotech Inc (G6.42), Pharmingen (polyclonal, G20–193), Research Diagnostics (6KA4G7), Sanbio/Monsan/Accurate (2B7), Zymed (HP6053).

Igλ

Accurate (AG7.47), Becton Dickinson (1–155–2), Biogenesis (polyclonal), Biosource (LOHL2), Caltag Laboratories/Sigma Chemical (HP6054), Cymbus Bioscience (24L6), Harlan Sera Lab/Accurate (Lam2.G4), Pharmingen (JDC12, polyclonal), Zymed (HP6054).

IgA

Accurate (GA1, SB14, A1–18), Accurate/Sigma Chemical (GA112), Becton Dickinson (1–155–1), Biodesign (polyclonal), Biogenesis (polyclonal, 15D6, 2E2), Biosource (LOHA8), Cymbus Bioscience (M24A), Dako 6E2C1, polyclonal), E-Y Labs (polyclonal), Immunotech Inc/Immunotech SA (NIF2), Pharmingen (polyclonal), Sanbio/Monsan/Accurate (MH14–1), Sigma Chemical (A1–18), Zymed (WAN741).

IgD

Becton Dickinson (TA4.1), Biogenesis (polyclonal), Biogenex (NI158, polyclonal), Biosource (LOHD11), Dako (IgD26, polyclonal), E-Y Labs (polyclonal), Harlan Sera Lab/Accurate (1AD86), Immunotech (JA11), Sera-Lab Ltd (12.1), Sigma Chemical (HJ9).

IgE

Accurate (GE1, AMD-E), Accurate/Sigma Chemical (GE1), Biodesign (polyclonal), Biogenesis (0257), Dako C!A-E-7.12, E1, polyclonal), E-Y Labs (polyclonal).

IgG

Accurate (polyclonal, 4.22D10, A57H, SL13), Accurate/Sigma Chemical (GG4), Becton Dickinson (C3–124), Becton Dickinson/Biodesign (polyclonal), Biodesign (polyclonal), Biogenesis (polyclonal, 2D7), Dako (A57H, polyclonal), E-Y Labs (polyclonal, NL16, GB7B), Harlan Sera Lab/Accurate (ISE503, C3–8–80, C27–15), Pharmingen (G7–18, G18–145, G18–21, G18–3, polyclonal), Sanbio/Monosan/Accurate (MH25–1, BL-G4–1), Sigma Chemical (SH21, SK44).

IgG F(ab)

Accurate/Sigma Chemical (SG16), E-Y Labs (HP6014).

IgM

Accurate (AMD-u, SB17), Accurate/Sigma Chemical (MB11), Becton Dickinson (145–8), Biogenesis (polyclonal), Dako (R1/69, polyclonal), E-Y Labs (polyclonal), Pharmingen (G20–127, polyclonal).

Fixation/preparation

Immunostaining of cytoplasmic immunoglobulin can be

performed in formalin-fixed paraffin-embedded sections, fresh frozen sections and cytologic preparations. Other fixatives and processing procedures such as AMEX (Sato et al, 1986) and freeze-drying (Stein et al, 1985) have been suggested to produce effective immunoglobulin staining.

Background

Surface membrane immunoglobulin (SIg) expression is the classical and specific marker of B-lymphocytes and serves as the antigen recognition molecule for this lymphocyte population. Each of the heavy chain classes of Ig can be expressed on the B cell membrane and more than one heavy chain class can be expressed on the same cell, the majority of peripheral B cells expressing IgM with or without IgD, less than 10% expressing IgM or IgA.

IgM is the first heavy chain class to appear in B cell ontogeny with the majority of immature B cells expressing IgM in high density. This decreases in density with maturation and increasing amounts of IgD appears on the cell membrane. The IgM and IgD molecules that co-exist in the same membrane cap exist independently but share the same idiotype and have the same light chain. Following B cell activation and differentiation, there is loss of IgM and IgD as the result of a productive isotype gene rearrangement switch. With the progression to antibody-forming plasma cells, different subpopulations of SIgM and/or SIgG bearing memory B cells may appear.

Clonality of a given B cell population can be inferred from the uniformity of light chain class expression as individual B cell can express either κ or λ light chains but not both; the ratio of κ:λ bearing B cells being 2:1. A vast predominance of κ or λ light chain bearing B cells indicates monoclonality, generally implying a neoplastic proliferation, whereas a mixture of light chain bearing cell types suggests polyclonality and a reactive or non-neoplastic proliferation of B cells.

Direct immunofluorescent staining with heterologous antisera raised against whole or Fab fragments of human Ig molecules is the simplest method of identifying SIg. Class specific anti-sera monospecific for individual heavy and light chain determinants (monovalent antisera) may be employed to determine the precise isotype of the SIg but these procedures require fresh cell preparations. Alternatively, immunoenzyme techniques can be used on cytocentrifuge preparations and imprints as well as frozen sections (Banks et al, 1983; Forbes & Leong, 1987). The latter procedures have suffered from the high level of background staining which can make interpretation difficult.

Ideally, the aim would be to be able to perform consistent staining of immunoglobulin in fixed, paraffin-embedded, allowing the advantage of retrospectivity as well as optimal cytomorphology. While many attempts have been made with special fixatives such as B5 and other mercury-based fixatives, and the application of various enzymatic digestions, they have not been met with much success.

Coupled with the recent introduction of HIER, the use of 4 M urea as the retrieval solution as produced consistent results, with the claim that the procedure not only allows the demonstration of cytoplasmic Ig but also surface Ig (Merz et al, 1993). We have taken the method further and employed HIER in 4 M urea solution in combination with proteolytic digestion prior to antigen retrieval (Leong et al 2002). This has resulted in the consistent demonstration of cellular immunoglobulin in routinely fixed, paraffin-embedded sections revealing a number of patterns of immunoglobulin localization. Peri-nuclear staining of endoplasmic reticulum was the most consistent pattern often with associated staining of the golgi. Membrane staining was also possible as was cytoplasmic staining, the latter as distinct globular heterogenous deposits of immunoglobulin rather than the homogenous staining seen in false positive staining. Stringent washing in between each incubation step result in a clean background in the case of follicular lymphomas.

Applications

About 80% of non-Hodgkin's lymphoma in western countries are of B cell lineage and the majority express monotypic SIg (Lukes et al, 1978; Tubbs et al, 1983). The examination of lymphoid proliferations for the presence and clonal nature of Sig expression is a common practice and forms the basis for traditional immunophenotypic analysis (Leong and Forbes, 1982). By convention, it is inferred that monoclonal B cell proliferations are neoplastic. This analysis has traditionally been carried out by flow cytometry on cell suspensions, in cytospin preparations of disaggregated cells, or in frozen tissue sections. The SIg isotypes expressed by B cell non-Hodgkin's lymphoma and lymphoid leukemias parallel those of normal B cells. The most common heavy chain class is IgM, with or without associated IgD, and IgG and IgA are expressed much less frequently. The ratio of Igκ to Igλ-bearing lymphomas is about 2:1.

Comments

When staining terminally-differentiated B cells such as plasma cells, it is important to remember that unlike SIg, which is detectable in viable cells in suspension or in minimally fixed frozen sections, the staining of CIg requires permeabilization of the cell membrane by the fixative to allow penetration of the anti-Ig reagents. Therefore, sections fixed by a gentle fixative such as acetone will not allow the demonstration of CIg and plasma cells may show false-negative staining. Alcohol and formalin are suitable fixatives for the demonstration of CIg in cell preparations and tissue sections respectively. We have found that fixation of freshly prepared or air-dried smears and cell preparations followed by HIER in 4 M urea produces excellent staining of CIg in lymphoid cells through a wide range of differentiation. Formalin-fixed, paraffin-embedded sections also show consistent staining for both CIg as well as SIg following a combination of trypsin digestion and HIER in 4 M urea.

References

Banks PM, Caron BL, Morgan TW. Use of imprints for monoclonal antibody studies: Suitability of air-dried preparations from lymphoid tissues with an immunohistochemical method. American Journal of Clinical Pathology 1983;79:438–42.

Forbes IJ, Leong AS-Y. Essential oncology of the lymphocyte. London: Springer-Verlag, 1987, pp184–8.

Merz H, Rickers O, Schrimel S, et al. Constant detection of surface and cytoplasmic immunoglobulin heavy and light chain expression in formalin-fixed and paraffin-embedded material. Journal of Pathology 1993;170:257–64.

Leong AS-Y, Forbes IJ. Immunological and histochemical techniques in the study of the malignant lymphomas: A review. Pathology 1982;14:247–54.

Leong AS-Y, Yin H, Hafajee Z, et al. Patterns of immunoglobulin staining in fixed, paraffin-embedded tissue in the lymphoproliferative disorders. Applied Immunohistochemistry and Molecular Morphology 2002;10:110–4.

Lukes RJ, Parker JW, Taylor CR, et al. Immunologic approach to non-Hodgkin's lymphomas and related leukemias. Analysis of the results of multiparameter studies of 425 cases. Seminars in Hematology 1978;15:322–35.

Sato Y, Mukai K, Watanabe S, et al. The AMEX method. A simplified technique of tissue processing and paraffin-embedding with improved preservation of antigens for immunostaining. American Journal of Pathology 1986;125:431–5.

Stein H, Gatter K, Asbahr H, Mason DY. Use of freeze-dried paraffin-embedded sections for immunohistologic staining with monoclonal antibodies. Laboratory Investigation 1985;52:676–83.

Tubbs RR, Fishleder A, Weiss RA, et al. Immunohistologic cellular phenotypes of lymphoproliferative disorders. Comprehensive evaluation of 564 cases including 257 non-Hodgkin's lymphomas classified by the International Formulation. American Journal of Pathology 1983;113:207–21.

NOTES

Inhibin

Sources/clones

Biogenesis (monoclonal 16Ba), Biodesign (monoclonal E4), Santa Cruz (polyclonal), Serotec (R1, E4).

Fixation/preparation

Antibodies to inhibin may be applied to paraffin-embedded tissues fixed in formalin; however, microwave pretreatment in citrate buffer is essential for optimum immunostaining.

Background

Inhibin is a peptide hormone produced by ovarian granulosa cells, which selectively inhibits the release of follicle stimulating hormone (FSH) from the pituitary gland (McLachlan et al, 1987), acting as a modulator of folliculogenesis (Findlay et al, 1993). A peak of its serum levels is reached during the follicular phase of the menstrual cycle; being undetectable in the serum of menopausal women (Lappöhn et al, 1989). It is produced and overexpressed by granulosa cell tumors, thus being an early marker for tumor growth. Hence, its usefulness pertains to being that of a marker of tumor recurrence before clinical manifestation (Lapp''hn et al, 1989). Several inhibin subunits can be detected by immunostaining in the granulosa cell layers of the human ovary and in neighbouring theca cells. Clone R1 was raised against a synthetic peptide corresponding to the 1–32 peptide of the alpha subunit of 32 kD human inhibin and reacts specifically with this molecule (Isotype: IgG2b) (Groome et al, 1990). Clone E4 was raised against a synthetic peptide corresponding to the 84–114 peptide sequence of the beta A subunit of 32 kD human inhibin A and activin A (Isotype 2b) (Groome and Lawrence, 1991). E4 reacts with both the beta A and beta B subunits of human inhibin and activin.

Applications

Using monoclonal antibody to human inhibin 32-kD alpha subunit, follicle epithelia in 6/6 samples of ovarian tissue (under 40 years), 6/6 adult granulosa cell tumors and three late metastases from granulosa cell tumors in females showed positive immunoreaction (Fleming et al, 1995). No staining was found in hemangiopericytomas, leiomyosarcoma, and malignant melanoma. This would be useful in distinguishing the sarcomatoid growth pattern of granulosa cell tumors from soft tissue tumors. Further, no reaction was observed in 10 ovarian carcinomas, whilst in two of these cases single cells of the specialized ovarian stroma stained positively with inhibin.

In another study inhibin immunostaining was also detected in stromal hyperthecosis, juvenile granulosa cell tumors and Sertoli-Leydig cell tumors (Stewart et al, 1997); proving that inhibin is a sensitive immunohistochemical marker of a wide range of gonadal stromal tumors. In Sertoli-Leydig cell tumors, inhibin stained more intensely the gonadal stromal component compared to the retiform areas that stained more for keratin (Mooney et al, 2002).

Alpha-inhibin is a good marker of syncytiotrophoblastic cells but does not stain cytotrophoblastic cells. It can therefore be employed for the identification of placental site nodule or of a trophoblastic tumor such as choriocarcinoma, placental site trophoblastic tumor or epithelioid trophoblastic tumor (McCluggage 2002).

Strong cytoplasmic staining of 17/19 cases of hepatocellular carcinoma, including pleomorphic and glandular variants has been demonstrated (McCluggage et al, 1997). Focal weak luminal staining of glands of adenocarcinoma was also present. Hence, immunostaining with anti-inhibin antibody may be of value in the differentiation of hepatocellular carcinoma from adenocarcinoma involving the liver.

Together with calretinin, inhibin can be employed to identify adrenocortical tumors (Appendix 1.18). Inhibin was demonstrated in 73% of tumors and in combination with calretinin identified 94% of adrenocortical tumors with no difference in staining patterns in normal adrenal cortex, adrenocortical adenomas and adenocarcinomas (Jorda et al, 2002).

Comments

Inhibin antibody is useful to confirm the diagnosis of both adult and juvenile granulosa cell tumors, especially tumors with unusual growth patterns and in metastatic sites. A cautionary note with this application is that uterine tumors resembling ovarian sex cord tumors may have been shown to immunoexpress inhibin rarely (1/7 cases) (Oliva et al, 2002). It is also helpful in distinguishing hepatocellular carcinoma from adenocarcinomas in the liver. The recent demonstration of alpha-inhibin in granular cell tumors of the gallbladder and extra hepatic bile ducts (Murakata & Ishak, 2001) adds to the existing list of inhibin-positive lesions that includes sex cord stromal tumors (granulosa cells tumors, luteinised thecomas, Leydig cell tumors), placental and gestational trophoblastic lesions, and adrenal cortical tumors.

References

Findlay JK. An update on the roles of inhibin, activin and follistatin as local regulators of folliculogenesis. Biology of Reproduction 1993;48:15–23.

Flemming P, Wellman A, Hansjörg Maschek, Lang H, Georgii A. Monoclonal antibodies against inhibin represent key markers of adult granulosa cell tumors of the ovary even in their metastases. A report of three cases with late metastasis, being previously misinterpreted as haemangiopericytoma. American Journal of Surgical Pathogy 1995;19:927–33.

Groome N, Lawrence M. Preparation of monoclonal antibodies to the beta A subunit of ovarian inhibin using a synthetic peptide immunogen. Hybridoma 1991;10:309–16.

Groome N, Hancock J, Betteridge A, Lawrence M, Craven R. Monoclonal and polyclonal antibodies reactive with the 1–32 amino terminal sequence of the alpha subunit of human 32K inhibin. Hybridoma 1990;9:31–42.

Jorda M, De MB, Nadji M. Calretinin and inhibin are useful in separating adrenocortical neoplasms from pheochromocytomas. Applied Immunohistochemistry and Molecular Morphology 2002;10:67–70.

Lapp"hn RE, Burger HG, Bouma J, et al. Inhibin as a marker for granulosa-cell tumors. New England Journal of Medicine 1989;321:790–3.

McCluggage WG, Maxwell P, Patterson A, Sloan JM. Immunohistochemical staining of hepatocellular carcinoma with monoclonal antibody against inhibin. Histopathology 1997;30:518–22.

McCluggage WG. Recent advances in immunohistochemistry in gynecological pathology. Histopathology 2002;40:309–26.

McLachlan RI, Robertson DM, Burger HG, de Kretser DM. Circulating immunoreactive inhibin levels during the normal menstrual cycle. Journal of Clinical Endocrinology and Metabolism 1987;65:954–61.

Murakata LA, Ishak KG. Expression of inhibin-alpha by granular cell tumors of the gallbladder and extrahepatic ducts. American Journal of Surgical Pathology 2001;25:1200–3.

Mooney EE, Nogales FF, Bergeron C, Tavassoli FA. Retiform Sertoli-Leydig cell tumours: clinical, morphological and immunohistochemical findings. Histopathology 2002;41:110–7.

Oliva E, Young RH, Amin MB, Clement PB. An immunohistochemical analysis of endometrial stromal and smooth muscle tumors of the uterus: a study of 54 cases emphasizing the importance of using a panel because of overlap in immunoreactivity for individual antibodies. American Journal of Surgical Pathology 2002;26:403–12.

Stewart CJR, Deffers MD, Kennedy A. Diagnostic value of inhibin immunoreactivity in ovarian gonadal stromal tumors and their histological mimics. Histopathology 1997;31:67–74.

Ki-67 (MIB1, Ki-S5)

Sources/clones

Accurate (MM1), Biogenex (Ki-67, MIB1), Boehringer Mannheim (Ki-67, Ki-S5), Cymbus Bioscience (Ki67), Dako (Ki-67, polyclonal), Diagnostic Biosystems (Ki-67, polyclonal), Dako (Ki-67, polyclonal), Immunotech (MIB1), Novocastra (MM1), RDI (Ki67), Serotec (Ki67), Zymed (7B11).

Fixation/preparation

Monoclonal Ki-67 is immunoreactive in frozen sections but not in paraffin sections (although there are claims of reactivity following HIER, the results are not consistent). MIB1, Ki-S5 and polyclonal Ki-67 are all immunoreactive in routinely fixed, paraffin-embedded tissues. Immunoreactivity is enhanced following HIER combined with proteolytic digestion. Best results are obtained with retrieval solutions of low pH and at neutral and high pHs.

Background

The Ki-67 antibody was generated against a Hodgkin's disease cell line and was found to identify a nuclear antigen expressed in all non-G_0 phases of the cell cycle, ie, all proliferating cells. The antigen recognized by Ki-67 is a 345–395 kD non-histone protein complex which is highly susceptible to protease treatment (Gerdes, et al 1991). The gene encoding the Ki-67 protein is localized on chromosome 10 and organized in 15 exons. The center of the gene is formed by an extraordinary 6845 bp exon containing 16 successively repeated homologous segments of 366 bp, the "Ki-67 repeats", each containing a highly conserved new motif of 66 bp, the "Ki-67 motif". The deduced peptide sequence of this central exon is associated with high turnover proteins such as other cell cycle-related proteins, oncogenes and transcription factors. Like the latter, the Ki-67 antigen plays a pivotal role in maintaining cell proliferation because Ki-67 protein antisense oligonucleotides significantly inhibit 3H-thymidine uptake in human tumor cell lines in a dose-dependant manner (Duchrow et al, 1995).

There is a good correlation between the percentage of Ki-67 positive cells in normal tissues and cell kinetic parameters such as ^{3}H-thymidine labeling indices although generally, Ki-67 immunostaining give a higher proliferative index than the S-phase fraction, as defined by flow cytometric analysis or by ^{3}H-thymidine incorporation.

Until recently, the limitation of the Ki-67 antibody was its requirement for frozen tissue. Several antibodies to the Ki-67 antigen are now available which are immunoreactive in routinely fixed sections, namely, MIB1, Ki-S5, polyclonal Ki-67 and Ki-S1 (not commercially available to our knowledge). The proliferation indices obtained with all these five antibodies correlated well with that obtained with monoclonal Ki-67 in frozen sections, indicating that they are suitable substitutes with the advantage of being immunoreactive in fixed paraffin-embedded sections (Leong et al 1995). This was not the case with the antibodies to proliferating cell nuclear antigens PC10 and 19A2, both of which have been demonstrated to be fixation dependant (Leong et al 1993).

Applications

Numerous studies have compared the Ki-67 proliferation indices in frozen sections with other prognostic parameters such as tumor grade, hormone receptor status and p53 expression. In general, Ki-67 indices have been shown to be of prognostic relevance (Brown and Gatter 1990, Raymond and Leong 1988,1989). Similar studies have now been performed in wax-embedded archival tissues with some of the new antibodies, particularly MIB1, confirming their relevance as prognostic markers (Wintzer et al 1991; Sahin et al 1991, Healy et al 1995; Kindblom et al 1995; Nawa et al 1996). Ki-67 counts have also been useful in distinguishing between benign and malignant liver proliferations (Grigioni et al 1995) and to predict progress of granulosa cell tumors (Costa et al 1996), Barrett's dysplasia (Polkowski et al 1995) and ovarian serous tumors (Garzetti et al 1995). More recently, MIB1 has been applied to brain tumors as predictors of survival (Verstegen et al, 2002; Torp & Granli, 2001). Delays in fixation do not appear to affect Ki-67 counts (using a polyclonal antibody) in intracranial malignant tumors (Di Tommaso et al, 1999).

Comments

In many cells the Ki-67 antigen appears to be localized to the nucleoli or peri-nucleolar region, with lighter diffuse nuclear staining in both frozen and fixed sections. When assessing proliferation indices, notable intratumoral heterogeneity will be observed and counts should be taken from the areas of highest proliferation, usually at the periphery of the tumor. MIB1 is the antibody of choice when assessing proliferation indices. PCNA produces a high

background and is fixation sensitive.

References

Brown DC, Gatter KC. Monoclonal antibody Ki-67: Its use in histopathology. Histopathology 1990;17:489–503.

Costa MJ, Walls J, Ames P, Roth LM. Transformation in recurrent ovarian granulosa cell tumors: Ki67 (MIB1) and p53 immunohistochemistry demonstrates a possible molecular basis for the poor histopathologic prediction of clinical behavior. Human Pathology 1996;27:274–81.

Di Tommaso L, Kapucuoglu N, Losi L, et al. Impact of delayed fixation on evaluation of cell proliferation in intracranial malignant tumors. Applied Immunohistochemistry and Molecular Morpholgy 1999;7:209–13.

Duchrow M, Schluter C, Key G, et al. Cell proliferation-associated nuclear antigen defined by antibody Ki-67: a new kind of cell cycle-maintaining proteins. Archives of Immunology, Therapy and Experimentation 1995;43:117–21.

Garzetti GG, Ciavattini A, Goteri G, et al. Ki67 antigen immunostaining (MIB1 monoclonal antibody) in serous ovarian tumors: index of proliferative activity with prognostic significance. Gynecologic Oncology 1995;56:169–74.

Gerdes J, Li L, Schlueter DM. Immunohistochemical and molecular biologic characterization of the cell proliferation-associated nuclear antigen that is defined by monoclonal antibody Ki-67. American Journal of Pathology 1991;138:867–73.

Grigioni WF, Fiorentino M, D'Errico A, et al. Overexpression of c-met proto-oncogene product and raised Ki67 index in hepatocellular carcinomas with

respect to benign liver conditions. Hepatology 1995;21:1543–1546.

Healy E, Angus B, Lawrence CM, Rees JL. Prognostic value of Ki67 antigen expression in basla cell carcinomas. British Journal of Dermatology 1995;133:737–41.

Kindblom LG, Ahlden M, Meis-Kindblom JM, Stenman G. Immunohistochemical and molecular analysis of p53, MDM2, proliferating cell nuclear antigen and Ki67 in benign and malignant peripheral nerve sheath tumours. Virchows Archives 1995;427:19–26.

Leong AS-Y, Milios J, Tang SK. Is immunolocalization of proliferating cell nuclear antigen (PCNA) in paraffin sections a valid index of cell proliferation? Applied Immunohistochemistry 1993;1:127–35.

Leong AS-Y, Vinyuvat S, Suthipintawong C, Milios J. A comparative study of cell proliferation markers in breast carcinomas. Journal of Clinical Pathology: Molecular Pathology 1995;48:M83-M87.

Nawa G, Ueda T, Mori S, et al. Prognostic significance of Ki67 (MIB1) proliferation index and p53 over-expression in chondrosarcomas. International Journal of Cancer 1996;69:86–91.

Polkowski W, van Lanschot JJ, Ten Kate FJ, et al. The value of p53 and Ki67 as markers for tumor progression in the Barrett's dysplasia-carcinoma sequence. Surgical Oncology 1995;4:163–71.

Raymond WA, Leong AS-Y, Bolt JW, et al. Growth fractions in human prostatic carcinoma determined by Ki-67 immunostaining. Journal of Pathology 1988;156:161–7.

Raymond WA, Leong AS-Y. The relationship between growth fractions and oestrogen receptors in human breast carcinoma, as determined by immunohistochemical staining. Journal of Pathology 1989;158:203–11.

Sahin AA, Ro J, Ro JY, et al. Ki-67 immunostaining in node-negative stage I/II breast carcinoma. Significant correlation with prognosis. Cancer 1991;68:549–57.

Torp SH, Granli US. Proliferation activity in human glioblastomas assessed by various techniques. APMIS 2001;109:865–9.

Verstegen MJ, Leenstra DT, Ijlst-Keizers H, Bosch DA. Proliferation and apoptosis-related proteins in intracranial ependydomas: an immunohistochemical analysis. Journal of Neurooncology 2002;56:21–8.

Wintzer HO, Zipfel I, Schulte-Monting J, et al. Ki-67 immunostaining in human breast tumours and its relationship to prognosis. Cancer 1991;67:421–8.

NOTES

Laminin

Sources/clones

Becton Dickinson (4C12.8), Biogenesis (2D8–39, 2D8–30, 2D8–33), Biogenex (LAM1), Dako (polyclonal, 4C7), EY Laboratories (polyclonal), Euro-Diagnostics (polyclonal), Immunotech (4C12), Monosan (polyclonal).

Fixation/preparation

Most available antibodies are immunoreactive in cryostat sections and fixed, embedded tissues but require antigen retrieval in the form of HIER or proteolytic digestion or both.

Background

Laminin, a glycoprotein of about 900 kD, is secreted by fibroblasts, epithelial, myoepithelial, endothelial and smooth muscle cells, and together with type IV collagen, form the two principal components of basal lamina. There are three genetically distinct chains of laminin, α-, β-, and γ-chains, which are held together by disulfide bonds and by a triple-stranded coiled-coil structure. Ultrastructurally, the basal lamina is composed of a lamina lucida of low electron density, adjacent to the parenchymal cells, and a basal lamina densa of high electron density, adjacent to the connective tissue matrix. By rotary shadowing, laminin has a cross-like shape, consisting of three short arms of 200 kD and one long arm of 400 kD. Laminin is exclusively localized to the basal lamina, predominantly to the lamina lucida, and is invariably present in basal lamina surrounding muscle, nerve, fat and decidua cells, and separating epithelial and endothelial cells from adjacent connective tissues. Laminins are potent modulators of numerous biological processes in development, including cell proliferation, migration, and differentiation. In adult tissues, laminins influence the maintenance of specific gene expression and are involved in various pathological situations, including fibrosis, carcinogenesis, and metastasis.

Clone 4D7 reacts with the terminal globular domain of the A-chain of laminin, whereas polyclonal antibodies were generated to laminin isolated from rat yolk sac tumor cell line.

Applications

Laminin has been shown to play a role in cell adhesion and attachment to the basal lamina, both *in vivo* and *in vitro*. The basal lamina is generally extremely stable, but in certain pathological states, may undergo local dissolution. This process is likely to play a crucial role in the invasiveness and progression of malignant tumors (Liotta 1984). Loss or defective organization of the basal lamina matrix in malignant neoplasms may be the result of increased breakdown by tumor-derived degradative enzymes, decreased synthesis, or decreased or abnormal assembly of the secreted basal lamina components (Pujuguet et al, 1994). In human breast carcinoma, there is suggestion that overexpression of the nm23-H1 gene, a putative metastasis supressor gene, leads to the formation of basal lamina and growth arrest (Howlett et al, 1994). Antisera to type IV collagen and laminin, the major components of basal lamina allow the study of the organization of the basal lamina in various benign and malignant tumors (Autio-Harmainen et al, 1988; Havenith et al, 1989, Nair et al 1997; Kuwano et al, 1997). Laminin immunostaining with the immunogold-silver technique in resin embedded sections allows exquisite demonstration of the basal lamina in a variety of tissues (Leong 1993). The majority of invasive carcinomas are recognized to synthesize varying amounts of basal lamina material, but the basal lamina surrounding the tumor nests are generally fragmented, and in many cases, completely absent. Benign and *in situ* lesions appear to be circumscribed by intact basal lamina.

Diagnostic applications of collagen type IV immunostaining have mostly centered on the demonstration of basal lamina in invasive tumors, particularly epithelial tumors, and their changes with tumor invasion and metastasis. In particular, the demonstration of an intact basal lamina has been used to distinguish benign glandular proliferations such as microglandular adenosis and sclerosing adenosis from well-differentiated carcinoma like tubular carcinoma of the breast (Raymond & Leong, 1991; Tavassoli & Bratthauer, 1993). Distinctive patterns of basal distribution were recently demonstrated in various types of soft tissue tumors, adding to the diagnostic armamentarium for this group of neoplasms, which are often difficult to separate histologically and with existing immunological markers (Leong et al, 1997). While the presence of basal lamina cannot be used as an absolute discriminant for blood vessels and lymphatic spaces, the latter do not display the reduplication of the basal lamina characteristic of blood vessels and generally show thin and discontinuous staining of basal lamina (Suthipintawong et al, 1995). The distinctive staining observed around blood vessels has been employed as a marker when performing capillary density measurements (Madsen & Holmskov, 1995). Laminin immunostaining together with collagen type IV was employed to demonstrate frequent breaches in the basal lamina of the mucosa of patients with celiac disease, suggesting that interaction between gliadin and components of the extracellular matrix may have a role in the genesis of mucosal epithelial damage (Verbeke et al, 2002).

A recent study suggests that the presence of basal lamina as demonstrated with laminin immunostaining may be a clue to the identification of hepatocellular carcinoma as non-malignant hepatocytes lack basal lamina (Yoshida et al, 1996).

Comments

The use of proteolytic digestion following HIER further enhances immunoreactivity. With the polyclonal antibodies we employ Protease at 0.25 mg/ml for 2 minutes (Leong et al 1996).

References

Autio-Harmainen H, Karttunen T, Apaja-Sarkkinen M, et al. Laminin and tyope IV collagen in different histological stages of Kaposi's sarcoma and other vascular lesions of blood vessels or lymphatic vessel origin. American Journal of Surgical Pathology 1988;12:469–76.

Havenith MG, Van Zandvoort EHM, Cleutjens JPM, Bosman FT. Basement membrane deposition in benign and malignant naevomelanocytic lesions: An immunohistochemical study with antibodies to type IV collagen and laminin. Histopathology 1989;15:137–46.

Howlett AR, Petersen OW, Steeg PS, Bissell MJ. A novel function for the nm23-H1 gene: overexpression in human breast carcinoma leads to the formation of basement membrane and growth arrest. Journal of the National Cancer Institutes 1994;86:1838–44.

Kuwano H, Sonoda K, Yasuda M, et al. Tumor invasion and angiogenesis in early esophageal squamous cell carcinoma. Journal of Surgical Oncology 1997;65:188–93.

Leong AS-Y. Immunohistochemistry – theoretical and practical aspects. In: Leong AS-Y (editor) Applied immunohistochemistry for the surgical pathologist. London: Edward Arnold, 1993, pp 1–22.

Leong AS-Y, Milios J, Leong FJ. Epitope retrieval with microwaves. A comparison of citrate buffer and EDTA with three commercial retrieval solutions. Applied Immunohistochemistry 1996;4:201–7.

Leong AS-Y, Vinyuvat S, Suthipintawong C, Leong FJ. Patterns of basal lamina immunostaining in soft-tissue and bony tumors. Applied Immunohistochemistry 1997;5:1–7.

Liotta LA. Tumor invasion and metastases: Role of the basement membrane. Warner-Lambert Parke-Davis Award Lecture. American Journal of Pathology 1984;117:339–48.

Madsen K, Holmskov U. Capillary density measurements in skeletal muscle using immunohistochemical staining with anti-collagen type IV antibodies. European Journal of Applied Physiology 1995;71:472–4.

Nair SA, Nair MB, Jayaprakash PG, et al. The basement membrane and tumor progression in the uterine cervix. General Diagnostic Pathology 1997;142:297–303.

Pujuguet P, Hammann A, Martin F, Martin M. abnormal basement membrane in tumors induced by rat colon cancer cells. Gastroenterology 1994;107:701–11.

Raymond WA, Leong AS-Y. Assessment of invasion in breast lesions using antibodies to basement membrane components and myoepithelial cells. Pathology 1991;23:291–7.

Suthipintawong C, Leong, AS-Y, Vinyuvat S. A comparative study of immunomarkers for lymphangiomas and hemangiomas. Applied Immunohistochemistry 1995;3:239–44.

Tavassoli FA, Bratthauer GL. Immunohistochemical profile and differential diagnosis of microglandular adenosis. Modern Pathology 1993;6:318–22.

Verbeke S, Gotteland M, Fernandez M, et al. Basement membrane and connective tissue proteins in intestinal mucosa of patients with celiac disease. Journal of clinical Pathology 2002;55:440–5.

NOTES

Lysozyme (muramidase)

Sources/clones

Axcel/Accurate (polyclonal), Biodesign (polyclonal), Biogenesis (6C6/8, polyclonal), Biogenex (polyclonal), Biomedia (polyclonal), Calbiochemical (polyclonal), Chemicon (polyclonal), Dako (polyclonal), Diagnostic Biosystems (polyclonal), Fitzgerald (polyclonal), Milab (polyclonal), Zymed (polyclonal).

Fixation/preparation

Lysozyme (muramidase) is resistant to fixation and immunoreactivity is enhanced following proteolytic digestion and HIER. The antibodies are immunoreactive in frozen sections and cytological preparations.

Background

Lysozyme (muramidase) is a 14.5 kD strongly basic protein which is a mucolytic enzyme found in saliva, gastrointestinal secretions, tears, urine, and serum. Lysozyme has been localized in granulocytes, histiocytes and some epithelial cells. The protein has been localized ultrastructurally in the secretory granules of Paneth cells and the brush border of granular mucus cells of the small intestine. It has also been localized to the granules of alveolar type II pneumocytes as well as the lysosomal granules of multi-nucleated histiocytes. In the lymph node, lysozyme is found in the tingible body macrophages of the germinal centers and in macrophages scattered in the paracortex. Dendritic reticulum cells, interdigitating reticulum cells, lymphocytes and plasma cells generally lack lysozyme. Langerhans cells and sinus macrophages may show stainable lysozyme.

Applications

Lysozyme has been employed as a marker of histiocytes/macrophages and of myeloid differentiation. It is a useful marker in both paraffin-embedded trephine biopsies and bone marrow clot preparations allowing distinction of acute myeloid leukemia from acute lymphoblastic leukemia (Davey et al, 1990; Horny et al, 1994;); as well as in the identification of extramedullary myeloid cell tumors (Trawcek et al, 1993). The combination of myeloperoxidase and lysozyme was found to be reliable marker of myeloid lineage (Quintanilla-Martinez et al, 1995).

Lysozyme has been described in Langerhans histiocytosis (Thompson et al, 1996), follicular dendritic cell tumors (Masunaga et al, 1997), granular cell tumors, malignant fibrous histiocytoma, and various alleged histiocytic tumors.

Lysozyme combined with GCDFP15 had great specificity for apocrine differentiation in adnexal tumors of the skin; whereas eccrine tumors stained only for GCDFP15 (Ansai et al, 1995; Meybehm & Fischer, 1997) (Appendix 1.19).

Comments

While a useful marker of lysosomal inclusions in a variety of cell types including histiocytes/monocytes, this marker is not specific and must be employed in the context of a panel which includes other histiocytic markers such as CD68, alpha-1-antitrypsin, alpha-1-antichymotrypsin.

References

Ansai S, Koseki S, Hozumi Y, Kondo S. An immunohistochemical study of lysozyme, CD15,(LeuM1), and gross cystic disease fluid protein-15 in various skin tumors. Assessment of the specificity and sensitivity of markers of apocrine differentiation. American Journal of Dermatopathology 1995;17:249–55.

Davey FR, Elghetany MT, Kurec AS. Immunophenotyping of hematologic neoplasms in paraffin-embedded tissue sections. American Journal of Clinical Pathology 1990;93: S17–S26.

Horny HP, Wehrmann M, Steinke B, Kaiserling E. Assessment of the value of immunohistochemistry in the subtyping of acute leukemia on routinely processed bone marrow biopsy specimens with particular reference to macrophage-associated antibodies. Human Pathology 1994;25:810–4.

Masunaga A, Nakamura H, Katata T, et al. Follicular dendritic cell tumor with histiocytic characteristics and fibroblastic antigen. Pathology International 1997;47:707–12.

Meyhehm M, Fischer HP. Spiradenoma and dermal cylindroma: comparative immunohistochemical analysis and histogenetic considerations. American Journal of Dermatopathology 1997;19:154–61.

Quintanilla-Martinez L, Zukerberg LR, Ferry JA, Harris NL. Extramedullary tumors of lymphoid or myeloid blasts. The role of immunohistology in diagnosis and classification. American Journal of Clinical Pathology 1995;104:431–43.

Thompson LD, Wenig BM, Adair CF, et al. Langhans cell histiocytosis of the thyroid: a series of seven cases and a review of the literature. Modern Pathology 1996;9:145–9.

Traweek ST, Arber DA, Rapapport H, Brynes RK. Extramedullary myeloid cell tumors. An immunohistochemical and morphologic study of 28 cases. American Journal of surgical Pathology 1993;17:1011–19.

MAC 387 (Macrophage marker)

Sources/clones

Dako (MAC 387)

Fixation/preparation

Applicable to formalin-fixed paraffin sections, acetone-fixed cryostat sections or fixed cell smears. Requires enzymatic pretreatment for optimum immunostaining and immunoreactivity is not enhanced by HIER.

Background

MAC 387 (IgG1, Kappa) was raised against purified peripheral blood monocytes (Flavell et al, 1987). The antibody recognizes the leukocyte antigen L1 or calprotectin (Steinbakk et al, 1990). The L1 antigen consists of three non-covalently bound polypeptide chains with a total molecular mass of 365 kD. L1 was discovered more than 15 year ago as a major cytosol protein fraction (50–60%) of neutrophilic granulocytes (Fagerhol et al, 1990). This antigen is expressed in neutrophil granulocytes, monocytes, certain reactive tissue macrophages, squamous epithelia and reactive epidermis (Brandtzaeg et al, 1988). This antigen is also reputed to be

expressed in *early* inflammation and is present only in cells of the mononuclear-phagocyte system and *not* dendritic system. In vitro experiments have shown the purified composite molecule to exhibit striking antimicrobial properties (Steinbakk et al, 1990).

Applications

MAC 387 antibody produces a cytoplasmic labeling pattern in many myelomonocytic cells. Apart from identifying reactive macrophages, MAC 387 also highlights macrophages in several histiocytoses including hemophagocytic syndrome, Rosai-Dorfman disease and Langerhans' cell histiocytoses (Malone, 1991; Brandtzaeg et al, 1992). True histiocytic lymphomas should be MAC 387 positive, whilst a small number of large cell anaplastic lymphomas may show immunopositivity (Norton & Isaacson, 1989). Squamous cell carcinomas of the skin, bronchus, bladder and oral cavity may show immunoreactivity (Brandtzaeg et al, 1992), helping us to distinguish from other types of carcinoma. MA387 was employed to characterize mammary foam cells. Together with in situ hybridization and other

immunomarkers including epithelial membrane antigen, cytokeratin (CK) and gross cystic disease fluid protein 15 (GCDFP-15), it was shown that mammary foam cells were of three types: epithelial cells with apocrine differentiation that were EMA+CK+GCDFP-15+, macrophage-like cells that were MAC387+CK-GCDFP-15- and a group with intermediate profile between an epithelial cell and macrophage (Damiani et al, 1998).

Comments

MAC 387 is a good broad-spectrum macrophage marker but is less specific for cells of the mononuclear-phagocyte system than other markers like CD68 and HAM56. Tissues rich in macrophages are suitable as a positive controls.

References

Brandtzaeg P, Jones DB, Flavell DJ, Fagerhold MK. Mac 387 antibody and detection of formalin resistant myelomonocytic L1 antigen. Journal of Clinical Pathology 1988;41:963–70.

Brandtzaeg P, Dale I, Gabrielsen T-Ø. The leucocyte protein L1 (calprotectin): usefulness as an immunohistochemical marker antigen and putative biological function. Histopathology 1992;21:191–6.

Damiani S, Cattani MG, Buonamici L, Eusebi V. Mammary foam cells. Characteristion by immunohistohemistry and in situ hybridization. Virchows Archives 1998;432:433–40.

Fagerhol MK, Andersson KB, Naess-Andresen C-F, Brandtzaeg P, Dale I. Calprotectin (The L1 leukocyte protein). In: Smith NL, Dedman TR (eds). Stimulus Response Coupling: The Role of Intracellular Calcium-Binding Proteins. Boca Raton, Florida. CRC Press. 1990:187–210.

Flavell DJ, Jones DB, Wright DH. Identification of tissue histiocytes on paraffin sections by a new monoclonal antibody. Journal of Histochemistry and Cytochemistry 1987;35:1217–26.

Malone M. The histiocytoses of childhood. Histopathology 1991;19:105–19.

Norton AJ & Isaacson PG. Lymphoma phenotyping in formalin-fixed and paraffin wax-embedded tissues: II. Profiles of reactivity in the various tumour types. Histopathology 1989;14:557–69.

Steinbakk M, Naess-Andresen CF, Linghaas E et al. Antimicrobial actions of calcium binding leucocyte L1 protein, calprotectin. Lancet 1990;336:763–5.

MART-1/Melan-A

Sources/clones

Dako (clone A103), Biogenex (clone A103), Novocastra (clone A103)

Fixation/preparation

The antibodies are suitable for immunohistochemical analysis of fresh frozen and formalin-fixed paraffin-embedded tissue. For best results on archival material, antigen heat-induced retrieval methods are essential.

Background

The Melan-A gene was cloned from the human melanoma cell line SK-Mel29 (Coulie et al, 1994). Independently, the same gene was found by another group using a different cell line and named MART-1 (melanoma antigen recognized by T-cells) (Kawakami et al, 1994). Both clones are recognized by most HLA-A$_2$-restricted tumor-specific tumor infiltrating lymphocytes harvested from patients with melanoma. MART-1 (clone M2–7C10) and Melan-A (clone A103) are two different antibody clones generated by separate groups but recognize the same antigen. The Melan-A/MART-1 protein comprises 118 amino acids with a molecular weight of 20–22kD (Chen et al, 1996). Although not fully characterized regarding subcellular localization, it is nevertheless thought to be associated with melanosomes and endoplasmic reticulum.

In normal tissue mRNA expression is limited to melanocytes in the skin and retina (Coulie et al, 1994). Immunopositivity for Melan-A/MART-1 has been demonstrated in both primary and metastatic malignant melanoma (Jungbluth et al, 1998; Fetsch et al, 1999) with a range of positivity in 81–90% of tumors. These positive rates are slightly better than HMB-45 (75–80%). Unlike HMB-45, Melan-A/MART-1 are purported to yield a homogeneous cytoplasmic staining pattern in both melanomas and melanocytic nevi, with a stronger intensity and greater percentage of tumor cell immunopositivity. In contrast, HMB-45 stains mainly the intraepidermal and superficial dermal component of compound nevi. Melan-A/MART-1 has a limited role in the differential diagnosis of desmoplastic melanoma (Busam & Jungbluth, 1999). In a study of 22 cases of HMB45- melanomas including 8 desmoplastic melanomas, Melan A was positive in 9, but not in any cases of desmoplastic melanoma (Xu et al, 2002). The epithelioid melanomas (primary and metastatic) show a better frequency of expression with these antibodies than in spindle cell and desmoplastic melanomas (Blessing et al, 1998).

Strong, diffuse granular staining of Melan-A has been demonstrated in adrenocortical adenomas and carcinomas (primary and metastatic) and Leydig/Sertoli-Leydig cell tumors of the ovary and testes (Busam et al, 1998). Clone A103 was shown to stain 21 adrenal cortical tumors but none of 16 metastatic carcinomas in the adrenal, 10 pheochromocytomas and only one of 269 extra-adrenal carcinomas (Loy et al, 2002). Although regarded as being not specific, the recognition of steroid hormone-producing tumors was a consistent finding with Melan-A, but not with MART-1 (Fetsch et al, 1999). This may reflect differences in the antigenic epitopes or purity of the two clones (Fetsch et al, 1999). Alternatively, cross-reactivity with a similar epitope of a different gene may explain the positive staining of steroid tumors with Melan-A (Busam & Jungbluth,

1999). However, immunopositivity with both antibodies has been demonstrated in tumors of perivascular epithelioid cells (PEComas, e.g., angiomyolipoma, lymphangioleiomyomatosis and "sugar" tumors of the lung) capable for both myoid and melanocytic differentiation (Busam & Jungbluth, 1999).

Applications

The antibodies are useful for the detection of primary and metastatic melanomas, especially with an epithelioid morphology; but with a limited value in spindle and desmoplastic melanomas. It should be noted that MART-1 has been better studied on cytologic material, whilst Melan-A has been more extensively studied on archival material.

In assessing metastatic tumors of unknown primary/origin, Melan-A is useful to distinguish adrenocortical carcinoma from renal cell and hepatocellular carcinomas. In such instances, other melanoma markers would be essential to rule out metastatic melanomas, reinforcing the importance of a panel of antibodies for immunohistological investigation. Melan A is also a useful marker to identify adrenal cortical tumors from other tumors in the adrenals and retroperitoneum

(Appendix 1.18). Both antibodies have demonstrated usefulness in the confirmation of PEComas.

References

Blessing K, Sanders DSA, Grant JJH: Comparison of immunohistochemical staining of the novel antibody melan-A with S100 protein and HMB-45 in malignant melanoma and melanoma variants. Histopathology 1998;32:139–46.

Busam K, Iversen K, Coplan K, et al. Immunoreactivity for A103, and antibody to Melan-A (Mart-1), in adrenocortical and other steroid tumors. American Journal of Surgical Pathology 1998;22:57–63.

Busam KJ, Jungbluth AA. Melan-A, a new melanocytic differentiation marker. Advances in Anatomical Pathology 1999;6:182–7.

Chen YT, Stockert E, Jungbluth A, et al. Serologic analysis of Melan-A (MART-1), a melanocytic-specific protein homogeneously expressed in human melanomas. Proceedings of the National Academy of Sciences 1996;93:5915–9.

Coulie PG, Brichard V, van Pel A, et al. A new gene coding for a differentiation antigen recognized by autologous cytologic T lymphocytes on HLA-A2 melanomas. Journal of Experimental Medicine 1994;180:35–42.

Cramer SF: The new melanoma markers: MART-1 and Melan-A (The NIH Experience). American Journal of Surgical Pathology 1999;23:607–13.

Fetch PA, Marincola FM, Filie A, et al. Melanoma-associated antigen recognized by T cells (MART-1): the advent of a preferred immunocytochemical antibody for the diagnosis of metastatic malignant melanoma with fine-needle aspiration. Cancer 1999;87:37–42.

Jungbluth AA, Busam KJ, Gerald WL, et al. A103, an anti-Melan-A monoclonal antibody for the detection of malignant melanoma in paraffin-embedded tissues. American Journal of surgical Pathology 1998;22:595–602.

Kawakami Y, Eliyahu S, Delgado CH, et al. Cloning of the gene coding for a shared human melanoma antigen recognized by autologous T-cells infiltrating into tumor. Proceedings of the National Academy of Sciences USA 1994;91:3515–9.

Loy TS, Phillips RW, Linder CL. A103 immunostaining in the diagnosis of adrenal cortical tumors: an immunohistochemical study of 316 cases. Archives of Pathology and Laboratory Medicine 2002;126:170–2.

Shin SJ, Hoda ES, Ying L, DeLellis RA. Diagnostic utility of the monoclonal antibody A103 in fine-needle aspiration biopsies of the adrenal. American Journal of Clinical Pathology 2000;113:295–302.

Xu X, Chu AY, Pasha TL, et al. Immunoprofile of MiTF, tyrosinase, Melan A and MAGE-1 in HMB45-negative melanomas. Applied Immunohistochemistry and Molecular Morphology 2002;26:82–7.

Maspin

Sources/clones

BDPharM (15781A monoclonal)

Fixation/preparation

The antibody reacts with human maspin and is applicable to both frozen and formalin-fixed tissues. HIER is necessary to enhance immunoreactivity; otherwise a highly sensitive detection system such as EnVision is required.

Background

Maspin is a unique member of the serpin family, which inhibits tumor invasion and metastasis of human breast and prostate cancers. This inhibitory protease harbours tumor suppressor, tumor invasiveness-supression and anti-angiogenic properties. Maspin has also been shown to inhibit cell motility and appears to be down regulated during cancer progression from benign to invasive and metastatic states (Maas et al, 2001). It is consistently expressed by mammary myoepithelial cells as well as many other human epithelial cells and is a cytoplasmic protein that associates with secretory vesicles and is present on the cell surface (Pemberton et al, 1997).

Applications

To date most of the work done with maspin has been in the human breast myoepithelial cells. Maspin has been employed as a marker of myoepithelial cells comparing well with other markers of these cells including alpha-smooth muscle actin and S100 but producing no staining of stomal, neural or vascular elements (Reis-Filho et al, 2001). It has been employed to distinguish radial scar from tubular carcinoma of the breast (Lele et al, 2000). Maspin has also been demonstrated in mammary epithelial cells, the strongest immunoexpression being found in normal breast and fibrocystic change with a significant stepwise decrease in maspin staining occurring with the ductal carcinoma-in-situ – invasive cancer – lymph node metastasis sequence. A subset of infiltrating carcinomas showed strong maspin immunostaining and was significantly associated with lower rate of nodal metastasis, independent of tumor size and grade (Maass et al, 2001).

Maspin immunostaining has been applied to distinguish pancreatic neoplasms with the demonstration of this protein in ductal adenocarcinomas, intraductal papillary mucinous tumors, mucinous cystic tumors but not in acinar cell carcinomas, pancreatic endocrine tumors, solid-pseudopapillary tumors and serous cystadenomas (Oh et al, 2002). It has been suggested that decreased immunoexpression of maspin may be a significant factor associated with the metastatic potential of stage I and stage II oral squamous cell carcinomas (Yasumatsu et al, 2001) and may be of prognostic relevance also in prostatic carcinoma (Machtens et al, 2001).

Comments

Antigen retrieval is necessary for immunoreactivity of this antibody in fixed sections. Myoepithelial cells show both nuclear and cytoplasmic staining; the protein is localised to the cytoplasm in epithelial cells.

References

Lele SM, Graves K, Gatalica Z. Immunohistochemical detection of maspin is a useful adjunct in distinguishing radial sclerosing lesion from tubular carcinoma of the breast. Applied Immunohistochemistry and Molecular Morphology 2000;8:32–6.

Maass N, Teffner M, Rosel F, et al. Decline in the expression of the serine proteinase inhibitor maspin is associated with tumor progression in ductal carcinomas of the breast. Journal of Pathology 2001;195:321–6.

Machtens S, Serth J, Bokemeyer C, et al. Expression of the p53 and maspin protein in primary prostatic carcinoma: correlation with clinical features. International Journal of Cancer 2001;95:337–42.

Oh YL, Song SY, Ahn G. Expression of maspin in pancreatic neoplasms: application of maspin immunohistochemistry to the differential diagnosis. Applied Immunohistochemistry and Molecular Morphology 2002;10:62–6.

Pemberton PA, Tipton AR, Pavloff N, et al. Maspin is an intracellular serpin that partitions into secretor vesicles And is present at the cell surface. Journal of Histochemistry and Cytochemistry 1997;45:1697–706.

Reis-Fiho JS, Milanezi F, silva P, Schmitt FC. Maspin expression in myoepithelial tumors of the breast. Pathology Research and Practice 2001;197:817–21.

Yasumatsu R, Nakashima T, Hirakawa N, et al. Maspin expression in stage I and stage II oral tongue squamous cell carcinoma. Head and neck 2001;23:962–6.

MDM-2 protein

Sources/clones

Accurate (19E3), Dako (SMP14), Novocastra (1B10, polyclonal), Oncogene (1F2).

Fixation/preparation

Several of the antibodies are immunoreactive in fixed paraffin-embedded tissue sections besides fresh tissue and cell preparations.

Background

The MDM-2 protein encodes for a nuclear phosphoprotein that binds p53 and inhibits its ability to activate transcription by concealing the p53 activation domain. It has been suggested that MDM-2 overexpression might represent an alternative mechanism by which p53-mediated pathways are inactivated in human tumors, thus having a possible role in oncogenesis. MDM-2 overexpression as a result of gene amplification and/or increased mRNA expression can be detected by immunohistochemical analysis.

Applications

The ability to stain for MDM-2 protein in fixed tissue sections has stimulated a great deal of interest in its expression in various neoplasms. The correlation of MDM-2 protein levels with p53 may provide insights into oncogenesis and has the potential of providing prognostic information. Several studies have included the detection of p21/waf1 protein together with MDM-2 as both these oncoproteins are downstream effectors of p53, p21 playing a major role in negatively regulating cell cycle progression, while MDM-2 inhibits the effects of p53.

Current results of immunohistochemical analyses of MDM-2 and p53 protein are far from conclusive, although many support an inverse correlation between the two oncoproteins. Such studies have included uterine sarcoma (Seki et al, 1997), breast carcinoma (Jiang et al, 1997), thymoma (Stefanki et al, 1997), osteogenic sarcoma (Lonardo et al, 1997), glioblastoma (Biernat et al, 1997), lung carcinoma (Higashiyama et al, 1997), oral carcinoma (Matsumura et al, 1996), malignant melanoma (Gelsleichter et al, 1995), thyroid carcinoma (Jennings et al, 1995) and rhabdomyosarcoma (Keletti et al, 1966).

More recent studies that support the role of MDM-2 protein in tumorigenesis include tumors such as oral squamous cell carcinoma (Shwe et al, 2001), malignant fibrous histiocytoma of the jejunum (Jiao et al, 2002), non-small cell carcinoma of the lung (Eymin et al, 2002), adult medulloblastoma (Giordana et al, 2002), carcinoma of the breast (Hori et al, 2002), oral ameloblastoma (Sandra et al, 2002) and carcinoma of the urinary bladder (Uchida et al, 2002). Interestingly, MDM-2 protein was confined to follicular adenomas of the thyroid compared to p53 protein that was not immunoexpressed in such tumors (Czyz et al, 2001).

Comments

Immunostaining for MDM-2 has also been successfully conducted on cytological preparations (Dowell et al, 1996).

References

Biernat W, Kleihaues P, Yonekawa Y, Ohgaki H. Amplification and overexpression of MDM2 in primary (de novo) glioblastomas. Journal of Neuropathology and Experimental Neurology 1997;56:180–5.

Czyz W, Kuzdak K, Pasieka Z, et al. p53, MDM2, bcl-2 staining in follicular neoplasms of the thyroid gland. Folia Histochemistry and

Cytobiology 2001;39 (Suppl 2):167–8.

Dowell SP, McGoogan E, Picksley SM, et al. Expression of p21waf1/Cip1, MDM2 and p53 in vivo: analysis of cytological preparations. Cytopathology 1996;7:340–51.

Eymin B, Gasseri S, Brambilla C, Brambilla E. MDM2 overexpression and p14 (ARF) inactivation are two mutually exclusive events in primary lung tumors. Oncogene 2002;21:2750–61.

Gelsleichter L, Gown AM, Zarbo RJ, et al. P53 and mdm-2 expression in malignant melanoma: an immunocytochemical study of expression of p53, mdm-2, and markers of cell proliferation in primary versus metastatic tumors. Modern Pathology 1995;8:530–5.

Giordana MT, Duo D, Gasverde S, et al. MDM2 overexpression is associated with short survival in adults with medulloblastoma. Neruo0oncology 2002;4:115–22.

Higashiyama M, Doi O, Kodama K, et al. MDM2 gene amplification and expression in non-small cell lung cancer: immunohistochemical expression of its protein is a favourable prognostic marker in patients without p53 protein accumulation. British Journal of Cancer 1997;75:1302–8.

Hori M, Shimasaki J, Inagawa S, et al. Overexpression of MDM2 oncoprotein correlates with possession of estrogen receptor alpha and lack of MDM2 mRNA splice variants in human breast cancer. Breast Cancer Research and Treatment 2002;71:77–83.

Jiao YF, Nakamura S, Sugai T, et al. p53 gene mutation and MDM2 overexpression in a case of primary malignant fibrous histiocytoma of the jejunum. APMIS 2002;110:165–71.

Jennings T, Bratslavsky G, Gerasimov G, et al. Nuclear accumulation of MDM2 protein in well-differentiated papillary thyroid carcinoma. Experimental and Molecular Pathology 1995;62:199–206.

Jiang M, Shao ZM, Wu J, et al. P21/waf1/cip1 and mdm-2 expression in breast carcinoma patients as related to prognosis. International Journal of Cancer 1997;74:529–34.

Keletti J, Quezado MM, Abaza MM, et al. The MDM2 oncoprotein is overexpressed in rhabdomyosarcoma cell lines and stabilizes wild-type p53 protein. American Journal of Pathology 1996;149:143–51.

Lonardo F, Ueda T, Huvos AG, et al. P53 and MDM2 alterations in osteosarcomas: correlation with clinicpathologic features and proliferative rate. Cancer 1997;79:1541–7.

Matsumura T, Yoshihama Y, Kimura T, et al. P53 and MDM2 expression in oral squamous cell carcinoma. Oncology 1996;53:308–12.

Sandra F, Nakamura N, Kanematsu T, et al. The role of MDM2 in the proliferative activity of amelobalstoma. Oral Oncology 2002;38:153–7.

Seki A, Kodaman J, Miyagi Y, et al. Amplification of the mdm-2 gene and p53 abnormalities in uterine sarcomas. International Journal of Cancer 1997;73:33–7.

Shwe M, Chiguchi G, Yamada S, et al. p53 and MDM2 co-expression in tobacco and betel nut chewing associated oral squamous cell carcinomas. Journal of Medical and Dental Science 2001;48:113–9.

Stefanaki K, Rontogianni D, Kouvidou CH, et al. Expression of p53, mdm2, p21/waf1 and bcl-2 proteins in thymomas. Histopathology 1997;30:549–55.

Uchida T, Minei S, Gao JP, et al. Clinical significance of p53, MDM2 and bbcl-2 expression in transitional cell carcinoma of the bladder. Oncology Reports 2002;9:253–9.

Measles

Sources/clones

Biogenex (1.3, polyclonal), Chemicon (polyclonal), Seralab.

Fixation/preparation

This antibody is applicable to formalin-fixed paraffin-wax embedded tissue. The number of positive cells are increased significantly with microwave pretreatment (McQuaid et al, 1995).

Background

Measles, an acute febrile eruption, has been one of the most common diseases of civilization. Despite the development of an effective vaccine, it remains a worldwide health problem.

The measles virion is composed of a central core of ribonucleic acid with a helically arranged protein coat surrounded by a lipoprotein envelope with spike-like structures. The virion is 120–200 nm in diameter and is classified as a morbillivirus in the paramyxovirus family.

Applications

Subacute sclerosing panencephalitis (SSPE) is a rare, fatal disease of children caused by a persistent measles virus infection of the central nervous system. Immunodetection of viral proteins using antibodies raised to measles is useful to confirm the diagnosis of SSPE in brain biopsies and post-mortem CNS tissue (McQuaid et al, 1995).

Using microwave antigen retrieval systems, increased immunoreactivity was seen in neuronal processes, suggesting that this may represent virus spreading from cell to cell (McQuaid et al, 1995). Attempts to demonstrate the M-protein in the brain of an SSPE patient using immunohistochemistry proved futile, even though nucleotide sequences coding for M protein were detected (Brown et al, 1987). This suggested either diminished synthesis and/or rapid degradation of M.protein in the SSPE brain.

Persistence of infection and ability to induce chronic inflammation have been used to argue for a role for measles in the etiology of Crohn's disease. Immunostaining using both measles virus-specific monoclonal and polyclonal antibodies was positive within endothelial cells in areas of granulomatous vasculitis. In situ hybridization for measles virus genomic RNA also produced positive signals in a similar location; but also showed strongly positive cells in the secondary lymphoid follicles (Wakefield et al, 1993). By employing an immunogold method, ultrastructural studies have shown significantly higher levels of anti-measles antigen in Crohn's disease compared to ulcerative colitis, tuberculous lymphadenitis and non-granulomatous areas of bowels with Crohn's disease but no significant difference between Crohn's disease and SSPE (Daszak et al, 1997). An epidemiological association between Crohn's disease and measles virus exposure in early life has been suggested in case-control studies (Ekbom et al, 1996). It is therefore suggested that Crohn's disease may be a chronic granulomatous vasculitis in reaction to a persistent infection with measles virus within the vascular endothelium (Wakefield et al, 1995). Recent RT-PCR studies have suggested a link between measles virus and a new variant inflammatory bowel disease (ileocolonic lymphonodular hyperplasia) in children (Uhlmann et al, 2002).

Comments

Application of antibodies to measles virus would be useful in developing countries where SSPE is more frequently seen. Both polyclonal and monoclonal antibodies give good immunoreactivity following microwave pretreatment (Rahman et al, 1996; Allen et al, 1996)

References

Allen IV, McQuaid S, McMahon J, et al. The significance of measles virus antigen and genome distribution in the CNS in SSPE for mechanisms of viral spread and demyelination. Journal of Neuropathology and Experimental Neurology 1996;55:471–80.

Brown HR, Goller NL, Thormar H, et al. Measles virus matrix protein gene expression in a subacute sclerosing panencephalitis patient brain and virus isolate demonstrated by cDNA hybridization and immunocytochemistry. Acta Neuropathology (Berl) 1987;75:123–30.

Daszak P, Purcell M, Lewin J, et al. Detecction and comparative analysis of persistent measles virus infection in Crohn's disease by immunogold electron microscopy. Journal of clinical Pathology 1997;50:299–304.

Ekbom A, Daszak P, Kraaz W, Wakefield AJ. Crohn's disease after in-utero measles virus exposure. Lancet 1996;348:515–7.

McQuaid S, McConnell R, McMahon J, Herron B. Microwave antigen retrieval for immunocytochemistry on formalin-fixed, paraffin-embedded post-mortem CNS tissue. Journal of Pathology 1995;176:207–16.

Rahman SM, Eto H, Morshed SA, Itakura H. Giant cell pneumonia: light microscopy, immunohistochemical, and ultrastructural study of an autopsy case. Ultrastructural Pathology 1996;20:585–91.

Uhlmann V, Martin CM, Sheils O, et al. Potential viral pathogenic mechanism for new variant inflammatory bowel disease. Modern Pathology 2002;55:84–90.

Wakefield AJ, Pittilio RM, Sim R, et al. Evidence of persistent measles virus infection in Crohn's disease. Journal of Medical Virology 1993;39:345–53.

Wakefield AJ, Ekbom A, Dhillon AP, et al. Crohn's disease: pathogenesis and persistent measles virus infection. Gastroenterology 1995;108:911–6.

Mel-CAM (CD146)

Source/clone

Alexis (polyclonal COM7A4);
Biocytex (monoclonal F435H7).

Fixation/preparation

This antibody is applicable to
formalin-fixed paraffin-embedded
tissue. Antigen retrieval with
citrate buffer is recommended
(Shih and Kurman, 1998).

Background

Melanoma cell adhesion
molecule (Mel-CAM) is a cell
adhesion molecule that belongs
to the immunoglobulin
supergene family. Mel-CAM was
originally designated MUC18
and was discovered by differential
screening of a cDNA library
from a human melanoma cell
line (Lehmann et al, 1989; Sers et
al, 1993). Mel-CAM is a 113-kd
single chain molecule containing
five immunoglobulin-like
domains, a transmembrane
stretch, and a short cytoplasmic
tail with several potential
phosphorylation sites. It
functions by binding to an
unidentified counter-receptor on
the surface of adjacent cells (Shih
et al, 1994). In addition to its
action as a cell-cell adhesion
molecule, the extracellular

domain of Mel-CAM contains a
potential proteoglycan-binding
motif that may facilitate cell-
extracellular matrix adhesion
(Albelda et al, 1991).

Mel-CAM expression has
been detected in a variety of
tissues, including hair follicles,
cerebellar cortex, endothelium,
and smooth muscle (Lehmann et
al, 1987; Shih et al, 1994; Kuzu et
al, 1993). Mel-CAM is expressed
in more than 90% of cutaneous
melanomas (Shih et al, 1994) and
has also been detected in
angiosarcomas and
leiomyosarcomas (Shih et al,
1996). Other neoplasms,
including hematopoietic tumors,
glial tumors, and a variety of
carcinomas and sarcomas, have
failed to demonstrate Mel-CAM
immunoreactivity (Shih et al,
1994; Lehmann et al, 1987).

Mel-CAM has also been
reported to be a specific cell
surface marker for intermediate
trophoblasts (IT) (Shih and
Kurman, 1996). In contrast,
chorion-type intermediate
trophoblasts, endometrial
glandular and surface epithelium,
and inflammatory cells in the
implantation site were Mel-CAM
immunonegative or only focally
and weakly positive. Hence, Mel-
CAM is a specific and sensitive
marker for IT differentiation in

normal placentas, implantation
sites and in gestational
trophoblastic tumors (Shih and
Kurman, 1996). A double-staining
technique with MIB-1 antibody
to determine the proliferative
index in Mel-CAM defined IT
was found to be useful in the
differential diagnosis of
exaggerated placental versus
placental site trophoblastic tumor
and placental site trophoblastic
tumor versus choriocarcinoma
(Shih and Kurman, 1998).

Applications

Gestational trophoblastic tumors
and tumor-like lesions can be
confused with a variety of non-
trophoblastic tumors. Since this
distinction is important for
management purposes, using an
IT-specific marker like Mel-
CAM would be useful in
resolving this differential
diagnosis (Appendix 1.34).

References

Albelda SM, Muller WA, Buck CA,
  Newman PJ. Molecular and
  cellular properties of PECAM-1
  (endoCAM/CD31): A novel
  vascular cell-cell adhesion
  molecule. Journal of Cellular
  Biology 1991;114:1059–68.
Kuzu I, Bicknell R, Fletcher CDM,
  Gatter KC. Expression of
  adhesion molecules on the

endothelium of normal tissue vessels and vascular tumors. Laboratory Investigation 1993;69:322–8.

Lehmann JM, Holzmann B, Breibart EW, et al. Discrimination between benign and malignant cells of melanocytic lineage by two novel antigens, a glycoprotein with a molecular weight of 113,000 and a protein with molecular weight of 76,000. Cancer Research 1987;47:841–5.

Lehmann JM, Riethmuller G, Johnson JP. Muc18, a marker of tumor progression in human melanoma, shows sequence similarity to the neural cell adhesion molecules of the Ig superfamily. Proceedings of the National Academy of Sciences of the United States of America 1989;86:9891–5.

Sers C, Kirsch K, Rothbacher U, et al. The gene encoding the melanoma-associated glycoprotein MUC18 displays a unique structure among the members of the immunoglobulin superfamily. Proceedings of the National Academy of Sciences of the United States of America 1993;90:8514–8.

Shih IM, Elder DE, Speicher D, et al. Isolation and functional characterization of the A32 melanoma-associated antigen. Cancer Research 1994;54:2514–20.

Shih IM, Kurman RJ. Expression of melanoma cell adhesion molecule in intermediate trophoblast. Laboratory Investigation 1996;75:377–88.

Shih IM, Kurman RJ. Ki-67 labeling index in the differential diagnosis of exaggerated placental site, placenta site trophoblastic tumor, and choriocarcinoma: A double immunohistochemical staining technique using Ki-67 and Mel-CAM antibodies. Human Pathology 1998;28:27–33.

Shih IM, Kurman RJ. The pathology of intermediate trophoblastic tumors and tumor-like lesions. International Journal of Gynecological Pathology 2001;20:31–47.

Metallothioneins

Sources/clones

Dako (E9).

Fixation/preparation

Immunoreactive in fixed paraffin-embedded tissue sections as well as cell preparations and frozen sections. Immunoreactivity is enhanced following HIER.

Background

Metallothioneins (MTs) are low molecular weight, heavy-metal-binding proteins whose expression is induced by heavy metals as well as other factors such as stress, glucocorticoids, lymphokines and xenobiotics (Kagi 1993). MTs have been described in most vertebrate and invertebrate species. Two major isoforms, MT-I and MT-II, are distributed in most adult mammalian tissues. Recently, another isoform MT-0 has been recognized and genes for MT-III and MT-IV with restriction to brain neurons and stratified epithelium have been described (Jasani & Schmid 1997). Interest in MTs has focussed on its overexpression and susceptibility to carcinogenic and anticarcinogenic effects of cadmium, spontaneous

mutagenesis and anti–cancer drugs, and tumor resistance to chemotherapeutic agent (see Jasani & Schmid 1997).

Applications

The ability to stain for MTs with immunohistochemical methods has produced a large amount of data concerning their expression at different stages of development and progression of a wide variety of tumors. Briefly, overexpression of MT has been associated with the type and grade of some tumors such as ductal breast carcinoma (Oyama et al, 1996), skin carcinoma (Zelger et al, 1994), cervical carcinoma (Lim et al, 1996), pancreatic carcinoma (Ohshio et al, 1996), prostatic carcinoma (Zhang et al 1996) melanoma (Zelger et al, 1993), bladder carcinoma (Ioachim et al, 2001), renal cell carcinoma (Tuzel et al, 2001), small carcinoma of the lung (Joseph et al, 2001), and ovarian carcinoma (Hengstler et al, 2001). While overexpression of MTs appears to be mostly associated with locally invasive carcinomas of poor histological type and grade, reduced overall survival and local recurrence of tumor (but not lymph node or distant metastases), this is not true of all tumors. In colonic (Giuffre

et al, 1996), bladder (Saika et al, 1994; Bahnson et al, 1994) and fibroblastic skin tumors (Zelger et al, 1994), overexpression of MTs is associated with lower grade, better differentiated tumors. In squamous cell carcinoma of the esophagus, overexpression of MT appears to predict tumors that benefit from chemotherapy (Kishi et al, 2002). The reason for this apparent discrepancy is not clear. It has been suggested that current antibodies for immunostaining are unable to distinguish between MT-I and MT-II isoforms, or metal-bound and metal-free (apoMT) forms of the protein. Furthermore, they are also unable to detect overexpression of MT-0, MT-III and MT-IV isoforms accounting for the apparently conflicting observations (Jasani & Schmid 1997). The use of MT expression to predict response to chemotherapy is another avenue that requires further study (Saika et al, 1994; Giuffre et al, 1996).

MT has been described as a marker of deep penetrating dermatofibroma, allowing its distinction from dermatofibrosarcoma protuberans, which was consistently negative by immunostaining (Zelger et al, 1994). Increased immunoexpression of MT has been demonstrated in fibroblasts of all ulcerative lesions of ulcerative colitis and Crohn's disease, and suggested a protective role for MT. It was also immunoexpressed in a lower percentage of epithelial cells in these diseases (Bruwer et al, 2001).

Comments

MT staining is found in nucleus, cytoplasm and cell membrane, and the proliferating edges of tumors show most intense staining (Cherian 1994; Tuzel et al, 2001).

References

Bahnson RR, Becich M, Ernstoff MS, et al. Absence of immunohistochemical metallothionein staining in bladder tumor specimens predicts response to neoadjuvant cisplatin, methotrexate and vinblastine chemotherapy. Journal of Urology 1994;152:2272–5.

Bruwer M, Schmid KW, Metz KA, et al. Increased expression of metallothionein in inflammatory bowel disease. Inflammation Research 2001;50:289–93.

Cherian MG. The significance of the nuclear and cytoplasmic localization of metallothionein in human liver and tumor cells. Environmental Health Perspectives 1994;102:131–5.

Gauffre G, Barresi G, Sturniolo GC, et al. Immunohistochemical expression of metallothionein in normal human rectal mucosa, in adenomas, and in adenocarcinomas and their associated metastases. Histopathology 1996;29:347–54.

Iochim EE, Charchanti AV, Stavropoulos NE, et al. Localisation of metallothionein in urological carcinoma of the human urinary bladder: an immunohistochemical study including correlation with HLA-DR antigen, p53, and proliferation indices. Anticancer Research 2001;21:1757–61.

Jasani B, Schmid KW. Significance of metallothionein overexpression in human tumors. Histopathology 1997;31:211–4.

Joseph MG, Banerjee D, Kocha W, et al. Metallothionein expression in patients with small cell carcinoma of the lung: correlation with other molecular markers and clinical outcome. Cancer 2001;92:836–42.

Kagi JHR. Overview of methallothionein. Metallobiochemistry Part B: metallothionein and related molecules. Methods in Enzymology 1993;205:613–26.

Kishi K, Doki Y, Miyata H, et al. Prediction of the response to chemoradiation and prognosis in oesophageal squamous cancer. British Journal of Surgery 2002;89:597–603.

Lim K, Evans A, Adams M, et al. Association of immunohistochemically detectable metallothionein (IDMT) expression with malignant transformation in cervical neoplasia. Journal of Pathology 1996;178 (suppl):48A.

Ohshio G, Imamura T, Okada N, et al. Immunohistochemical study of metallothionein in pancreatic carcinomas. Journal of Cancer Research and Clinical Oncology 1996;122:351–5.

Oyama T, Take H, Hikino T, et al. Immunohistochemical expression of metallothionein in invasive breast cancer in relation to proliferative activity, histology and prognosis. Oncology 1996;53:112–7.

Saika T, Tsushima T, Ochi J, et al. Over-expression of metallothionein and drug-resistance in bladder cancer. International Journal of Urology 1994;1:135–9.

Tuzel E, Kirkali Z, Yorukoglu K, et al. Metallothionein expression in renal cell carcinoma: subcellular localization and prognostic significance. Journal of Urology 2001;165:1710–3.

Zhang XH, Jin L, Sakamoto T, Takenaka I. Immunohistochemical localization of metallothionein in human prostate cancer. Journal of Urology 1996;156:1679–81.

Zlger B, Sidoroff A, Hopfl R, et al. Metallothionein expression in nonmelanoma skin cancer. Applied Immunohistochemistry 1994;2:254–60.

Zlger B, Hittmair A, Schir M, et al. Immunohistochemically demonstrated metallothionein expression in malignant melanoma. Histopathology 1993;23:257–64.

Micropthalmia transcription factor (MiTF)

Sources/clones

Neomarker/Lab Vision (D5, monoclonal antibody recognizes only human MiTF; C5, recognizes both mouse and human Mitf, D5+C5).

Fixation/preparation

These antibodies are applicable to formalin-fixed, paraffin-embedded tissues and require heat-induced antigen retrieval.

Background

The microphthalmia (*Mi*) gene is located on chromosome 3p (Tachibana et al, 1994) and encodes a basic-helix-loop-helix zipper protein (Moore, 1995). This DNA-binding protein regulates transcription of genes involved in melanin synthesis, such as tyrosinase (Yasumoto et al, 1994). Studies in mice have shown that MiTF is essential for pigment synthesis, and embryogenesis and postnatal survival of melanocytes (Hemesath et al, 1994). In humans, MiTF comprises four isoforms that differ at their amino-termini and expression patterns (Carreira et al, 2000). Isoforms A and B are present in retinal pigment epithelium, cervical cancer cells and

melanoma cells. Isoform H is present in the retinal pigment epithelium and cervical cancer cells but not melanoma cells; whilst isoform M is present only in melanoma cells (Udono et al, 2000). Humans with heterozygous mutations of Mitf have Waardenburg syndrome 2a, which is characterized by the presence of a white forelock and deafness (Tassabehji et al, 1994). Knockout mice with homozygous deletions of Mitf also show disruption of osteoclastogenesis, resulting in osteopetrosis (Kawaguchi and Noda, 2000).

In a study of 76 consecutive melanomas, 100% of tumors were reported to be positive with antibody D5, which recognizes both mouse and human MiTF (King et al, 1999). This high sensitivity and specificity for melanocytic differentiation was also duplicated for cutaneous nevi (King et al, 2001) and in 88% of metastatic melanoma (Miettinen et al, 2001). These results compare favorably with HMB-45, Melan-A and tyrosinase (Chang & Folpe, 2001). However, the situation is less defined with the utility of MiTF in the diagnosis of desmoplastic malignant melanoma. Differences in the rates of immunopositivity in the latter tumor have ranged

from 3–55% (Chang & Folpe, 2001). This may be related to the size of the tumor, as MiTF expression appears to be less common in small dermal desmoplastic melanomas than in those that form a distinct mass (Chang & Folpe, 2001).

MiTF immunoexpression has also been demonstrated in a rare group of neoplasms that display combined features of melanocytic and myoid differentiation, the perivascular epithelioid cell family of tumors or PEComas, e.g. angiomyolipoma and related tumors. The efficacy appears to approximate HMB-45 and Melan-A for the diagnosis of PEComas (Chang & Folpe, 2001). An advantage of MiTF in small biopsies is that a greater number (>50%) of cells are positive. Other soft tissue neoplasms with melanocytic differentiation have also been demonstrated to show MiTF expression, namely, melanotic schwannomas, cellular blue nevi and clear cell sarcomas (Koch et al, 2001; Granter et al, 2001).

Applications

MiTF appears to be the most sensitive marker for melanocytic nevi and typical epithelioid melanomas (Appendix 1.10).

However, like other markers for melanoma including HMB45 and Melan A, it does not appear to show sensitivity for desmoplastic melanoma (Xu et al, 2002). MiTF has a definite role in soft tissue neoplasms with a melanocytic differentiation, e.g. PEComas, clear cell sarcoma and melanotic schwannoma. As a nuclear marker, MiTF is largely free of the cytoplasmic artifacts that plague biotin-rich and/or peroxidase-rich tissues such as kidney and liver (Chang and Folpe, 2001).

References

Busam KJ, Iversen K, Coplan KC, Jungbluth AA: Analysis of microphthalmia transcription factor expression in normal tissues and tumors, and comparison of its expression with S-100 protein, gp100, and tyrosinase in desmoplastic malignant melanoma. American Journal of Surgical Pathology 2001;25:197–204.

Carreira S, Lui B, Goding CR. The gene encoding the T-box factor Tbx2 is a target for the microphthalmia-associated transcription factor in melanocytes. Journal of Biological Chememistry 2000;275:21920–7.

Chang KL, Folpe AL. Diagnostic utility of microphthalmia transcription factor in malignant melanoma and other tumors. Advances in Anatomical Pathology 2001;5:273–5.

Granter SR, Weilbaecher KN, Quigley C, et al. Clear cell sarcoma shows immunoreactivity for microphthalmia transcription factor: further evidence for melanocytic differentiation. Modern Pathology 2001;14:6–9.

Hemesath TH, Steingrimsson E, McGill G, et al. Microphthalmia, a critical factor in melanocyte development, defines a discrete transcription factor family. Genes Development 1994;8:2770–80.

Kawaguchi N, Noda M: Mitf is expressed in osteoclast progenitors in vitro. Experimental Cellular Research 2000;260:284–91.

King R, Googe PB, Weilbaecher KN, et al. Microphthalmia transcription factor expression in cutaneous benign, malignant melanocytic, and nonmelanocytic tumors. American Journal of Surgical Pathology 2001;25:51–7.

King R, Weilbaecher KN, McGill G, et al. Microphthalmia transcription factor: a sensitive and specific marker for melanoma diagnosis. American Journal of Pathology 1999;155:731–8.

Koch MB, Shih IM, Weiss SW, et al. Microphthalmia transcription factor and melanoma cell adhesion molecule expression distinguish desmoplastic/spindle cell melanoma from morphologic mimics. American Journal of Surgical Pathology 2001;25:58–64.

Miettinen M, Fernandez M, Franssile K, Gatalica Z, Lasota J, Sarlomo-Rikala M: Microphthalmia transcription factor in the immunohistochemical diagnosis of metastatic melanoma: comparison with four other melanoma markers. American Journal of Surgical Pathology 2001;25:205–11.

Moore KJ: Insight into the microphthalmia gene. Trends in Genetics 1995;11:442–8.

Tachibana M, Perez-Juardo LA, Nakayama A, et al. Cloning of MITF, the human homolog to the mouse microphthalmia gene and assignment to chromosome 3p14.1-p12.3. Human Molecular Genetics 1994;3:553–7.

Tassabehji M, Newton VE, Read AP. Waardenburg syndrome type 2 caused by mutations in the human microphthalmia transcription (MITF) gene. Nature and Genetics 1994;8:251–5.

Udono T, Yasumoto K, Takeda K, et al. Structural organization of the human microphthalmia-associated transcription factor gene containing four alternative promoters. Biochemistry Biophysics Acta 2000;1491:205–19.

Versategui C, Bille K, Ortonne JP, et al. Regulation of the microphthalmia-associated transcription factor gene by the Waardenburg syndrome type 4 gene, SOX10. Journal of Biology and Chemistry 2000;275:30757–60.

Xu X, Chu AY, Pasha TL. Immunoprofile of MiTF, tyrosinase, Melan A, and MAGE 1 in HMB45-negative melanomas. American Journal of Surgical Pathology 2002;26:82–7.

Yasumoto K, Yokoyama K, Shibata K, et al: Microphthalmia-associated transcription factor as a regulator for melanocyte-specific transcription of the human tyrosinase gene. Molecular and Cell Biology 1994;14:8058–70.

Mitochondria

Source/clone

Biogenex (113–1), Chemicon International (MAB 1273).

Fixation/preparation

Monoclonal antibody 113–1 is designed for the specific localization of mitochondria in formalin-fixed, paraffin-embedded tissue sections, or 2% formaldehyde/acetone-fixed cell preparations. Antigen retrieval pretreatment is recommended prior to the immunohistochemical procedure.

Background

Monoclonal antibody clone 113–1 recognizes a 60-kD nonglycosylated protein component of mitochondria in human cells. This marker may be useful in the identification of mitochondria in cells, tissues, and biochemical preparations. It produces a cytoplasmic granular "spaghetti-like" staining pattern in the cytoplasm of human cells (Biogenex product insert).

Antimitochondrial antibody 113–1 has been shown to be a useful discriminatory adjunct in the complex differential diagnosis of granular renal cell tumors (Tickoo et al, 1997). Distinctive staining patterns were observed with chromophobe RCC showing a peripheral accentuation of coarse cytoplasmic granules, a diffuse and fine granularity in renal oncocytomas, and an irregular cytoplasmic distribution of coarse granules in the granular variant of clear cell RCC. In addition, staining was most intense in the eosinophilic variant of papillary RCC with irregular cytoplasmic distribution of coarse granules.

In the salivary gland, immunohistochemistry using the anti-mitochondria antibody proved to be a highly sensitive and specific method for light microscopic identification of mitochondria and superior to routine H&E or PTAH stains for the detection of normal and metaplastic oncocytic cells. This was also useful in the demonstration of neoplastic cells rich in mitochondria: Warthin's tumor, benign oncocytoma and oncocytic carcinoma (Shintaku and Honda, 1997) and deciduoid mesothelioma (Serio et al, 2002), all of which show an intense, finely granular immunoreactivity in the cytoplasm.

Antimitochondrial antibody is also useful in the confirmation/identification of poorly differentiated oxyphilic (Hurthle cell) carcinomas of the thyroid; showing selective marking of oxyphilic, mitochondria-rich cells (Papotti et al, 1996).

Oncocytic (mitochondria-rich) differentiation identifying a subset of meningiomas that behave aggressively may also be accomplished with the use of this antibody. Six so-called oncocytic meningiomas all successfully showed an immunopositive reaction with antimitochondrial antibody (Roncaroli, 1997).

Application

Antimitochondrial antibody clearly has a role in the identification of oncocytic tumors on both paraffin sections and cell preparations. It is also applicable to the differential diagnosis of granular cell tumors of the kidney, with distinctive cytoplasmic immunopositive patterns delineating the various tumors. It is also helpful in the identification of oncocytic meningiomas (in conjunction with a panel including EMA and vimentin), which have a potential aggressive behavior.

References
Biogenex Laboratories. Monoclonal antibody to mitochondrial antigen (data sheet).

Papotti M, Torchio B, Grassi L, et al. Poorly differentiated oxyphilic (Hurthle cell) carcinomas of the thyroid. The American Journal of Surgical Pathology 1996;20:686–94.

Roncaroli F, Riccioni L, Cerati M, et al. Oncocytic meningioma. The American Journal of Surgical Pathology 1997;21:375–82.

Serio G, Scattone A, Pennella A, et al. Malignant deciduoid mesothelioma of the pleura: report of two cases with long survival. Histopathology. 2002;40:348–52.

Shintaku M, Honda T. Identification of oncocytic lesions of salivary glands by anti-mitochondrial immunohistochemistry. Histopathology 1997;31:408–11.

Tickoo SK, Amin MB, Linden MD, et al. Antimitochondrial antibody (113–1) in the differential diagnosis of granular renal cell tumors. The American Journal of Surgical Pathology 1997;21:922–30.

MOC-31

Source/clones

Dako (monoclonal, MOC-31).

Fixation/preparation

This antibody may be applied to both paraffin-embedded tissue sections and cytological material.

Background

MOC-31 is a monoclonal antibody generated with the use of neuramidase-treated cells from a small cell lung carcinoma cell line (GLS-1) being the immunogen (De Leij et al, 1984). In 1987, MOC-31 was clustered as a SCLC-cluster 2 antibody during the First International Workshop on Small-Cell Lung Cancer Antigens in London (Souhami et al, 1987). The SCLC-cluster 2 antibodies detect a 38-kDa epithelial-associated transmembrane glycoprotein which is also named "epithelial glycoprotein 2" or EGP-2, since it only occurs in epithelial cells (De Leij et al, 1994). The latter was derived from the strong expression of EGP-2 in non-squamous carcinomas and its absence in lymphomas, melanomas and neuroblastomas. Hence, MOC-31 is a monoclonal antibody that recognizes a

glycoprotein of unknown function present in the membrane of epithelial cells.

In 1994, it was reported that 98% of acetone-fixed cytological preparations of adenocarcinomas from a variety of sites stained positively with MOC-31 but mesotheliomas did not (Ruitenbeek et al, 1994). This was subsequently confirmed in paraffin-embedded tissue sections (Edwards & Oates, 1995). Whilst others have indicated that this marker provided no value in separating mesotheliomas from adenocarcinoma (also in cytological material), Ordonez (1998) provided conclusive evidence for the role of MOC-31. Reactivity was obtained in 100% pulmonary adenocarcinomas and 85% non-pulmonary adenocarcinomas but only in 5% of mesotheliomas. The latter was restricted to a few positive cells in contrast to the adenocarcinomas where it was strong and diffuse. More recently, a study combining MOC-31 and HBME-1 demonstrated a diagnostic efficiency of 76.1% for the distinction between metastatic carcinoma and mesothelioma in the pleura (Gonzalez-Lois et al, 2001). These authors have reviewed the literature on MOC-31 showing

the range of specificity to be 97.7% to 80% (which lowers to 12.5% with cytology samples). The sensitivity ranged from 100% to 61.2%.

The role of MOC-31 has been expanded and shown to distinguish between hepatocellular carcinoma and adenocarcinoma (both metastatic and cholangiocarcinoma) being negative in primary hepatomas (Porcell et al, 2000).

Applications

MOC-31 may be helpful as part of a panel of antibodies to distinguish between mesotheliomas and adenocarcinoma. There appears to be sufficient evidence to validate its inclusion in a panel to distinguish hepatomas from adenocarcinoma (both primary and secondary) in the liver.

References

De Leij L, Helrich W, Stein T, et al: SCLC-cluster-2 antibodies detect the pancarcinoma/epithelial glycoprotein EGP-2. International Journal of Cancer 1994;8 (Suppl):60–3.

De Leij L, Poppema S, Klein Nulend J, et al: Immunoperoxidase staining on frozen sections as a first screening assay in the preparation of monoclonal antibodies directed against small cell carcinoma of the lung. European Journal of Cancer and Clinical Oncology 1984;20:123–8.

Edwards C, Oates J: OV 632 and MOC 31 in the diagnosis of mesothelioma and adenocarcinoma: An assessment of their use in formalin fixed and paraffin wax embedded material. Journal of Clinical Pathology 1995;48:626–30.

Gonzalez-Lois C, Ballestin C, Sotelo MT, Lopez-Rios F, Garcia-Prats MD, Villena V: Combined use of novel epithelial (MOC-31) and

mesothelial (HBME-1) immunohistochemical markers for optimal first line diagnostic distinction between mesothelioma and metastatic carcinoma in pleura. Histopathology 2001;35:528–34.

Ordonez NG: Value of the MOC-31 monoclonal antibody in differentiating epithelial pleural mesothelioma from lung adenocarcinoma. Human Pathology 1998;29:166–9.

Porcell AI, De Young BR, Proca DM, Frankel WL: Immunohistochemical analysis of hepatocellular and adenocarcinoma in the liver:

MOC31 compares favorably with other putative markers. Modern Pathology 2000;13:773–8.

Ruitenbeek T, Gouw ASH, Poppema S: Immunocytology of body cavity fluids: MOC-31, a monoclonal antibody discriminating between mesothelial and epithelial cells. Archives of Pathology and Laboratory Medicine 1994;118:265–9.

Souhami RL, Beverley PCL, Bobrow LG: Antigens of small-cell lung cancer: First International Workshop. Lancet 1987;2:325–6.

Muscle Specific Actin (MSA)

Sources/clones

Biogenex (HHF35), Dako (HHF35), Diagnostic Biosystems (HHF35), Enzo (HHF35), Biogenesis, Sanbio (SA1C1), Zymed (ZMSA-5, ZCA34, ZSA-1).

Fixation/preparation

The antibody HHF35 is immunoreactive in fixed paraffin-embedded tissue sections and staining is enhanced following HIER.

Background

There are at least six different actin isotypes in mammals. They are four isotypes found exclusively in muscular tissues and include alpha-skeletal, alpha-cardiac, and alpha and gamma smooth muscle actins; and two other isotypes, beta and gamma cytoplasmic actin, found in most cell types, including nonmuscle cells of the body. Early antiactin antibodies were polyclonal and did not distinguish among various actin isotypes and were of low sensitivity and specificity. Various monoclonal antibodies have now been described and the most widely used is clone HHF35, available commercially, which recognizes a common epitope of alpha-skeletal, alpha-cardiac, and alpha and gamma smooth muscle actin isotypes (Tsukada et al, 1987). This antibody labels myoepithelial and smooth muscle cells as well as leiomyomas and leiomyosarcomas. Muscle specific actins (MSA) have also been described in pericytes, reactive myofibroblasts, and skeletal and cardiac muscle. Positive staining cells have been reported in the deep ovarian cortical stroma and theca externa of secondary ovarian follicles, alveolar soft part sarcoma, epithelioid sarcoma, infantile digital fibromatosis, ovarian sclerosing stromal tumors and Kaposi's sarcoma, representing either myofibroblasts or pericytes in these conditions. Glomus tumors stain positive for MSA, a finding that supports a smooth muscle derivation of these tumors (Dervan Et al, 1989), and the variable extent of MSA staining observed in malignant mesothelioma (Kung et al, 1995) and malignant fibrous histiocytoma has been attributed to myofibroblastic differentiation in these tumors. Actin staining of unequivocal tumor cells has been reported in occasional cases of metastatic endometrial stromal sarcoma and malignant peripheral nerve sheath tumor but it has not been ascertained if these findings represent aberrant actin expression of tumor cells or cross-reactivity of anti-actin antibodies. MSA has also been observed in the cells of the capsule of the liver, kidney and spleen and in decidual cells, some stromal cells of chorionic villi and the so-called fibroblastic reticulum cells of lymph nodes and spleens.

Applications

The increased sensitivity and specificity of newer monoclonal antibodies allow the use of anti-MSA antibodies in the identification of pleomorphic spindle cell tumors. Because of varying sensitivities, it is best to employ MSA with other myogenic markers such as smooth muscle actin and desmin when examining tumors, which potentially confuse with rhabdomyosarcoma (RMS), leiomyosarcoma (LMS) and myofibroblastic tumors (Azumi et al, 1988). Much of the current controversy as to which of these markers is the most sensitive for myogenic differentiation stems from the fact that the expression of the individual markers varies with the site of origin of the tumor (Rangdaeng & Truong, 1991). For example, most soft tissue and uterine LMS contain predominantly alpha smooth muscle actin but those from the gastrointestinal tract show only beta and gamma non-muscle actins and would thus be negative for HHF35. Myofibroblasts show heterogeneous immunophenotype and may be positive for vimentin only; for vimentin and alpha smooth actin; for vimentin and desmin; or for vimentin, desmin and alpha smooth muscle actin (Skalli et al, 1989). Myofibroblastic proliferations such as nodular fasciitis may display characteristic peripheral/subplasmmalemal staining for muscle actin, yielding a "tram track" appearance (Leong & Gown, 1993). Increased expression of MSA has been correlated with mesangial cell injury and proliferation in both rats and humans, and can be employed as a marker of mesangial cell injury, activation and proliferation (Alpers et al, 1992).

Comments

Zenker's fixative appears to cause a marked decreased in the intensity of MSA staining. False-positive reactivity with clones HHF35 and 1A4 has been reported in non-Hodgkin's lymphoma, a problem attributed to contaminating antibodies, partial antibody degradation or excess antibody concentration which may occur with ascitic fluid preparations of anti-MSA (Sheehan & O'Brian, 1995). The problem was not observed in tissue culture supernatant antibodies and was abolished by the addition of 50mmol/L of EDTA to the prediluted antibody. MSA remains a well-used marker for contractile cells. Other myogenic markers include desmin, smooth muscle actin, and the actin-binding proteins calponin and h-caldesmon. A recent study of atypical fibroxanthoma and benign fibrous histiocytoma of the skin showed immunoreactivity respectively for calponin (3/10; 11/17), desmin (3/10; 1/17), SMA (3/10; 13/17) and MSA (HHF35) (1/10; 5/17), with no staining for h-caldesmon in any of the cases. In contrast leiomyosarcoma had high immunoreactivity for calponin (17/17), desmin (13/17), SMA (16/17), MSA (16/17) and h-caldesmon (11/17) (Sakamoto et al, 2002)

References

Alpers CE, Hudkins KL, Gown AM, Johnson RJ. Enhanced expression of "muscle-specific" actin in glomerulonephritis. Kidney International 1992;41:1134–42.

Azumi N, Ben-Erza J, Battifora H. Immunophenotypic diagnosis of leiomyosarcomas and rhabdomyosarcomas with monoclonal antibodies to muscle specific actin and desmin in formalin-fixed tissue. Modern Pathology 1988;1:469–74.

Dervan PA, Tobbia IN, Casey M, et al. Glomus tumors: an immunohistochemical profile of 11 cases. Histopathology 1989;14:483–91.

Kung IT, Thallas V, Spencer EJ, Wilson SM. Expression of muscle actins in diffuse mesotheliomas. Human Pathology 1995;26:565–70.

Rangdaeng S, Truong LD. Comparative immunohistochemical staining for desmin and muscle specific actin. A study of 576 cases. American Journal of Clinical Pathology 1991;96:32–45.

Leong AS-Y, Gown AM. Immunohistochemistry of "solid" tumours: poorly differentiated round cell and spindle cell tumors I. IN: Leong AS-Y (ed). Applied Immunohistochemistry for the Surgical Pathologist. London: Edward Arnold, 1993, pp24–72.

Sakamoto A, Oda Y, Yamamoto H, et al. Calponin and h-caldesmon expression in atypical fibroxanthoma and superficial leiomyosarcoma. Virchows Archives 2002;440:404–9.

Sheehan M, O'Brian DS. False-positive immunoreactivity with muscle-specific actins in non-Hodgkin's lymphoma. Archives of Pathology and Laboratory Medicine 1995;119:225–8.

Skalli O, Schurch W, Seemeyer TA, et al. Myofibroblasts from diverse pathologic settings are heterogenous in their content of actin isoforms and intermediate filament protein. Laboratory Investigation 1989;60:275–85.

Tsukada T, Tippens D, Gordon D, et al. HHF35, a muscle-specific actin-specific monoclonal antibody. I. Immunocytochemical and biochemical characterisation. American Journal of Pathology 1987;126:51–60.

Mycobacterial Antigen

Source/clone

Polyclonal rabbit anti–BCG (Dako)

Fixation/preparation

These antibodies are applicable to formalin-fixed paraffin-embedded tissue sections.

Background

The identification of mycobacteria in tissue sections and smears is the most rapid method of detection compared with culture and polymerase chain reaction. This is underscored by the fact that mycobacterial infections carry a significant morbidity and mortality, emphasizing the need for rapid identification in tissue sections. The yield of acid-fast stains for the detection of mycobacteria may be less than one organism per tissue section and acid-fast stains require relatively intact organisms with retained capsular integrity.

The polyclonal rabbit anti–BCG (bacille Calmette–Guerin) was raised against an attenuated strain used to immunize against *Mycobacterium tuberculosis* infections, containing a substantial number of shared antigens with other mycobacterial species. Hence, this antibody is capable of detecting antigen in debris and fragmented organisms that retain their antigenicity and immunoreactivity (Hove et al, 1998). Using immunohistochemistry, Higuchi et al (1981) demonstrated that fragments and wall components of BCG persisted in inoculation sites long after acid-fact stains could no longer detect bacilli. In clinical material, eight of 10 cases of culture-proven infection in which acid-fast stains were negative, immunoreactivity with anti–BCG was demonstrated in organisms and/or antigen (Wiley et al, 1990). These authors detected immunoreactive clumps of mycobacterial debris, cells and cell fragments in caseating granulomata. In histiocytic granulomata of mycobacterial infections, the cytoplasm of epithelioid cells contained both organisms and debris (Wiley et al, 1990). Furthermore, this immunostaining reaction was evident at low-power (scanning) magnification.

However, immunohistochemical detection of mycobacterial antigen has a limited utility in cases where many of the organisms are viable and abundant; having no advantage over established procedures (acid-fast stains) in these circumstances (Humphrey and Weiner, 1987).

Applications

Anti–BCG has a role in detecting mycobacterial organisms/antigens in fixed paraffin-embedded sections, especially in cases in which acid-fast stains are negative and a high index of suspicion exists on morphological interpretation. Further, the cross-reactivity of polyclonal anti–BCG with a wide variety of mycobacterial species allows for the detection of organisms in a wide range of clinical settings. Immunohistochemical staining with the Dako antibody compared to mycobacterial culture is reported to show a sensitivity of 52%, specificity of 76%, positive predictive value of 61% and negative predictive value of 69%.

References
Carabias E, Palenque E, Serrano R, et al. Evaluation of an immunohistochemical test with polyclonal antibodies raised against mycobacteria used in formalin-fixed tissue compared with mycobacterial specific culture. APMIS 1998;106:385–8.

Higuchi S, Moritaka S, Dannenberg AM, et al. Persistence of protein, carbohydrate and wax components of tubercle bacilli in dermal BCG lesions. American Review of Respiratory Disease 1981;123:397–401.

Hove MGM, Smith MB, Hightower B, Pencil SD. Detection of mycobacteria with use of immunohistochemistry in granulomatous lesions staining negative with routine acid-fast stains. Applied Immunohistochemistry 1998;6:169–72.

Humphrey DM, Weiner MH. Mycobacterial antigen detection by immunohistochemistry in pulmonary tuberculosis. Human Pathology 1987;18:701–8.

Wiley EL, Mulhollan TJ, Beck B, et al. Polyclonal antibodies raised against bacillus Calmette-Guerin Mycobacterium Duvalii and Mycobacterium Paratuberculosis used to detect mycobacteria in tissue with the use of immunohistochemical techniques. American Journal of Clinical Pathology 1990;94:307–12.

Myelin Basic Protein (MBP)

Sources/clones

Axcel/Accurate (polyclonal), Biogenesis, Biogenex (130–137), Biomedia/Accurate (MAB3), Biosource, Biotec, Boehringer Mannheim, Cymbus (MIG-MI9), Dako, Research Diagnostics (MIG-MI9), Serotec, Zymed (polyclonal).

Fixation/preparation

The antigen is formalin resistant and its immunoreactivity is enhanced by proteolytic digestion or HIER. The antibody can be applied to frozen sections.

Background

Myelin basic protein (MBP) is found in the central and peripheral system. It is found in oligodendrocytes and myelin of white matter in the brain and spinal cord, and to a lesser extend in grey matter. It also is found in peripheral nerve.

Applications

MBP is useful in research but has limited applications in diagnostic immunohistochemistry where its use is largely in the diagnosis of soft tissue tumors. It has been demonstrated in neuromas, neurofibromas, ganglioneuromas, and tumors with neural differentiation and neural elements but is not present in glial tissues. The protein has been employed in a panel of antibodies to identify palisaded encapsulated neuromas of the skin (Argenyi 1990) and is useful for the distinction of neurofibromas from neurotized melanocytic nevi. Neurofibromas showed focal staining for CD57 (Leu 7), glial fibrillary acidic protein and MBP whereas neurotized nevi failed to express these markers (Gray et al, 1990). MBP (together with CD57) has also been demonstrated in some granular cell tumors (Mazur et al, 1990), suggesting neural differentiation in some of these lesions. MBP is a useful marker of ganglioneuroblastomas, ganglioneuromas and gangliocytic paraganglioma (Furihata et al, 1996; Molenaar et al, 1990).

Comments

The use of MBP as a marker of schawannomas is well established (Wick et al, 1987) although some studies have failed to find MBP in Schwann cell neoplasms (Clark et al, 1985; Johnson et al, 1988; Sharma et al, 1990) and both immunohistochemical and Western blot analyses have failed to demonstrate MBP in oligodendrogliomas and Schwann cell tumors (Schwechheimer et al, 1992). Other markers such as S100, fibrillary acidic protein and CD57 are preferred for the characterization of nerve sheath differentiation.

References

Argenyi ZB. Immunohistochemical characterization of palisaded encapsulated neuroma. Journal of Cutaneous Pathology 1990;7:329–35.

Clark HB, Minesky JJ, Agrawal D, Agarawal HC. Myelin basic protein and P2 protein are not immunohistochemical markers for Schwann cell neoplasms. A comparative study using antisera to S100, P2, and myelin basic proteins. American Journal of Pathology 1985;121:96–101.

Furihata M, Sonobe H, Iwata J, et al. Immunohistochemical characterization of a case of duodenal gangliocytic paraganglioma. Pathology International 1996;46:610–3.

Gray MH, Smoller BR, McNUtt NS, Hsu A. Neurofibromas and neurotized melanocytic nevi are immunohistochemcally distinct neoplasms. American Journal of Dermatopathology 1990;12:234–41.

Johnson MD, Glick AD, Davis BW. Immunohistochemical evaluation of Leu 7, myelin basic protein,

S100- protein, glial fibrillary acidic-protein, and LN3 immunoreactivity in nerve sheath tumors and sarcomas. Archives of Pathology and Laboratory Medicine 1988;112:155–60.

Mazur MT, Schultz JJ, Myers JL. Granular cell tumor – immunohistochemical analysis of 21 benign and one malignant tumor. Archives of Pathology and Laboratory Medicine 1990;114:692–6.

Molenaar WM, Baker DL, Pleasure D, et al. The neuroendocrine and neural profiles of neuroblastomas, ganglioneuroblastomas, and ganglioneuromas. American Journal of Pathology 1990;136:375–82.

Schwechheimer K, Gass P, Berlet HH. Expression of oligodendroglia and Schwann cell markers in human nervous system tumors. An immunomorphological study and western blot analysis. Acta Neuropathologica (Berlin) 1992;83:283–91.

Sharma S, Sarkar C, Mathur M, et al. Benign nerve sheath tumors: a light microscopic, electron microscopic and immunohistochemical study of 102 cases. Pathology 1990;22:191–5.

Wick MR, Swanson PE, Scheithauer BW, Manival JC. Malignant peripheral nerve sheath tumor: an immunohistochemical study of 62 cases. American Journal of Clinical Pathology 1987;87:425–33.

Myeloperoxidase

Sources/clones

Accurate (CLBMPO.1), Axcel/Accurate (MPO-7, polyclonal), Biodesign (polyclonal), Dako (MPO-7, polyclonal), Research Diagnostics (CLB-MPO1–1).

Fixation/preparation

May be applied to formalin-fixed, paraffin-embedded tissue sections. This antibody may also be used to label acetone-fixed, frozen sections and fixed cell smears. The rabbit polyclonal antibody reacts with myeloperoxidase in a variety of fixatives including Zenker's-acetic acid solution, B5 solution and formalin (Pinkus and Pinkus, 1991). Pretreatment with trypsin is essential before immunostaining. HIER does not appear to enhance immunoreactivity but is not deleterious. The monoclonal antibodies do not work on formalin-fixed tissues and should only be used on frozen sections.

Background

Myeloperoxidase is the major constituent of primary granules of myeloid cells. It therefore serves as a reliable marker for myeloid cells, including early (immature) and mature forms. The appearance of myeloperoxidase precedes neutrophil elastase during myeloid cell differentiation. Further, myeloperoxidase antibody does not react with lymphoid or epithelial cells (Pinkus and Pinkus, 1991). The myeloperoxidase immunogen was isolated from human granulocytes.

Other immunohistochemical markers for myeloid cells, eg. lysozyme, CD15. Mac 387 and CD 68, despite being sensitive, lack specificity in that they also stain histiocytes and other cell types including epithelium (Mason and Taylor, 1975). CD43 and CD45RO also stain myeloid cells frequently, but demonstrate T cells and histiocytes as well (Traweek et al, 1993).

Applications

Immunostaining for myeloperoxidase on paraffin sections is helpful in confirming the myeloid nature of the primitive cells that infiltrate marrow tissue. Positive reaction excludes lymphoblastic leukemia and malignant lymphoma and is therefore crucial for patient management. Skin infiltrates with acute myeloid leukemia, which may be subtle, benefits from the application of antimyeloperoxidase antibody to highlight the neoplastic population (Wong & Chan, 1995).

Granulocytic sarcoma presenting as a tumor mass may occur in isolation or in association with myeloid disorders (Nieman et al, 1981). In the absence of a history of a haematological malignancy, an erroneous diagnosis of lymphoma may lead to an inappropriate treatment being instituted. Hence a high index of suspicion and the use of antibodies (including myeloperoxidase) for the demonstration of the myeloid nature of the cellular proliferation avoids a misdiagnosis. A study of 22 cases of granulocytic sarcoma on archival material proved myeloperoxidase immunostaining to be the most sensitive for demonstrating neoplastic myeloid cells, being positive in all cases (Wong and Chan, 1995). Chloroacetate esterase and lysozyme was positive in only 68% and 86% of case respectively. Lysozyme may show a strong reaction in some cases of granulocytic sarcoma, complicating acute myelomonocytic leukemia. The advantage of myeloperoxidase is the reduced background staining. Various other studies (Pinkus and Pinkus, 1991; Traweek et al, 1993) have also demonstrated myeloperoxidase to be a highly sensitive tool for the confirmation of neoplastic myeloid cells in granulocytic sarcoma. Other markers of myeloid cells include CD43, CD15 and histochemical staining for chloroacetate-esterase.

Comments

Antimyeloperoxidase should be included in the immunohistochemical panel for lymphoma investigation. Any "lymphoma" that cannot be classified with confidence should raise the suspicion of a granulocytic sarcoma. Furthermore, tumor cells marking with only T-cell markers CD43 or CD45RO, but not the specific T-marker CD3, or alternatively stain only for histiocytic markers such as CD68 or CD15, should raise the alarm for a possible granulocytic sarcoma (Wong & Chan, 1995). Myeloperoxidase is not only specific but by far the most sensitive of the myeloid markers (Menasce et al, 1999).

References

Mason DY, Taylor CR. The distribution of muramidase (lysozyme) in human tissues. Journal of Clinical Pathology 1975;28:124–32.

Menasce LP, Banerjee SS, Beckett E, Harris M. Extra-medullary myelioid tumour (granulocytic sarcoma is often misdiagnosed: A study of 26 cases. Histopathology 1999;34:391–8.

Neiman RS, Barcos M, Berard C, et al. Granulocytic sarcoma: a clinicopathologic study of 61 biopsied cases. Cancer 1981;48:1426–37.

Pinkus GS, Pinkus JL. Myeloperoxidase: a specific marker for myeloid cells in paraffin sections. Modern Pathology 1991;4:733–41.

Traweek ST, Arber DA, Rappaport H, Brynes RK. Extramedullary myeloid cell tumors: an immunohistochemical and morphologic study of 28 cases. American Journal of Surgical Pathology 1993;17:1011–9.

Van der Schoot CE, Daams GM, Pinkster J, et al. Monoclonal antibodies against myeloperoxidase are valuable immunological reagents for the diagnosis of acute myeloid leukaemia. British Journal of Haematology 1990;74:173–8.

Wong KF, Chan JKC. Antimyeloperoxidase: Antibody of choice for labeling of myeloid cells including diagnosis of granulocytic sarcoma. Advances in Anatomic Pathology 1995;2:65–8.

MyoD1

Sources/clones

Accurate/Novocastra (5.8A), Dako (5.8A).

Fixation/preparation

Anti-MyoD1 can be used on formalin-fixed, paraffin-embedded tissue sections. Deparaffinised tissue sections require heat pretreatment in citrate buffer prior to immunohistochemical staining procedure. Sialinized slides are recommended to improve adherence of tissue sections to glass slides. Ideally, this antibody requires fresh frozen tissue for optimum results.

Background

The differentiation of skeletal muscle at the molecular level requires activation and transcription of genes encoding muscle specific proteins and enzymes such as desmin and creatine kinase. These activities are controlled by a set of genes including *MyoD1,* myogenin, myf-5 and myf-6 (Funk et al, 1991; Tonin et al, 1991). It is thought that *MyoD1* activation is an early event that commits the cell to skeletal muscle lineage (Hosoi et al, 1992). Transfection

of the *MyoD1* gene into non-muscle cells has been shown to induce conversion of fibroblasts into myoblasts (Davis et al, 1987). Similarly, muscle-specific genes in tumor cell lines may be activated by forced expression of exogeneously introduced Myod1 (Weintraub et al, 1989). The *MyoD1* gene has been localized to the short arm of chromosome 11 (Gressler et al, 1990). The activation of MyoD1 gene, as reflected in the detection of mRNA or protein product represents a stage of skeletal muscle differentiation that is earlier than that of currently available immunohistochemical markers, such as desmin and myoglobin.

The MyoD1 protein is a 45 kD nuclear phosphoprotein, (5.8A reacts with an epitope between amino acid residues 170 and 209), with nuclear expression restricted to skeletal muscle tissue. Monoclonal anti-MyoD1 strongly stains nuclei of myoblasts in developing skeletal muscle whilst the majority of adult skeletal muscle has been found to be negative (Wang et al, 1995), including a wide variety of normal tissue. However, weak cytoplasmic staining has been observed in non-muscle tissue, including

glandular epithelium (Wang et al, 1995).

Applications

MyoD1 nuclear immunostaining has been demonstrated in the majority of rhabdomyosarcomas of various histological subtypes (Appendix 1.27). In fact it has been shown that the MyoD1 expression in rhabdomyosarcomas is inversely related to the degree of cellular differentiation of tumor cells (Wang et al, 1995). This phenomenon is useful to distinguish embryonal rhabdomyosarcomas from other small blue round cell tumors of childhood, viz, Ewing's sarcoma/peripheral primitive neuroectodermal tumor, neuroblastoma and childhood lymphomas. Wilm's tumors and ectomesenchymoma with rhabdomyosarcomatous foci also show nuclear expression of MyoD1 (Dias et al, 1992) (Appendix 1.3). It has also been shown that the sensitivity and specificity of the MyoD1 antibody in the differential diagnosis of adult pleomorphic soft tissue sarcomas approaches that of pediatric rhabdomyosarcomas (Wesche et al, 1995). The demonstration of MyoD1 protein in four cases of alveolar soft part sarcoma was initially used as evidence for its rhabdomyosarcomatous differentiation (Rosai et al, 1991); however, subsequent studies have not confirmed the presence of this regulatory protein in the tumor (Ordonez & Mackay, 1998; Gomez et al, 1999). Other evidence of myogenic differentiation in alveolar soft part sarcoma include the demonstration of desmin and/or myoglobin (Ordonez, 1999; Tornoczky et al, 2001)

Comments

A note of caution worthy of mention is that granular cytoplasmic immunoreactivity for MyoD1 has been demonstrated in most neuroblastomas and occasional Ewing's sarcomas/PNETs (Wang et al, 1995) and alveolar soft part sarcomas. Only nuclear staining should be considered as evidence of skeletal myogenic differentiation, although our own experience has been that nuclear expression occurs in the primitive skeletal tumors, whilst tumors with cytoplasmic/myogenic differentiation have demonstrated cytoplasmic immunopositivity; the. The cytoplasmic immunostaining with anti-MyoD1 (clone 5.8A) has been suggested to represent cross-reactivity with an unknown cytoplasmic antigen. In their study of 12 cases of alveolar soft part sarcoma, Wang et al (1960) found positivity for desmin in six tumors but no specimen showed nuclear expression of MyoD1 or myogenin. However, there was considerable cytoplasmic staining with the anti-MyoD1, a phenomenon observed with

various nonmuscle and neoplastic tissues with this antibody. Biochemical analysis of fresh frozen tumor tissue showed no specific band corresponding to the 45 kD MyoD1. The cytoplasmic and non-specific background staining and reactivity for nonmyoid tissues can hinder the practical utility in paraffin-embedded sections (Cessna et al, 2001). Staining seems to be more consistent in alveolar rhabdomyosarcomas, especially in tumor cells lining fibrous septae and perivascular areas and embryonal rhabodomyosarcomas showing more variable staining (Cessna et al, 2001). Another study suggested that MyoD1 was generally expressed in small, primitive tumors cells and larger cells exhibiting morphologic evidence of skeletal muscle differentiation failed to stain for the protein (Cui et al, 1999). It was suggested that an earlier claim of a high level of sensitivity of MyoD1 in fixed tissue may not be so as only 35% of rhabdomyosarcomas were positive in paraffin sections compared to 60% positivity in frozen sections of the same tumors (Mukunyadzi et al, 1999)

References

Cessna MH, Zhou H, Perkins SL, et al. Are myogenin and myoD1 expre4ssion specific for rhabdomyosarcoma? A study of 150 cases, wioth emphasis on spindle cell mimics. American Journal of surgical Pathology 2001;25:1150–7.

Cui S, Hano H, Harada T, et al. Evaluation of new monoclonal anti-MyoD1 and anti-myogenin antibodies for the diagnosis of rhabdomyosarcoma. Pathology International 1999;49:62–8.

Davis RL, Weinbtraub H, Lassar AB. Expression of a single transfected cDNA converts fibroblasts to myoblasts. Cell 1987;51:987–1000.

Dias P, Parham DM, Shapiro DN, et al. Monoclonal antibodies to the myogenic regulatory protein MyoD1: Epitope mapping and diagnostic utility. Cancer Research 1992;52:6431–9.

Funk WD, Ouellette M, Wright WE. Molecular biology of myogenic regulatory factors. Molecular Biology Medicine 1991;8:185–93.

Gressler M, Hameister H, Henry I, et al. The human MyoD1 (MYF3) gene maps on the short arm of chromosome 11 but is not associated with the WAGR locus on the region for the B-W syndrome. Human Genetics 1990;86:135–8.

Gomez JA, Amin MB, Ro JY, et al. Immunohistochemical profile of myogenin and MyoD1 does not support skeletal muscle origin of alveolar soft part sarcoma. Archives of Pathology and Laboratory Medicine 1999;123:503–7.

Hosoi H, Sugimoto T, Hayashi Y, et al. Differential expression of myogenic regulatory genes, *MyoD1* and myogenin in human rhabdomyosarcoma sublimes. International Journal of Cancer 1992;50:977–83.

Mukunyadzi P, Dias P, Houghton PJ, Pharham DM. Comparison of MyoD1 immunostaining of pediatric tumors using frozen opr paraffin-embedded sections. Applied Immunohistochemistry and Molecular Morphology 1999;7:260–5.

Ordonez NG. Alveolar soft part sarcoma: a review and update. Advances in Anatomical Pathology 1999;6:125–39.

Ordonez NG, Mackay B. alveolar soft part sarcoma: a review of the pathology and histogenesis. Ultrastructural Pathology 1998;22:275–92.

Rosai J, Dias P, Parham DM, Shapiro DN, Houghton P. MyoD1 protein expression in alveolar soft part sarcoma as confirmatory evidence of its skeletal muscle nature. American Journal of Surgical Pathology 1991;15:974–81.

Tonin PN, Scrable H, Shimada H, Cavence WK. Muscle-specific gene expression in rhabdomyosarcomas and stages of human fetal skeletal muscle development. Cancer Research 1991;51:100–6.

Tornoczky T, Kalman E, Sapi Z, et al. Cytogenetic abnormalities of alveolar soft part sarcomas using interphase fluorescent in situ hybridization: trisomy for chromosome 7 and monosomy for chromosomes 8 and 18 seem to be characteristic of the tumor. Virchows Archives 2001;438:173–80.

Wang NP, Marx J, McNutt MA, et al. Expression of myogenic regulatory proteins (Myogenin and MyoD1) in small blue round cell tumors of childhood. American Journal of Pathology 1995;147:1799–1810.

Wang NP, Bacchi CE, Jiang JJ, et al. Does alveolar soft-part acrcoma exhibit skeletal muscle differentiation? An immunohistochemical and biochemical study of myogenic regulatory protein expression. Modern Pathology 1996;9:495–506.

Weintraub H, Tapscott SJ, Davis RL, et al. Activation of muscle-specific gene in pigment, nerve, fat, liver and fibroblast cell lines by forced expression of MyoD. Proceedings of the National Academy of Science USA. 1989;86:5434–8.

Wesche WA, Fletcher CDM, Dias E, et al. Immunohistochemistry of MyoD1 in adult pleomorphic soft tissue sarcomas. American Journal of Surgical Pathology 1995;19:261–9.

NOTES

Myogenin

Sources/clones

Dako (F5D), Pharmingen (5FD), Santa Cruz (polyclonal).

Fixation/preparation

F5D is immunoreactive in fixed, paraffin-embedded tissue sections and HIER enhances immunoreactivity.

Background

Myogenin belongs to a family of regulatory proteins essential for muscle development. Studies in mice indicate that myogenin is not required for the initial aspects of myogenesis, including myotome formation and the appearance of myoblasts, but late stages of embryogenesis are more dependent on myogenin (Venuti et al, 1995). Expression levels in fetal skeletal muscle were found to be 20-fold higher than that of adult rat skeletal muscle. Chickens appear to show the same pattern of myoblast development with fetal myoblasts expressing both MyoD and myogenin within the first day of culture whereas adult myoblasts are essentially negative for both proteins at the same period of culture and subsequently express first MyoD and myogenin before expressing sarcomeric myosin

(Yablonka–Reuveni & Paterson, 2001). Expression of myogenin is restricted to cells of skeletal muscle origin and appears to be inversely related to the degree of cellular differentiation making it a potentially useful marker for skeletal muscle differentiation in the identification and typing of anaplastic round cell tumors in childhood (Appendix 1.3 & 1.11).

Applications

F5D recognizes an epitope located in the amino acid region 138–158 of the myogenin protein and has been found to label nuclei of myoblasts of human fetus but no reactivity was observed in adult skeletal muscle (Wang et al, 1995). The antibody to F5D labels nuclei of the majority of human rhabdomyosarcomas (Folpe et al, 1997) and Wilm's tumors. The extent of staining for myogenin has been reported to be inversely related to degree of cellular differentiation in rhabdomyosarcoma tumor cells (Wang et al, 1995). Strong immunostaining for myogenin in significantly associated with tumors of the alveolar subclass of rahbdomyosarcoma (Dias et al, 2000). Although all rhabdomyosarcomas show staining for myogenin, the alveolar variant

showed strongest nuclear staining even in cases with subtle alveolar architecture in which myogenin highlighted and enhnaced visualization of the alveolar pattern. Embryonal rhabdomyosarcomas, in contrast, showed greater variability in staining pattern and intensity (Cessna et al, 2001). No reactivity was reported with Ewing's sarcoma/peripheral primitive neuroectodermal tumor, neuroblastoma or adult skeletal muscle (Wang et al, 1995), nodular fasciitis, malignant fibrous histiocytoma, malignant peripheral nerve sheath tumor, leiomyosarcoma or alveolar soft part sarcoma. Focal nuclear staining was rarely seen in desmoid, synovial sarcoma, infantile fibromatosis and infantile fibrosarcoma (Cessana et al, 2001). The same study concluded that in contrast to myogenin, MyoD1 staining was much less useful in the identification of rhabdomyosarcoma because of cytoplasmic and non-specific background staining and reactivity of non-myoid tissues (Appendix 1.27).

Comments

Only nuclear staining should be regarded as positive. Clone F5D

M

Myogenin

shows strong reactivity in paraffin sections following HIER. Myogenin has proven to be a better and more sensitive marker of skeletal muscle differentiation in poorly differentiated rhabdomyosarcoma than MyoD1, given that the latter displays non-specific cross-reactivity with an unknown cytoplasmic antigen in non-muscle cells and tumors (Wang et al, 1995; Cessna et al, 2001; Folpe, 2002). Pleomorphic rhabdomyosarcoma also stain for myogenin (Furlong et al, 2001). The absence of immunoexpression of myogenin in alveolar soft part sarcoma casts doubts on its alleged skeletal muscle lineage (Gomez et al, 1999).

References

Cessna MH, Zhou H, Perkins SL, et al. Are myogenin and myoD1 expression specific for rhabdomyosarcomas? A study of 150 cases, with emphasis on spindle cell mimics. American Journal of Surgical Pathology 2001;25:1150–7.

Folpe AL, Patterson K, Gown AM. Antibodies to desmin identify the blastemal component of nephroblastoma. Modern Pathology 1997;10:895–900.

Flope AL. MyoD1 and myogenin expression in human neoplasia: A review and update. Advances in Anatomical Pathology 2002;9:198–203.

Furlong MA, Mentzel T, Fanburg-Smith JC. Pleomorphic rhabdomyosarcoma in adults: a clinicopathologica study of 38 cases with emphasis on morphologic variants and recent skeletal muscle-specific markers. Modern Pathology 2001;14:595–603

Gomez JA, Amin MB, Ro JY, et al. Immunohistochemical profile of myogenin and MyoD1 does not support skeletal muscle lineage in alveolar soft part sarcoma. Archives of Pathology and Laboratory Medicine 1999;123:503–7.

Venuti JM, Morris JH, Vivian JL, et al. Myogenin is required for late but not early aspects of myogensis during mouse development. Journal of Cell Biology 1995;128:563–576.

Wang NP, Marx J, McNutt MA, et al. Expression of myogenic regulatory proteins (myogenin and MyoD1) in small blue round cell tumors of childhood. American Journal of Pathology 1995;147:1799–1810.

Yablonka–Reuveni Z, Paterson BM. MyoD and myogenin expression patterns in cultures of fetal and adult chicken myoblasts. Journal of Histochemistry and Cytochemistry 2001;49:455–62.

Myoglobin

Sources/clones

Accurate (M-2–167, M-3–416), American Research Products (1B4, 1F6, 4G8, 8H5), Axell/Accurate (polyclonal), Biogenesis (DA2, polyclonal), Biogenex (MG-1, polyclonal), Chemicon (polyclonal), Dako (polyclonal), Sera Lab (polyclonal), Sigma Chemical (MG-1), Zymed (Z001).

Fixation/preparation

Myoglobin is resistant to formalin fixation. Immunoreactivity is not significantly enhanced by proteolytic digestion and is not responsive to HIER.

Background

Myoglobin, a 17.8 kD protein is the oxygen carrier hemoprotein, a specific marker for striated muscle cells. It is also present in cardiac muscle. The antibodies do not cross react with hemoglobin. Cross-reactivity with myoglobins of other mammalian species may occur with some antibodies.

Applications

Anti-myoglobin has been used to indicate early myocardium

necrosis and skeletal muscle trauma and necrosis. Myoglobin was one of the earliest markers of striated muscle differentiation but its expression appears to be linked to the differentiation of rhabdomyosarcoma cells, so that a sizeable number of such tumors, particularly the poorly differentiated ones, exhibit no staining. In our experience, morphologically recognizable rhabdomyoblasts express myoglobin, whereas poorly differentiated tumors fail to stain so that this marker is not helpful when it is actually required (Leong et al, 1989; Gruchala et al, 1997). Its application as a marker of early ischemic myocardium appears to be less reliable than cytoskeletal proteins such as vinculin, desmin and alpha-actinin (Zhang and Riddick, 1996). Myoglobin immunostaining has been employed in the study of ragged-red fiber of patients with mitochondrial encephalomyopathy (Kunishige et al, 1996).

Staining for myoglobin can also be performed in renal biopsies of patients with myoglobin-containing casts due to conditions such as necrotizing myopathy or rhabdomyolysis (Helliwell et al, 1991).

Comments

Myoglobin is obviously not a dependable marker of striated muscle differentiation, especially in poorly differentiated rhabdomyosarcoma. Other markers such as desmin, muscle-specific actin and MyoD1 should be employed for the identification of striated muscle differentiation. The use of myoglobin as a marker of skeletal muscle tumors has been surplanted by myogenin and to a lesser extent, MyoD1 (Cessna et al, 2001; Furlong et al, 2001; Dias et al, 2000) The protein released from necrotic muscle may be phagocytosed by macrophages which should not be mistaken for rhabdomyoblasts.

References

Cessna MH, Zhou H, Perkins SL, et al. Are myogenin and myoD1 expression specific for rhabdomyosarcoma? A study of 150 cases, with emphasis on spindle cell mimics. American Journal of Surgical Pathology 2001;25:1150–7.

Dias P, Chen B, Dilday B, et al. Strong immunostaining for myogenin in rhabdomyosarcoma is significantly associated with tumors of the alveolar subclass. American Journal of Pathology 2000;156:399–408.

Furlong MA, Mentzel T, Fanburg-Smith JC. Pleomorphic

rhabdomyosarcoma in adults: a clinicopathologic study of 38 cases with emphasis on morphologic variants and recent skeletal muscle-specific markers. Modern Pathology 2001;14:595–603.

Guruchala A, Niezabitowski A, Wasilewska A, et al. Rhabdomyosarcoma. Morphologic, immunohistochemical and DNA study. General Diagnostic Pathology 1997;142:175–84.

Helliwell TR, Choakley JH, Walgenmakers AJ, et al. Necrotizing myopathy in critically-ill patients. Journal of Pathology 1991;164:307–14.

Kunishige M, Mitsui T, Akaike M, et al. Localisation and amount of myoglobin and myoglobin mRNA in ragged-red fiber of patients with mitochondrial encephalomyopathy. Muscle and Nerve 1996;19:175–82.

Leong AS-Y, Kan AE, Milios J. Small round cell tumours in childhood: Immunohistochemical studies in rhabdomyosarcoma, neuroblastoma, Ewing's sarcoma, and lymphoblastic lymphoma. Surgical Pathology 1989;2:5–17.

Zhang JM, Riddick L. Cytoskeleton immunohistochemical study of early ischemic myocardium. Forensic Science International 1996;80:229–38.

Neurofilaments

Sources/clones

Neurofilament triplet proteins

Antibodies are available from
Accurate (A286), Biogenex
(2F11, NF01), Dako (2F11,
NR4), Diagnostic, E Y Labs,
Enzo, Labsystems, Sera Lab (BIO-
51H, 2F11).

Neurofilament 70 kD

Antibodies are available from
Accurate, Biodesign (NR4,
DP5–1–12), Biogenesis NF01),
Boehringer Mannheim (N52),
Calbiochem, Chemicon, Cymbus
Bioscience (NR4), Immunotech
(DP5–1–12), Novocastra,
Oncogene (NR4), Sera Lab
(NR4), Serotec (DP5–1–12),
Sigma (NR4, N52), Zymed
(RMS12).

Neurofilament 150 kD

Antibodies are available from
Accurate (NN18, RNF403),
Amersham, American Research
(NF403), Chemicon, Cymbus
Bioscience (BF10), Biodesign
(DP43.16), Biogenesis (BIO-
46H, polyclonal), Boehringer
Mannheim (BF10, NN18),
Immunotech (DP43.16), Medac,
Milab (NF403), Novocastra
(BF10), Oncogene (NN-18),
RDI (BF10), Saxon (403), Sera

Lab (NN18), Sigma (NN18),
Zymed (RM0270, RM0281,
FNP7).

Neurofilament 200 kD

Antibodies are available from
Accurate (N52.1.7), Amersham,
American Research (NF402),
Biodesign (RT97), Biogenesis
(BIO-66H), Boehringer
Mannheim (RT97, NE14),
Calbiochem, Chemicon, Cymbus
Bioscience (RT97), ICN (402),
Immunotech (DP12.10), Medac,
Milab, Novocastra (RT97), RDI
(RT97), Oncogene (NE-14),
Pierce (NE14), Saxon (402), Sera
Lab (NE14), Serotec, Sigma
(NE14), Zymed (RM024, TA51).

Fixation/preparation

Most antibodies available are
immunoreactive in routine
processed tissues but the
neurofilament triplet proteins are
fixation dependent and
immunostaining is enhanced
following HIER.

Background

Neurofilaments NF) are distinct
from other intermediate filaments
(IF) in that they are composed of
three different subunits of distinct
but related proteins of 70, 150

and 200 kD as compared to other
IFs which range from 40 to 70
kD in molecular weight. The
antigenic determinants of each of
the subunits may be unique or
shared and each NF protein is a
separate gene product. NFs are
found in neurons and the
neuronal processes of the central
and peripheral nervous tissue. It is
likely that nearly all neurons can
constitutively express all three NF
genes and reports of absence of
subunits of NF in certain neurons
probably reflect technical
limitations, as the proteins are
fixation dependent. It is likely
that neurofilaments play an
important role in the health of
the neuron with recent evidence
that overexpression of NF 200kd
resulted in severe neurological
disorder while elimination of this
intermediate filament appeared to
impart resistance to some
neurotoxic agents (Gotow, 2000)

Applications

The antibodies to NFs stain all
neurons and axonal processes of
the central and peripheral
nervous system. The only
exception seems to be the
olfactory sensory neurons, which
contain only vimentin IFs and are
unique in that they die and are
replenished throughout the life

span of the mammal. The immunostaining of NF is employed for the study of neuronal distribution and innervation in normal and abnormal tissues (Krammer et al, 1994; Oki et al, 1995), and neuronal differentiation in neoplasms. The detection of NF helps identify neurons and axonal processes in cases of suspected Hirschsprung's disease. NFs are found in a variety of tumors including, neuroblastoma, ganglioglioma, medulloblastoma, retinoblastoma, pineal parenchymal tumors (Appendix 1.7, 1.37), and in neuroendocrine and neuroepithelial tumors such as Merkel cell carcinoma (Leong et al, 1986), carcinoid (Kimura et al, 1989), esthesioneuroblastoma, ganglioneuroblastoma, ganglioneuroma, neuroblastoma, oat cell carcinoma, paraganglioma, pheochromocytoma, and in teratomas with neuronal differentiation. NF may also be expressed in primitive/peripheral neuroectodermal tumors (PNETs) (Llombart-Bosch et al, 1989; Papierz et al, 1995). Anti-NF is useful in the separation of neuroblastoma and PNET from other small round cell tumors in childhood (Leong et al, 1989), which include rhabdomyosarcoma, lymphoblastic leukemia and small cell osteogenic sarcoma (Appendix 1.3). Immunohistochemical analysis for neural differentiation in Ewing sarcoma/PNET of bone and soft tissues showed good concordance with ultrastructural findings (Franchi et al, 2001).

Comments

As all neurons express all three subunits of NF, antibodies to the triplet protein should be employed in diagnostic workups for intracranial tumors and small round cell tumors in childhood.

References

Franchi A, Pasquinelli G, Cenacchi G, et al. Immunohistochemical and ultrastructural investigation of neural differentiation in Ewing sarcoma/PNET of bone and soft tissues. Ultrastructural Pathology 2001;25:219–25.

Gotow T. Neurofilaments in health and disease. Medical Electron Microscopy 2000;33:173–99.

Kimura N, Sasano N, Namiki T. Coexpression of cytokeratin, neurofilament and vimentin in carcinoid tumors. Virchows Archives (A Pathology and Anatomy) 1989;415:69–77.

Krammer HJ, Karahan ST, Sigge W, Kuhnel W. Immunohistochemistry of markers of the enteric nervous system in whole-mount preparations of the human colon. European Journal of Pediatric Surgery 1994;4:274–8.

Leong AS-Y, Phillips GE, Pieterse AS. Criteria for the diagnosis of primary neuroendocrine carcinoma of the skin (Merkel cell carcinoma). A histological, immunohistochemical and ultrastructural study of 13 cases. Pathology 1986;18:393–9.

Leong AS-Y, Kan AE, Milios J. Small round cell tumors in childhood: Immunohistochemical studies in rhabdomyosarcoma, neuroblastoma, Ewing's sarcoma, and lymphoblastic lymphoma. Surgical Pathology 1989;2:5–17.

Llombart-Bosch A, Terrier-Lancombe MJ, Peydro-Olaya A, Contesso G. Peripheral neuroectodermal sarcoma of soft tissue (peripheral neuroepithelioma): a pathologic study of ten cases with differential diagnosis regarding other small round cell sarcomas. Human Pathology 1989;20:273–80.

Oki T, Fukuda N, Kawano T, et al. Histopathologic studies of innervation of normal and prolapsed mitral valves. Journal of heart Valve Disease 1995;4:496–502.

Papierz W, Alwasiak J, Kolasa P, et al. Primitive neuroectodermal tumors: ultrastructural and immunohistochemical studies. Ultrastructural Pathology 1995;19:147–66.

Neuron-Specific Enolase (NSE)

Sources/clones

Accurate (BBSNCU1), American Research (5G10, NH3), Axcel, Biodesign (MIG-N3, 5E2), Biogenesis (BG10), Biogenex (MIG-N3), Biotec (XNE12), Cymbus Bioscience (5E2), Dako (BBS-NC, VI-H14), Immunotech, Novocastra (VI-H14, SE2), Research Diagnostics (5E2, 5G10, 5A4), Sanbio (MIG-N3), Sera-Lab (MIG-N3), Serotec (MIG-N3), Shandon (BBS-NC, VI-H14), and Zymed.

Fixation/preparation

Both polyclonal and monoclonal antibodies are immunoreactive in routinely prepared tissue sections. HIER enhances Immunostaining.

Background

Neuron-specific enolase (NSE) is the glycolytic isoenzyme of the enolase gamma-gamma dimer specifically detected in neurons and neuroendocrine cells, and their corresponding tumors (Wich et al, 1983; Venores et al, 1984). In addition, NSE has been demonstrated in the non-neoplastic cells of the pituitary, peptide secreting tissues, pinealocytes, neuroendocrine cells of the lung, thyroid, parafollicular cells, adrenal medulla, islets of Langerhans, Merkel cells of the skin (Leong et al, 1986) and melanocytes. NSE immunostaining is also positive in normal striated muscle, hepatocytes and, to a lesser extent, smooth muscle (Cooper, 1994).

While highly sensitive, NSE has low specificity. Antibodies to NSE enjoyed great popularity in the earlier days of diagnostic immunohistochemistry as a marker of neural and neuroendocrine differentiation. However, it was soon realized that most anti-NSE preparations showed a high rate of unwanted cross-reactivity even among the monoclonal antibodies, and a high level of background staining often made interpretation difficult. NSE has since become known facetiously as "non-specific enolase" (Bjerkehagen et al, 1994). While its application in immunohistochemistry is limited, assays for NSE are being increasingly performed as diagnostic and prognostic markers in the serum, pleural effusions and cerebrospinal fluid in cases of head injury, status epilepticus, small cell carcinoma of the lung, neuroblastoma, various neuroendocrine tumors, germ cell tumors and malignant melanoma.

Applications

NSE is still a useful marker to identify peripheral nerves (Leonard et al, 1995). In the context of desmoplastic melanomas, which are often negative for the melanoma-specific markers HMB45 and NKIC3, NSE and S100 are sensitive markers (Abstey et al, 1994). S100-positive spindle cells were found in the scars of previously biopsied cases of atypical nevi and melanomas (20/20) and non-nevomelanocytic lesions (9/10). NSE diffusely stained the fibroblast population in the two cases of non-nevomelanocytic lesions that were further studied with a number of other melanocytic markers, which were all negative (Chorny & Barr, 2002). When used for the identification of neuroendocrine differentiation, it is necessary that it be employed in a panel with more specific markers such as chromogranin, PHE 5 and synaptophysin. NSE positivity has been demonstrated in a many as 83% of testicular carcinoma-in-situ as well as in overt testicular germ cell tumors including seminomas, non-seminomas and mixed germ cell tumors (Kang et al, 1996).

Pyothorax-associated lymphoma is also diffusely positive for NSE (71%) and NSE is less frequently positive in other lymphomas (15%) (Nakatsuka et al, 2002).

Comments

Monoclonal antibodies to NSE produce less background staining; however, specificity is only slightly increased. PGP 9.5 stains a very similar spectrum of cells and tumors. As PGP 9.5 shows greater sensitivity it would serve as a suitable substitute for NSE; however, either marker should be used in isolation especially when employed for the identification of neuroendocrine differentiation.

References

Anstey A, Cerio R, Ramnarain N, et al. Desmoplastic malignant melanoma. An immunocytological study of 25 cases. American Journal of Dermatopathology 1994;16:14–22.

Bjerkehagen B, Fossa SD, Raabe N, et al. Transitional cell carcinoma of the renal pelvis and its expression of p53 protein, c-erbB-2 protein, neuron-specific enolase, Phe 5, chromogranin, laminin and collagen type IV. European Urology 1994;26:334–9.

Chorny JA, Barr RJ. S100-positive spindle cells in scars: a diagnostic pitfall in the re-excision of desmoplastic melanoma. American Journal of Dermatopathology 2002;24:309–12.

Cooper EH. Neuron-specific enolase. International Journal of Biological Markers 1994;9:205–10.

Kang JL, Meyts ER, Skakkeback NE. Immunoreactive neuron-specific enolase (NSE) is expressed in testicular carcinoma-in-situ. Journal of Pathology 1996;178:161–5.

Leonard N, Hourihane DO, Whelan A. Neuroproliferation in the mucosa is a feature of coeliac disease and Crohn's disease. Gut 1995;37:763–5.

Leong AS-Y, Phillips GE, Pieterse AS. Criteria for the diagnosis of primary endocrine carcinoma of the skin (Merkel cell carcinoma). A histological, immunohistochemical and ultrastructural study of 13 cases. Pathology 1986;18:393–9.

Leong AS-Y, Kan AE, Milios J. Small round cell tumors in childhood: Immunohistochemical studies in rhabdomyosarcoma, neuroblastoma, Ewing's sarcoma and lymphoblastic lymphoma. Surgical Pathology 1989;2:5–17.

Nakatsuka S, Nishiu M, Tomita Y, et al. Enhanced expression of neuron specific enolase (NSE) in pyothorax-associated lymphoma (PAL). Japanese Journal of Cancer Research 2002;93:411–6.

Venores SA, Bonnin JM, Rubinstein LF. Immunohistochemical demonstration of NSE in neoplasms of the CNS and other tissues. Archives of Pathology and Laboratory Medicine 1984;108:536–40.

Wick MR, Sheithauer BW, Kovacs E. NSE in neuroendocrine tumors of the thymus, bronchus and skin. American Journal of Clinical Pathology 1983;29:703–7.

Neutrophil elastase

Sources/clones

Axcel/Accurate (MP57),
Biogenesis (AHN-10),
Calbiochem (polyclonal),
Chemicon (AHN10), Dako
(NP57).

Fixation/preparation

NP57 may be used on both
formalin-fixed paraffin-embedded
sections and frozen sections. If
other fixatives are used, eg,
acetone or methanol, there is a
tendency for the antigen to
diffuse from the myeloid cell
cytoplasm and to localize in the
cell nucleus.

Background

Neutrophil elastase is a neutral
protease, which plays a major role
in the killing of micro-organisms
and in the initiation of tissue
injury during inflammatory
reactions. The enzyme is present
in the primary (azurophilic)
granules of myeloid cells.
Neutrophil elastase consists of
three isoenzymes with similar
molecular masses (approximately
30 kD) (Ohlsson & Olsson,
1974). Monoclonal anti-
neutrophil elastase (NP57) was
raised against human neutrophil
granule proteins (Pulford et al,

1988). This antibody labels
neutrophils in routinely processed
histological specimens and also
reacts (although more weakly)
with a minor population of
normal blood monocytes. Other
cell types, including epithelial
cells, are NP57 negative (Pulford
et al, 1988).

Applications

Neoplastic cells in 27/37 (73%)
bone marrow specimens of acute
myeloid leukemia were NP57
positive (Ralfkiaer et al, 1989).
The number of positive cells
varied from few (5–10%) to
virtually all of the cells. In
routinely processed biopsy
specimens from lymphoid organs
with extramedullary
haematopoiesis or infiltrates of
chronic myeloid leukemia, NP57
was confined to neutrophils and
their precursors (Ralfkiaer et al,
1989). Other studies (van der
Schoot et al, 1990; Traweek et al,
1993) have demonstrated NP57
positivity in 53% of acute
myeloid leukemia and 54% of
extramedullary myeloid cell
tumors respectively. These
percentages appear to be slightly
lower than that obtained when
staining for myeloperoxidase. This
probably indicates that elastase is
synthesized later during myeloid

maturation than myeloperoxidase.
Leukemias of lymphoid origin
are not stained.

Comments

The detection of elastase with
monoclonal NP57 forms a useful
supplement to other
immunohistochemical markers
for myeloid disorders. However, a
recent study that compared a
variety of markers for myeloid
precursors in granulocytic
sarcoma concluded that CD43,
lysozyme, myeloperoxidase and
CD15 were the most sensitive
markers staining a large
proportion of the cells of the
majority of well-differentiated
tumors and a smaller proportion
of poorly differentiated/blastic
tumors. Neutrophil elastase was
the least sensitive of the markers
of myeloid differentiation
including chloroacetate esterase
histochemical staining (Menasce
et al, 1999).

References

Menasce LP, Banerjee SS, Beckett E,
    Harris M. Exgtra-medullary
    myeloid tumor (granulocytic
    sarcoma) is often misdiagnosed: a
    study of 26 cases. Histopathology
    1999;34:391–8.
Ohlsson K, Olsson I. The neutral
    proteases of human granulocytes.
    Isolation and partial

characterization of granulocyte elastases. European Journal of Biochemistry 1974;42:519–27.

Pulford KAF, Erber WN, Crick JA, Olsson I, Gatter KC, Mason DY. Monoclonal antibody against human neutrophil elastase for the study of normal and leukaemic myeloid cells. Journal of Clinical Pathology 1988;41:853–60.

Ralfiaier E, Pulford KAF, Lauritzen AF, Armstrom S, Guldhammer B, Mason DY. Diagnosis of acute myeloid leukaemia with the use of monoclonal anti-neutrophil elastase (NP-57) reactive with routinely processed biopsy samples. Histopathology 1989;14:637–43.

Traweek ST, Arber DA, Rappaport H, Brynes RK. Extramedullary myeloid cell tumors: an immunohistochemical and morphologic study of 28 cases. American Journal of Surgical Pathology 1993;17:1011–19.

Van der Schoot CE, Daams GM, Pinkster J, Vet R, von dem Borne AEG. Monoclonal antibodies against myeloperoxidase are valuable immunological reagents for the diagnosis of acute myeloid leukaemia. British Journal of Haematology 1990;74:173–8.

nm23/NME1

Sources/clones

Accurate (NM301),
Accurate/Novocastra (37.6),
Dako (polyclonal), Novocastra
(nm23–301, polyclonal),
Oncogene (NM301, polyclonal),
Pharmingen (NM301).

Fixation/preparation

Some of the available antibodies
are immunoreactive in fixed,
paraffin-embedded sections.
HIER is required.

Background

The nm23 gene family was
originally identified in a murine
melanoma cell-line and nm23 H1
was found to be transcribed at a
10-fold higher rate in cells of
lower metastatic potential. Two
highly homologous human genes
have subsequently been identified
– nmE1 and nmE2, located on
chromosomes 17q, and coding
for the 18.5 and 17 kD proteins
nm23 H1 and nm23 H2
respectively. nm23 is mainly
cytoplasmic, but nuclear and
membrane localisation has also
been seen (Urano et al 1993).

Applications

The nm23 gene product was
believed initially to play a role in
suppressing tumor metastasis. This
may be too simplistic a view,
with both metastasis suppression
and disease progression being
linked to elevated gene
expression in different tumors.
Isotype-specific studies on breast
neoplasms have indicated that it is
nm23 H1 and not nm23 H2 that
correlates with metastases (Royds
et al 1993). A recent report found
statistical correlation between
nm23-H1 and tenascin
immunoexpression and a
statistical correlation between
nm23-H1 immunoexpression and
lymph node metastases (Kaya et
al, 2002). Somatic allelic deletions
of nm23 H1 have been reported
in some human neoplasms such
as breast, kidney, colon, and lung
cancer; in some cases associated
with an increased incidence of
metastases (Leone et al 1991).
The loss of nm23 function
appears to correlate with
phenotypic markers of metastatic
potential in some human tumors.

However, there is no strong
evidence of direct involvement of
the nm23 in metastasis, and a
bystander effect rather than a
causative role for nm23 cannot
be ruled out, the reduced nm23
level being a reflection of a more
dedifferentiated state of the
tumor. nm23 expression
correlates inversely with
metastatic potential in in vitro
and experimental animal systems,
with transfection of the nm23
gene into melanoma K1735 cells
resulting in a reduction of tumor
metastases.

Preliminary studies in
esophageal carcinoma (Patel et al
1997) indicate that failure to
express p53 and nm23 may be
related to an unfavorable
prognosis in patients with
advanced esophageal carcinoma.
Similarly, there is reduced staining
of nm23-H1 in laryngeal
squamous cell carcinoma
compared with laryngeal polyps
(Lee CS et al 1996b). In contrast,
progression of ovarian carcinoma
is accompanied by overexpression
of nm23 protein (Harlozinska et
al 1996; Srivatsa PJ et al 1996).
While some studies suggest that
overexpression of nm23-H1 is an
early event in the development of
prostatic adenocarcinoma (Myers
et al 1996; Igawa et al 1994),
others show elevated levels of
nm23-H1 and H2 in benign
prostatic hyperplasia and postulate
a role in the suppression of
malignancy (Konishi et al 1993).

In pituitary adenoma, strong
expression of nm23 H2 is
associated with noninvasive
adenomas, and may restrain
tumor aggression (Takino et al
1995). Expression in uveal

melanoma appears to be inversely proportional to the depth of scleral invasion (Greco et al 1997), however, in melanoma of the skin, there are conflicting studies. Lee et al (1996a) found reduced nm23-H1 immunohistological expression to be associated with melanomas that have high metastatic potential and poorer prognosis. Kanitakis et al (1997) found nm23 does not have a direct correlation with metastatic potential.

In transitional cell carcinoma of the bladder (Shiina et al 1996) and FIGO Stage IB cervical carcinoma (Kristensen et al 1996), nm23 protein immunoreactivity is not an independent prognostic factor. Staining for nm23 has little value in testicular seminoma, where expression of both the nm23-H1 and nm23-H2 proteins was found not to be associated with metastatic or invasive status of the tumor (Hori et al 1997).

Expression of nm23 protein (and c-ras products) was significantly decreased in complete hydatidiform moles that progressed to gestational trophoblastic tumors compared to those that remitted spontaneously after evacuation. The decreased expression of nm23 protein and increased expression of c-erbB-2 protein were strong predictors for the malignant transformation of complete mole (Yang et al, 2002). Similar studies have shown nm23 to be a significant factor for predicting a favourable prognosis in non-small cell carcinoma of the lung (Katakura et al, 2002; Graham et al, 2002), and laryngeal squamous cell carcinoma (Sikorska et al, 2002).

Comments

Polyclonal antiserum to nm23 produces strong cytoplasmic staining after HIER.

References

Graham AN, Maxwell P, Mulholland K, et al. Increased nm23 immunoreactivity is associated with selective inhibition of systemic tumour cell dissemination. Journal of Clinical Pathology 2002;55:184–9.

Greco IM, Calvisi G, Ventura L, Cerrito F. An immunohistochemical analysis of nm23 gene product expression in uveal melanoma. Melanoma Research 1997;7:231–6.

Harlozinska A, Bar JK, Gerber J. nm23 expression in tissue sections and tumor effusion cells of ovarian neoplasms. International Journal of Cancer 1996;69:415–9

Hori K, Uematsu K, Yaswoshima H, et al. Immunohistochemical analysis of the nm23 gene products in testicular seminoma. Pathology International 1997;47:288–92.

Igawa M, Rukstalis DB, Tanabe T, Chodak GW. High levels of nm23 expression are related to cell proliferation in human prostate cancer. Cancer Research 1994;54:1313–8.

Kanitakis J, Euvrard S, Bourchany D, et al. Expression of the nm23 metastasis-suppressor gene product in skin tumors. Journal of Cutaneous Pathology 1997;24:151–6.

Katakura H, Tanaka F, Oyanagi H, et al. Clinical significance of nm23 expression in resected pathologic stage 1, non-small cell lung cancer. Annals of Thoracic Surgery 2002;73:1060–4.

Kaya H, Hucumenoglu S, Bozkurt SU, et al. Expression of nm23 and tenascin in invasive ductal carcinomas of the breast. European Journal of Gynecologic Oncology 2002;23:261–3.

Konishi N, Nakaoka S, Tsuzuki T, et al. Expression of nm23-H1 and nm23-H2 proteins in prostate carcinoma. Japanese Journal of Cancer Research 1993;84:1050–4.

Kristensen GB, Holm R, Abeler VM, Trope CG. Evaluation of the prognostic signifcance of nm23/NDP kinase protein expression in cervical carcinoma: an immunohistochemical study. Gynecological Oncology 1996;61:378–83.

Lee CS, Pirdas A, Lee MW. Immunohistochemical demonstration of the nm23-H1 gene product in human malignant melanoma and Spitz nevi. Pathology 1996a;28:220–4.

Lee CS, Redshaw A, Boag G. nm23-H1 protein immunoreactivity in laryngeal carcinoma. Cancer 1996b;77:2246–50.

Leone A, McBride OW, Weston A. Somatic allelic deletion of nm23 in human cancer. Cancer Research 1991;51:2490–3.

Myers RB, Srivastava S, Oelschlager DK, et al. Expression of nm23-H1 in prostatic intraepithelial neoplasia and adenocarcinoma. Human Pathology 1996;27:1021–4.

Patel DD, Bhatavdekar JM, Chikhlikar PR et al. Clinical significance of p53, nm23, and bcl-2 in T3–4N1M0 oesophageal carcinoma: an immunohistochemical approach. Journal of Surgical Oncology 1997;65:111–6.

Royds JA, Stephenson TJ, Rees RC. nm23 protein expression in ductal in situ and invasive human breast carcinoma. Journal of the National Cancer Institute 1993;85:727–31.

Shiina H, Igawa M, Nagami H, et al. Immunohistochemical analysis of proliferating cell nuclear antigen, p53 protein and nm23 protein, and nuclear DNA content in transitional cell carcinoma of the bladder. Cancer 1996;78:1762–74.

Sikorska B, Danilewicz M, Wagrowska-Danilewicz M. Prognostic significance of

CD44v6 and nm23 protein immunoexpression in laryngeal squamous cell carcinoma. Polish Journal of Pathology 2002;53:17–24.

Srivatsa PJ, Cliby WA, Keeney GL, et al. Elevated nm23 protein expression is correlated with diminished progression-free survival in patients with epithelial ovarian carcinoma. Gynecological Oncology 1996;60:363–72.

Takino H, Herman V, Weiss M, Melmed S. Purine-binding factor

(nm23) gene expression in pituitary tumors: marker of adenoma invasiveness. Journal of Clinical Endocrinology and Metabolism 1995;80:1733–8.

Urano T, Furukawa K, Shiku H. Expression of nm23/NDP kinase proteins on the cell surface. Oncogene 1993;8:1371–6.

Yang X, Zhang Z, Jia C, et al. The relationship between expression of c–ras, c–erbB-2, nm23 and p53 gene products and development of trophoblastic tumor and their

predictive significance for the malignant transformation of complete hydatidiform mole. Gynecological Oncology 2002;85:438–44.

NOTES

Osteopontin

Source/clone

Santa Cruz (OPN (K-20): SC-10591, goat polyclonal antibody), National Institute for Dental Research (OPN LF7, rabbit polyclonal antibody).

Fixation/preparation

OPN LF7 is applicable to formalin-fixed, paraffin-embedded tissue sections.

Background

Osteopontin (OPN, also designated Bone Sialoprotein 1, Urinary Stone Protein, spp-1, eta-1, nephropontin, uropontin) is an extracellular matrix cell adhesion phosphoglycoprotein (Butler, 1989). OPN is produced predominantly by osteoblasts but is also synthesized by brain and kidney cells. OPN is deposited into unmineralized matrix at the cement lines before calcification, and between collagen fibrils of fully matured tissue (McKee and Nanci, 1996). OPNs isolated from or secreted by various tissues have molecular weights between 44 and 75 kD, due to post-translational modifications (Butler, 1995). OPN exists in multiple forms, such as glycosylated, phosphorylated and cleaved mature forms of approximately 66–68 kD molecular weight protein suggestive of diverse functions in various tissues.

OPN functions as a substrate for transglutaminase and is involved in cell adhesion (Denhardt & Guo, 1993). OPN (K-20) is an affinity-purified goat polyclonal antibody raised against a peptide mapping near the carboxy terminus of osteopontin of human origin.

Whilst OPN was originally extracted from bone extracellular matrix stroma, it has also been detected in normal epithelia of various organs with luminal epithelial surfaces (Brown et al, 1992). OPN has been detected in breast, endometrial and renal adenocarcinomas where it has been postulated to function in adhesive interaction of cancer cells with the extracellular matrix, influencing biological behavior (Bellahcene & Castronovo, 1995; Brown et al, 1994). A study of primary ovarian tumors and their metastases from 30 patients demonstrated weak or absent immunoexpression in the majority of ovarian adenocarcinomas and their metastases. In contrast, the majority of borderline ovarian tumors were OPN immunopositive, suggesting a potential importance in the pathogenesis of ovarian BOTs (Tiniakos et al, 1998). Lung, gastrointestinal, prostate, bladder and other human carcinomas do not express OPN (Brown et al, 1994). OPN was detected in the cytoplasm of infiltrating leukocytes, granulation tissue cells, fibroblasts and mast cells in the peritoneum of patients with peritoneal calcification following long-term continuous peritoneal dialysis (Nakasato et al, 2002) and was also found in all calcified vessels in patients with calciphylaxis or calcific uremic arteriopathy (Ahmed et al, 2001).

Applications

OPN currently has no diagnostic applications. It may have a role in the genesis of some cancers as has been suggested with hepatocellular carcinoma (Gotoh et al, 2002) and squamous cell carcinoma of the lung (Zhang et al, 2001).

References

Ahmed S, O'Neill KD, Hood AF, et al. Calciphylaxis is associated with hyperphosphatemia and increased osteopontin expression by vascular smooth muscle cells. American Journal of Kidney Diseases 2001;37:1267–76.

Bellahcene A, Castronovo V. Increased expression of osteonectin and osteopontin, two bone matrix proteins, in human breast cancer. The American Journal of Pathology 1995;146:95–100.

Brown LF, Berse B, Van De Water L, et al. Expression and distribution of osteopontin in human tissues: widespread association with luminal epithelial surfaces. Molecular Biology of the Cell 1992;3:1169–80.

Brown LF, Papadopoulos-Sergiou A, Berse B, et al. Osteopontin expression and distribution in human carcinomas. The American Journal of Pathology 1994;145:610–23.

Butler WT. The nature and significance of osteopontin. Connective Tissue Research 1989;23:123–36.

Butler WT. Structural and functional domains of osteopontin. Annals of the New York Academy of Sciences 1995;760:6–11.

Denhardt T, Guo X. Osteopontin: a protein with diverse functions. The FASEB Journal 1993;7:475–82.

Gotoh M, Sakamoto M, Kanetaka K, et al. Overexpression of osteopontin in hepatocellular carcinoma. Pathology International 2002;52:19–24.

McKee MD, Nanci A. Osteopontin at mineralized tissue interfaces in bone, teeth and osseointegrated implants: ultrastructural distribution and implications for mineralized tissue formation, turnover, and repair. Microscopy Research & Technique 1996;33:141–64.

Nakazato Y, Yamaji Y, Oshima N, et al. Calcification and osteopontin localization in the peritoneum of patients on long-term continuous ambulatory peritoneal dialysis therapy. Nephrology, Dialysis and Transplantation 2002;17:1293–303.

Tiniakos DG, Yu H, Liapis H. Osteopontin expression in ovarian carcinomas and tumors of low malignant potential (LMP). Human Pathology 1998;29:1250–4.

Zhang J, Takahashi K, Takahashi F, et al. Differential osteopontin expression in lung cancer. Cancer Letters 2001;171:215–22.

Osteopontin

P27kip1

Sources/clones

Lab Vision Corp (DCS70), Pharmingen (G173–524), Transduction Laboratory.

Fixation/preparation

The anti-p27 antibody is immunoreactive in fixed paraffin-embedded sections but only following HIER in citrate buffer at neutral pH.

Background

The p27kip1 (p27) gene encodes an inhibitor of cyclin-dependent kinase (CDK) activity. Two families of proteins that generally inhibit cell cycle progression regulate the activity of cyclin-dependent kinase complexes. These are the INK4 group of p16, p15, p18 and p19 which may have suppressor functions and whose activities are dependent on a normal retinoblastoma protein and show maximal expression during S-phase, and the group of CDK inhibitors which include p21/WAF1/CIP1, p27kip1 and p57/kip2. Overexpression of the latter group inhibits kinase activities of several cyclins and causes cell cycle arrest. The role of kip protein in regulating cell cycle progression in normal and neoplastic cells has not been elucidated although p27-deficient mice develop multiple organ hyperplasia suggesting that this CDK inhibitor has anti-proliferative activity in vivo (Toyoshima & Hunter, 1994; Hengst & Reed, 1996).

Applications

Several studies have revealed a marked decrease in the percentage of cells expressing p27 in benign and malignant neoplasms compared to normal tissues, with an inverse relationship to Ki-67 antigen, a marker of cell proliferation. Studies with transgenic knockout mice deficient in p27 have shown that p27 protein inhibits proliferation in tissues such as the thymus, pituitary and spleen, leading to hyperplasias of these organs. The exact role of p27 abnormalities in tumor development remains uncertain. Mutations are relatively uncommon in the p27 gene and other mechanisms such as translational control with decreased p27 or down-regulation of p27 by specific mitogens may occur during tumor development. The observations that p27 levels are markedly decreased in highly malignant tumors such as anaplastic thyroid carcinomas compared with normal thyroid and benign adenomas suggests that loss of p27 expression may be associated with tumor progression.

Evaluation of p27 protein has the potential of predicting the biological behavior of various neoplasms and can be employed to study cell cycle regulation during tumor progression. Recent data show loss or low immunoexpression of p57 with poor prognosis or lymph node metastasis in patients with astrocytoma (Sxhiffer et al, 2002), cervical carcinoma (Huang et al, 2002), rectal carcinoma (Schwandner et al, 2002), papillary thyroid carcinoma (Khoo et al, 2002), renal cell carcinoma (Migita et al, 2002), and gastric carcinoma (Liu et al, 2001). The results in breast carcinoma have been conflicting and describe decreased immunoexpression to be associated with lymph node metastasis in one study in men (Anderson et al, 2002), and high levels in tumors with nodal metastasis in another study of women (Kouvaraki et al, 2002). Parodoxical overexpression of p27 has been described in endometrioid adenocarcinoma of the uterus with lymph node metastasis, myometrial invasion and advanced stage disease (Watanabe et al, 2002).

Comments

The antibody from Transduction Laboratory, Lexington, KY, is immunoreactive in routine-fixed paraffin-embedded tissues (Lloyd et al, 1997). The antigen is located in the nucleus.

References

Anderson J, Reddy VB, Green L, et al. Role of expression o cell cycle inhibitor p27 and MIB-1 in predicting lymph node metastasis in male breast carcinoma. Breast Journal 2002;8:101–7.

Huang LW, Chao SL, Hwang JL, Chou YY. Down-regulation of p27 is associated with malignant transformation and aggressive phenotype of cervical neoplasms. Gynecologic Oncology 2002;85:524–8.

Kouvaraki M, Gorgoulis VG, Rassidakis GZ, et al. High expression levels of p27 correlate with lymph node status in a subset of advanced invasive breast carcinomas: relation to E-cadherin alterations, proliferative activity, and ploidy of the tumors. Cancer 2002;94:2454–65.

Lloyd RV, Jin L, Qian X, Kulig E. Aberrant p27^{kip1}expression in endocrine and other tumors. American Journal of Pathology 1997;150:401–7.

Toyoshima H, Hunter T. p27, a novel inhibitor of G1 cyclin-Cdk protein kinase activity is related to p21. Cell 1994;78:67–74.

Hengst L, Reed SI. Translational control of p27^{kip1} accumulation during the cell cycle. Science 1996;271:1861–4.

Khoo ML, Beasley NJ, Ezzat S, et al. Overexpression of cyclin D1 and underexpression of p27 predict lymph node metastases in papillary thyroid carcinoma. Journal of Clinical Endocrinology and Metabolism 2002;87:1814–8.

Liu XP, Kawauchi S, Oga A, et al. Combined examination of p27 (Kip1), p21 (Waf1/Cip1) and p53 expression allows precise estimation of prognosis in patients with gastric carcinoma. Histopatholopgy 2001;39:603–10.

Migita T, Oda Y, Naito S, Tsuneyoshi M. Low expression of p27 (Kip1) is associated with tumor size and poor prognosis in patients with renal cell carcinoma. Cancer 2002;94:973–9.

Schiffer D, Cavalla P, Fiano V, et al. Inverse relationship between p27/kip 1 and the F-box protein Skp2 in human astrocytic gliomas by immunohistochemistry and Western blot. Neuroscience Letters 2002;328:125–8.

Schwandner O, Bruch HP, Broll R. p21, p27, cyclin D1, and p53 in rectal cancer: immunohistology with prognostic significance? International Journal of Colorectal Diseases 2002:17:11–9.

Watanabe J, Sato H, Kanai T, et al. Paradoxical expression of cell cycle inhibitor p27 in endometrioid adenocarcinoma of the uterine corpus – correlation with proliferation and clinicopathological parameters. British Journal of Cancer 2002;87:81–5.

p53

Sources/clones

Antibodies to both wild type and mutant p53 are available from Accurate, Biodesign (Pab1801, 53–12), BioSource, Bioprobe (BP53–12), Chemicon, Cymbus Bioscience, Medac (CM-1), Dako (DO-7), Immunotech, Novocastra, Oncogene (Pab1801, Pab421, Pab122), Oncor, Pharmingen (G59–12), Serotec (Pab1801, BP53–12) and Signet.

Antibodies to mutant p53

Biogenesis, Chemicon and Oncogene (Pab240).

Antibodies to wild type p53

Biodesign (Pab246), Oncogene (Pab1620) and Serotec (Pab246).

Fixation/preparation

Fresh or frozen tissues, clones Pab1801 and DO7 effective in formalin fixed tissue and with best results following MW epitope retrieval.

Background

In the current constellation of oncogenes and recessive tumor suppressor genes, the p53 molecule represents one of the most common genetic changes associated with human cancer, being implicated in a wide range of malignancies. The p53 gene displays several unusual features, the most important of which is the ability to act as either a dominant oncogene or a recessive tumor-suppressor gene. A combination of genetic events that affect both alleles of the gene results in the loss of expression of wild-type (WT) p53. This may occur as a complete loss of one allele of the gene as a result of a large chromosomal deletion combined with a point missense mutation on the other allele. Mutation leads to the loss of DNA binding and transcriptional regulatory activities of the p53 phosphoprotein with a corresponding loss of its growth suppressive activity and its role as "the guardian of the genome". The mutated protein has abnormal conformation, impaired DNA-binding, and a prolonged or stabilized half-life, the latter resulting in immunohistochemically stainable levels within nuclei in nearly all tumors showing p53 gene mutation. While a loss of transformation-suppression activity and a gain of transforming potential often accompany mutation of p53, not all p53 mutants are equal in terms of their biological activity. Mutations at different hot spots manifest different and distinct phenotypes and there is geographic variation in the sites of mutations thought to reflect the effects of different environmental and regional carcinogens and co-factors.

The p53 gene is located on the short arm of human chromosome 17 and the majority of mutations in the gene are clustered in the most highly conserved domains spanned by 4–9 axons. An important relationship exists between DNA damage hot spots and the capacity to repair the DNA as mutation abolishes the arrest or delay seen in the normal cellular response to DNA damage. Although the WT p53 gene product is not essential for progress of cells through the cell cycle, it does negatively regulate cell growth or division. By binding to specific DNA sequences, the p53 WT product is able to inhibit adjacent gene transcription and serves to prevent uncontrolled cellular proliferation. Thus loss of WT p53 activity induces a release from G1-S cell cycle checkpoint control following DNA damage, increasing genomic instability and promoting gene amplification. Binding of WT p53 to a variety of viral proteins such as protein E6, a product of the human papilloma virus, Simian virus 40 T-antigen and the Epstein-Barr nuclear antigen, as well as to cellular proteins such as heat-shock protein 70 and MDM-2 replication protein, may result in an inactivated complex and a loss of transformation-suppression activity (Chang et al, 1993; Batsakis & El-Naggar, 1995).

Applications

Immunohistochemical detection of nuclear p53 protein is based on the increase in concentration of the protein to detectable levels, secondary to an increased synthesis and a lower degradation with longer half-life. In general, there is good agreement between the frequency of positive immunostaining and the frequency of tumors with mutations detected by direct DNA sequencing. However, there are discrepancies between these findings and analysis at the protein level. There is also a danger in assuming positive staining to be an indication of an underlying mutation as p53 protein can be stabilized by other means such as sequestration of normal nuclear protein in the cytoplasm with inactivation of its tumor suppressor function or by binding with the cellular proteins previously mentioned (Hall &

Lane, 1994). Also, the use of anti-p53 antibodies that do not react with all mutant forms and other events may lead to failure to detect p53 in neoplasms. The analysis of p53 in neoplastic and pre-neoplastic states is a powerful tool which provides molecular information on the oncogenic process and the ability to stain for abnormal forms of the protein in tissue sections, particularly those fixed in formalin, allows an important avenue of investigation. Furthermore, there is evidence to suggest that the expression of abnormal p53 may be a prognostic parameter in some neoplasms (Batsakis & El-Naggar, 1995) including phyllodes tumor of the breast (Tse et al, 2002), high-risk breast cancer patients undergoing high dose chemotherapy (Hensel et al, 2002), and thyroid neoplasms (Hosal et al, 1997).

Comments

Immunostaining of p53 can be affected by degradation of antigen during tissue processing and it is important to recognize the fixation conditions and the nature of the antibody employed (Fisher et al, 1994). Monoclonal antibody PabI801 (Biogenesis, Gibco BRL and Medac) recognizes most of the mutant and wild-types of p53 but 1801 is not suitable for paraffin-embedded tissues. Our own experience is largely with DO7 (Medac, Biogenex, Dako) which

identifies both wild-type and mutant protein in formalin-fixed paraffin-embedded sections and best results are obtained after MW epitope retrieval.

References

Batsakis JG, El-Naggar AK. p53: 15 years after discovery. Advances in Anatomic Pathology 1995;2:71–88.

Chang F, Syrjanen S, Tervahauta A, Syrjanen K. Tumorigenesis associated with the p53 tumour suppressor gene. British Journal of Cancer 1993;68:653–61.

Fisher DJ, Gillett CE, Vojtesek B, et al. Problems with p53 immunohistochemical staining: the effect of fixation and variation in the methods of evaluation. British Journal of Cancer 1994;69:26–31.

Hall PA, Lane DP. p53 in tumour pathology: can we trust immunohistochemistry? – Revisited. Journal of Pathology 1994;172:1–4.

Hensel M, Schneeweiss A, Sinn HP, et al. p53 is the strongest predictor of survival in high-risk primary breast cancer patients undergoing high-dose chemotherapy with autologous blood stem cell support. International Journal of Cancer 2002;100:290–6.

Hosal SA, Apel RL, Freeman JL, et al. Immunohistochemical localisation of p53 in human thyroid neoplasms: correlation with biological behavior. Endocrine Pathology 1997;8:21–8.

Tse GM, Putti TC, Kung FY, et al. Increased p53 protein expression in mammary phyllodes tumors. Modern Pathology 2002;15:734–40.

Pancreatic Hormones (insulin, somatostatin, vasoactive intestinal polypeptide, gastrin, glucagon, pancreatic polypeptide)

Pancreatic endocrine tumors have been associated with several distinct clinical syndromes, such as hypoglycaemia, glucagonoma syndrome, Zollinger-Ellison syndrome, and WDHA (watery diarrhoea, hypokalaemia and achlorhydria) syndrome (Mukai et al, 1982). Routine histological examination usually fails to predict the behavior and endocrine manifestations of these neoplasms (Creutzfeldt, 1980). Immunohistochemistry permits the specific demonstration of various pancreatic hormones in tissue sections.

Sources/clones

Insulin

Accurate (K36AC10), Axcel/Accurate (polyclonal), Biodesign (MAb 1, E2-E3, polyclonal), Biogenesis (E6E5, D4B8, IN05, C7C9, polyclonal), Biogenex (AE9D6, polyclonal), Caltag Laboratories (polyclonal), Cymbus Bioscience (MAB1), Research Diagnostics (MAB1), Dako (polyclonal), E-Y Labs, Fitzgerald (M91284, M91285, M322212, M322213, polyclonal), Immunotech Inc/Immunotech SA (E2E3), Novocastra (polyclonal), Research Diagnostics, Sanbio/Monosan (N-05, polyclonal), Sigma Chemical (K36AC10), Zymed (Z005, Z006, polyclonal).

Somatostatin

Accurate (YC7, BM17), Axcel/Accurate (polyclonal), Biogenesis (170.3, polyclonal), Biogenex (polyclonal), Caltag Laboratories (polyclonal), Dako (polyclonal), Fitzgerald (polyclonal), Novocastra (polyclonal), Pharmingen (YC7), Sanbio/Monosan (polyclonal), Zymed (polyclonal).

Vasoactive intestinal polypeptide (VIP)

Accurate, Biodesign (polyclonal), Biogenesis (VIP-001), Biogenex (polyclonal), Immunotech (103.10), Serotec, Zymed (polyclonal).

Gastrin

Axcel/Accurate (polyclonal), Biodesign (polyclonal), Biogenesis (polyclonal), Biogenex (polyclonal), Caltag Laboratories (polyclonal), Dako (polyclonal), Fitzgerald (M28046, M28047, polyclonal), Immunotech Inc (4C7A1), Novocastra, Sanbio/Monosan (polyclonal), Zymed (polyclonal).

Glucagon

Accurate/Sigma Chemical (K79bB10), Axcel/Accurate (polyclonal), Biodesign (polyclonal), Biogenesis (polyclonal), Biogenex (polyclonal), Caltag Laboratories (polyclonal), Dako (polyclonal), Fitzgerald (polyclonal), Immunotech (polyclonal), Sanbio/Monosan (polyclonal), Zymed (polyclonal).

Pancreatic polypeptide (PP)

Axcel/Accurate (polyclonal), Becton Dickinson, Biodesign (polyclonal), Biogenesis (polyclonal), Biogenex (polyclonal), Dako (polyclonal), Eli Lilly (polyclonal), Zymed (polyclonal).

Fixation/preparation

These antibodies are applicable to formalin-fixed paraffin embedded tissue as well as frozen sections. No pretreatment or antigen unmasking is necessary for any of the antibodies.

Background

The antigens used as immunogens to raise rabbit antibodies against the pancreatic hormones were as follows: insulin – porcine pancreatic insulin; somatostatin – synthetic peptide somatostatin – 14; VIP – natural porcine VIP, conjugated to glutaraldehyde as carrier protein; gastrin – synthetic human gastrin-17 non-sulphated form conjugated to bovine serum albumin; glucagon – porcine glucagon.

Although there are at least eight different cell types identified in the pancreatic islets (Dayal & O'Brian, 1981), only the resident four major cell types (A-, B-, D- and PP- cells) and G- and VIP-cells (in neoplastic conditions) will be considered here. In the normal adult islet, insulin containing B-cells account for 60–80 % of endocrine cells (Erlandsen et al, 1976) and occupy the central portion of the islets. Glucagon containing A-cells constitute 20–30 % and somatostatin containing D-cells, 5–11 %. A- and D-cells are mostly present in the periphery of the islets and are also scattered within the islets along capillaries. Physiologically, glucagon increases hepatic glucose production and opposes hepatic glucose storage; insulin increases peripheral glucose uptake and opposes glucagon-mediated hepatic glucose production. Hence, the delicate balance of these two hormones maintains blood glucose homeosotasis. Somatostatin has inhibitory actions on both A- and B-cells through a "paracrine" effect, thereby regulating the balance of A- and B-cell functions. PP-cells are the least numerous and are present both within and outside the islets. The function of pancreatic polypeptide is not fully understood. PP-cells have a

variable distribution in the pancreas, with PP-cell rich islets being occasionally present in the posterior lobe of the pancreatic head. Hence, caution should be exercised when evaluating hyperplastic changes of PP-cells (Mukai, 1983).

Although the presence of gastrin in D-cells has been disputed, recent studies indicate that gastrin is not present in normal adult islets (Dayal & O'Brian, 1981). VIP has been localized in human islets but the exact cellular origin is not fully understood (Said, 1980). In the rat, diabetes mellitus induced by streptozotocin resulted in a reduction of the number of insulin-positive cells in the islet of Langerhans while that of VIP and neuropeptide-Y increased significantly after the onset of diabetes. Both these hormones evoked large and significant increases in insulin release from pancreatic tissue fragments of normal rats (Adeghate et al, 2001).

In the gastro-duodenal segment gastrin has been immunolocalized to the G-cells of the gastric antrum, whilst somatostatin has been found in endocrine cells and nerves of the intestinal wall digestive mucosa.

Applications

Endocrine tumors of the gastrointestinal tract and pancreas may demonstrate a wide variety of histomorphological patterns: (I) solid (nodular solid nests with peripheral invading cords), (ii) solid and glandular (with focal glandular formation), (iii) gyriform (trabecular or ribbon-like structures forming anastomosing pattern) and (iv)

glandular (tubular or acinar structures), (Mukai et al, 1982). With the availability of antibodies to the secretory products, specific designation of these neoplasms has led to terms such as insulinoma, glucagonoma, gastrinoma, somatostatinoma and VIPoma. However, small tumors found incidentally at autopsy may be clinically silent and do not necessarily cause clinical symptoms. Further, many pancreatic endocrine tumors are multihormonal (Mukai et al, 1982). Hence, the designation of pancreatic endocrine tumor followed by the description of the hormone(s) demonstrated in situ (e.g. insulin-producing) whenever this can be ascertained is the preferred terminology. Pancreatic endocrine tumors, which do not cause clinically apparent endocrine syndromes, are usually labeled as nonfunctioning tumors. However, with the acceptance of hormone production as a sign of function, the number of nonfunctioning tumors decrease with application of immunohistochemical staining procedures using antibodies to specific hormones.

In general, most insulin-producing tumors associated with hypoglycemia are benign. Conversely, endocrinologically active gastrin-producing tumors, glucagons-producing tumors, VIP-producing tumors and somatostatin-producing tumors are often malignant. However, there are no definite morphologic criteria to predict hormonal activity or behavior. Metastasis is the only sign of malignancy. Therefore, all pancreatic endocrine tumors should be regarded as potentially malignant, even though metastasis may not be apparent at the time of initial surgery (Mukai, 1983).

The common clinical syndromes and their causative hormones are as follows: hypoglycemia (insulin), Zollinger-Ellison syndrome (gastrin), Glucagonoma syndrome (glucagon), WDHA syndrome (Verner-Morrison syndrome) (vasoactive intestinal pancreatic polypeptide) and Somatostatinoma syndrome (somatostatin). Apart from the first two syndromes which are relatively frequent, the remaining three are either infrequent or rare (Larsson, 1978). Occasionally, pancreatic endocrine tumors fail to demonstrate immunoreaction in the presence of clinical syndromes. Explanations for this aberrant phenomenon include abnormal peptides (although biologically active) which may not react with specific anti-hormone antibodies, fixation artifact, or alternatively rapid turnover in tumor cells resulting in only minute amounts being stored (Mukai et al, 1982).

Tumors from some patients with WDHA syndrome have been found to secrete PP (Lundqvist et al, 1978). PP also appears to be the most commonly found in hormone silent/nonfunctioning tumors (Mukai et al, 1982). Whilst the physiologic function of PP is not yet fully understood, PP cells are nevertheless a component often demonstrated in multihormonal tumors (Larsson, 1978). The frequency of multihormone production by islet cells tumors has been stated to be as high as 50% (Owyang & Go, 1980). These tumors usually cause only one clinical syndrome, and a

combination of syndromes is extremely rare. In fact, the predominant cell type in a tumor does not necessarily cause the corresponding syndrome (Larsson et al, 1975). Any combination of cell types is possible in pancreatic endocrine tumors, the most striking example being the high frequency of PP cells in tumors secreting VIP and causing the WDHA syndrome (Schwartz, 1979). The most likely explanation for the common presence of several cell types in pancreatic endocrine tumors is that they derive from a multipotential stem cell that may differentiate in various directions (Mukai et al, 1982).

Antibodies to pancreatic hormones may also be applied to the diagnosis of islet cell hyperplasia seen in the non-neoplastic pancreas of patients with islet cell tumors (Larsson, 1977) and primary G-cell hyperplasia (gastrin producing) in the antrum of the stomach. The latter is clinically indistinguishable from Zollinger-Ellison's syndrome due to gastrinoma (Lewin et al, 1984). The demonstration of an increase in number and size of the β cell mass in the ductulo-insular complexes in neonatal hyperinsulinaemic hypoglycemia is another application of pancreatic hormone immunohistochemistry (Jaffe et al, 1980). An immunohistochemical study of 100 pancreatic tumors in 28 patients with multiple endocrine neoplasia, type I demonstrated a predominant hormonal secretion in 83 tumors (with 50–90% of the same cell type), including 37 glucagon, 27 insulin, 11 PP, 1

gastrin and 1 VIP cell tumors (Le Bodic et al 1996).

Duodenal (periampullary) somatostatin-rich carcinoid tumors (psammomatous somatostatinoma) need to be distinguished from adenocarcinoma, because the prognosis is better in the former even though lymph node metastases may occur with carcinoids (Chetty et al, 1993). Other neuroendocrine tumors of the duodenum that require immunohistochemistry for their recognition include gastrinomas (most common), gangliocytic paraganglioma (Hamid et al, 1986), serotonin-/calcitonin-/pancreatic polypeptide-producing tumors and poorly differentiated neuroendocrine carcinomas. A characteristic feature of MEN-associated gastrinoma is their frequent multicentricity (Pipeleers-Marichal et al, 1990).

Gastrointestinal carcinoid tumors have also benefited from the development of immunohistochemical technology: gastrin, VIP, PP and glucagon have been demonstrated (apart from serotonin in cases of carcinoid syndrome). In children, WDHA syndromes have been reported in association with VIP-secreting ganglioneuromas and ganglioneuroblastomas (Long et al, 1981). A recent study showed that carcinoid tumors of the ampulla of Vater differed immunohistochemically from carcinoid tumors elsewhere in the duodenum (Makhlouf et al, 1999). Two-thirds of the ampullary tumors expressed somatostatin, whilst over half of the duodenal carcinoid tumors expressed gastrin. Another study also confirmed the gastrin expression in duodenal carcinoids (75% immunopositive) with only 20% of ampullary carcinoids expressing gastrin (Bornstein-Quevedo & Gamboa-Dominguez, 2001). Somatostatin, pancreatic polypeptide and gastrin has also been demonstrated albeit in less than a third of carcinoid tumors of the extrahepatic bile ducts (Maitra et al, 2000).

Increased neuroproliferation in the appendix is associated with an increase in VIP, substance P and growth-associated protein-43 in adults with acute right lower quadrant abdominal pain. Recently, this finding was also demonstrated in children by immunostaining. Increased neuroproliferation was demonstrated in the appendiceal lamina propria and muscularis of children who presented with abdominal pain compared with appendices removed incidentally. The VIP immunoexpression in these children was higher or similar to those appendices that showed histological inflammatory changes (Bouchard et al, 2001).

Comments

Immunohistochemistry has contributed extensively to the understanding of the morphofunctional relationship of pancreatic (and related) endocrine tumors. Apart from the cellular localization of secretory products in these tumors, prediction of biological behavior has also been possible. Positive control tissue for this panel of pancreatic hormones include: normal pancreas (insulin, glucagon, somatostatin and PP), gastric antrum (gastrin) and colon (VIP).

References

Adeghate E, Ponery AS, Pallot DJ, Singh J. Distribution of vasoactive intestinal polypeptide, neuropeptide-Y and substance P and their effects on insulin secretion from the in vitro pancreas of normal and diabetic rats. Peptides 2001;22:99–107.

Bouchard S, Russo P, Radu AP, Adzick NS. Expression of neuropeptides in normal and abnormal appendices. Journal of Pediatric Surgery 2001;36:1222–6.

Bornstein-Quevedo L and Gamboa-Dominguez A. Carcinoid tumors of the duodenum and Ampulla of Vater; A clinicomorphologic, immunohistochemical and cell kinetic comparison. Human Pathology 2001;32:1252–6.

Chetty R, Silvester AC, Pitson GA. Duodenal (periampullary) somatostatin-rich carcinoid in a patient with type 1 neurofibromatosis. Pathology 1993;25:354–5.

Creutzfeldt, W. Endocrine tumors of the pancreas: Clinical chemical and morphological findings. In *The Pancreas*, P.J. Fitzgerald and A.B. Morrison, Eds. Williams & Wilkins, Baltimore, 1980, pp 208–30.

Dayal Y, O'Brian DS. The pathology of the pancreatic endocrine cells. In DeLellis RA (ed). *Diagnostic Immunohistochemistry,* New York, Masson, USA, 1981, pp 111–35.

Erlandsen SL, Hegre OD, Parsons JA, et al. Pancreatic islet cell hormones: Distribution of cell types in the islet and evidence for the presence of somatostatin and gastrin within the D-cell. Journal of Histochemistry and Cytochemistry 1976;24:883–7.

Hamid QA, Bishop AE, Rode J, et al. Duodenal gangliocytic paraganglioma: A study of 10 cases with immunocytochemical neuroendocrine markers. Human Pathology 1986;17:1151–7.

Jaffe RM, Hashida Y, Yunis EJ. Pancreatic pathology in hyperinsulinaemic hypoglycaemia of infancy. Laboratory Investigation 1980;42:356–65.

Larsson L.-I. Two distinct types of islet abnormalities associated with endocrine pancreatic tumours. Virchows Archives (Pathologic Anatomy) 1977;376:209–19.

Larsson L.-I., Grimelius L, H†kanson R, et al. Mixed endocrine pancreatic tumors producing several peptide hormones. American Journal of Pathology 1975;79:271–84.

Larsson L.-I. Classification of pancreatic endocrine tumors. Scandinavian Journal of Gastroenterology 1978;14(Suppl 53):15–8.

Le Bodic MF, Heymann MF, Lecomte M, et al. Immunohistochemical study of 100 pancreatic tumors in 28 patients with MEN type I. American Journal of Surgical Pathology 1996;20:1378–84.

Lewin KJ, Ulich T, Walsh JH. Primary gastrin cell hyperplasia of the gastric antrum. American Journal of Surgical Pathology 1984;8:821–32.

Long RG, Bryant MG, Mitchell SJ, et al. Clinicopathological study of pancreatic and ganglioneuroblastoma tumors secreting vasoactive intestinal polypeptide (vipomas). British Medical Journal 1981;282:1767–71.

Lundqvist G, Krause U, Larsson L.-I, et al. A pancreatic-polypeptide-producing tumour associated with the WDHA syndrome. Scandinavian Journal of Gastroenterology 1978;13:715–8.

Maitra A, Krueger JE, Tascilar M, et al. Carcinoid tumors of the extrahepatic bile ducts: a study of 7 cases. American Journal of Surgical Pathology 2000;24:1501–10.

Maklouf HR, Burke AP, Sobin LH. Carcinoid tumors of the Ampulla of Vater: a comparison with duodenal carcinoid tumors. Cancer 1999;85:1241–9.

Mukai K, Greider MH, Grotting JC, Rosai J. Retrospective study of 77 pancreatic endocrine tumors using the immunoperoxidase method. American Journal of Surgical Pathology 1982;6:387–99.

Mukai K. Functional pathology of pancreatic islets: Immunocytochemical exploration. Pathology Annual 1983;2:87–107.

Owyang C and Go VL. Multiple hormone-secreting tumors of the gastrointestinal tract. In *Gastrointestinal Hormones*. G.B.J. Glass, Ed. Raven Press, New York, 1980, pp 741–8.

Pipeleers-Marichal M, Somers G, Willems G et al. Gastrinomas in the duodenum of patients with multiple endocrine neoplasia type 1 and the Zollinger-Ellison syndrome. New England Journal of Medicine 1990;322:723–7.

Said SI. Vasoactive intestinal peptide (VIP): Isolation, distribution, biological actions, structure-function relationships, and possible functions. In Glass GBJ (ed), *Gastrointestinal Hormones*, New York, Raven Press, 1980, pp 245–73.

Schwartz TW. Pancreatic-polypeptide (PP) and endocrine tumours of the pancreas. Scandinavian Journal of Gastroenterology 1979;14 (Supp 53):93–100.

NOTES

Parathyroid Hormone-Related Protein (PTHrP)

Sources/clones

Biogenesis (polyclonal), Calbiochem (212–10.7), Fitzgerald (polyclonal).

Fixation/preparation

Applicable to both frozen sections and formalin-fixed paraffin-embedded tissue sections.

Background

Humoral hypercalcaemia of malignancy (HHM) is a syndrome characterized by low levels of PTH, few/absent bone metastases and hypophosphatemia. Parathyroid hormone-related protein (PTHrP) has been isolated from tumors with HHM and shown to be responsible for the PTH-like effects and disruption of calcium homeostasis (Ralston et al, 1991; Roskams & Desmet, 1997) The amino acid sequence of PTHrP bears homology to PTH from amino acid 1–13, but is unique thereafter (Burtis et al, 1990). Although functioning via PTH receptor, PTHrP is the product of a separate gene located on the short arm of chromosome 12 (Suva et al, 1987). Antibody to PTHrP

(Ab-1) reacts with amino acid residues 38–64 of human PTHrP and shows no cross reactivity with human parathyroid hormone.

In addition to being produced by malignant tumors, PTHrP is found in normal keratinocytes, lactating mammary tissue, placenta, parathyroid glands, the central nervous system and a number of other sites, suggesting that it may have a widespread physiologic role (Burtis et al, 1990; Kramer et al, 1991). PTHrP is thought to act in an autocrine and paracrine manner in various tissues to modulate other functions in addition to regulating calcium mobilization.

Through studies of osteoblast turnover in vitro it was suggested that PTHrP and the PTH-1 receptor might play an important role in exerting both pro- and anti-apoptotic effects in mesenchymal cells (Chen et al, 2002).

Immunostaining for PTHrP suggests that production of the peptide by stromal cells and giant cells may be involved in the formation of osteoclast-like cells in giant cell tumor of tendon sheath by acting in an autocrine/paracrine fashion (Nakashima et al., 1996).

Applications

Most squamous cell carcinomas from a variety of sites synthesize PTHrP irrespective of the calcium status of the patient (Lloyd, 1994). Using a polyclonal antibody to PTHrP (1–130), 93% of 40 invasive squamous cell carcinomas were found to be immunopositive (Liapis et al, 1993). Interestingly the strongest immunoreactivity for PTHrP in the squamous carcinomas was in areas of invasion and with desmoplasia. Adenocarcinomas (smaller percentage than squamous cancers) of breast, lung and kidney, hepatocellular carcinoma, mesothelioma, neuroendocrine tumors and T-cell leukemias are other neoplasms that may express PTHrP (Lloyd, 1994). The presence of PTHrP and its receptor has been demonstrated in normal breast epithelium and breast carcinomas suggesting that most breast tumors are able to respond to PTHrP (Downey et al, 1997).

Cholangiocarcinomas may be immunopositive for PTHrP (and chromogranin A), whilst all hepatocellular carcinomas were negative (Roskams et al, 1993). Mixed primary liver tumors contained PTHrP immunoreactivity only in areas of cholangiocellular differentiation. Moreover, all metastatic adenocarcinomas (especially from GIT) were negative except for 2/5 metastatic breast carcinomas.

Using polyclonal antibodies against synthetic PTHrP peptides, immunopositivity was demonstrated in primary parathyroid adenomata and hyperplastic glands from patients with chronic renal failure, whilst primary hyperplastic glands were negative (Danks et al, 1990).

Comments

The frequency of expression of PTHrP is so great and widespread, that it may be useful as a tumor marker in the histological diagnosis of certain cancers, e.g., squamous cell carcinoma of the lung. The protein has been shown to be a potential marker of pancreatic adenocarcinoma (Bouvet et al, 2002) and the co-expression of PTHrP and PTH/PTHrP receptor in chondrosarcomas may be of value in differentiating between benign and malignant cartilaginous lesions (Kunisada et al, 2002). Furthermore, the role of PTHrP in distinguishing between primary hepatocellular carcinoma and cholangiocarcinoma in the liver appears to be fairly reliable. Reactive bile ductules or squamous epithelium of epidermis are recommended control tissue. PTHrP has also been demonstrated in uterine tumors resembling ovarian sex-cord tumors (Suzuki et al, 2002), multiple myeloma (Kitazawa et al, 2002), endometrium (Hoshi et al, 2001) and salivary glands (Seidel et al, 2001).

References

Burtis WJ, Brady TG, Orloff JJ, et al. Immunochemical characterization of circulating parathyroid hormone-related protein in patients with humoral hypercalcemia of cancer. New England Journal of Medicine 1990;322:1106–12.

Bouvet M, Nardin SR, Burton DW, et al. Parathyroid hormone-related protein as a novel tumor marker in pancreatic adenocarcinoma. Pancreas 2002;24:284–90.

Chen HL, Demiralp B, Schneider A, et al. Parathyroid hormone and parathyroid hormone-related protein exert both pro- and anti-apoptotic effects in mesenchymal cells. Journal of Biology and Chemistry 2002;277:19374–81.

Danks JA, Ebeling PR, Hayman JA, et al. Immunohistochemical localization of parathyroid hormone-related protein in parathyroid adenoma and hyperplasia. Journal of Pathology 1990;161:27–33.

Downey SE, Hoyland J, Freemont AJ, et al. Expression of the receptor for parathyroid hormone-related protein in normal and malignant breast tissue. Journal Pathology 1997;183:212–7.

Hoshi, Morimoto T, Saito H, et al. PTHrP and PTH/PTHrP receptor expression in human endometrium. Endocrinology Journal 2001;48:219–25.

Kitazawa R, Kitazawa S, Kajimoto K, et al. Expression of parathyroid hormone-related protein (PTHrP) in multiple myeloma. Pathology International 2002;52:63–8.

Kramer S, Reynolds FH Jr., Castillo M, et al. Immunological identification and distribution of parathyroid hormone-like protein polypeptides in normal and malignant tissues. Endocrinology 1991;128:1927–37.

Kunisada T, Moseley JM, Slavin JL, et al. Co-expression of parathyroid hormone-related

protein (PTHrP) and PTH/PTHrP receptor in cartilaginous tumours – a marker for malignancy? Pathology 2002;34:133–7.

Liapis H, Crouch EC, Roby J, Rader JS. In situ localization of parathyroid hormone-like protein and Mrna in intraepithelial neoplasia and invasive carcinoma of the uterine cervix. Human Pathology 1993;24:1058–66.

Lloyd RV. Parathyroid hormone-related protein: Role in hypercalcemia of malignancy. Advances in Anatomic Pathology 1994;1:82–6.

Ralston SH, Danks J, Hayman J, et al. Parathyroid hormone-related protein of malignancy: Immunohistochemical and biochemical studies in normocalcaemic and hypercalcaemic patients with cancer. Journal of Clinical Pathology 1991;44:472–6.

Roskams T, Willems M, Campos RV et al. Parathyroid hormone-related peptide expression in primary and metastatic liver tumours. Histopathology 1993;23:519–25.

Roskams T, Desmet V. Parathyroid-hormone-related peptides. A new class of multifunctional proteins. American Journal of Pathology 1997;150:779–85.

Nakashima M, Ito M, Ohtsuru A, et al. Expression of parathyroid hormone (PTH) –related peptide (PTHrP) and PTH/PTHrP receptor in giant cell tumour of tendon sheath. Journal of Pathology 1996;180:88–94.

Seidel J, Zabel M, Surdyk-Zasada J, et al. Immunocytochemical localisation of PTHrP in human and rat salivary glands. Folia Histochemistry and Cytochemistry 2001;39:171–2.

Suva LJ, Winslow GA, Wettenhall REH, et al. A parathyroid hormone-related protein implicated in malignant hypercalcemia: cloning and expression. Science 1987;237:893–6.

Suzuki C, Matsumoto T, Fukunaga M, et al. Uterine tumor resembling ovarian sex-cord tumors producing parathyroid hormone-related protein of the uterine cervix. Pathology International 2002;52:164–8.

NOTES

Parathyroid hormone

Sources/clones

Binding Site (polyclonal), Biodesign (polyclonal), Biogenesis (polyclonal), Biogenex (polyclonal), Dako (polyclonal), Fitzgerald (polyclonal), Novocastra (polyclonal).

Fixation/preparation

This antibody is applicable to formalin-fixed paraffin-embedded tissue, frozen sections and cytologic preparations. Although not always required, enzyme pretreatment before immunodetection may improve results on paraffin-embedded.

Background

The parathormone gene, closely linked to that of β-globin, is located on the short arm of chromosome 11 in humans (as are the genes for calcitonin and insulin). The initial form in which parathormone is synthesized within the cell is a single-chain polypeptide of 115 amino acid residues, preproparathyroid hormone. This is cleaved within the cell to form a proparathyroid hormone, from which a further 6 amino acids are split, leaving the 84-amino acid chain of parathormone. (Habener

et al, 1984). The rate of parathormone secretion is directly responsive to the level of calcium in the serum, and indeed the cytoplasm, of parathyroid cells, as has been shown by studies both *in vivo* and *in vitro*. (Brown et al, 1982). Recent in vitro studies of osteoclast turnover suggest that both PTH and PTH-related protein exert both pro- and anti-apoptotic effects in mesenchymal cells (Chen et al, 2002).

Applications

Surgical pathologists are familiar with the ability of parathyroid proliferations to assume a variety of histological guises, posing difficulty to categorize any given lesion as hyperplastic, adenomatous or carcinomatous in nature (Wick et al, 1997). This is usually resolved with the macroscopic appearance of the remaining parathyroid glands as assessed by the surgeon. The role of the surgical pathologist is to identify the lesion as parathyroid in nature and to assess whether it is normocellular or hypercellular. Although easily accomplished in the majority of instances, rare examples of parathyroid hyperplasia/adenoma showing a follicular/trabecular arrangement

may cause concern over the alternative diagnosis of a thyroid adenoma. This becomes more pertinent when the parathyroid lesion abuts into the thyroid gland or lies within the thyroid capsule. Immunodetection for thyroglobulin and parathyroid hormone (PTH) is especially useful to resolve the problem (Permanetter et al, 1983). Nevertheless, caution should be exercised since parathyroid cells often discharge their hormonal product almost as soon as it is packaged in the cytoplasm, resulting in false-negative PTH immunostaining, although the cells are biologically synthetic (Wick et al, 1997).

PTH antibody is also useful to distinguish cell parathyroid hyperplasia/neoplasms from thyroid and metastatic neoplasms (Wick et al, 1997); although the pathologist is typically aware of the preoperative hypercalcaemic status. Occasionally when the surgeon does not supply this information, PTH immunohistochemistry is essential. Even more problematic, are situations in which clear cell parathyroid carcinomas are nonsecretory, without an abnormality in mineral metabolism (Aldinger et al, 1982). In such situations, metastatic renal cell carcinoma or metastatic clear cell carcinoma of the lung is evident, warranting PTH immunohistochemistry to arrive at the correct diagnosis (Wick et al, 1997). The other instance in which PTH antibodies are useful, is in the consideration of parathyroid carcinomas located primarily in the anterior mediastinum (intrathymically). In this situation distinction from primary thymic metastatic carcinomas, non-Hodgkin's lymphoma and germ cell tumors is necessary (Murphy et al, 1986).

Comments

The diagnosis of the majority of parathyroid proliferation may be accomplished with an adequate history, biochemistry profile and histomorphological assessment.

However, rare instances in which the tumors have an abnormal location, clear cell morphology or are non-secretory may result in erroneous diagnoses, warranting PTH immunohistochemistry. Normal parathyroid glands are adequate for positive control tissue.

References

Aldinger KA, Hickey RC, Ibanez ML, Samaan NA. Parathyroid carcinoma: A clinical study of seven cases of functioning and two cases of nonfunctioning parathyroid cancer. Cancer 1982;49:388–97.

Brown EM. PTH secretion in vivo and in vitro. Regulation by calcium and other secretagogues. Mineral Electrolyte Metal 1982;8:130–50.

Chen HL, Demiralp B, Schneider A, et al. Parathyroid hormone and parathyroid hormone-related protein exert both pro- and anti-apoptotic effects in mesenchymal cells. Journal of Biology and Chemistry 2002;277:19374–81.

Habener JF, Rosenblatt M, Potts JT. Parathyroid hormone; biochemical aspects of biosynthesis, secretion, action and metabolism. Physiology Reviews 1984;64:985–1053.

Murphy MN, Glennon PG, Diocee MS, et al. Nonsecretory parathyroid carcinoma of the mediastinum. Cancer 1986;58:2468–76.

Permanetter W, Nathrath WBJ, Lohrs U. Immunohistochemical analysis of thyroglobulin and keratin in benign and malignant thyroid tumors. American Journal of Surgical Pathology 1983;7:535–46.

Wick MR, Ritter JH, Humphrey PA, Nappi O. Clear cell neoplasms of the endocrine system and thymus. Seminars in Diagnostic Pathology 1997;14:183–202.

P-glycoprotein (P-170), Multi-Drug Resistance (MDR)

Sources/clones

Accurate (MRPr1), Biodesign (JSB-1), Coulter (UIC1), Dako (C494, 4E3, C219), Immunotech (MRK-16, UIC2), Monosan (JSB-1, MRPm6, LRP-56), Novocastra, Oncogene, Sanbio (MRPr1), Sera-Lab (JSB-1), Signet (C219, C494, JSB-1), Zymed (JSB-1).

Fixation/preparation

Most antibodies available are immunoreactive in frozen sections and some react in fixed paraffin-embedded sections, enhanced by HIER treatment.

Background

P-glycoprotein (P-170) is a transmembrane protein of 170 kD molecular weight. It has been associated with both intrinsic and acquired resistance to certain chemotherapeutic agents, particularly anthracyclines and vinca alkaloids. It is an energy-dependent pump which functions in drug efflux, reducing intracellular accumulation of chemotherapeutic agents, thus conferring the so-called multi-drug resistance (MDR) phenomenon on cells expressing increased levels of this protein

Kartner & Ling, 1989; Gottesman et al, 1991). One of the most perplexing problems encountered in chemotherapy is the resistance of certain tumors to all chemotherapeutic regimens, while other tumors, which are initially chemo-sensitive to a particular agent, show resistance to treatment over time and with disease progression. Furthermore, tumor cells which are resistant to one drug often show cross-resistance to a wide variety of other, structurally unrelated drugs. For example, tumor cells resistant to Adriamycin can show cross-resistance to diverse drugs to which it has never been exposed, including vinca alkaloids and mitomycin C, but not to other drugs such as alkylating agents. This is known as the MDR phenomenon (Leong & Leong, 1997). A family of so-called MDR genes encodes the P-glycoprotein, apparently with only the protein encoded by the MDR 1 gene inducing the MDR phenotype.

There is extensive evidence from *in vitro* studies, especially with non-human cell lines, that over-expression of P-glycoprotein results in reduced accumulation of drug within the cell. Recently, mice have been generated with knockout of

MDR 1 and these animals show abnormalities of transport at the blood-brain barrier and are more sensitive to drugs.

Applications

Molecular and immunohistochemical studies of P-glycoprotein reveal that it is over-expressed in a number of intrinsically resistant tumors such as carcinomas of the liver, pancreas, colon, adrenal cortex and kidney, and appears to vary according to the differentiation of the cells. Interestingly, in these cases, high levels of the protein have also been demonstrated in the normal tissues from which the tumors are derived. The physiologic function of P-glycoprotein can be deduced from its normal tissue distribution in that high levels of expression are seen in endothelial cells of the blood-brain barrier and in renal proximal tubules, both cell types having the primary function of moving toxic molecules across cell membranes (Schinkel et al, 1994).

P-glycoprotein expression has been found significantly more frequently in soft tissue sarcomas, neuroblastomas and hepatoblastomas and generally in disseminated tumors but not in malignant brain tumors and nephroblastoma (Kucerova et al, 2001). Tumors responsive to chemotherapy generally show low levels of P-glycoprotein expression and solid tumors that are most responsive to systemic chemotherapy such as seminomas and embryonal carcinomas, rarely display detectable levels of the protein. Tumors from patients previously treated with chemotherapy show frequent elevation of P-glycoprotein, suggesting that the MDR phenotype is induced by exposure to chemotherapy. The detection of elevated levels of P-glycoprotein expression has the potential to identify tumors likely to be resistant to conventional chemotherapy and may provide a rational for the use of alternative treatments for such patients. Immunohistological evaluation appears to be the method of choice for the assessment of P-glycoprotein, largely because it allows morphological correlation and discrimination from that in non-tumor cells (Ramani & Dewchand, 1995). However the published results are conflicting with immunoexpression of p-glycoprotein and other multi-drug resistance-related proteins not changing significantly after chemotherapy (Lazaris et al, 2002). It was recently shown that there was no significant correlation between p-glycoprotein expression in tumor cells with clinical course, stage and grade of nephroblastoma. However, positivity in tumor capillary endothelial cells correlated significantly with unfavorable outcome, suggesting that chemoresistance depended on an active blood-tumor barrier (Camassei et al, 2002).

Comments

Only two MDR genes are know to be present in man, namely MDR 1 and MDR 3, but only the MDR 1 gene product confers the MDR phenotype. One of the most widely used antibodies to P-glycoprotein is clone C219 that reacts with both the MDR 1 and MDR 3 gene products. Several other antibodies specific to the MDR 1 gene product have now been described. They include HYB-241 and HYB-612, and C494. While earlier studies were conducted on frozen sections, HIER has improved the immunoreactivity in fixed paraffin-embedded sections. Renal proximal tubules are used as the standard positive control because of the high levels of expression of P-glycoprotein in the epithelial cells. The antigen is localized to the cell membrane and shows specific polarization in some cell types, e.g., the apical and basolateral membranes of pulmonary epithelium (Scheffer et al, 2002) and the trabecular structures resembling canalicular membrane or in the luminal membrane in hepatocellular carcinoma cells (Nies et al, 2001).

References

Camassei FD, Arancia G, Cianfriglia M, et al. Nephroblastoma: multi-drug resistance P-glycoprotein expression in tumor cells and introtumoral capillary endothelial cells. American Journal of Pathology 2002;117:484–90.

Cordon-Cardo C, O'Brien JP, Boccia J, et al. Expression of the multidrug resistance gene product (P-glycoprotein) in human normal and tumor tissues. Journal of Histochemistry and Cytochemistry 1990;38:1277–87.

Gottesman MM, Goldstein LJ, Fojo A, et al. Expression of the multidrug resistance gene in human cancer. In: Ronison IB (ed). Molecular cellular biology of multi-drug resistance in tumor cells. New York: Plenum Press, 1991, pp291–301.

Kartner N, Ling V. Multidrug resistance in cancer. Science 1989;260:44–51.

Kucerova H, Sumerauer D, Drahokoupilova E, et al. Significance of P-glycoprotein expression in childhood malignant tumors. Neoplasma 2001;48:472–8.

Lazaris AC, Kavantzas NG, Zorzos HS, et al. Markers of drug resistance in relapsing colon cancer. Journal of Cancer Research and Clinical Oncology 2002;128:114–8.

Leong AS-Y and Leong FJ. Cancer genetics – what you need to know. Diagnostic Cytopathology 1998;18:33–40.

Lopes JM, Bruland OS, Bjekehagen B, et al. Synovial sarcoma: Immunohistochemical expression of P-glycoprotein and glutathione S transferase-pi and clinical drug resistance. Pathology Research and Practice 1997;193:21–36.

Nies AT, Konig J, Pfannschmidt M, et al. Expression of the multidrug resistance proteins MRP2 and MRP3 in human hepatocellular carcinoma. International Journal of Cancer 2001;94:492–9.

Ramani P, Dewchand H. Expression of mdr 1/P-glycoprotein and P110 in neuroblastoma. Journal of Pathology 1995;175:13–22.

Schinkel AH, Smith JJM, van Telingen O. Disruption of the mouse mdr1AP-glycoprotein gene leads to a deficiency in the blood-brain barrier and to increased sensitivity to drugs. Cell 1994;77:491–502.

Scheffer GL, Pijnenborg AC, Smit EF, et al. Multidrug resistance related molecules in human and murine lung. Journal of Clinical Pathology 2002;55:332–9.

Pituitary Hormones (ACTH, FSH, HGH, LH, PRL, TSH)

Sources/clones

Anti-adrenocorticotropin (ACTH)

Axcel/Accurate (polyclonal), Biodesign (polyclonal), Biogenesis (polyclonal), Biogenex (polyclonal), Caltag Laboratories (polyclonal), Chemicon (polyclonal), Dako (02A3, polyclonal), Fitzgerald (polyclonal), Milab (polyclonal), Novocastra, Sanbio/Monosan (polyclonal), Seralab, Serotec (A1H5, A5B12), Sigma (polyclonal), Zymed (polyclonal).

Anti-follicle stimulating hormone (FSH)

Axcel/Accurate (polyclonal), Biodesign (301,1801,29; 701, 702, 706, 709, S1, polyclonal), Biogenesis (754, 143, BIO–FSHb-00, polyclonal), Biogenex (78/74 1F11, polyclonal), Dako (polyclonal), Fitzgerald (polyclonal, M27301, M210201, M26092, M94166, M94163, M94164).

Anti-human growth hormone (HGH)

Accurate (12), Biodesign (901,902, polyclonal), Biogenesis (2F10, Rt, polyclonal), Biogenex (54/9 2A2, polyclonal), Dako (polyclonal), Fitzgerald

(M94168, M94169, M32222, polyclonal), Novocastra (polyclonal), Seralab (polyclonal) Serotec (B008, E1, G1), Sigma Chemical (GHC2), Zymed (ZMGH2, polyclonal).

Anti-human luteinizing hormone (LH)

American Research Products (1561–18), Axcel/Accurate (polyclonal), Biodesign (2004, 6101, 6102, 6103, [6206,6207,62], polyclonal), Biogenesis (1C10, 3D7, 4E3, G11, polyclonal), Biogenex (3LH 5B6 YH4, polyclonal), Cymbus Bioscience (6101), Dako (polyclonal), Fitzgerald (polyclonal), Serotec (INNbLH1), Zymed (ZMLH2, ZSL11).

Anti-prolactin (PRL)

Axcel/Accurate (polyclonal), Biodesign (164.22.12, [6201–6204,62], [ME.121,ME.1], S2, [2605,2606]), Biogenesis (1D5, 626/02, 633/1, polyclonal), Dako (polyclonal), Fitzgerald (M94192, M94193, M94194, M31031, M31032, M31033, M310110, M310111, M310112, polyclonal), Immunotech (164.22.16), Zymed (ZMPL1).

Anti-human thyroid stimulating hormone (TSH)

American Research Products (25TH7G12), Axcel/Accurate (polyclonal), Biodesign (9001–90010), Biogenesis (TSH-03, polyclonal), Biogenex (5404, polyclonal), Dako (polyclonal), Fitzgerald (polyclonal), Novocastra (QB2.6, polyclonal), Seralab (JOS2.2, polyclonal), Zymed (ZMTS2, ZMTS4).

Fixation/preparation

All of the antibodies against the pituitary hormones are applicable to formalin-fixed paraffin-embedded sections. Although not essential, enzyme antigen retrieval pretreatment with Target Unmasking Fluid (TUF, Signet) or trypsin may improve immunoreaction on paraffin-embedded and frozen sections.

Background

In all instances antibodies against the pituitary hormones were raised using purified extract from human pituitary glands as immunogen respectively. The adenohypophysis comprises approximately 75% of the normal pituitary gland. It consists of the pars distalis, pars intermedia, and pars tuberalis. The pars distalis is roughly divided into a midline zone (PAS-positive mucosubstance containing ACTH [15–20%], FSH/LH [10%] and TSH [5%] cells) and two lateral portions that stain positively with acidic dyes (PRL 15–20% and GH 50%). It should be noted that cells are not strictly limited in their geographic distribution. Trichrome stains such as the PAS-orange G method serve to highlight the PAS-positive basophils and the orange-G-positive acidophils. Since this reactivity correlates only crudely with hormonal function, it is therefore necessary to resort to immunohistochemical characterization for proper identification. The cells are arranged in cords, and are encircled by well-formed basement membrane. These cells lie in the immediate proximity to a capillary to facilitate the secretory process. The general, histochemical and immunohistochemical characteristics of normal adenohypophyseal cells are summarized in Table 1. (for review see Scheithauer, 1984).

Applications

The major role of antibodies to pituitary hormones is that it serves as the primary basis of adenoma classification. A study comprising a surgical series (Robert, 1979) showed 80% of pituitary adenomas to be functional whilst a combined surgical/autopsy series found only 50% to be hormonally functional (Earle and Dillard, 1973). In adults, adenomas may present with hyperfunction (amenorrhoea-galactorrhoea, Cushing's disease, Nelson's syndrome, and acromegaly or gigantism), hypofunction (insufficiency of gonadal, thyroidal or adrenal function) or with compressive signs (visual disturbance, headache, or raised intracranial pressure) (Scheithauer, 1984). Aggression of pituitary adenomas is based on the radiological assessment: Grade I, microadenomas (<10 mm); grade 2, intrasellar adenoma; grade 3, diffuse adenomas with erosion of sellar floor, and grade 4, invasive adenomas with widespread sellar erosion and destruction (Hardy and Vezina, 1976).

The conventional tinctorial classification of adenomas, based on affinity of tumor cells for acid or basic dyes correlated crudely with the functional characteristics. Acidophil adenomas were presumed to produce growth hormone, whilst basophilic adenomas were considered synonymous with ACTH secretion and Cushing's disease. Chromophobe adenomas, in contrast were considered non-functioning, with symptoms being attributed to local destructive or compressive effects (Scheithauer, 1984). Hence, with the advent of commercially available specific antisera to pituitary hormones, a functional classification has emerged (Table 2).

Comments

Histopathology laboratories servicing neurosurgical units need to provide a comprehensive functional characterization of pituitary adenomas. The use of the normal pituitary gland will suffice as a positive control for the six hormones.

References

Earle KM, Dillard SH Jr. Pathology of adenomas of the pituitary gland. Exerpta Medica International Congress Series No. 303, 1973, pp 3–16.

Hardy J, Vezina JL. Transsphenoidal neurosurgery of intracranial neoplasm. Advances in Neurology 1976;15:261–5.

Robert F. Electron microscopy of human pituitary tumors. In: Tindall GT, Collins WF eds. *Clinical Management of Pituitary Disorders*. New York, Raven Press, 1979, pp 113–31.

Scheithauer BW. Surgical Pathology of the Pituitary: The Adenomas. Part 1. Pathology Annual 1984;pp 317–69.

Table 1 Normal cellular composition of the pituitary gland: morphological, functional and immunohistochemical characteristics (modified from Scheithauer, 1984).

Cell	Product	Location/Percentage	Immuno-histochemistry
Somatotroph	GH 21 kD polypeptide	Lateral 50%	GH
Lactotroph	PRL 23.5 kD polypeptide	Posterolateral 15–20%	PRL
Corticotroph	ACTH 4.5 kD polypeptide	Midline 15–20%	ACTH
Gonadotroph	FSH 35 kD and LH 28.2 kD glycoproteins	Generalized 10%	FSH and LH
Thyrotroph	TSH 28 kD glycoprotein	Anterior midline 5%	TSH

Table 2 Functional classification of pituitary hormones (Modified from Sheithauer, 1984).

Adenoma type	H & E	PAS	Immuno-Histochemistry
Prolactin cell	C, A	–	PRL
Growth hormone cell	A, C	–	GH
Mixed GH cell and PRL cell	A, C	–	GH and PRL
Mammosomatotroph cell	A	–	GH, strong +
			PRL, weak +
Acidophil stem cell	C	–	PRL+, GH (variable)
Corticotroph cell	B, C	+	ACTH
Gonadotroph cell	B, C	+	Both or either FSH, LH
Thyrotroph cell	B, C	+	±TSH
Null cell	C	–	None
Null cell, oncocytic	A	–	None

NOTES

Placental Alkaline Phosphatase (PLAP)

Sources/clones

Accurate (8B6, polyclonal),
American Research (polyclonal),
Biogenesis (PLAP001,
polyclonal), Biogenex
(polyclonal), Dako (8B6, 8A9,
polyclonal), Novocastra
(polyclonal), Sanbio (MIG-P),
Sigma (8B6), Zymed
(polyclonal).

Fixation/preparation

The antigen is resistant to
fixation and both polyclonal and
monoclonal antibodies are
immunoreactive in fixed paraffin-
embedded sections. HIER
enhances staining.

Background

The alkaline phosphatases (AP)
are a heterogenous group of
glycoproteins, which are usually
confined, to the cell surface
(Stolbach et al, 1969). The
isoenzymes differ in terms of
their biochemical properties,
anatomical sites of production
and reactivity with different
antibodies. APs probably have a
role in cellular transport,
regulation of metabolism, gene
transcription and cellular
differentiation. At least three
genes encode the human AP

isoenzymes, one for tissue-
nonspecific AP present in the
liver, bone and kidney, one for
the synthesis of intestinal AP, and
one or more genes for the
placental isoenzyme (PLAP). The
different isoenzymes differ in
molecular weight and amino
acid composition and have
different properties. The tissue-
nonspecific and intestinal
variants are heat-sensitive
whereas the PLAP isoenzymes
are heat-resistant. PLAP occurs
only in higher primates and
displays a high degree of genetic
polymorphism. It is a dimer of
65 kD subunits and is
synthesized during the G_1 phase
of the cell cycle The enzyme is
produced by trophoblasts and is
responsible for the
hyperphosphatemia observed
during pregnancy. Biochemically,
immunologically and
electrophoretically, PLAP can be
separated into three distinct
subtypes (Fishman, 1995). The
phase 1 isoenzyme corresponds
to that produced by 6–8 week
trophoblasts, the second is a
mixture of the early phase and
term-placental isoenzymes, and
the phase 3 corresponds to the
13 weeks-term gestation AP
isoenzymes. PLAP-like reactivity
has been reported in the serum
of about 5% of patients with

tumors that included carcinoma
of the lung, ovary, breast, colon
and endometrium, as well as
malignant lymphoma and
multiple myeloma. Raised levels
of serum PLAP were found in
25% of patients with seminoma.
Several isoenzymes of AP have
been specifically named. The
Regan isoenzyme was named
after a patient with lung cancer
whose serum had the phase 3-
type isoenzyme. It was also
found in 4–14% of patients with
a variety of neoplasms including
testicular germ cell tumors and
carcinomas of the breast, ovary,
lung, stomach and pancreas as
well as in the serum of patients
with ulcerative colitis, familial
polyposis and cirrhosis of the
liver. The Nagao isoenzyme was
named after a patient with
pleural carcinomatosis and bears
some similarities to the phase 3
PLAP. The Nagao AP has been
found in the serum and tumor
cells of patients with
adenocarcinoma of the bile ducts
and pancreas. The Kashahara
variant was detected in tumor
extracts of hepatocellular
carcinoma and possesses some of
the properties of the placental
isoenzyme. Other non-Regan
isoenzymes have been described
in patients with gastrointestinal
cancer, benign gynecological

disease and female genital cancer, testicular teratomas and lung tumors.

Applications

Antibodies to PLAP are primarily used as a diagnostic discriminator of germ cell tumors in the context of separation from somatic carcinomas and mediastinal tumors (Appendix 1.5, 1.12). It is also useful for the identification of intraventricular germ cells tumors (Appendix 1.35). Membrane-based PLAP has been documented immunohistochemically in seminoma, embryonal carcinoma, gonadoblastoma, endodermal sinus tumor and choriocarcinoma (Manivel et al, 1987) and metastatic deposits of seminoma (Koshida et al, 1996), making this marker an important one for the identification of germ cell tumors (Appendix 1.37). Spermatocytic seminoma and immature teratomas were negative (Koshida et al, 1996; Kraggerud et al, 1999). Epithelial neoplasms of the ovary (Nakopoulou et al, 1995) and Intratubular neoplastic germ cells also labeled for PLAP. It has been suggested that PLAP immunostaining may help separate partial and complete hydatidiform moles and choriocarcinoma. Partial moles show weak hCG and strong PLAP, complete moles show strong expression of hCG (human chorionic gonadotrophin) and weak PLAP, whereas choriocarcinoma display strong expression of hCG and weak PLAP and hPL (human placental lactogen) (Losch & Kainz, 1996) (Appendix 1.34). A recent paper suggests that intermediate trophoblasts do not express PLAP (Santos et al, 1999), an observation that requires confirmation. PLAP has also been observed in cell lines from human bladder cancer and in somatic tumors such as tumors of the female genital tract, intestine, lung and less frequently in breast and renal carcinomas (Wick et al, 1987). Epithelial membrane antigen (EMA) is said to help the distinction of germ cell tumors from these somatic tumors, which express EMA, whereas germ cell tumors do not.

References

Fishman WH. The 1993 ISOBM Abbott Award Lecture: Isoenzymes, tumor markers and oncodevelopmental biology. Tumour Biology 1995;16:394–402.

Kraggerud SM, Berner A, Bryne M, et al. Spermatocytic seminomas as compared to classical seminomas: an immunohistochemical and DNA flow cytometric study. APMIS 1999;107:297–302.

Koshida K, Uchibayashi T, Yamamoto H, et al. A potential use of a monoclonal antibody to placental alkaline phosphatase (PLAP) to detect lymph node metastases of seminoma. Journal of Urology 1996;155:337–41.

Losch A, Kainz C. Immunohistochemistry in the diagnosis of the gestational trophopblastic disease. Acta Obstetrics Gynecology Scandinavia 1996;75:753–6.

Manivel JC, Jessurun J, Wick MR, Dehner LP. Placental alkaline phosphatase immunoractivity in testicular germ cell neoplasms. American Journal of Surgical Pathology 1987;11:21–9.

Nakopoulou L, Stefanaki K, Janinis J, Mastrominas M. Immunohistochemical expression of placental alkaline phosphatase and vimentin in epithelial ovarian neoplasms. Acta Oncologica 1995;34:511–5.

Santos LD, Fernando SS, Yong JL, et al. Placental site nodules and plaques: a clinicopathological and immunohistochemical study of 25 cases with ultrastructural findings. Pathology 1999;31:328–36.

Stolbach LL, Krant MJ, Fishman WH. Ectopic production of an alkaline phosphatase isoenzyme in patients with cancer. New England Journal of Medicine 1969;281:757–62.

Wick MR, Swanson PE, Manivel JC. Placental-like alkaline phosphatase reactivity in human tumors: An immunohistochemical study of 520 cases. Human Pathology 1987;18:946–54.

Pneumocystis carinii

Sources/clones

Accurate (3F6), Axcel/Accurate (3F6), Biodesign (092, 093), Biogenesis (0G1/1), Biogenex (3F6), Chemicon, Dako (3F6).

Fixation/preparation

The DAKO antibody reacts with an antigenic epitope of human Pneumocystis carinii, which is resistant to fixation in formalin and picric acid, paraffin embedding, and extraction with ethanol and xylene. This antibody may also be used to detect P. carinii in smears prepared from bronchoalveolar lavage fluid and sputum samples (Elvin et al, 1988). However, enzymatic digestion of smears (e.g. trypsin) must be performed before staining.

Background

The DAKO antibody (IgM, Kappa) reacts with an 82kD parasite-specific component of human Pneumocystis carinii (Linder et al, 1987). No cross reactivity was found with a number of parasites and fungi (Elvin et al, 1988).

Applications

The AIDS epidemic brought about an increased need for specific markers that recognize Pneumocystis carinii. Newly developed antibodies mark cyst and/or trophozoites (Linder and Radio, 1989). While the sensitivity of the immunohistochemical method appears to be greater than the Giemsa stain, it is only slightly better than the GMS stain, warranting the use of immunostaining in sputum, where identification of the pathogen is more difficult than in bronchoalveolar lavage (Linder and Radio, 1989). The other advantage of immunostaining is that both cyst wall and trophozoites are stained whereas the silver stain only labels the cyst wall (Amin et al, 1992). However, the former staining pattern may appear amorphous or focally granular, which may be confused with non-specific staining of mucin or intracellular/free particulate material (Amin et al, 1992). The 3F6 monoclonal antibody has been found to be consistently more sensitive at detecting cysts of pneumocystis in both sputum and bronchoalveolar lavage specimens (Elvin et al, 1988; Wazir et al 1944b).

Comments

Immunohistochemistry for Pneumocystis carinii is a useful adjunct to traditional Giemsa and silver stains, particularly in cytopathology laboratories that examine a large number of respiratory specimens from HIV-positive patients.

References

Amin MB, Mezger E, Zarbo RJ. Detection of Pneumocystis carinii. Comparative study of monoclonal antibody and silver staining. American Journal of Clinical Pathology 1992;98:13–8.

Elvin KM, Björkman A, Linder E, Heurlin N, Hlorpe A. Pneumocystis carinii pneumonia: detection of parasites in sputum and bronchoalveolar lavage fluid by monoclonal antibodies. British Medical Journal 1988;297:381–4.

Linder E, Lundin L, Vorma H. Detection of *Pneumocystis carinii* in lung-derived samples using monoclonal antibodies to an 82kDa parasite component. Journal of Immunological Methods 1987;98:57–62.

Linder J, Radio SJ. Immunohistochemistry of Pneumocystis carinii. Seminars in Diagnostic Pathology 1989;6:238–44.

Wazir JF, Brown I, Martin-Bates E, Coleman DV. EB9, a new antibody for the detection of trophozoites of Pneumocystis carinii in bronchoalveolar lavage specimens in AIDS. Journal of Clinical Pathology 1994;47:1108–11.

Wazir JF, Macrorie SG, Coleman DV. Evaluation of the sensitivity, specificity, and predictive value of monoclonal antibody 3F6 for the detection of Pneumocystis carinii pneumonia in bronchoalveolar lavage specimens and induced sputum. Cytopathology 1994;5:82–9.

Pregnancy-specific β-1-glycoprotein (SP1)

Sources/clones

Axcel/Accurate, Biodesign
(BD4D8), Biogenesis
(polyclonal), Biogenex (4E4,
polyclonal), Chemicon
(polyclonal), Dako (polyclonal),
Fitzgerald (M32236), Research
Diagnostics (BB4E4), Zymed
(polyclonal).

Fixation/preparation

The antigen is fixation resistant
and immunoreactivity may be
improved with proteolytic
digestion or HIER.

Background

Pregnancy specific beta-1
glycoprotein (SP1) together with
human chorionic gonadotrophin
(hCG) and placental alkaline
phosphatase (PLAP) are three
major proteins produced by the
trophoblasts of the human
placenta. Immunohistochemical
studies suggest that SP1 and hCG
are also present in the human
amnion. Recent molecular
cloning studies indicate that the
human SP1s form a group of
closely related placental proteins
that, together with the
carcinoembryonic antigen family
members comprise a subfamily
within the immunoglobulin

superfamily. The main source of
SP1 is the syncytiotrophoblast but
it has been demonstrated that
amniotic as well as chorionic
membranes express low levels of
SP1 genes, although only certain
subpopulations of SP1 transcripts
were expressed, with differences
in species expression between
amnion, chorion and trophoblasts
(Plouzek et al, 1993). The
function of the SP1s is largely
unknown. Recent information
suggests that the SP1 family
induce secretion of anti-
inflammatory cytokines in
mononuclear phagocytes and the
tetraspanin, CD9 has been
identified as a receptor of murine
SP1 (Waterhouse et al, 2002).

Applications

The immunohistochemical
applications of SP1 have been
mainly in the study of placental
elements and their corresponding
tumors. Differing levels of
expression of hCG, human
placental lactogen (hPL) and SP1
were observed in the feto-
maternal tissues throughout
pregnancy. hCG was strongly
localized in the cytoplasm of the
syncytiotrophoblast in the 12 day
blastocysts, remaining strong until
8–10 week before decreasing and
becoming almost negative at

term. hCG showed variable
staining in the implantation site.
hPL and SP1 appeared later than
hCG in the syncytiotrophoblast,
increasingly rapidly by week 8
and remaining strong until term
(Sabet et al, 1989).
Immunolocalization studies of
SP1 in syncytiotrophoblasts
suggest a secretory pathway
including synthesis in the
endoplasmic reticulum,
processing by the Golgi and
exocytic release into maternal
blood in the intervillous space
(Schlafke et al, 1992).

The presence of SP1,
vimentin, cytokeratin and PLAP,
particularly the first three
antigens, has been used to
identify intermediate trophoblasts
in the placental site nodule
(Shibata & Rutgers, 1994)
(Appendix 1.34).

Comments

SP1 is not specific to placental
cells. It is expressed in a variety
of non-placental tumors. In an
immunoelectron microscopic
study of colonic carcinomas, SP1
and carcinoembryonic antigen
were found in all seven tumors
studied; none of the tumors
showing morphologic evidence
of choriocarcinoma. PLAP and
hCG was found in two tumors

(Haynes et al, 1985). In urothelial tumors, immunoreactive SP1 were observed in five of 47 high-grade tumors. HCG and hPL were found in nine and seven cases respectively. These findings suggested that morphologic and functional trophoblastic differentiation evolved from transitional cell carcinoma (Campo et al, 1989). Earlier studies suggested that SP1 expression was a poor prognostic factor in breast carcinoma but this has not been substantiated (Wright et al, 1987). SP! has been employed in the panel for the distinction of mesothelioma from adenocarcinoma, being positive in almost 60% of adenocarcinomas. However, SP1 is also expressed in mesotheliomas, albeit, in lower frequency (6%) (Pfaltz et al, 1987). In lung carcinomas, SP1 was immunostained in 87% of non-small cell carcinomas and in 51% of small cell carcinomas with a significant negative correlation of both SP1 and CEA immunoexpression with grade of differentiation inf adenocarcinoma (Slodkowska et al, 1998).

References

Campo E, algaba F, Palacin A, et al. Placental proteins in high-grade urothelial neoplasms. An immunohistochemical study of human chorionic gonadotropin, human placental lactogen, and pregnancy-specific beta 1-glycoprotein. Cancer 1989;63:2497–504.

Haynes WD, Shertock KL, Skinner JM, Whitehead R. The ultrastructural immunohistochemistry of oncofetal antigens in large bowel carcinomas. Virchows Archives A Pathology Anatomy and Histopathology 1985;405:263–75.

Pfaltz M, Odermatt B, Christen B, Ruttner JR. Immunohistochemistry in the diagnosis of malignant mesothelioma. Virchows Archives A Pathology Anatomy and Histopathology 1987;411:387–93.

Plouzek CA, Leslie KK, Stephens JK, Chou JY. Differential gene expression in the amnion, chorion, and trophoblast of the human placenta. Placenta 1993;14:277–85.

Sabet LM, Daya D, Stead R, et al. Significance and value of immunohistochemical localization of pregnancy specific proteins in feto-maternal tissue throughout pregnancy. Modern Pathology 1989;2:227–32.

Schlafke S, Lantz KC, King BF, Enders AC. Ultrastructural localization of pregnancy-specific beta 1-glycoprotein (SP1) and cathepsin B in villi of early placenta of the macaque. Placenta 1992;13:417–28.

Shibata PK, Rutgers JL. The placental site nodule: an immunohistochemical study. Human Pathology 1994;25:1295–1301.

Slodkowska J, Szturmowitcz M, Rudzinski P, et al. Expression of CEA and trophoblastic cell markers by lung carcinoma in association with histological characteristics and serum marker levels. European Journal of Cancer Prevention 1998;7:51–60.

Waterhouse R, Ha C, Dvcksler GS. Murine CD9 is the receptor for pregnancy-specific glycoprotein 17. Journal of Experimental Medicine 2002;195:277–82.

Wright C, Angus B, Napier J, et al. Prognostic factors in breast cancer: immunohistochemical staining for SP1 and NCRC 11 related to survival, tumour epidermal growth factor receptor and oestrogen receptor status. Journal of Pathology 1987;153:325–31.

Progesterone Receptor (PR)

Sources/clones

Abbott (PgR-ICA), Becton
Dickinson (PR33, PR4–12),
Biogenesis (1A6), Biogenex
(PgR-1A), Dako (1A6,
polyclonal), Immunotech
(PR10A9), Novocastra (1A6),
Zymed (1A6).

Fixation/preparation

Most antibody clones currently
available are immunoractive in
routinely fixed paraffin embedded
tissues and enhanced after HIER.
Enzymatic predigestion is not
required (Leong & Milios, 1993).

Background

In selected target tissues,
estrogens have been found to
stimulate not only mitogenesis
but also the synthesis of specific
proteins. One of these estrogen-
induced proteins is the
progesterone receptor (PR).
Progesterone and synthetic
progestins activate the receptor,
provoke its phosphorylation and
DNA-binding ability and induce
its regulatory activities. Since the
PR is an estrogen-inducible
protein, its expression is
indicative of an intact estrogen
receptor pathway and may
identify tumors that are
hormonally responsive to
estrogen, thereby improving the
overall predictive value of steroid
receptor assays in selected tumors
such as breast carcinoma.

The PR displays the typical
three-domain structure of the
steroid-thyroid receptor family.
the central domain contains two
"zinc finger" structures
responsible for the specific
recognition of the cognate DNA
sequences. The carboxyl-
terminal domain contains the
hormone and anti-hormone
binding sites. The complete
organization of the human PR
gene has been determined. It
spans over 90 kb and contains
eight exons. The first exon
encodes the N-terminal part of
the receptor, the DNA binding
domain is encoded by two
exons, each corresponding to
one zinc finger and the steroid
binding domain is encoded by
five exons.

The signal responsible for the
nuclear localization of the PR is
a complex one. The receptor
continuously shuttles between the
nucleus and cytoplasm. The
receptor diffuses into the
cytoplasm and is constantly and
actively transported back into the
nucleus similar to the
phenomenon for estradiol and
glucocorticosteroid receptors.
Immunolocalization of PR is
confined to the nucleus.

Applications

The value of estrogen and
progesterone receptor assays in
predicting response to hormonal
treatment in advanced breast
cancer patients has been well
supported by both studies
employing cytosol-based ligand
binding methods and
immunohistochemical assays, the
prognostic utility being strongest
in premenosausal women.
Approximately 50% of breast
cancers are ER+ PR+, 20%
ER+ PR-, 5% ER- PR+, and
25% ER- PR-.

Those women whose cancers
express both ER and PR show
the greatest likelihood of
responding to endocrine
treatment. Using conventional
biochemical assays, the response
rate is about 77% for ER+ PR+
tumors, 46% for ER- PR+, 27%
for ER+ PR-, and 11% for ER-
PR- tumors. However, it is
clinically recognized that a small
proportion of women with
tumors, which are receptor
negative, will show a positive
response to hormonal therapy,
and as many as one third of those
with receptor positive tumors
may fail to respond to such

treatment. The significance of breast carcinomas biochemically negative for estrogen receptor (ER), but positive for PR, is poorly understood. It has been proposed that these tumors, more common in younger women, contain ER whose presence is masked in a biochemical binding assay by endogenous estrogen. Such tumors should be positive for ER by immunocytochemical assay but this was not proven in one study, which found that ER–PR+ tended to have larger tumor size and higher histologic grade and S-phase fractions compared to ER+PR+ tumors. It was concluded that biochemically ER–PR+ breast carcinomas are biologically different from ER+PR+ tumors (Keshgegian, 1994).

There has been some suggestion that PR may be a more important predictor as there are more responders among patients with ER–PR+ compared to ER+PR– tumors. In some series although this remains to be proven, the prognostic advantage of steroid receptor positivity was lost after 4–5 years of follow up (Lipponen et al, 1992). As with the estrogen receptor, there is increasing evidence that immunohistological assays provide more accurate prognostication than cytosol-based methods (Mohammed et al, 1986; Pertschuk et al, 1996).

Comments

We employ PgR-ICA, which is enhanced following HIER. Immunostaining is further enhanced following HIER in TRS (Dako) as compared to citrate buffer (Leong et al, 1996; MacGrogan et al, 1996). Consistent immunostaining is obtained in cytological preparations that have been fixed in 10% formalin following complete air-drying. HIER should be used (Suthipintawong et al, 1997).

Problems associated with reporting of results and the relevance of objective assessment of immunostains with image analysis equipment is discussed under the section on "estrogen receptor". Interestingly, in a recent study of hormone receptors in rat brain, it was shown that while immunoreactivity for both androgen and estrogen receptors decreased after immersion fixation compared to perfused sections at time of removal of the brain, PR immunoreactivity was not affected. However, all three receptors decreased gradually with increasing postmortem interval (Fodor et al, 2002).

References

Fodor M, van Leeuwen FW, Swaab DF. Diffferences in postmortem stability of sex steroid receptor immunoreactivity in rat brain. Journal of Histochemistry and Cytochemistry 2002;50:641–50.

Guichon-Mantel A, Delabre K, Lescop P, Milgrom E. Intracellular traffic of steroid hormone receptors. Journal of Steroid Biochemistry and Molecular Biology 1996;56:3–9.

Keshgegian AA. Biochemically estrogen receptor-negative, progesterone receptor-positive breast carcinoma. Immunocytochemical hormone receptors and prognostic factors. Archives of Pathology and Laboratory Medicine 1994;118:240–4.

Leong AS-Y, Milios J, Leong FJ. Epitope retrieval with microwaves. A comparison of citrate buffer and EDTA with three commercial retrieval solutions. Applied Immunohistochemistry 1996;4:201–7.

Leong AS-Y, Milios J. Comparison of antibodies to estrogen and progesterone receptors and the influence of microwave antigen retrieval. Applied Immunohistochemistry 1993;1:282–8.

Lipponen P, Aaltomas S, Eskelinen M. The changing importance of prognostic factors in breast cancer during long term follow-up. International Journal of Cancer 1992;51:698–702.

MacGrogan G, Soubeyran I, De Mascarel I, et al. Immunohistochemical detection of progesterone receptors in breast invasive ductal carcinomas: A correlative study of 942 cases. Applied Immunohistochemistry 1996;4:219–27.

Mohammed RH, Lakatua DJ, Haus E, Yasmineh WJ. Estrogen and progesterone receptors in human breast cancer: correlation with histologic subtype and degree of differentiation. Cancer 1986;58:1076–81.

Pertschuk L, Feldman J, Kim Y-D et al. Estrogen receptor (ER) immunocytochemistry in paraffin with ER1D5 predicts breast cancer endocrine response more accurately that H222Sp in frozen sections or cytosol-based ligand binding assays. Cancer 1996;77:2541–9.

Suthipintawong C, Leong AS-Y, Chan KW, Vinyuvat S. Immunostaining of estrogen receptor, progesterone receptor, MIB1 and c-erbB-2 in cytological preparations – A simplified method. Diagnostic Cytopathology 1997;17:127–33.

Proliferating Cell Nuclear Antigen (PCNA)

Sources/clones

Biodesign (PC10), Biogenesis (PC10), Biogenex (19A2), Boehringer Mannheim (PC10), Camon (19A2), Chemicon, Coulter (19A2), Dako (PC10), Diagnostic Biosystems (PC10), Medac (PC10), Oncogene (PC10, 19F4), 19A2), Serotec (19.A2), Signet (PC10), Zymed (ZO49).

Fixation/preparation

Both the main clones, PC10 and 19A2 to proliferating cell nuclear antigen (PCNA) are immunoreactive in fixed embedded tissues. However, the antigen is fixation dependent and HIER produces significant enhancement of immunostaining. HIER in 1% zinc sulfate is reported to produce the best staining (Shin et al, 1994), although we have found citrate buffer at pH 6.0 to be sufficiently effective.

Background

PCNA, formerly called cyclin (now recognized to be a much wider class of proteins associated with cell proliferation), represents a component of DNA polymerase-δ (Bravo & Macdonald-Bravo, 1987) and is a

36 kD intranuclear proliferation associated antigen. An antibody to this antigen was first described in the blood of selected patients with systemic lupus erythematosus. This polypeptide has since been found in both normal and transformed cells and is tightly associated to the sites of DNA replication. Its expression is highest during S-phase of the cell cycle and there is generally a good correlation between expression of PCNA and the S-phase fraction determined by flow cytometry in a given tumor cell population. However, certain caveats apply to the use of anti-PCNA antibodies as marker of cell proliferation. In malignant cell lines such as HeLa, PCNA levels increase during S-phase but it is not zero during the other phases of the cell cycle. Indeed, in this cell line the levels of PCNA increase only by a factor of 2–3 during S-phase (Morris & Matthews, 1989). There are also at least two forms of PCNA, one associated with the "replicon" structure and the other, more loosely associated in the cell nucleus. Both proteins are retained by formalin fixation but only the former is retained by alcoholic fixatives such as methacarn (Bravo et al, 1987). Furthermore, the antigen persists in cells that are no longer in the cycling phase and

are in G_0. Generally PCNA counts obtained with clone PC10 have been higher that those obtained with Ki-67 (Leong et al, 1995) or S-phase fraction measured by flow cytometry, despite PCNA being considered to be primarily an S-phase-associated protein. PCNA has a relatively long half-life of 20 hours and may be immunohistochemically detected in cell that have recently left the cell cycle and may be in G_0. Discrepancies have also been demonstrated between PCNA counts obtained with PC10 and that of S-phase fraction by thymidine and bromodeoxyuridine uptake in a variety of tumors and in the experimental situation (Yu et al, 1991; Scott et al 1991). The PCNA index was found to be two to three times that of values obtained with DNA polymerase-alpha (Kawakita et al, 1992). There is ample evidence that the antigen is very fixation-dependent and different antibody clones show vastly different sensitivities for the antigen (Leong et al, 1993; Coltrera et al, 1993).

Applications

PCNA immunostaining offers an alternative to the well-established, but cumbersome methods of assessing tumor growth fractions, namely titriated thymidine or bromodeoxyuridine incorporation, or flow cytometry and has been enthusiastically employed in numerous publications, despite the limitations discussed above.

Comments

PC10 is the most sensitive of the antibody clones available but bearing in mind the fixation dependency of PCNA, comparisons between laboratories are invalid unless fixation protocols are standardized. Furthermore, because of the long half-life of the antigen, only strongly stained cells should be counted and weakly stained cells show poor correlation with the S-phase fraction (Yu et al, 1995). Methanol is the fixative of choice (Burford-Mason et al, 1994). Despite these reservations, PCNA immunostaining has remained a very method of assessing proliferating tumor cells and has been used as a predictive marker of tumor outcome in a variety of tumors (Kayaselcuk et al, 2002; Kolar et al, 2002; Preethi et al, 2002; Qin et al, 2002; Kouvaraki et al, 2002). Without standardization of fixation and tissue processing such results should be viewed with a great deal of circumspect. Ki-67 is by far a better marker for cycling cells and the inhibitors of cyclin-dependent kinases such as $p21^{WAF1}$ and $p27^{kip1}$ provide immunohistological assessment of non-cycling cells.

References

Bravo R, Macdonald-Bravo H. Existence of two populations of cyclin/proliferating cell nuclear antigen during the cell cycle: Association with DNA replication sites. Journal of Cell Biology 1987;105:1549–54.

Burford-Mason AP, MacKay AJ, Cummins M, Dardick I. Detection of proliferating cell nuclear antigen in paraffin-embedded specimens is dependent on preembedding tissue handling and fixation. Archives of Pathology and Laboratory medicine 1994; 118:1007–13.

Coltrera MD, Skelly M, Gown AM. Anti-PCNA antibody PC10 yields unreliable proliferation indexes in routinely processed, deparaffinized, formalin-fixed tissue. Applied Immunohistochemistry 1993;1:193–200.

Kawakita N, Seki S, Yanani A, et al. Immunocytochemical identification of proliferating hepatocytes using mononuclear antibody to proliferating nuclear cell antigen (PCNA/cyclin). Comparison with immunocytochemical staining for DNA polymerase-alpha. American Journal of Clinical Pathology 1992;97 (Suppl 1):S14–20.

Kayaselcuk F, Zorludemir S, Gumurduhu D, et al. PCA and Ki-67 in central nervous system tumors: correlation with the histological type and grade. Journal of Neurooncology 2002;57:115–21.

Kolar Z, Murray PG, Zapletalova J. Expression of c-erbB-2 in node negative breast cancer does not correlate with estrogen receptor status, predictors of hormone responsiveness, or PCNA expression. Neoplasma 2002;49:110–3.

Kouvaraki M, Gorgoulis VG, Rassidakis GZ, et al. High expression levels of p27 correlate with lymph node status in a subset of advanced invasive breast carcinomas: relation to E-cadherin alterations, proliferative activity, and ploidy of the tumors. Cancer 2002;94:2454–65.

Leong AS-Y, Milios J, Tang SK. Is immunolocalization of proliferating cell nuclear antigen (PCNA) in paraffin sections a valid index of cell proliferation? Applied Immunohistochemistry 1993;1:127–35.

Leong AS-Y, Vinyuvat S, Suthipintawong C. A comparative study of cell proliferation markers in breast carcinomas. Journal of Clinical Pathology: Molecular Pathology 1995;48:M83-M87.

Preethi TR, Chacko P, Kesari AL, et al. Apoptosis in epithelial ovarian tumors. Pathology Research and Practice 2002;198:273–80.

Qin LX, Tang ZY, Ma ZC, et al. P53 immunohistochemical scoring: an independent prognostic marker for patients after hepatocellular carcinoma resection. World Journal of Gastroenterology 2002;8:459–63.

Scott RJ, Hall PA, Haldane JS. A comparison of immunohistochemical markers of cell proliferation with experimentally determined growth fraction. Journal of Pathology 1991;165:173–8.

Shin HJ, Shin DM, Shah T, Ro JY. Optimization of proliferating cell nuclear antigen immunohistochemical staining by microwave heating in zinc sulfate solution. Modern Pathology 1994;7:242–8.

Yu CC-W, Hall PA, Fletcher CDM, et al. Hemangiopericytomas: the prognostic value of immunohistochemical staining with a monoclonal antibody to proliferating cell nuclear antigen (PCNA). Histopathology 1991;19:29–33.

Yu CC-W, Dublin EA, Camplejohn RS, Levison DA. Optimization of immunohistochemical staining of proliferating cells in paraffin sections of breast carcinoma using antibodies to proliferating cell nuclear antigen and the Ki-67 antigen. Annals of Cell Pathology 1995;9:45–52.

Prostate-Specific Antigen (PSA)

Sources/clones

Accurate (ER-PR8), Biodesign (8), Biogenesis (PSA-001, 07), Biogenex (8), Dako (ER-PR8, polyclonal), Enzo, Hybritech, Immunotech, Oncogene (OS94.3), Oxoid (PSB535), Sanbio (8), Serotec (SC.5), Zymed (2009).

Fixation/preparation

The antigen is resistant to formalin fixation and immunostaining is enhanced by heat-induced epitope retrieval.

Background

Prostate-specific antigen (PSA) is a chymotrypsin-like, 33kD single chain glycoprotein with selective serine protease activity for cleaving specific peptides. The PSA gene is a member of the human kallikrein gene family and is located on the 13q region of chromosome 19. PSA is selectively produced by the epithelial cells of the acini and ducts of the prostatic gland and is secreted into the semen where it is directly involved in the liquefaction of the seminal coagulum that is formed at ejaculation. The sequence of PSA shows extensive homology with γ-nerve growth factor (56%), epidermal growth factor-binding protein (53%), and α-nerve growth factor (51%). This feature together with its ability to digest insulin growth factor-binding protein-III (IGFBP-3) to release biologically active IGF-I, makes PSA a candidate growth factor or a cytokine or modulator of cell growth. PSA has also recently been suggested to be capable of being produced by cells bearing steroid hormone receptors under conditions of steroid hormone stimulation (Diamandis & Yu, 1995).

Applications

PSA is a useful biochemical marker as any disruption of the normal architecture of the prostate allows diffusion of PSA into the stoma where it gains access to the peripheral blood through the microvasculature. Elevated serum PSA levels are thus seen with prostatitis, infarcts, benign hyperplasia, and transiently after manipulation and biopsy. Most importantly, significant elevations are seen with prostatic adenocarcinoma, making it an important tool for diagnosis as well as monitoring response to treatment. Although cancer produce less PSA per cell than normal prostatic epithelium, the greater number of malignant cells and the disruption of stroma in the malignant gland accounts for the elevated serum PSA levels.

Immunostaining for PSA has proven to be an effective method of identifying cells of prostatic origin, however, the presence of PSA cannot be used to differentiate between benign and malignant. Antibodies to PSA show high sensitivity although very occasion carcinomas have been reported to be negative for PSA. Correlations of PSA tissue reactivity with Gleason's grade of prostatic cancer have shown that high-grade tumors may be entirely negative by immunolabelling. There was initial suggestion that the presence of PSA-negative cells in a prostatic carcinoma correlates with a more aggressive clinical course but this has not been confirmed and most tumors display very heterogeneous staining (Bostwick, 1994).

Comments

As the occasional case of prostatic carcinoma and metastatic deposit may show only weak or no staining for PSA, it is best to use this marker in conjunction with other markers of prostatic tissue such as prostatic acid phosphatase and CD57 (Leu 7). A combination of these three markers gives the highest diagnostic yield (Appendix 1.15). Furthermore, immunoreactivity to PSA has been shown in a variety of extra-prostatic tissues including the epithelium of the urethra, periurethral glands of both males and females, urachal remnants, endometrium (Clements & Mukhtar, 1994) transitional epithelium of the bladder and in cystitis cystica and glandularis, anal mucosa and anal glands (Stein et al, 1982), ductal cells of the normal pancreas and normal salivary glands. PSA immunoreactivity is also seen in urethral and periurethral gland adenocarcinoma, extramammary Paget's disease of the penis and pleomorphic adenoma and carcinoma of the salivary gland (Elgamal et al, 1996). PSA has been found in breast carcinoma cells and was initially suggested to confer a positive prognosis but more recent controlled studies have not confirmed this earlier finding (Miller et al, 2001).

Neutrophils and some neuroendocrine tumors also stain for PSA.

Small, closely apposed Cowper's glands can mimic neoplastic prostatic glands especially in core biopsies and can be distinguished by the absence of prostatic markers such as PSA, prostatic acid phosphatase and carcinoembryonic antigen. While Cowper's glands like malignant prostatic glands do not stain for high molecular weight cytokeratin they show a peripheral layer of attenuated myoepithelial cells which can be highlighted by staining for smooth muscle actin (Saboorian et al, 1997).

Specificity is improved by using the monoclonal antibodies. We have had consistent results with clone ER-PR8 from Dako when used with MW-induced retrieval.

References

Bostwick DG. Prostate-specific antigen. Current role in diagnostic pathology of prostatic cancer. American Journal of Clinical Pathology 1994;102 (Suppl1):S31–S37.

Clements A, Mukhtar A. Glandular kellikreins and prostate specific antigen are expressed in the human endometrium. Journal of Endocrinology and Metabolism 1994;78:1536–9.

Diamandis EP, Yu H. New biological functions of prostate-specific antigen? Journal of Clinical endocrinology and Metabolism 1995;80:1515–6.

Elgamal AA, Ectors NL, Sunardhi-Widyaputra S, et al. Detection of prostate specific antigen in pancreas and salivary glands: A potential impact on prostatic carcinoma overestimation. Journal of Urology 1996;156:464–8.

Miller MK, Unger PD, Bleiweiss IJ. Immunohistochemical analysis of prostate specific antigen in breast cancer. Breast Cancer Research and Treatment 2001;68:111–6.

Saboorian MH, Huffman H, Ashfaq R, et al. Distinguishing Cowper's glands from neoplastic and pseudoneoplastic lesions of prostate: immunohistochemical and ultrastructural studies. American Journal of Surgical Pathology 1997;21:1069–74.

Stein BS, Peterson RO, Vangore S, Kendall AR. Immunoperoxidase localization of prostate specific antigen. American Journal of Surgical Pathology 1982;2:553–7.

Prostatic Acid Phosphatase (PAP)

Sources/clones

Accurate (P-29, 4LJ, SB19), Biodesign, Biogenesis (501, 503, 504), Biogenex (045), Camon, Chemicon, Dako (PASE/4LJ, polyclonal), Diagnostic, Immunotech (PAP29), Milab/Med, Novocastra, Oxoid (PAY376), Sanbio (4LJ), Saxon, Sera Lab (8), Serotec, Sigma (PAP12, PAP29) and Zymed (ZMPAP4).

Fixation/preparation

Both poly-and monoclonal antibodies are immunoreactive in fixed, paraffin-embedded tissues and staining is enhanced by heat-induced epitope retrieval.

Background

Acid phosphatases hydrolyze phosphoric acid esters at acid pH. They are found in a variety of tissues and differences in electrophoretic patterns or sensitivity to isoenzyme inhibitors allowed the distinction of isoforms of the enzyme to specific tissues. Normal prostatic tissue contains several isoforms but only two are secreted in the seminal fluid. Acid phosphatase activity is mainly localized to the lysozomes of prostatic epithelial cells and ultrastructurally is identified within microvilli of the apical cell membranes and in the secretory granules at the supranuclear or apical regions of benign cells. Although synthesized in rough endoplasmic reticulum, PAP is not demonstrable in this site and because it is only recognized in lysozomes it is assumed that antibodies recognize PAP only when packaged into granules. Basal cells are negative for PAP. Serum levels of the enzyme reflect the amount of enzyme released into the circulation and is dependent on the tumor mass and also the rate of synthesis and access to the intravascular space. Low levels of the enzyme have been suggested to represent low rates of synthesis by poorly differentiated tumors.

Applications

PAP immunostaining is a useful discriminator for prostatic tissue and its diagnostic specificity and sensitivity is increased when used in a panel in conjunction with PSA and CD57 (Leu 7). Like PSA, immunoreactivity for PAP is more intense and homogenous in benign prostatic tissue than in prostatic carcinoma. PAP is localized within prostatic acini and ducts, although the latter tend to show weaker and more heterogeneous staining (Leong & Gown, 1993).

Rare cases of squamous metaplasia of the prostatic epithelium show staining for PAP. There is weak positivity in seminal vesicle epithelium and like PSA, periurethral glands in both men and women are positive for the enzyme. Other non-prostatic tissues that may show PAP immunostaining are anal glands in men, neuroendocrine cells of the rectum, transitional epithelium and von Brun's nests of the bladder, renal tubular epithelium, pancreatic islet cells, hepatocytes gastric parietal cells and mammary ductal epithelium. Neutrophils show the strongest concentration of PAP among non-prostatic tissues. Neoplasms that show cross-reactivity are mainly those derived from the cloaca, such as urinary bladder, periurethral glands and colon and neuroendocrine tumors (Wahol & Longtime, 1985; Epstein, 1993).

Comments

In general, PAP is relatively specific for prostatic neoplasms. However, because of the cross-reactivity of both PAP and prostate specific antigen (PSA) with the tissues listed above, it is still best to use PAP in conjunction with PSA, particularly in the context of a tumor in the perineum whose differential diagnosis includes prostatic carcinoma, transitional carcinoma and adenocarcinoma of the bladder and rectal carcinoma (Leong et al, 1996). Besides PAP and PSA, the panel should include an antibody to high molecular weight cytokeratin, CK 20 and CK 7 (Appendix 1.15). Cowper's glands may mimic prostatic adenocarcinoma because they are small closely packed acini lined by a single cell layer and do not stain for high molecular weight cytokeratin. However, these glands do not stain for prostatic markers such as PAP, prostate specific antigen and carcinoembryonic antigen and show an attenuated myoepithelial cell layer in the periphery, staining with smooth muscle actin (Saboorian et al, 1997).

Acid phosphatase consists of several isoenzymes and polyclonal antibodies to PAP cross react with isoenzyme 4, which is present in small amounts in most human tissues. Furthermore, polyclonal antibodies recognize several antigenic sites and may produce weak background staining but this is not seen with monoclonal antibodies that recognize only one antigenic site. Clone PASE/4LJ from Dako produces satisfactory results.

References

Epstein JI. PSA and PAP as immunohistochemical markers in prostatic cancer. Urologic Clinics of North America 1993;20:757–70.

Leong AS-Y, Gown AM. Immunohistochemistry of "solid" tumors: poorly differentiated round cell and spindle cell tumors – I. IN: Leong AS-Y (ed) Diagnostic Immunohistochemistry for the Surgical Pathologist. London: Edward Arnold, 1993, pp24–72.

Leong FJ, Leong AS-Y, Swift J. Signet ring carcinoma of the prostate. Pathology, Research and Practice 1996;192:1232–8.

Saboorian MH, Huffman H, Ashfaq R, et al. Distinguishing Cowper's glands from neoplastic and pseudoneoplastic lesions of prostate: immunohistochemical and ultrastructural studies. American Journal of Surgical Pathology 1997;21:1069–74.

Wahol MJ, Longtime JA. The ultrastructural localization of prostate specific antigen and prostatic acid phosphatase in hyperplastic and neoplastic human prostates. Journal of Urology 1985;134:607–11.

Protein Gene Product 9.5 (PGP 9.5)

Sources/clones

Accurate (31A3, 13C4),
Biogenesis (31A3, 13C4).

Fixation/preparation

HIER enhances Immunostaining
in paraffin-embedded sections in
citrate buffer at pH 6.0.

Background

Protein gene product 9.5 (PGP
9.5) is a ubiquitin carboxyl-
terminal hydrolase whose gene is
mapped to chromosome 4p14,
spans 10 kb and contains nine
exons (Edwards et al, 1991). It
displays 5' features some common
to many genes and others
common with neurofilament
neuron-specific enolase and Thy-
1-antigen gene 5' regions
(Wilkinson et al, 1989). PGP 9.5 is
a 27 kD soluble protein which has
been shown by immunostaining
in all levels of the central and
peripheral nervous system, many
neuroendocrine cells, in part of
the renal tubule, spermatogonia
and non-pregnant corpus luteum
(Wilson et al, 1988). Benign and
neoplastic follicular center
lymphoid cells also stain for the
antigen (Langlois et al, 1995).

There is some evidence from
studies in glioma cell lines that
the protein is maximally
expressed during the growth
phase and that it may play a role
in glial cells during brain
development, in reactive gliosis,
or in tumorigenesis of the glial
lineage (Giambanco et al, 1991).
PGP 9.5 has been demonstrated
in pituitary adenoma, medullary
carcinoma of thyroid, pancreatic
islet cell tumor, paraganglioma,
neuroblastoma, carcinoid tumors
from a variety of sites and Merkel
cell carcinoma (Rode et al, 1985;
Gosney et al, 1995).

PGP9.5 is now thought to be
a neurospecific peptide that
functions to remove ubiquitin
from ubiquitinated proteins and
prevents them from targeted
degradation by proteasomes.
Thus, in neoplasms, the increased
deubiquitination of cyclins by
PGP9.5 could contribute to
uncontrolled growth of somatic
cells that is the hallmark of
cancer. PGP9.5 overexpression
has been negatively correlated
with outcome in pancreatic
(Tezel et al, 2002) and colorectal
carcinoma (Yamazaki et al, 2002).
Interestingly, the examination of
gene expression with the SAGE
method demonstrated the
presence of PGP9.5 transcripts in
normal lung epithelium, lung
tumor cell lines as well as
ressected primary non-small cell
lung carcinoma, suggesting that
increased expression of PGP9.5
may have a role in carcinogenesis
(Hibi et al, 1999).

Applications

PGP 9.5 is distinct from neuron-
specific enolase (NSE) and is
largely employed as a marker of
nervous and neuroendocrine
differentiation. However, it is of
low specificity as shown in a
study of bronchial carcinomas
where, like NSE, PGP 9.5
actually labeled more cases of
non-small cell tumors than small
cell lesions. PGP 9.5 has the
advantage of producing a more
intense stain with less
background compared to NSE
but if used as a marker of neural
and neuroendocrine
differentiation, it must be
employed in conjunction with
chromogranin and synaptophysin
which are more specific markers
for this purpose. Other
applications of PGP 9.5 include
the study of unmyelinated nerve
fibers in the skin and colonic
mucosa, atrial myxomas, and
inclusion bodies in the central
nervous system (Wilson et al,
1988; Gosney et al, 1995).

PGP9.5 may also be a useful
marker for the identification of
malignant peripheral nerve sheath

tumors as such tumors often display a lack of stainable S100 protein, especially in the epithelioid variant, PGP9.5 showing a sensitivity of 94% compared to 38% for S100. However, PGP9.5 also showed low specificity as it was found in 4/6 synovial sarcomas and 3/9 leiomyosarcomas (Hoang et al, 2001).

Comments

Before the advent of HIER, it was recommended that fresh tissues be fixed in a solution of 95% alcohol-5% acetic acid for 2–3 hrs to obtain optimal results. This is no longer necessary as HIER produces marked enhancement of immunoreactivity compared to other methods of antigen unmasking, with both increase in number of positive-staining cells as well as increased intensity of reaction within individual cells and their processes (McQuaid et al, 1995).

References

Edwards YH, Fox MF, Povey S, Hinks LJ. The gene for human neuron specific ubiquitin C-terminal hydrolase (UCHL1, PGP9.5) maps to chromosome 4p14. Annals of Human Genetics 1991;55:273–8.

Giambanco I, Bianchi R, Ceccarelli P, et al. "Neuron-specific" protein gene product 9.5 (PGP 9.5) is also expressed in glioma cell lines and its expression depends on the cellular growth state. FEBS Letters 1991;290:131–4.

Gosney JR, Gosney MA, Lye M, Butt SA. Reliability oif commercially available immunocytochemical markers for identification of neuroendocrine differentiation in bronchoscopic biopsies of bronchial carcinoma. Thorax 1995 50:116–20.

Hibi K, Westra WH, Borges M, et al. PGP9.5 as a candidate tumor marker for non-small cell lung cancer. American Journal of Pathology 1999;155:711–5.

Hoang MP, Sinkre P, Albores-Sasvedra J. Expression of protein gene product 9.5 in epithelioid and conventional malignant peripheral nerve sheath tumors. Archives of Pathology and Laboratory Medicine 2001;125:1321–5.

Langlois NE, King G, Herriot R, Thompson WD. An evaluation of the staining of lymphomas and normal tissues by the rabbit polyclonal antibody to protein gene product 9.5 following non-enzymatic retrieval of antigen. Journal of Pathology 1995;175:433–9.

McQuaid S, McConnell R, McMahon J, Herron B. Microwave antigen retrieval for immunocytochemistry on formalin-fixed, paraffin-embedded post-mortem CNS tissue. Journal of Pathology 1995;176:207–16.

Rode J, Dhillon AP, Doran JF, et al. PGP 9.5, a new marker for human neuroendocrine tumors. Histopathology 1985;9;147–58.

Tezel E, Hibi K, Nagasaka T, Nakao A. PGP9.5 as a prognostic factor in pancreatic cancer. Clinical Cancer Research 2000;6:4764–7.

Wilkinson KD, Lee KM, Deshpande S, et al. The neuron-specific protein PGP 9.5 is a ubiquitin carboxyl-terminal hydrolase. Science 1989;246:670–3.

Wilson PO, Barber PC, Hamid QA, et al. The immunolocalization of protein gene product 9.5 using rabbit polyclonal and mouse monoclonal antibodies. British Journal of Experimental Pathology 1988;69:91–104.

Yamazaki T, Hibi K, Takase T, et al. PGP9.5 as a marker for invasive colorectal carncer. Clinical Cancer Research 2002;8:192–5.

pS2

Sources/clones

Biogenex (PS2.1), Dako (BC04), Labvision Corp (PS2.1, R47–94).

Fixation/preparation

The antigen survives formalin fixation and is enhanced by HIER.

Background

pS2 is a 6660 Dalton, 60 amino acid secretory polypeptide protein that was isolated from the breast carcinoma cell line MCF-7. It belongs to a recently-described family of trefoil-shaped growth factors which includes human intestinal trefoil factor (hITF) and human spasmolytic polypeptide (hSP). Although its exact function is unknown, it is believed to be part of a steroid-dependent stimulatory pathway. An estrogen-regulated protein, it has been studied as a marker of an intact estrogen pathway, and hence marker hormone sensitivity and favorable prognosis in breast carcinoma. There is growing evidence that members of the trefoil peptide family are involved in active maintenance of the integrity of gastrointestinal mucosa and facilitating its repair (Poulsom 1996; May & Westley 1997).

Applications

pS2 positivity is preferentially expressed in hormone-dependent cells in breast cancer. Low concentrations of the protein have been associated with a poor prognosis (Foekens et al 1990; Predin et al 1992) while strong expression predicted responsiveness to endocrine treatment (Racca et al 1995). The 5-year recurrence-free survival and overall survival were 85% and 95% respectively for estrogen receptor (ER)+/progesterone receptor (PR)+/pS2+ tumors, but only 50% and 54% for patients with ER+/PR+/pS2- tumors (Foekens et al 1990).

In another study of 72 advanced breast cancer cases, 76% of pS2+ cases had stable disease, complete remission, or partial remission as compared with 37% of the pS2- cases. The authors proposed that pS2 may help differentiate the 35–50% of ER+ breast cancer patients who do not clinically respond to hormone therapy, and the rare ER- patients who do (Schwartz et al 1991). However, further studies have found that while pS2 immunostaining correlates with age, estrogen receptor and progesterone receptor status, it is not an independent prognostic factor and is not an indicator of increased survival in breast cancer (Speiser et al 1994; Wysocki et al 1994). pS2 is thus best viewed as an estrogen receptor associated protein and not an independent prognostic marker (Elledge et al, 2000). It has been suggested that pS2 expression in breast cancers with BRCA1 mutation was significantly lower that sporadic breast cancer (Charafe-Jauffre et al, 2001).

pS2 is widely distributed throughout the gastrointestinal tract, particularly adjacent to damaged mucosa (Collier et al 1995; Poulsom 1996). It is consistently expressed in superficial and foveolar epithelium of non-neoplastic gastric mucosa and in 66% of gastric carcinomas, but has little value as a prognostic indicator (Machado et al 1996). Colorectal carcinoma stains with pS2 to a lesser extent but this too lacks statistical significance (Shousha et al 1993).

Expression in normal pancreas is usually absent however, it can be seen focally within occasional ducts in chronic pancreatitis and it is prominent in pancreatic adenocarcinoma and ampullary tumours (Collier et al 1995).

Comments

We employ clone PS2.1.

References

Charafe-Jauffre E, Eisinger F, Mathoulin-Portier MP, et al. pS2 expression in BRCA1-associated breast cancers. Anticancer Research 2001;21:2877–81.

Collier JD, Bennet MK, Bassendine MF, Lendrum R. Immunolocalization of pS2, a putative growth factor, in pancreatic carcinoma. Journal of Gastroenterology and Hepatology 1995;10:394–400.

Elledge RM, Green S, Pugh R, et al. Estrogen receptor (ER) and progesterone receptor (PR), by ligand-binding assay compared with ER, PgR and pS2, by immunohistochemistry in predicting response to tamoxifen in metastatic breast cancer: a Southwest Oncology Group Study. International Journal of Cancer 2000;89:111–7.

Foekens JA, Riol M-C, Seguin P. Prediction of relapse and survival in breast cancer patients by pS2 protein status. Cancer Research 1990:50;3832–7.

Machado JC, Carneiro F, Ribeiro P. pS2 protein expression in gastric carcinoma. An immunohistochemical and immunoradiometric study. European Journal of Cancer 1996;32A:585–90.

May FE, Westley BR. Trefoil proteins: their role in normal and malignant cells. Journal of Pathology 1997;183:4–7.

Poulsom R. Trefoil peptides. Baillieres Clinical Gastroenterology 1996;10:113–134.

Predine J, Spyratos F, Prud'homme JF. Enzyme-linked immunosorbent assay of pS2 in breast cancers, benign tumours, and normal breast tissues: correlation with prognosis and adjuvant hormone therapy. Cancer 1992:69;2116–23.

Racca S, Conti G, Pietribiasi F. Correlation between pS2 protein positivity, steroid receptor status and other prognostic factors in breast cancer. International Journal of Biological Markers 1995;10:87–93.

Schwartz LH, Koerner FC, Edgerton SM. pS2 expression and response to hormonal therapy in patients with advanced breast cancer. Cancer Research 1991;51;624–8.

Shousha S, Luqmani YA, Sannino P et al. pS2 immunostaining of colorectal carcinoma. Modern Pathology 1993;6:446–8.

Speider P, Stolzlechner J, Haider K et al. pS2 protein status fails to be an independent prognostic factor in an average breast cancer population. Anticancer Research 1994;14:2125–30.

Wysocki SJ, Iacopetta BJ, Ingram DM. Prognostic significance of pS2 mRNA in breast cancer. European Journal of Cancer 1994;30A:1882–4.

Rabies

Sources/clones

Accurate (HYB-3R7), Biodesign, Biogenesis (RAB50), Chemicon International (C4–62–15–2), Research Diagnostics (RV7C5).

Fixation/preparation

Anti-rabies monoclonal antibody may be applied to acetone fixed samples. It is also potentially applicable to formalin-fixed paraffin embedded tissue sections, although optimisation will be necessary with some form of antigen retrieval.

Background

Rabies is a rod or bullet shaped virus with a single stranded RNA genome, and belongs to the family Rhabdoviridae. It is a highly fatal disease of humans and warm-blooded vertebrates; usually transmitted via infected saliva following the bite of a diseased animal, most commonly dogs. Virus introduced into the bite wound enters the peripheral nerves and following an incubation of weeks to months, spreads to the spinal cord and brain. It produces a neurological derangement, lasting a few days to weeks and resulting in death.

Antibody C4–62–15–2 to rabies virus is specific to the N-nucleoprotein. It enjoys a wide range of species reactivity and includes mouse, raccoon, skunk, dog/coyote and bats (Smith, 1989).

Applications

During prolonged incubation periods, the sensory neurons of the dorsal root ganglia may be the site of viral sequestration. Efferent spread of virus in the nervous system may extend terminally to the eye and nerve fibers surrounding hair follicles. Hence, demonstration of antigen in corneal impression smears or skin biopsies may be used for confirmation of diagnosis in a live patient. Unless the diagnosis is confirmed during life, an autopsy must be performed with $10–20^3$ mm blocks of cerebrum, cerebellum, hippocampus, medulla, thalamus and brain stem being taken in duplicate: 50% glycerol-saline for virological examination and 10% buffered formalin for immunohistological examination.

Comments

Antibody to Rabies is useful in locating the Negri bodies in sections of brain. In one study of naturally infected domestic and wild animals, rabies antigen was detected in 62% of the brain areas in which inclusion bodies were not found (Palmer et al, 1985). The antigen is not limited to the Negri bodies but also traceable in the cytoplasm (Feiden et al, 1985; Sinchaisri et al, 1992). Most of the work with rabies antibodies has been performed on fresh tissue with direct immunofluorescence techniques (Bingham & van der Merwe, 2002) although recent application to formalin-fixed tissue has met with good success (Jogai et al, 2000).

References

Bingham J, van der Merwe M. Distribution of rabies antigen in infected brain material: determining th reliability of different regions of the brain for the rabies fluorescent antibody test. Journal of Virological Methods 2002;101:85–94.

Feiden W, Feiden U, Gerhard L, et al. Rabies encephalitis: immunohistochemical investigations. Clinical Neuropathology 1985 4:156–64.

Jogai S, Radotra BD, Banerjee AK. Immunohistochemical study of human rabies. Neuropathology 200;20:197–203.

Palmer DG, Ossent P, Suter MM, Ferrari E. Demonstration of rabies viral antigen in paraffin tissue sections: comparison of the immunofluorescence technique with the unlabeled antibody enzyme method. American Journal of Veterinary Research 1985;46:283–6.

Sinchaisri TA, Nagata T, Yoshikawa Y, et al. Immunohistochemical and histopathological study of experimental rabies infection in mice. Journal of Veterinary Medical Science 1992;54:409–16.

Smith JS. Rabies virus epitopic variation: use in ecologic studies. Advances in Virus Research 1989,36:215–53.

Retinoblastoma Gene Protein (P110ᴿᴮ, Rb protein)

Sources/clones

Accurate (84B3–1), Biodesign (RB1, 1F8), Biogenesis (RB), Dako (Rb1), Lab Vision (1F8), Novocastra (Rb1), Oncogene Research (AF11, LM95.1), Pharmingen (245), Santa Cruz Lab (C-15)

Fixation/preparation

The antibodies are mostly immunoreactive only in fresh frozen sections although some antibodies stain fixed paraffin-embedded sections but only after HIER.

Background

The Rb gene is located on chromosome 13q14 and spans a region of more than 200 kb, including 27 exons. The Rb gene is the only tumor suppressor that has been shown to directly suppress tumor formation. It is a cell cycle regulator preventing cells from entering the S-phase. The Rb protein has a molecular mass of 105 kD and a number of antibodies which recognize specific parts of this protein have been developed. Besides loss of function due to chromosomal abnormalities including chromosomal deletion,

translocation and point mutation, as with p53, phosphorylation may inactivate the Rb protein. In addition, a variety of viral oncoproteins including simian virus 40 T antigen, E1A from adenovirus and E6 from human papilloma virus, may bind and inactivate the Rb protein.

Immunostaining may be a valid way to assess the presence of normal Rb protein but several factors affecting staining should be considered before accepting the relevance of the technique. Firstly, it has been observed that the level of expression of Rb protein is not the same in all cells in any individual tissue, e.g., in the epithelium of the cervix, there are low or undetectable levels of staining in the basal layers and staining increases with cell maturation. In contrast, low or absent anti-Rb protein staining was observed in the well-differentiated epithelial cells of the gastric mucosa such as the foveolar and mucus cells compared to the cells in the crypts and neck of the glands. Astrocytes and microglia do not show detectable Rb protein by immunostaining and other subsets of normal cells such as some stromal cells do not display demonstrable Rb protein. The reasons for failure to demonstrate

the protein at an equivalent level in all cells may relate to variations in expression as a function of cell cycling activity, cell differentiation and protein phosphorylation. More importantly, there is a large subset of cells which include endothelial cells, lymphocytes and stromal cells, in which the ability to demonstrate p110ᴿᴮ expression is critically dependent on the method of staining used (Cordon-Cardo & Richon, 1994).

Applications

The p53 and retinoblastoma (Rb) gene products must be the two most-studied tumor suppressor genes. While alterations in the p53 tumor suppressor gene have been recognized as the most frequent genetic alterations in human neoplasia, the extent of Rb gene alterations is less-well known. P53 alterations are mostly detected as overexpression of the protein and can easily be done with immunostaining, whereas most normal cells do not contain stainable wild-type p53 protein. In contrast, the Rb protein is detectable immunohistochemically in normal nontransformed cells, although whether this is so for all normal cells and tissues are currently unknown. As abnormality is based on the absence of stainable Rb protein, it is critical that techniques of maximal sensitivity must be employed and internal positive controls must be present in the sections (Skelly et al, 1996).

Alterations in the RB gene have been described in a number of human tumors including retinoblastoma, osteosarcoma, other sarcomas, leukemias, lymphomas, and certain carcinomas including those from the breast, prostate, lung, bladder, kidney and testis (Geradis et al, 1994). Rb gene alterations have been associated with increasing tumor grade and stage in a variety of tumors and there are increasing evidence that alterations of this gene are associated with increased risk for metastasis (Xu et al, 1991; 1993). In breast carcinoma there is some evidence of association with other signs of progression and loss of hormonal receptor expression (Drobnak et al, 1993). A downregulation of the Rb gene has been shown in the progression of melanocytic tumors, loss of expression correlated with increase in Clark level and shorter survival rates. All naevi with and without dysplasia showed high expression, and a large percentage of primary melanomas showing Rb-positive cells (Korabiowska et al, 2001). There was loss of immunostaining for Rb protein in ovarian carcinomas compared to benign and borderline tumors and this loss correlated with a higher proliferative index and loss of heterozygosity at the Rb-1 locus (Gras et al, 2001). In clear cell renal carcinoma increased Rb protein and decreased p27 immunoexpression are claimed to be powerful and independent poor prognostic factors (Haitel et al, 2001).

Comments

It was recently demonstrated that HIER in citrate buffer at pH 6.0 with overnight antibody incubation produced maximal sensitivity when staining fixed paraffin-embedded sections. Fixation in methacarn also requires HIER treatment and the use of DNAse produced variable results. The use of low pH buffers can produce false-positive results. Thus, in the assessment of Rb protein, as with other fixation-sensitive antigens, it is clear that the findings of individual laboratories cannot be generalized owing to differences in fixation and immunolabelling techniques. However, these factors do not preclude the assessment of the Rb protein in laboratories where fixation and other variables are strictly controlled.

References

Cordon-Cardo C, Richon VM. Expression of the retinoblastoma protein is regulated in normal human tissues. American Journal of Pathology 1994;144:500–10.

Drobnak M, Cote RJ, Saad AD, et al. P53 and Rb alterations in primary breast carcinoma: correlation with hormone receptor expression and lymph node metastases. International Journal of Oncology 1993;2:173–8.

Geradis J, Hu SX, Lincoln CE, et al. Aberrant RB gene expression in routinely processed, archival tumor tissues determined by three different anti-RB antibodies. International Journal of Cancer. 1994;58:161–7.

Gras E, Pons C, Machin P, et al. Loss of heterozygosity at the RB-1 locus and pRB immunostaining in epithelial ovarian tumors: a molecular, immunohistochemical and clinicopatholgic study. International Journal of Gyncologic Pathology 2001;20:335–40.

Haitel A, Wiener HG, Neudert B, et al. Expression of the cell cycle proteins p21, p27, and pRb in clear cell renal carcinoma and their prognostic significance. Urology 2001;58:477–81.

Korabiowska M, Ruschenburg I, Betke H, et al. Downregulation of the retinoblastoma gene expression in the progression of malignant melanoma. Pathobiology 2001;69:274–80.

Skelly M, Coltrera MD. Gown AM. Immunohistochemical analysis of p110ᴿᴮ expression in human cells and tissues. A reappraisal and critical review of the literature. Applied Immunohistochemistry 1996;4:16–24.

Xu HJ, Cagle PT, Moore GE, Benedict WF. Absence of retinoblastoma protein expression in primary non-small cell lung carcinomas. Cancer Research 1991;52:2735–9.

Xu HJ, Cairns P, Hu SX, et al. Loss of RB protein expression in primary bladder cancer correlates with loss of heterozygosity at the RB locus and tumor progression. International Journal of Cancer 1993;53:781–4.

S100

Sources/clones

Accurate (polyclonal), Biodesign (polyclonal), Biogenesis (15E2E2, polyclonal), Biogenex (15E2E2, polyclonal), Chemicon (monoclonal, polyclonal), Cymbus Bioscience (MIG5), Dako (polyclonal), ICN (polyclonal), Immunotech (polyclonal), Medac (S1/61/69), Novocastra (polyclonal), Oncogene (OS94.5), RDI (MIG-5), Sera Lab (polyclonal), Serotec (polyclonal), Sigma (polyclonal), Zymed (polyclonal).

Fixation/preparation

Formalin-fixed tissues are ideally suited for S100 immunostaining and the antigen is resistant to long durations of fixation in formalin. Its reactivity can still be enhanced by heat-induced antigen retrieval but not by proteolytic digestion.

Background

S100 protein, so named because of its solubility in a saturated ammonium sulfate solution, occurs as three biochemically distinct forms. Each is a protein dimer of two subunits, designated α and β. The three dimers are S100A$_o$ (α-α), S100A (α-β), and S100B (β-β). The α and β subunits each have a molecular weight of approximately 10.5 kD with extensive amino acid sequence homology between the two subunits. They both have amino acid sequences known to code for the calcium binding sites of the calmodulin family of proteins. S100 is highly acidic and water-soluble with varying affinities for calcium, zinc and manganese. These properties are related to many basic cell functions such as cation diffusion across lipid membranes, microtubule assembly and stability, calcium and cyclic nucleotide regulation and increased activity of RNA polymerase, drug-protein interactions, the plasma membrane function of neurons and interaction with chromosomes and synaptosomes. S100 protein is conserved in nature and is present within the cells of all three germ layers in humans a reflection of its important role in basic cell function.

Applications

S100 has been demonstrated in a wide variety of normal and abnormal tissues. Formalin fixation and paraffin embedding may alter antigenic sites and aldehyde fixation may prevent diffusion of the highly soluble antigen that can produce artefactual immunolocalization patterns. Indeed, one study has reported granular staining of virtually every cell type when fresh frozen tissue was stained with a monoclonal S100 antibody.

Normal and neoplastic cartilaginous tissue including benign and malignant chondroid tumors express S100 protein and is useful for the distinction of non-cartilaginous bone tumors, which are mostly negative for the antigen. Cartilaginous tumors can be distinguished from chordomas by the presence of cytokeratin and EMA in the latter and their absence in the former. S100 is also useful for the labeling of myoepithelial cells in mammary ducts particularly when distinguishing sclerosing adenosis from tubular carcinomas, the former displaying a distinct layer of myoepithelial cells. Sustentacular or satellite cells of the adrenal medulla and paraganglia and their corresponding tumors are labeled by S100 antibodies, as are the folliculo-stellate cells of the anterior pituitary (Nakajima et al, 1982; Takahashi et al, 1984; Loeffel et al, 1985).

The S100 antigen is a useful marker of peripheral nerve cells. The protein is present in the nuclei and cytoplasm of Schwann cells and satellite cells in parasympathetic and sympathetic ganglia (Daimaru et al, 1985). The β-subunit has been reported in these cells but not in neurons, the latter contain the α-subunit that is not expressed in Schwann cells or satellite cells. Pacinian corpuscles also contain S100 protein. While S100 protein is expressed in the majority of benign nerve sheath tumors, as many as 40–50% of malignant Schwann cells do not stain. A population of S100-positive Schwann cells can be demonstrated in neurofibromas but variable numbers of perineural and intermediate cells within these tumor do not stain for S100 protein. Correspondingly, neurogenic sarcomas arising in patients with neurofibromatosis show a spectrum of expression of S100 protein. Both benign and malignant granular cell tumors contain S100 protein expressed as the β-subunit, a feature used to support an origin from Schwann cells.

The other group of cells which are labeled by S100 antibodies are the histiocytes. The interdigitating reticulum cells of the paracortical areas in the lymph node are stained by S100 protein antibodies, as are dendritic reticulum cells of the lymphoid follicles. Langerhans' cells of the skin, mucous membranes and other sites are also positive for S100 protein, expressing S100B activity (β-β). As such, S100 protein is a useful marker for the identification of Langerhans' cell histiocytosis.

One of the most useful applications of the S100 protein is its use as a marker of nevus cells and melanomas. Virtually all benign melanocytic lesions contain S100 protein which is also observed in over 95% of malignant melanomas. When used in conjunction with a panel comprising cytokeratin, vimentin and LCA, it allows the identification of malignant melanoma from its common mimics, namely, anaplastic carcinoma and large cell lymphoma. Similarly, the inclusion of anti-CEA forms a useful panel to distinguish Bowen's disease, Paget's disease of the skin and superficial spreading malignant melanoma. Because a small number of melanomas may fail to express S100 protein, antibodies to HMB45 and the melanoma-associated antigen NKI/C3 are useful additional markers for melanoma.

S100 protein is expressed by adipocytes and a proportion of liposarcomas also stains positive. Tumors of the cutaneous adnexae and salivary glands also express S100 protein.

Comments

Although S100 protein is a useful marker for the identification of melanoma, Langerhans' cell histiocytosis and peripheral nerve tumor, the antibodies should be used in the context of the differential diagnosis derived from morphologic and clinical appearances. A wide variety of carcinomas including those from the lung, pancreas, female genitourinary tract as well as *Mycobacteria ulcerans* organisms have been reported to show positivity so that S100 antibodies should not be used or interpreted in isolation. We have also observed the staining of benign skeletal and smooth muscle cells with some anti-S100 antibodies.

The use of S100 to identify residual melanoma cells in re-excision biopsies is fraught with problems as S100-positive spindle cells are often present in the scar tissue. These spindle cells may stain for neuron-specific enolase but do not label with HMB45, Melan A or CD57 (Chorny & Barr, 2002). These cells may occur in re-excisions of non-melanoma tumors and stain with the Schwann cell differentiation markers p75NGFR, CD56/N-CAM and GAP-43 suggesting that they represent reactive proliferating Schwann cells (Trejo et al, 2002)

References

Chorny JA, Barr RJ. S100-positive cells in scars: a diagnostic pitfall in the re-excision of desmoplastic melanoma. American Journal of Dermatopathology 2002;24:309–12.

Daimaru Y, Hashimoto H, Enjoji M. Malignant peripheral nerve sheath tumours (malignant schwannomas). An immunohistochemical study of 29 cases. American Journal of Surgical Pathology 1985;9:434–44.

Loeffel SC, Gillespie GY, Mirmiran SA, et al. Cellular immunolocalisation of S100 protein within fixed tissue sections by monoclonal antibodies. Archives of Pathology and Laboratory Medicine 1985;109:117–22.

Nakajima T, Watanabe S, Sato Y, et al. An immunoperoxidase study of S100 protein distribution in normal and neoplastic tissues. American Journal of Surgical Pathology 1982;6:715–27.

Takahashi K, Isobe T, Ohtsuki Y, et al. Immunohistochemical study on the distribution of α and β subunits of S100 protein in human neoplasm and normal tissues. Virchow's Archives (Cellular Pathology) 1984;45:385–96.

Trejo O, Reed JA, Prieto VG. Atypical cells in human cutaneous re-excision scars for melanoma express p75NGFR, CD56/N-CAM and GAP-43: evidence of early Schwann cell differentiation. Journal of Cutaneous Pathology 2002;29:397–406.

NOTES

Serotonin

Sources/clones

Accurate (5HTH209, YC5/45, polyclonal), Axcel/Accurate (5HT-H209), American Qualex (polyclonal), Biodesign (polyclonal), Biogenesis (polyclonal), Biogenex (polyclonal), Caltag Laboratories (polyclonal), Chemicon (polyclonal), Dako (5HT-H209), Fitzgerald (M09203), Immunotech (polyclonal), Pharmingen (YC5–45), Sanbio/Monosan (polyclonal), Serotec (polyclonal), Seralab (polyclonal), Zymed (polyclonal).

Fixation/preparation

The antibodies to serotonin are immunoreactive in formalin-fixed, paraffin-embedded tissue sections. HIER enhances immunoreactivity.

Background

Serotonin (5-hydroxytryptamine) is a neurotransmitter substance, which is found in a broad range of normal, hyperplastic and neoplastic tissues, including the gastrointestinal tract, central nervous system, adrenergic nerve fibers, platelets and basophils. The major use of this marker has been to identify serotonin-secreting carcinoid tumors, which mostly arise from the midgut (Westberg et al, 1997).

Applications

Immunostaining for serotonin has been employed as a marker of neuroendocrine differentiation. However, like other specific neuropeptides such as bombesin, ACTH, calcitonin and VIP, it is of low sensitivity and specificity and should only be employed in a panel of several antibodies with more specific markers such as chromogranin and synaptophysin. The major application of serotonin lies in the detection of carcinoid tumors (Zavala-Pompa et al, 1993; Zea-Iriarte et al, 1994; Burke et al, 199) particularly as such tumors may respond to specific therapy with the somatostatin analogue octreotide and alpha interferons (Wilander et al, 1989; Westberg et al, 1997). Serotonin may also be detected in scattered cells within other neuroendocrine tumors from a variety of sites (Le Bodie et al, 1996; Gilks et al, 1997; LaGuette et al, 1997; Lindberg et al, 1997). Whereas all tumors of the lung with dense core granules contained neuron-specific enolase, less contained serotonin (Wilson et al, 1985). In another study of 53 carcinoid tumors, 34 were argentaffin positive, 50 were argyrophil positive and 43 contained immunologically detectable serotonin (Shaw 1988).

Interestingly, using serotonin staining as a marker of neuroendocrine differentiation it was shown that androgen ablation promotes neuroendocrine cell differentiation in human and dog prostates. Replacement androgens and estrogens after castration restored this cell population to normal values and induced luminal differentiation and basal metaplasia respectively (Ismail et al, 2002).

Comments

Serotonin has limited application as a marker of neuroendocrine differentiation. If use for this purpose it should be employed with a panel of more specific and sensitive antibodies such as chromogranin and synaptophysin. Its main application today would be in a secondary panel to identify the specific neuropeptides produced in an established neuroendocrine tumor.

References

Burke AP, Thomas RM, Elsayed AM, Sobin LH. Carcinoids of the jejunum and ileum: an immunohistochemical and clinicopathologic study of 167 cases. Cancer 1997;79:1086–93.

Gilks CB, Young RH, Gersell DJ, Clement PB. Large cell carcinoma of the uterine cervix: a clinicopathologic study of 12 cases. American Journal of Surgical Pathology 1997;21:905–14.

Ismail AHR, Landry F, Aprikian AG, Chevalier S. Androgen ablation promotes neuroendocrine cell differentiation in dog and human prostate. Prostate 2002;51:117–25.

LaGuette J, Matias-Guiu X, Rosai J. Thyroid paraganglioma: a clinicopathologic and immunohistochemical study of three cases. American Journal of Surgical Pathology 1997;21:748–53.

Le Bodie MF, Heymann MF, Lecomte M, et al. Immunohistochemical study of 100 pancreatic tumors in 28 patients with multiple endocrine neoplasia, type I. American Journal of Surgical Pathology 1996;20:1378–84.

Linberg GM, Molberg KH, Vuitch MF, Albores-Saavedra J. Atypical carcinoid of the esophagus: a case report and review of the literature. Cancer 1997;79:1476–81.

Shaw PA. Comparison of immunological detection of 5-hydroxytryptamine by monoclonal antibodies with standard silver stains as an aid to diagnosing carcinoid tumours. Journal of Clinical Pathology 1988;41:265–72.

Westberg G, Ahlman H, Nilsson O, et al. Secretory patterns of tryptophan metabolites in midgut carcinoid tumor cells. Neurochemistry Research 1977;22:977–83.

Wilander E, Lundqvist M, Oberg K. Gastrointestinal carcinoid tumours. Histogenetic, histochemical, immunohistochemical, clinical and therapeutic aspects. Progress in Histochemistry and Cytochemistry 1989;19:1–18.

Wilson TS, McDowell EM, Marangos PJ, Trump BF. Histochemical studies of dense-core granulated tumors of the lung. Neuron-specific enolase as a marker for granulated cells. Archives of Pathology and Laboratory Medicine 1985;109:613–20.

Zavala-Pompa A, Ro JY, el-Naggar A, et al. Primary carcinoid tumor of testis. Immunohistochemical, ultrastructural, and DNA flow cytometric study of three cases with a review of the literature. Cancer 1993;72:1726–32.

Zea-Iriarte WL, Ito M, Naito S, et al. Goblet cell carcinoid of the appendix. Internal Medicine 1994;33:422–6.

Simian Virus 40 (SV40 T antigen)

Sources/clones

Biogenesis (0H9, 0G5), Chemicon, Oncogene (PAb416, PAb419, PAb280), Pharmingen (Pab101, Pab122), Santa Cruz (PAb101, Pab108)

Fixation/preparation

The use of this antibody was confined to the staining of fixed tissue culture cells (Montano and Lane, 1984) until the recent application of antigen retrieval (Baker-Cairns et al, 1996).

Background

SV40T antigen (Ab-3) is a mouse monoclonal antibody with specificity for antigenic determinants unique to the SV40 small T antigen and non-reactive with SV40 large T antigen (Montano & Lane, 1984). Both antigens are encoded by the early region of the SV40 genome (Tooze 1973).

Simian virus 40 (SV40) large T antigen is an 81 kD multifunctional viral phosphoprotein. Some of its functions are essential to the viral replication in monkey cells. Others contribute to its neoplastic transforming activity (Livingston & Bradley, 1987).

The large T antigen binds DNA and complexes with p53 protein (Lane and Crawford, 1979). It also forms a specific complex with the P105 product of the retinoblastoma susceptibility gene (De Caprio et al, 1988).

Applications

The use of this antibody has been confined to the research laboratory to define the cellular location of small t antigen in subcellular extracts of SV40 infected cells (Mantano and Lane, 1989). Pab280 reacted strongly with a cytoplasmic form of small t antigen that appears to be associated with the cytoskeleton. Small t was found to accumulate late in the SV40 lytic cycle and was localized in both the cytoplasm and the nucleus of cells infected with wild-type SV40 (Mantano and Lane, 1984). Research applications have centered around the use of SV40 as an effective gene transfer vector in vitro (Strayer 1996), the immortalization of cell lines and the stimulation of developmental abnormalities and tumorigenesis in transgenic mice (Kelley et al, 1991; Rudland et al, 1991; Kivela et al, 1991; Kon et al, 1997; Webber et al, 1997).

Comments

The recent demonstration that 60% of human mesotheliomas contain and express SV40 sequences stimulated a great deal of interest. It has also been shown that SV40 large T-antigen interferes with the normal expression of the tumor suppressor gene p53 in human mesotheliomas raises the possibility that SV40 may contribute to the development of human mesotheliomas (Carbone et al, 1997). The cell cycle inhibitor p21^{WAF1}, a downstream target of p53 was recently evaluated immunohistochemically and found to show a significant positive correlation with survival, further supporting the role of SV40 in the pathogenesis of mesothelioma (Baldi et al, 2002). One study has failed to demonstrate SV40 immunocytochemically in mesothelioma effusions and cell block preparations (Simsir et al, 2001). SV40 has been demonstrated in fixed tissue with the novel application of a DNA thermal cycler for antigen retrieval (Baker-Cairns et al, 1996).

The antigen is nuclear in location.

References

Baker-Cairns B, Meyers K, Hamilton R, et al. Immunohistochemical staining of fixed tissue using antigen retrieval and a thermal cycler. Biotechniques 1996;20:641–50.

Baldi A, Groeger AM, Esposito V, et al. Expression of p21 in SV40 large T antigen positive human pleural mesothelioma: relationship with survival. Thorax 2002;57:353–6.

Carbone M, Rizzo P, Grimley PM, et al. Simian virus-40 larg-T antigen binds p53 in human mesotheliomas. National Medicine 1997;3:908–12.

De Caprio JA, Ludlow JW, Figge, J, Shew J, Huang C, Lee W, Marsilio E, Paucha E, Livingston DM. SV40 large tumor antigen forms a specific complex with the product of the retinoblastoma susceptibility gene. Cell 1988;54:275–83.

Kelly KA, Agarwal N, Reeders S, Herrup K. Renal cyst formation and multifocal neoplasia in transgenic mice carrying the simian virus 40 early region. Journal of the American Society of Nephrology 1991;2:84–97.

Kivela T, Virtanen I, Marcus DM, et al. Neuronal and glial properties of a mucrine transgenic retinoblastoma model. American Journal of Pathology 1991;138:1135–48.

Kon Y, Miyoshi I, Maki K, et al. Morphological study of pituitary tumorigenesis in transgenic mice induced by hybrid oncogene of the thyrotropin beta-subunit and the simian virus 40 large T-antigen. Histology and Histopathology 1997;12:981–90.

Lane DP, Crawford LV. T antigen is bound to a host protein in SV40-transformed cells. Nature 1979;278:261–3.

Livingston DM, Bradley MK. The simian virus 40 large T antigen. A lot packed into a little. Molecular Biology and Medicine 1987;4:63–80.

Montano X, Lane DP. Monoclonal antibody to simian virus 40 small t. Journal of Virology 1984;51:760–7.

Montano X, Lane DP. Monoclonal antibody analysis of simian virus 40 small t-antigen expression in infected and transformed cells. Journal of Virology 1989;63:3128–34.

Rutland PS, Ollerhead GE, Platt-Higgins AM. Morphogenetic behavior of simian virus 40-transformed human mammary epithelial stem cells on collagen gels. In Vitro Cell Development Biology 1991;27A:103–12.

Simsir A, Fetsch P, Bedrossian CW, et al. Absence of SV-40 large T antigen (Tag) in malignant mesothelioma effusions: an immunocytochemical study. Diagnostic Cytopathology 2001;25:203–7.

Strayer DS. SV40 as an effective gene transfer vector in vivo. Journal of Biological Chemistry 1996;271:2741–6.

Tooze J. "Molecular biology of tumor viruses," Part 2, 2nd ed. Cold Spring Harbor Laboratory, Cold Spring Harbor, New York, 1973.

Webber MM, Bello D, Quander S. Immortalized and tumorigenic adult human prostatic epithelial cell lines: characteristics and applications Part 2. Tumorigenic cell lines. Prostate 1997;30:58–64.

Smooth muscle myosin-heavy chain

Sources/clones

Dako (clone SMMS-1).

Fixation/preparation

SMMS-1 may be used on formalin-fixed, paraffin-embedded tissue sections, cryostat sections or cell smears. For optimal results, deparaffinized tissue sections should be treated with a proteolytic enzyme followed by heat-induced antigen retrieval.

Background

Smooth muscle myosin-heavy chain (SMM-HC) is a cytoplasmic structural protein/component of smooth muscle cells. SMM-HC expression is developmentally regulated and appears early in smooth muscle development (Frid et al, 1992; Glukhova et al, 1990). Although specific for smooth muscle development, it is not a contractile regulatory protein. SMM-HC exists in two isoforms: MHC-1 (205 kD) and MHC-2 (200 kD) and is composed of dimerized heavy chains which then bind with two pairs of myosin light chains to form myosin polypeptide (Borrione et al, 1989; Sartore et

al, 1989). SMM-HC is encoded by a single gene through alternative splicing of mRNA (Babij, 1993; White et al, 1993). Both isoforms are specific for smooth muscle cells and are considered markers of "terminal" smooth muscle differentiation (Eddinger and Murphy, 1991).

Positive immunostaining in cryostat sections with SMM-HC antibody has been demonstrated in adult human visceral and vascular smooth muscle cells but not in epithelial cells, endothelial cells or connective tissue fibroblasts (Frid et al, 1992). In the normal breast tissue, SMM-HC highlights vascular smooth muscle and myoepithelial cells in lobules, duct and lactiferous sinuses in cryostat and routinely processed sections (Lazard et al, 1993). Similarly, periacinar and periductal myoepithelial cells of salivary gland are also immunopositive with SMM-HC, whereas all of the acinar/ductal epithelial cells were negative (Savera et al, 1997).

Anti-SMM-HC also labels intact myoepithelial cells in benign and *in situ* malignant breast lesions (Wang et al, 1997). Furthermore, while muscle actin-positive myofibroblasts were noted within the stroma of invasive carcinomas, SMM-HC

was expressed only on rare myofibroblasts in 7% of tumors. This predominantly negative immunostaining of myofibroblasts is helpful to avoid confusion between myoepithelial cells and the condensation of myofibroblasts around ducts. SMM-HC immunostaining has also proved to be useful for the demonstration of myoepithelial cells in salivary gland tumors (Savera et al, 1997) and lymphangioleiomyomatosis (Matsui et al, 2000).

Applications

Anti-SMM-HC may be of use for the demonstration of myoepithelial cells in the following more common histologic difficulties (Yaziji et al, 2000):
– radial scar versus infiltrating tubular carcinoma
– cancerization of adenosis by DCIS mimicking microinvasive carcinoma
– invasive cribriform carcinoma mimicking non-invasive lesions
– papillary carcinoma versus papilloma
– nipple adenoma and syringomatous nipple adenoma versus infiltrating duct carcinoma

Comments

Anti-SMM-HC has proved to be superior to muscle actin for the demonstration of myoepithelial cells in breast tissue as the latter also stains the vast number of myofibroblasts in the stroma.

References

Babij P. Tissue-specific and developmentally regulated alternative splicing of a visceral isoform of smooth muscle heavy chain. Nucleic Acids Research 1993;1:1467–71.

Borrione AC, Zanellato AM, Scannapieco G, et al. Myosin heavy-chain isoforms in adult and developing rabbit vascular smooth muscle. European Journal of Biochemistry 1989;183:413–7.

Eddinger TJ, Murphy RA. Developmental changes in actin and myosin heavy chain isoform expression in smooth muscle. Archives of Biochemistry and Biophysics 1991;284:232–7.

Frid MG, Shekhonin BV, Koteliansky VE, Glukhova MA. Phenotypic changes of human smooth muscle cells during development: late expression of heavy caldesmon and calponin. Developmental Biology 1992;153:185–93.

Glukhova MA, Frid MG, Koteliansky VE. Developmental changes in expression of contractile and cytoskeletal proteins inhuman aortic smooth muscle. Journal of Biological Chemistry 1990;265:13042–6.

Lazard D, Sastre X, Frid MG, et al. Expression of smooth muscle-specific proteins in myoepithelium and stromal myofibroblasts of normal and malignant human breast tissue: Proceedings of the National Academy of Sciences of the United States of America 1993;90:999–1003.

Matsui K, Tatsuguchi A, Valencia J, et al. Extrapulmonary lymphangioleiomyomatosis (LAM): clinicopathologic features in 22 cases. Human Pathology 2000;31:1241–8.

Sartore S, DeMarzo N, Borrione AC, et al. Myosin heavy-chain isoforms in human smooth muscle. European Journal of Biochemistry 1998;179:79–85.

Savera AT, Gown AM, Zarbo RJ. Immunolocalization of three novel smooth muscle-specific proteins in salivary gland pleomorphic adenoma: assessment of the morphogenetic role of myoepithelium. Modern Pathology 1997;10:1093–100.

Wang NP, Wan BC, Skelly M, et al. Antibodies to novel myoepithelium-associated proteins distinguish benign lesions and carcinoma in situ from invasive carcinoma of the breast. Applied Immunohistochemistry 1997;5:141–51.

White S. Martin AG, Periasamy M. Identification of a novel smooth muscle myosin heavy chain cDNA: isoform diversity in the S1 head region. American Journal of Physiology 1993;264:1252–8.

Yaziji H, Gown AM, Sneige N. Detection of stromal invasion in breast cancer: The myoepithelial markers. Advances in Anatomic Pathology 2000;7:100–9.

Spectrin/Fodrin

Sources/clones

Accurate (SB-SP1, SB-SP2), American Qualex (polyclonal), Biodesign (polyclonal), Biogenesis (B12G3, D4D7, 2C5, polyclonal), Calbiochem (polyclonal), Chemicon (polyclonal), ICN Immunologicals (AA6), Locus Genex, Helsinki (101AA6), Finland Novocastra (RBC1.5B1, RPC2.3D5), Serotec (D7A3, D4D7), Sigma Chemical (polyclonal), Zymed (Z068).

Fixation/preparation

The antibody is immunoreactive in fresh frozen tissue sections and in fixed paraffin-embedded sections following HIER.

Background

Spectrin is a flexible rod-shaped molecule of 200 nm length found in mammalian and avian erythrocytes. It is composed of two non-identical subunits, α and β, and linked to the plasma membrane by the protein ankyrin. Along with actin, ankyrin and band 4.1, spectrin forms a network or membrane skeleton that lies immediately beneath the plasma membrane. The main function of the spectrin cytoskeleton is that of structural support for the bi-lipid layer of the cell membrane and the spectrin-based membrane skeleton also controls lateral mobility of the erythrocyte membrane proteins (Bennett 1989, 1990a, 1990b). Thermal denaturation of spectrin leads to disintegration of the erythrocytes into vesicles and deficiencies or structural abnormalities of the membrane skeleton proteins leads to loss of shape or tensile strength of the erythrocytes resulting in fragmentation and destruction as they pass through the spleen. Defects of spectrin are associated with fragile erythrocytes in hemolytic anaemias such as hereditary elliptocytosis, pyropoikilocytosis and spherocytosis (Bennett & Gilligan 1993).

Non-erythroid cells also show a membrane skeleton which contains spectrin, although the molecular organization in such cells is less known. Non-erythroid spectrin is known as fodrin, molecular weight of 240 kD, exhibits many similarities to spectrin, including immunochemical cross-reactivity, and is found in virtually all non-erythroid cells. Besides the function of maintaining some specialized membrane domains, fodrin appears to be redistributed in a variety of cell surface events, suggesting that it acts as a dynamic mediator between the cell membrane, membrane skeleton and cytoskeleton. For example, there is significant reorganization of the spectrin network in cells treated with growth factors. In chromaffin cells, stimulation with a calcium ionophore results in secretion and a relocation of spectrin as cytoplasmic aggregates, antibody-induced capping of B lymphocyte surface immunoglobulin leads to redistribution of spectrin similar to the surface proteins and in A-431, an epidermoid carcinoma cell line, EGF induces cell surface remodeling and the accumulation of spectrin in membrane ruffles coincident with its phosphorylation. It is thought that calcium ions influence membrane skeleton assembly and maintenance by binding to spectrin, by calcium-regulated, calmodulin-mediated influence of the interactions between spectrin and other proteins, or by calcium-dependent protease cleavage of spectrin (Harris & Morrow, 1990; Davis & Bennett, 1994; Wallis, 1992). In skeletal muscle cells it has been shown that fodrin has a significant cytoskeletal role, lining the sarcolemma and remaining relatively uniform even when the cell changes in shape and shrinks (Herring et al, 2000).

Applications

Until recently, the antibody to spectrin/fodrin was employed only on fresh frozen tissue sections; however, with the use of microwave antigen retrieval, we were able to demonstrate immunoreactivity in fixed paraffin-embedded sections (Sormunen et al, 1997). The interest in fodrin lies in its role in cell adhesion during embryogenesis and in neoplasms. In comparison to their non-neoplastic counterparts, neoplastic epithelial cells show elevated levels of fodrin immunostaining regardless of tumor type. There was strong and fragmented and circumferential staining for fodrin, which often became accentuated with increasing grades of anaplasia, and loss of membrane staining corresponded with loss of tumor cell cohesiveness (Sormiunen et al 1997). More recent work suggests that fodrin is linked to E-cadherin and β-catenin, together having a role in cell-to-cell adhesion. The breakage of this complex is heralded by detachment of β-catenin and

associated with change in cell shape and cell adhesion in breast carcinoma (Sormunen et al, 1999). Earlier work with frozen tissue suggested that a number of cutaneous tumors show a diminished amount, or a total lack, of membrane-bound fodrin with increasing depolarization and proliferation of cells in solar keratosis and malignant melanoma. There was also accumulation of cytoplasmic fodrin in the invasive cells of squamous cell carcinoma and melanoma (Tuominen et al, 1996).

References

Bennett V. The spectrin–actin junction of erythrocyte membrane skeletons. Biochemia Biophysics Acta 1989;988:107–22.

Bennett V. Spectrin: a structural mediator between diverse plasma membrane proteins and the cytoplasm. Current Opinion in Cell Biology 1990a;2:51–6.

Bennett V. Spectrin-based membrane skeleton: A multipotential adaptor between plasma membrane and cytoplasm. Physiology Reviews 1990b;70:1029–65.

Bennett V, Gilligan DM. The spectrin-based membrane skeleton and micron-scale organization of the plasma membrane. Annual Reviews of Cell Biology 1993;9:27–66.

Davis LH, Bennett V. Identification of two regions of βG spectrin that bind to distinct sites in brain membranes. Journal of Biology and Chemistry 1994;269:4409–16.

Harris AS, Morrow JS. Calmodulin and calcium-dependent protease I coordinately regulate the interaction of fodrin with actin. Proceedings of the National Academy of Sciences USA 1990;87:3009–13.

Herring TL, Juranka P, Menally J, et al. The spectrin skeleton of newly-invaginated plasma membrane. Journal of Muscle Research and Cell Motility 2000;21:67–77.

Sormunen RT, Eskelinen S, Leong AS-Y. Fodrin immunolocalization in epithelial tumors. Applied Immunohistochemistry 1997;5:179–84.

Sormunen RT, Leong AS-Y, Vaaraniemi JP, et al. Fodrin, E-cadherin and beta-catenin immunolocalization in infiltrating ductal carcinoma of the breast correlated with selected prognostic indices. Journal of Pathology 1999;187:416–23.

Tuominen H, Sormunen R, Kallionen M. Non-erythroid spectrin (fodrin) in cutaneous tumours: diminished in cell membranes, incrased in the cytopl;asm. British Journal of Dermatology 1996;135:576–80.

Wallis CJ, Wenegieme EF, Babitch JA. Characterisation of calcium binding to brain spectrin. Journal of Biology and Chemistry 1992;267:4333–7.

Surfactant apoprotein-A

Sources/clones

Chemicon (polyclonal), Dako (PE10)

Fixation/preparation

The antibodies are immunoreactive in fixed, paraffin-embedded tissues and immunoreactivity is enhanced by heat induced antigen retrieval.

Background

Pulmonary surfactant apoproteins together with phospholipids play an essential role in maintaining the surface tension of intra-alveolar fluid and preventing the alveoli from collapsing at the end of expiration. Surfactant has been localised in two functionally distinct structures within alveolar type II pneumocytes, viz, the lamellar bodies and lysosomes, the former probably involved in surfactant secretion and the latter in degradation (Gibson & Widnell, 1991). Surfactant has also been demonstrated within tracheobronchial epithelial cells by immunostaining (Masuda et al, 1993).

Applications

Except for type II pneumocytes and pulmonary macrophages, and the walls and perivascular connective tissues of small to medium sized blood vessels of the lung, normal cells or tissues are generally not labelled by the PE10 antibody. In particular, it does not react with type I pneumocytes and mesothelial cells and has been shown to be negative in mesotheliomas so that it is a useful marker to distinguish pulmonary adenocarcinomas from mesotheliomas (Noguchi et al, 1989). A recent study demonstrated immunolabelling for surfactant apoprotein A in human normal and neoplastic breast epithelium, a finding confirmed by the demonstration of surfactant messenger RNA in both benign and neoplastic breast samples (Braidotti et al, 2001).

In a study of peripheral pulmonary adenocarcinomas, tumors could be divided into Type I or mucinous bronchioloalveolar adenocarcinomas, Type II or nonmucinous bronchioloalveolar adenocarcinomas and conventional peripheral adenocarcinomas with and without areas of Type I and Type II tumors. Immunostaining revealed that those adenocarcinomas without Type II morphology did not stain for surfactant (Ritter et al, 1998).

Surfactant immunoexpression does not appear to distinguish between Type II pneumocyte and Clara cell type adenocarcinomas, perhaps because of a common precursor (Mori et al, 1996). The protein, together with carcino-embryonic antigen and Clara cell antigen has been demonstrated in the so-called sclerosing hemangioma of the lung (Yousem et al, 1988).

Immunostaining for surfactant has found application in forensic autopsies in relation to the assessment of the severity and duration of respiratory distress from non-central nervous system or peripheral/alveolar damage. Those cases dying from hyaline membrane syndrome form various traumas, protracted death from drowning, mechanical asphyxia and fire death displayed intense granular staining of intra-alveolar surfactant apoprotein. In contrast, there was weak staining following death from alcohol intoxication, poisoning by hypnotics and carbon monoxide poisoning (Zhu et al, 2000). Surfactant immunoexpression has been shown to be significantly reduced in lungs from infants with pulmonary hypoplasia suggesting that there is also suppression or defect in functional maturity in such lungs

(Minowa et al, 2000). Immunoexpression of the protein A has been used as a marker to link rhabdoid tumor of the lung to origin from adenocarcinoma (Miyagi et al, 2000).

Comments

PE10 is a specific marker of Type II pneumocyte and Clara cells with a reasonable level of sensitivity. PE10 alone was not found to be useful in discriminating between primary pulmonary tumors and metastatic adenocarcinomas in fine needle aspiration biopsies because of low specificity and sensitivity and had to be employed in a panel with TTF-1, CK7 and CK20 to produce significant results (Chieng et al, 2001). The recent demonstration of surfactant apoprotein A and messenger RNA in both normal and neoplastic breast epithelium by immunolabelling and reverse transcriptase-polymerase chain reaction respectively (Braidotti et al, 2001) and the demonstration of the surfactant apoprotein A gene expression in a subgroup of epithelial cells in human large and small intestine (Lin et al, 2001) raises possibility of a wider role of this protein in the regulation of inflammatory processes and its tissue specificity.

References

Braidotti P, Cigala C, Graziani D, et al. Surfactant protein A expression in human normal and neoplastic breast epithelium. American Journal of Clinical Pathology 2001;116:721–8.

Chieng DC, Cangiarella JF, Zakowski MF et al. Use of thyroid transcription factor 1, PE-10, and cytokeratin 7 and 20 in discriminating between primary lung carcinomas and metastatic lesions in fine-needle aspiration biopsy specimens. Cancer 2001;93:330–6.

Gibson KF, Widnell CC. The relationship between lamellar bodies and lysosomes in type II pneumocytes. American Journal of Respiratory Cell Molecular Biology 1991;4:504–13.

Lin Z, deMello D, Phelps DS, et al. Both human SP-A1 and SP-A2 genes are expressed in small and large intestine. Pediatric Pathology and Molecular Medicine 2001;20:367–86.

Masuda T, Andoh Y, Shimura S, et al. Surfactant apoprotein A secretion by human tracheobronchial epithelial cells. Respiratory Physiology 1993;92:239–51.

Minowa H, Takahashi Y, Kawaguchi C, et al. Expression of intrapulmonary surfactant apoprotein-A in autopsies lungs: comparative study of cases with or without pulmonary hypoplasia. Pediatric Research 2000;48:674–8.

Mori M, Tezuka F, Chiba R, et al. Atypical adenomatous hyperplasia and adenocarcinoma of the human lung: their heterology in forma and analogy in immunohistochemical characteristics. Cancer 1996;77:665–74.

Myagi J, Tsuhako K, Kinjo T, et al. rhabdoid tumour of the lung is dedifferentiated phenotype of pulmonary adenocarcinoma. Histopathology 2000;37:37–44.

Noguchi M, Nakajima T, Hirohashi S, et al. Immunohistochemical distinction of malignant mesothelioma from pulmonary adenocarcinoma with anti-surfactant apoprotein, anti-Lewis and anti-Tn antibodies. Human Pathology 1989;20:53–7.

Ritter JH, Boucher LD, Wick MR. Peripheral pulmonary adenocarcinomas with bronchioloalveolar features: immunophenotypes correlate with histologic patterns. Modern Pathology 1998;11:566–72.

Yousem SA, Wick MR, singh G, et al. So-called sclerosing hemangioma fo lung. An immunohistochemical study supporting a respiratory epithelial origin. American Journal of surgical Pathology 1988;12:582–90.

Zhu BL, Ishida K, Quan L, et al. Immunohistochemistry of pulmonary surfactant apoprotein A in forensic autopsy: reassessment in relation to the causes of death. Forensic Science International 2000;113:193–7.

Synaptophysin

Sources/clones

Accurate (SVP-38, S5768), Biodesign (SY-38), Biogenesis (SY-38), Biogenex (SY-38), Boehringer Mannheim (SY-38), Calbiochem, Cymbus Bioscience (SY-38), Dako (SY 38, polyclonal), Sanbio/Monosan (SY-38), Seralab (SY-38), Sigma Chemical (SVP-38).

Fixation/preparation

Applicable to formalin-fixed paraffin embedded sections. Microwave antigen retrieval in citrate buffer improves the immunostaining of this antibody. Enzyme pretreatment is not recommended for the monoclonal antibody, which is applicable to frozen sections, and cell smears. The polyclonal antibody requires enzyme pretreatment before immunostaining.

Background

Synaptophysin is an integral-membrane glycoprotein (38 kD) of presynaptic vesicles (Jahn et al, 1985). The protein is a component of the classical, locally recycled small synaptic vesicle present in almost all neurons (Navone et al, 1986).

Synaptophysin is localized to "empty" vesicles and is both chemically and topographically different from chromogranin (68 kD), a membrane protein of the dense-core neuroendocrine granules (Lloyd et al, 1983).

Antibody (SY38) to synaptophysin has been raised against presynaptic vesicles from bovine brain. Hence, the antibody shows reactivity with neuronal presynaptic vesicles of brain, spinal cord, retina, neuromuscular junctions and small vesicles of adrenal medulla and pancreatic islets of human, bovine, rat and mouse origin (Navone et al, 1986). In normal tissues, neuroendocrine cells of the human adrenal medulla, carotid body, skin, pituitary, thyroid, lung, pancreas and gastrointestinal mucosa are labelled with this antibody (Wiedenmann et al, 1986).

The polyclonal antibody (Dako) was raised against the synthetic human synaptophysin peptide coupled to keyhole limpet hemocyanin.

Applications

Antibody to synaptophysin allows specific staining of neuronal, adrenal and neuroepithelial tumors: these include pheochromocytoma, paraganglioma, pancreatic islet cell tumors, medullary thyroid carcinoma, pulmonary/gastrointestinal/mediastinal carcinoid tumors and pituitary/parathyroid adenomas. Other neural tumors like neuroblastomas, ganglioneuroblastomas, ganglioneuromas, central neurocytoma and ganglioglioma also demonstrate immunoreactions with this antibody (Gould et al, 1988; Chejfec et al, 1987; Stefaneanu et al, 1988). The DAKO-rabbit anti-human synaptophysin is also useful for the identification of normal and neoplastic neuroendocrine cells.

The so-called pigmented "black" tumor in the pancreas has been shown to be of neuroendocrine origin with definite staining for synaptophysin and chromogranin but not HMB-45, S100, glucagon or insulin (Smith et al, 2001).

Comments

Synaptophysin is a specific and fairly sensitive marker for neural/neuroendocrine tumors of low and high grades of malignancy. While earlier antibodies were sensitive to formalin fixation and worked best in alcohol fixed material, many of the currently available antibodies are immunoreactive in formalin-fixed paraffin-embedded section after heat-induced antigen retrieval. Synaptophysin is an excellent marker of neuroendocrine cells and should be used together with chromogranin in the detection of neuroendocrine differentiation. The recommended positive control tissue is pancreas (islets).

References

Chejfec G, Falkmer S, Grimelius L, et al. Synaptophysin. A new marker for pancreatic neuroendocrine tumors. American Journal of Surgical Pathology 1987;11:241 7.

Gould VE, Lee I, Wiedenmann B et al. Synaptophysin: a novel marker for neurons, certain neuroendocrine cells, and their neoplasms. Human Pathology 1986;17:979–83.

Navone F, Jahn R, Di Gioia G, et al. Protein p38: an integral membrane protein specific for small vesicles of neurons and neuroendocrine cells. Journal of Cell Biology 1986;103:2511–27.

Jahn R, Schiebler W, Ouimet C, et al. A 38 000-dalton membrane protein (P38) present in synaptic vesicles. Proceedings of the National Academy of Science USA 1985;82:4137–41.

Lloyd LV, Wilson BS. Specific endocrine tissue marker defined by a monoclonal antibody. Science 1983;222:628–30.

Smith AE, Levi AW, Nadasdy T, et al. The pigmented "black" neuroendocrine tumor fo the pancreas: a question of origin. Cancer 2001;92:1984–91.

Stefaneanu L, Ryan N, Kovacs K. Immunocytochemical localization of synaptophysin in human hypophyses and pituitary adenomas. Archives of Pathology and Laboratory Medicine 1988;112:801–4.

Wiedenmann B, Franke WW, Kuhn C, et al. Synaptophysin: a marker protein for neuroendocrine cells and neoplasms. Proceedings of the National Academy of Science USA 1986;83:3500–4.

TAG 72 (B72.3)

Sources/clones

Biogenesis, Biogenex, Lab Vision Corp, Medac, Signet.

Fixation/preparation

This antibody is applicable to formalin-fixed, paraffin-embedded tissue sections and cell blocks prepared from pleural and ascitic fluids.

Background

Clone B72.3 represents the monoclonal antibody to tumor-associated glycoprotein (TAG-72) (Isotype: IgT1). The immunogen is a membrane-enriched fraction of a breast carcinoma derived from liver metastases. This antibody recognizes a tumor-associated oncofetal antigen (TAG-72) expressed by a wide variety of human adenocarcinomas (Szpak et al, 1986; Muraro et al, 1988). It reacts with a sialyl-Tn epitope (72 kD) expressed on mucins (Gold et al, 1988). TAG-72 expression in fetal tissue is only observed in tissues of the gastrointestinal tract, including the colon, esophagus and stomach. Although weak reaction with some tissues of adults has been observed, no reactivity is seen with tissue from organ systems including lymphoreticular, cardiovascular, hepatic, pulmonary, neural, muscular, skin, endocrine and genito-urinary tract.

Applications

Immunoreactivity of TAG-72 has been observed in 19 of 22 (86%) pulmonary adenocarcinomas (Szpak et al, 1986). In contrast, none of the 20 mesotheliomas studied showed reactivity with this antibody. Other studies have found that malignant mesotheliomas can react with this antibody, albeit, in a small percentage of cases (6/42 or 14.2%) (Comin et al, 2001). Alternatively, adenocarcinomas from a variety sites show strong, usually focal and predominantly cytoplasmic reactivity with TAG-72 (Sheibani et al, 1992). This antibody has shown immunoreaction with 84% of invasive ductal breast carcinomas and 85–95% of colon, pancreatic, gastric, esophageal, lung, ovarian and endometrial adenocarcinomas. Other workers have found this antibody to be less sensitive, labeling only 30–40% of adenocarcinomas (Sheibani et al, 1992).

Studies investigating TAG-72 staining of serous effusions have found similar high specificity but with variable sensitivity. Metastatic adenocarcinoma has been reported to be positive in 58–95% of cases from effusion specimens (Shield et al, 1994). Although rare cases of TAG-72 staining in reactive mesothelial cells have been reported (Esteban et al, 1990), other studies did not observed staining in benign, reactive or malignant mesothelial cells (Friedman et al, 1996).

There is recent suggestion that immunoexpression of TAG-72 in breast cancer cells is a marker of more aggressive phenotype (Galietta et al, 2002).

Comments

Strong reactivity for TAG-72 appears to be relatively specific for adenocarcinoma, but the utility of this antibody is somewhat limited by the variable sensitivity. Nevertheless, it is recommended that TAG-72 be included in an immunodiagnostic panel for evaluation of suspected cases of mesothelioma (Appendix 1.17).

References

Comin CE, Novelli L, Boddi V, et al. Calretinin, thrombomodulin, CEA, and CD15: a useful combination of immunohistochemical markers for differentiating pleural epithelial mesothelioma from peripheral pulmonary adenocarcinoma. Human Pathology 2001;32:529–36.

Esteban JM, Tokatar S, Husain S, Battifora H. Immunocytochemical profile of benign and carcinomatous effusions. A practical approach to difficult diagnosis. American Journal of Clinical Pathology 1990;94:698–705.

Friedman MT, Gentile P, Tarectecan A, Fuchs A. Malignant mesothelioma: immunohistochemistry and DNA ploidy analysis as methods to differentiate mesothelioma from benign reactive mesothelial cell proliferation and adenocarcinoma in pleural and peritoneal effusions. Archives of Pathology and Laboratory Medicine 1996;120:959–66.

Galietta A, Pizzi C, Pettinato G, et al. Differential TAG-72 epitope expression in breast cancer and lymph node metastases: a marker of a more aggressive phenotype. Oncology Reports 2002;9:135–40.

Gold DV, Mattes MJ. Monoclonal antibody B72.3 reacts with a core region structure of O-linked carbohydrates. Tumor Biology 1988;9:137–44.

Muraro R, Kuroki M, Wunderlich D, et al. Generation and characterization of B72.3 second generation monoclonal antibodies reactive with the tumor-associated glycoprotein 72 antigen. Cancer Research 1988;48:4588–96.

Sheibani K, Esteban JM, Bailey A, Battifora H, Weiss LM. Immunopathologic and molecular studies as an aid to the diagnosis of malignant mesothelioma. Human Pathology 1992;23:107–16.

Shield PW, Callan JJ, Devine PL. Markers for metastatic adenocarcinoma in serous effusion specimens. Diagnostic Cytopathology 1994;11:237–45.

Szpak CA, Johnston WW, Roggli V, et al. The diagnostic distinction between malignant mesothelioma of the pleura and adenocarcinoma of the lung as defined by a monoclonal antibody B72.3. American Journal of Pathology 1986;122:252–60.

Tau

Sources/clones

Accurate (TAU2, polyclonal), Accurate/Sigma, Biodesign (TAU2), Biosource (AT8, BT2, HT7), Calbiochem, Chemicon, Dako (polyclonal), Labvision Corp (TAU5), Pharmingen (TAU2.1), Sigma (TAU2, polyclonal), Zymed (T14, T46).

Fixation/preparation

Most of the antibodies are immunoreactive in fixed paraffin embedded sections.

Background

The major components of the neuronal cytoskeleton are alpha and beta tubulin, the microfilament associated proteins (MAPs), neurofilaments and actin. Tau is a neuronal microtubule-associated protein, which is the major antigenic component of neurofibrillary tangles and senile plaques in Alzheimer's disease (Joachim et al, 1987). Comparison of tau-immunoreactive lesions in three relatively uncommon neurodegenerative diseases, namely, supranuclear palsy, Pick's disease and corticobasal degeneration, demonstrated unexpected pathological

similarities, but also fundamental differences between these disorders (Feany & Dickson, 1996).

Tau2 was produced using bovine MAP as immunogen. It reacts exclusively with the chemically heterogenous tau in both the phosphorylated and non-phosphorylated form. Tau2 does not react with other MAPs or with tubulin and localises along microtubules in axons, dendrites, somata and astrocytes, and on ribosomes. Tau2 cross reacts with bovine, monkey and chicken tissue. A variety of antibodies to phosphorylated neurofilament proteins have been shown to cross-react with phosphorylated epitopes of tau (Perry et al, 1985; Cork et al, 1986).

Applications

Applications of tau are mainly in the field of neuropathological research in neurodegenerative disorders. In the diagnostic setting, conventional silver impregnation stains such as Bielchowsky or Bodian are used for the demonstration of neurofibrillary tangles. These can now also be detected with antibodies to phosphorylated tau epitopes and ubiquitin. Tau is

not only a basic component of neurofibrillary degeneration but is also an etiologic factor, as demonstrated by mutations on the tau gene responsible for frontotemporal dementias with parkinsonism linked to chromosome 17. The abnormal accumulation of tau protein in glial in many neurodegenerative diseases suggests that in some instances the disease process may also target the glial tau, with neuronal degeneration as a secondary consequence of this process. Prominent filamentous tau pathology and brain degeneration in the absence of extracellular amyloid deposition thus characterize a number of neurodegenerative disorders other than Alzheimer's disease including progressive supranuclear palsy, corticobasal degeneration, Pick's disease, collectively referred to as the tauopathies (Forman et al 2000; Berry et al 2001). Tau protein has also been demonstrated in gastrointestinal stromal tumors in an intense diffuse staining pattern in both epithelioid and spindle cell tumors in as many as 76% of both gastric and small bowel tumors. Tau also immunostained other intra-abdominal tumors including neuroendocrine carcinomas, paragangliomas and desmoplastic round cell tumors (Chambonniere et al, 2001).

Comments

Nil

References

Berry RW, Quinn B, Johnson N, Cochran EJ, et al. Pathological glial tau accumulations in neurodegenerative disease: review and case report. Neurochemistry International 2001;39:469–79.

Chambonniere ML, Mosnier-Damet M, Mosnier JF. Expression of microtuble-associated protein tau by gastrointestinal stromal tumors. Human Pathology 2001;32:1166–73.

Cork LC, Sternberger NH, Sternberger LA, et al. Phosphorylated neurofilament antigens in neurofibrillary tangles in Alzheimer's disease. Journal of Neuropathology and Experimental Neurology 1986;45:56–64.

Feany MB, Dickson DW. Neurodegenerative disorders with extensive tau pathology: a comparative study and review. Annals of Neurology 1996;40:139–48.

Forman MS, Lee VM, Trojanowski JQ. New insights into genetic and molecular mechanisms of brain degeneration in tauopathies. Journal of Chemistry and Neuroanatomy 2000;20:225–44.

Joachim CL, Morris JH, Kosik KS, Selkoe DJ. Tau antisera recognize neurofibrillary tangles in a range of neurodegenerative disorders. Annals of Neurology 1987;22:514–20.

Perry G, Rizzuto N, Autilio-Gambetti L, Gambetti P. Paired helical filaments from Alzheimer's disease patients contain cytoskeletal components. Proceedings of the National Academy of Sciences USA 1986;82:3916–20.

Tenascin

Sources/clones

Biogenex (DB7, monoclonal),
Dako (M636, rabbit anti-human),
Dako (TN2, monoclonal).

Fixation/preparation

These antibodies react positively
with tenascin in formalin-fixed,
paraffin-embedded tissue sections.
Enzyme pretreatment with pepsin
is recommended with the use of
the monoclonal antibodies prior
to the immunohistochemical
procedure.

Background

Tenascin is a large glycoprotein of
the extracellular matrix with a
unique six-armed multidomain
macromolecular structures
(Schenk, 1994). It is expressed in
fibroblasts and the extracellular
matrix during embryogenesis and
growth (Erickson and Bourdon,
1989). Tenascin is synthesized by
fibroblasts and is believed to have
active functions in epithelial-
mesenchymal interactions.

Tenascin expression is also
induced during wound healing
and inflammatory processes. The
amino acid sequence of tenascin
comprises epidermal growth
factor (EGF)-like repetitions,
which bind to EGF receptors of

tumor cells, implying that
tenascin may play a role in tumor
invasion and metastasis (Jones et
al, 1988). Tenascin has also been
demonstrated in the extracellular
matrix of mature tissue and
benign and malignant neoplasms
(Koukoulis et al, 1991).

Hence, tenascin has been
demonstrated to be a stromal
marker of malignancy in breast
carcinoma; with a positive
correlation between tenascin
expression, 5-year disease-free
survival and distant metastases in
breast carcinomas (Jahkola, 1996).
Increased tenascin
immunoexpression has also been
demonstrated in the stroma of
gastric (Ikeada, 1995),
endometrial (Sasano, 1993) and
colon (Iskaros, 1997) carcinomas.
In comparison to normal tissue
and benign tumors, increased
tenascin expression has therefore
been regarded as a stromal marker
of tumor progression.

Tenascin immunoexpression
has also been demonstrated in
mesenchymal tumors, including
schwannomas, leiomyosarcomas,
fibromas, liposarcomas and other
fibrohistiocytic tumors (Schnyder
et al, 1997). The corona-like
expression of tenascin around
lymphofollicular infiltrates
appears to be a distinctive feature
of lymphocytic thyroiditis (Back

et al, 1997). A similar pattern of
tenascin staining has been
described in lymphoid
hyperplasia of the thymus
associated with myasthenia gravis,
another autoimmune disorder.
This has been interpreted as the
lymphoid follicles
stimulating/activating the
surrounding mesenchyme to
produce tenascin as part of the
extracellular matrix (Back et al,
1997), during the course of the
autoimmune disease process.

Recently, it was demonstrated
that tenascin is an extracellular
matrix glycoprotein that plays a
role in endometrial proliferation
and possibly endometrial
carcinogenesis (Sedele et al,
2002).

Application

Tenascin immunopositivity at the
dermal-epidermal junction
overlying dermatofibroma but
not dermatofibrosarcoma
protuberans has been shown to
be useful to distinguish between
these skin tumors (Kahn et al,
2001). However, there was no
difference in staining patterns
within both tumors. Malignant
pheochromocytomas (defined by
the presence of metastases)
demonstrated strong stromal
tenascin positivity, whilst

pheochromocytomas that had not metastasized were negative (Salmenkivi et al, 2001); the adrenal medulla was negative. In contrast, paragangliomas showed a heterogeneous pattern with no difference between "benign" and malignant paragangliomas.

References

Back W, Heubner C, Winter J, et al. Expression of tenascin in lymphocytic autoimmune thyroiditis. The Journal of Clinical Pathology 1997;50:863–6.

Biogenex Laboratories. Monoclonal antibody to tenascin (data sheet).

Erickson HP, Bourdon MA. Tenascin: an extracellular matrix protein prominent in specialized embryonic tissues and tumors. Annual Review of Cell Biology 1989;5:71–92.

Ikeada Y, Mori M, Kajiyama K, et al. Immunohistochemical suppression of tenascin in normal stomach tissue, gastric carcinomas and gastric carcinoma in lymph nodes. British Journal of Cancer 1995;75:189–92.

Iskaros BF, Tanaka KE, Hu X, et al. Morphologic pattern of tenascin as a diagnostic biomarker in colon cancer. Journal of Surgical Oncology 1997;64:98–101.

Jahkola T, Toivonen T, von Smitten K, et al. Expression of tenascin in invasion border of early breast cancer correlates with higher risk of distant metastasis. International Journal of Cancer 1996;69:445–7.

Jones FS, Burgoon MP, Hoffman S, et al. cDNA clone for cytotactin contains sequences similar to epidermal growth factor-like repeats and segments of fibronectin and fibrinogen. Proceedings of the National Academy of Sciences of the United States of America 1988;85:2186–90.

Kahn HJ, Fekete E, From L. Tenascin differentiates dermatofibroma from dermatofibrosarcoma protuberans: comparison with CD34 and Factor XIIIa. Human Pathology 2001;32:50–6.

Koukoulis GK, Gould VE, Bhattacharyya A, et al. Tenascin in normal, reactive, hyperplastic and neoplastic tissues: biologic and pathologic implications. Human Pathology 1991;22:636–43.

Salmenkivi K, Haglund C, Arola J, et al. Increased expression of tenascin in pheochromocytomas correlates with malignancy. The American Journal of Surgical Pathology 2001;25:1419–23.

Sasano H, Nagura H, Watanabe K, et al. Tenascin expression in normal and abnormal human endometrium. Modern Pathology 1993;6:23–6.

Schenk S, Chiquet-Ehrismann R. Tenascins. Methods Enzymol 1994;245:52–61.

Schnyder B, Semadeni RO, Fischer RW, et al. Distribution pattern of tenascin-C in normal and neoplastic mesenchymal tissue. International Journal of Cancer 1997;72:217–24.

Sedele M, Karaveli S, Pestereli HE, et al. Tenascin expression in normal, hyperplastic and neoplastic endometrium. International Journal of Gynecological Pathology 2002;12:161–6.

Terminal Deoxynucleotidyl Transferase (TdT)

Sources/clones

Accurate (polyclonal), Biodesign (monoclonal), Biogenex (6A6.09), Chemicon, Dako (HT1, HT3, HT4, polyclonal), Gentrak, Immunotech (HTdT, polyclonal), Sera-Lab (HTdT-1, polyclonal), Sigma (8–1 E4).

Fixation/preparation

While both immunofluorescent and immunoenzyme techniques were initially applied to cryostat sections and cell suspensions, immunohistochemical staining of formalin-fixed, paraffin-embedded sections is now possible. Paraffin section immunostaining is greatly enhanced by heat-induced antigen retrieval so that terminal deoxynucleotidyl transferase (TdT) can be demonstrated on routine and archival specimens without the need for DNAse digestion and prolonged incubation previously necessary. Both 4 M urea and citrate buffer pH 6.0 are suitable retrieval solutions (Orazi et al, 1994). Polyclonal antibodies are preferable to monoclonal antibodies for formalin-fixed, paraffin-embedded sections.

Background

Terminal deoxynucleotidyl transferase (TdT) is a 58 kD protein encoded by a 35 kb gene on chromosome 10q23–25. It is a nuclear enzyme that catalyzes the random addition of deoxynucleotidyl residues on the 3'OH termini of single-stranded DNA and of oligo-deoxynucleotide primers and differs from other DNA polymerases by not requiring template instruction for polymerization.

TdT is recognized to exert its DNA polymerase function during the early variation of genes coding for T and B cells perhaps by resulting in the addition of non-germline-encoded nucleotides (N-regions) although it function is still debated.

TdT is normally present only in hematopoietic tissues such as thymus and bone marrow, where it is restricted to a proportion of multipotent cell precursors and immature T and B lymphocytes. TdT positivity is never observed in normal peripheral blood cells.

Approximately 1–2% (more in young individuals) of bone marrow cells show TdT positivity and these mostly express B cell precursor phenotype in cell suspension studies. In trephine biopsies, TdT-positive cells do not display preferential localization and are sparsely dispersed in interstitial spaces.

In the thymus, T lymphocytes can be defined into three maturation stages corresponding to their microenvironment. Stage I thymocytes, accounting for 0.5–5% of thymocytes, reside in the sub-capsular zone of the thymus and comprise large TdT blast cells which express CD7, CD2, CD5, and cCD3 (cytoplasmic). Stage II thymocytes, accounting for 60–80% of thymocytes, are TdT and express CD7, CD5, cCD3, CD2, CD1, CD4 and CD8. Stage II thymocytes, accounting for 15–20% of thymocytes, reside in the medulla, do not express TdT nor CD1 and show differentiation into either CD4+ or CD8+ cells.

Applications

TdT as a marker is mostly used in the diagnosis of lymphomas and leukemias. TdT activity is seen in acute lymphoblastic leukemias (ALL) of both B and T cell lineages so that TdT is a useful diagnostic marker for lymphoblastic leukemias (Chilosi & Pizzolo, 1995). In addition, as many as 30% of patients with chronic granulocytic leukemia develop a lymphoid blast crisis which is characterized by a lymphoblastic phenotype with nuclear TdT expression. These TdT lymphoblastic crisis have a better prognosis than TdT-nonlymphoid blast crisis and respond to ALL-like therapy.

There are about 20% of cases of acute non-lymphoid leukemias that also express TdT and in which the proportion of TdT blasts co-expressing various myeloid markers is variable. It has been suggested that the expression of TdT in such cases is a marker of poor prognosis but this is controversial. Such cases often show the phenomenon of phenotypic and genotypic "lineage infidelity" in which there is expression of lymphoid antigens such as CD7 and there is rearrangement of Ig and T cell receptor genes.

The L3 ALL in the FAB classification, which represents Burkitt-type leukemia, is an exception as the blast cells of this type of leukemia represents a "mature" B cell phenotype with surface immunoglobulin expression.

TdT is a reliable marker to distinguish lymphoblastic lymphoma (LL) from other lymphomas that are always TdT negative. LL are related to T-ALL and their distinction from the latter can be difficult, nevertheless, clinical and phenotypic differences have been observed with the latter tending to show a more immature immunophenotype. While LL is frequent in children, forming about one third of all non-Hodgkin's lymphoma, it also makes up about 5% of cases in adults, and cases of non-t, non-B or pre-B-cell LL have been reported in extranodal sites in both children and adults. TdT is particularly useful for the

separation of LL from the other small cell tumors of childhood (Leong 1999; Lucas et al, 2001) (Appendix 1.3).

TdT is thus a useful marker for diagnosis as well as for staging as it helps identify tumor cells from reactive lymphocytes. TdT staining can be used for the detection of early involvement and in staging, especially in extranodal sites such as the testes, CNS (through cerebrospinal fluid examination), skin, liver, kidney and other sites of extramedullary involvement, and for monitoring minimal residual disease following chemotherapy. In the assessment of residual LL, it should be noted that a small population of TdT+ lymphoblasts resides in benign lymph nodes and tonsils. In benign lymph nodes form 26 consecutive pediatric patient as TdT-positive cells were found adjacent to medullary and cortical sinuses in a frequency of 1 to 180 cells per high power field, as single cells or small clusters. These cells had a B precursor phenotype staining for CD79a, CD34 and CD10 (Onciu et al, 2001). In the tonsil, TdT-positive cells were demonstrated in all 15 adults and children studied by immunostaining, indicating that tonsils, like bone marrow and thymus are sites of lymphopoiesis (Strauchen & Miller, 2001).

In the identification of thymomas, particularly when sited in unusual sites such as the pleura, the presence of TdT-positive, CD1a+, Cd2+, CD99+ phenotype in the associated lymphoid population is supporting evidence of thymoma as is the aberrant expression of CD20 in the cytokeratin-positive neoplastic cells (Attanoos et al, 2002).

Comments

TdT represents a powerful tool in leukemia and lymphoma diagnosis but it should be used in the context of a complete panel of markers and relevant histochemical enzyme stains. The ability to stain for this DNA polymerase in paraffin embedded tissues, especially with polyclonal antibodies, following heat-induced antigen retrieval has greatly enhanced its diagnostic utility (Orazi et al, 1994). When immunostaining cryostat sections it is necessary to employ brief fixation in buffered formalin or Zamboni's fixative and to reduce diffusion of the enzyme the sections must be immersed in fixative immediately after cryosectoning (Chilosi et al, 1983). We employ the rabbit anti-TdT from Dako.

References

Attanoos RL, Galateau-Salle F, Gibbs AR, et al. Primary thymic epithelial tumours of the pleura mimicking malignant mesothelioma. Histopathology 2002;41:42–9.

Chilosi M, Pizzolo G. Review of terminal deoxynucleotidyl transferase. Biological aspects, methods of detection, and selected diagnostic applications. Applied Immunohistochemistry 1995;3:209–21.

Chilosi M, Pizzolo G, Fiore-Donati L et al. Routine immunofluorescent and histochemical analysis of bone marrow involvement of lymphoma/leukemia: the use of cryostat sections. British Journal of Cancer 1983;48:763–75.

Leong AS-Y. Immunohistology of small round cell tumors in childhood. Journal of Histotechnology 1999;22:239–46.

Lucas DR, Bentley G, Dan ME, et al. Ewing sarcoma vs lymphoblastic lymphoma. A comparative immunohistochemical study. American Journal of Clinical Pathology 2001;115:11–7.

Onciu M, Lorsbach RB, Henry EC, Behm FG. Terminal deoxynucleotidyl transferase-positive lymphoid cells in reactive lymph nodes from children with malignant tumor: incidence, distribution pattern, and immunophenotype in 26 patients. American Journal of Clinical Pathology 2002;118:248–54.

Orazi A, Cattoretti G, Joh K, Neiman RS. Terminal deoxynucleotidyl transferase staining of malignant lymphomas in paraffin sections. Modern Pathology 1994;7:582–6.

Strauchen JA, Miller LK. Terminal deoxynucleotidyl transferase-positive cells in human tonsils. American Journal of Clinical Pathology 2001;116:12–6.

NOTES

Thrombomodulin

Sources/clones

Advanced Immunochemical (polyclonal), American Diagnostic (polyclonal), Axcel (24FN, 3E2), Dako (1009).

Fixation/preparation

Antibodies to thrombomodulin is applicable to formalin-fixed paraffin embedded tissue.

Background

Thrombomodulin (TM) is a transmembrane glycoprotein composed of 575 amino acids (molecular weight 75 kD) with natural anticoagulant properties (Wen et al, 1987). It is normally expressed by a restricted number of cells, such as endothelial and mesothelial cells (Maruyama et al 1985). In addition, synovial lining and syncytiotrophoblasts of human placenta also express TM. Although TM contains six domains that are structurally similar to epidermal growth factor (EGF), there is no cross-reaction of anti-TM with EGF (Collins et al, 1992). The anticoagulant activity of TM results from the activation of protein C and the subsequent action on factors Va and VIIIa, and from the binding of thrombin (Suzuki et al, 1987).

Applications

Several immunohistochemical endothelial markers are currently available (Suthipintawong et al, 1995) and thrombomodulin serves as another marker, staining blood and lymphatic channels and their corresponding channels consistently. In a recent study, TM antibody stained 95% of benign lymphatic lesions (including lymphangioma and lymphangiectasia) (Appleton et al, 1996). In addition, TM demonstrated positivity in 100% benign vascular tumors (pyogenic granuloma and hemangioma) and 94% of malignant vascular tumors (Kaposi's sarcoma, angiosarcoma, and epithelioid hemangioendothelioma). Hence, TM serves as a sensitive marker for lymphatic endothelial cells and their tumors. There has also been recent interest in the use of TM as an immunohistochemical marker for mesothelial cells and malignant mesotheliomas. The results have been rather variable with some studies claiming high specificity whilst others were less specific in its role of distinguishing mesothelioma from adenocarcinoma. The table below illustrates the positivity rate for TM:

Based on these data, it appears that TM cannot be totally depended upon for the purpose of distinction between mesothelioma and pulmonary adenocarcinoma. TM may have a higher sensitivity for the small cell variant of mesothelioma (Attanoos et al, 2001).

TM has been immunohistochemically demonstrated in the endothelial cells of sinusoidal vessels in 93% (28/30 cases) of subdural hematomas. Together with demonstrable inhibition of the blood coagulation system in the hematoma, it has been postulated

Table 1		
	Mesothelioma %	Pulmonary Adenocarcinoma %
Collins et al, 1992	100	8
Brown et al, 1993	59	60
Attanoos et al, 1996	52	6
Doglioni et al, 1996	80	77

that continued production of TM results in the chronic subdural hematomas remaining liquefied and continuing to grow slowly. Transmitted pulsations in the hematoma cavity may generate sinusoidal vessel injury (Murakami et al, 2002). TM has been demonstrated in the surface cells and endothelium of neoplastic vessels in all 23 cases of cardiac myxoma studies with 82.6% showing TM in the stromal cells, 69.6% in perivascular cells. Calretinin was immunostained in 73.9% of tumors in stromal and perivascular cells (Acebo et al, 2001).

Thrombomodulin is immunoexpressed in a variety of tumors including squamous cell carcinomas of the lung, synovial sarcoma, angiosarcoma, transitional cell carcinoma, renal cell carcinomas and thymomas (Attanoos et al, 2002).

Comments

Clearly, the major role of TM remains in the confirmation of lymphatic and vascular tumors; although some advocate the use of TM as a mesothelioma-binding antibody in the standard panel of antibodies used for the evaluation of malignant mesothelioma (Ordonez, 1997).

References

Acebo E, Val-Bernal JF, Gomez-Roman JJ. Thrombomodulin, calretinin and c-kit (CD117) expression in cardiac myxoma. Histology and Histopathology 2001;16:1031–6.

Appleton MAC, Attanoos RL, Jasani B. Thrombomodulin as a marker of vascular and lymphatic tumors. Histopathology 1996;29:153–7.

Attanoos RL, Goddard H, Gibbs AR. Mesothelioma-binding antibodies: thrombomodulin, OV632 and HBME-1 and their use in the diagnosis of malignant mesothelioma. Histopathology 1996;29:209–15.

Attanoos RL, Webb R, Dojcinov SD, Gibbs AR. Malignant epithelioid mesothelioma: anti-mesothelial marker expression correlates with histological pattern. Histopathology 2001;39:584–8.

Attanoos RL, Galateau-Salle F, Gibbs AR, et al. Primary thymic epithelial tumours of the pleura mimicking malignant mesothelioma. Histopathology 2002;41:42–9.

Brown RW, Clark GM, Tandon AK, Allred DC. Multiple marker immunohistochemical phenotypes distinguishing malignant pleura mesothelioma from pulmonary adenocarcinoma. Human Pathology 1993;24:347–54.

Collins CL, Ordonez NG, Schaefer R, et al. Thrombomodulin expression in malignant pleural mesothelioma and pulmonary adenocarcinoma. American Journal of Pathology 1992;141:827–33.

Doglioni C, Dei Tos AP, Laurino L, et al. Calretinin: A novel immunocytochemical marker for mesothelioma. American Journal of Surgical Pathology 1996;20:1037–46.

Manuyama I, Bell C, Majerus P. Thrombomodulin is found on endothelium of arteries, veins, capillaries, and lymphatics, and on syncytiotrophoblasts of human placenta. Journal of Cellular Biology 1985;101:363–71.

Murakami H, Hirose Y, Sagoh M, et al. Why do chronic subdural hematomas continue to grow slowly and not coagulate? Role of thrombomodulin in the emchanism. Journal of Neurosurgery 2002;96:877–84.

Ordonez NG. Value of thrombomodulin immunostaining in the diagnosis of mesothelioma. Histopathology 1997;31:25–30.

Suthipintawong C, Leong AS-Y, Vinyuvat S. A comparative study of immunomarkers for lymphangiomas and hemangiomas. Applied Immunohistochemistry 1995;3:239–44.

Suzuli K, Kusumoto H, Deyashiki Y, et al. Structure and expression of human thrombomodulin, a thrombin receptor on endothelium acting as a cofactor for protein C activation. EMBO Journal 1987;6:1891–7.

Wen D, Dittman W, Ye R, Deaven L, Margerus P, Sadler J. Human thrombomodulins: Complete cDNA sequence and chromosome localization of the gene. Biochemistry 1987;26:4350–7.

Thyroglobulin

Sources/clones

Axcel/Accurate (polyclonal, DAK-Tg6), Biodesign (polyclonal, 101, 102, 103, 104), Biogenesis (polyclonal), Biogenex (polyclonal), Caltag Laboratories (14/14), Dako (polyclonal, DAK-Tg6), Chemicon (polyclonal), Fitzgerald (M370108, M310136, M310137, M310138, M310139), Immunotech SA (J7B49, J7C9–3, J7C76–20), Labvision Corp (2H11, 6E1), Novocastra (polyclonal, ID4), Sanbio/Monosan (14/14), Zymed (polyclonal).

Fixation/preparation

The antibodies to thyroglobulin are applicable to formalin-fixed paraffin sections, acetone-fixed cryostat sections and fixed cell smears.

Background

DAK-Tg6 (IgG1, Kappa) and 1D4 (IgG2a) were raised against purified human thyroglobulin. These antibodies react with thyroglobulin (300 kD) in normal, hyperplastic and neoplastic thyroid glands. Circulating iodide, derived from dietary sources and deiodination of thyroid hormones is selectively trapped by the thyroid gland. Oxidation of iodine to the organic form is then effected by a thyroid peroxidase enzyme (Magnusson et al, 1987), which is sited at the apical border of the follicular cell. This is now recognised as the antigen to thyroid antimicrosomal antibody in autoimmune disease (Portmann et al, 1988). Organic iodide is incorporated into mono- and di-iodotyrosine by binding to tyrosine residues on thyroglobulin stored in colloid. Thyroglobulin contains 140 tyrosine residues but not all of these are iodinated, and T4 and T3 synthesis occurs only at specific sites (Dunn et al, 1987). Hormone release is brought about by endocytosis of thyroglobulin at the apical pole of the follicular stem cell, fusion of endocytotic vesicles with lysosomes, and release of T3 and T4 by the proteolytic cleavage of thyroglobulin. These hormones are then secreted into the peripheral blood via the basal pole.

Applications

Apart from being immunoexpressed in all papillary and follicular carcinomas, thyroglobulin may also be useful in poorly differentiated and anaplastic carcinomas (Wilson et al, 1986; De Micco et al, 1987). Although both latter entities have been shown biochemically to synthesize 19S thyroglobulin, immunohistochemistry often fails to detect thyroglobulin in these tumors (Monaco et al, 1984). Hürthle cell tumors also demonstrate immunopositivity with thyroglobulin. The other major role of antibodies to thyroglobulin is in the identification of metastatic thyroid carcinomas. A note of caution is necessary, since thyroglobulin may be demonstrated in medullary carcinoma of the thyroid gland (Wilson et al, 1986). In such instances, attention to morphology as well as application of calcitonin antibodies would be crucial in avoiding an erroneous diagnosis. Antibodies to thyroglobulin do not react with epithelial cells from GIT, pancreas, kidney, lung and breast nor the malignancies that arise in these organs.

Comments

The main role of thyroglobulin antibody lies in the identification of poorly differentiated/anaplastic thyroid carcinomas and metastatic thyroid carcinoma. The development of antibodies to thyroid transcription factor (TTF-1) allows another relatively specific marker of comparable sensitivity to thyroglobulin for thyroid carcinoma. The use of thyroglobulin in an appropriate panel allows the distinction of thyroid follicular, papillary and medullary carcinoma and metastatic carcinoma (Appendix 1.30). Normal thyroid tissue may be used as positive controls. Because most antibodies are polyclonal care should be taken to titrate optimal dilutions to avoid background staining.

References

De Micco C, Ruf J, Carayon P, et al. Immunohistochemical study of thyroglobulin in thyroid carcinomas with monoclonal antibodies. Cancer 1987;59:471–6.

Dunn JT, Anderson PC, Fox JW, et al. The sites of thyroid hormone formation in rabbit thyroglobulin. Journal of Biology Chemistry 1987;262:16948–52.

Magnusson RP, Chazenbalk GD, Gestautas J, et al. Molecular cloning of the cDNA for human thyroid peroxidase. Molecular Endocrinology 1987;1:856–61.

Monaco F, Carducci C, De Luca M, et al. Human undifferentiated thyroid carcinoma synthesizes and secretes 19S thyroglobulin. Cancer 1984;54:79–83.

Portmann L, Fitch FW, Harvan W, et al. Characterisation of the thyroid microsomal antigen and its relationship to thyroid peroxidase, using monoclonal antibodies. Journal of Clinical Investigation 1988;81:1217–24.

Wilson NW, Pambakian H, Richardson TC, et al. Epithelial markers in thyroid carcinoma: an immunoperoxidase study. Histopathology 1986;10:815–29.

Thyroid Transcription Factor-1 (TTF-1)

Sources/clones

8G7G3/1 (Dako), 1–2.A5.9

Fixation/preparation

This antibody is applicable to formalin-fixed, paraffin-embedded tissue. However, heat-induced epitope retrieval is recommended prior to staining.

Background

TTF-1 is a 38kDa nuclear protein member of the *Nkx2* family of homeodomain transcription factors (Whitsett & Glasser, 1998). Human TTF-1 is a single polypeptide of 371 amino acids encoded by a single gene locus (Bingle, 1997).

TTF-1 expression was originally demonstrated in follicular cells of the thyroid gland (Civitareale et al, 1989) and subsequently in respiratory epithelial cells (Ghaffari et al, 1997). In the thyroid gland, TTF-1 activates the transcription of thyroglobulins and regulates the synthesis of calcitonin in C-cells (Suzuki et al, 1998). In the lung, TTF-1 binds and activates promoters of surfactant proteins and Clara cell secretory protein genes (Bruno et al, 1995; Zhang L et al, 1997). TTF-1 is expressed at the onset of lung and thyroid organogenesis and is essential for the normal development of these organs.

Exclusive expression in epithelial cells of the thyroid gland and lung allows TTF-1 to be a useful diagnostic antibody for tumors arising in these organs. In normal lung, TTF-1 is expressed in Type II cells and Clara cells. Whilst TTF-1 is expressed largely in pulmonary neoplasms, it is not specific for adenocarcinoma, being also immunopositive in squamous carcinoma, large cell carcinoma and carcinoid tumors (albeit to a lesser degree). However, a wider immunopositivity has been demonstrated in large cell neuroendocrine carcinoma, atypical carcinoid, and small cell carcinoma (Ordonez, 2000). Nevertheless, TTF-1 appears to be a sensitive marker for pulmonary adenocarcinoma, being positive in the majority of these tumors. In addition, squamous carcinoma of the lung was negative using the 8G7G3/1 anti-TTF-1 monoclonal antibody. In cytologic preparations, TTF-1 is also a highly selective marker for pulmonary adenocarcinoma (Hecht et al, 2001). Nonmucinous bronchioloalveolar adenocarcinomas (BACs) are strongly immunoreactive with TTF-1, whilst the mucinous BACs are negative (Goldstein and Thomas, 2001). Pulmonary sclerosing hemangioma has also been demonstrated to express TTF-1, suggesting an origin from respiratory epithelium (Devouassoux-Shisheboran et al, 2000; Chan & Chan, 2000).

Thyroid neoplasms, including papillary and follicular carcinomas (including medullary and insular carcinomas) are TTF-1 immunopositive (Katoh et al, 2000; Ordonez, 2000). However, anaplastic carcinomas are negative. Some focal TTF-1 immunoreactivity has been observed in 1/66 gastric adenocarcinomas and 1/8 endometrial adenocarcinomas (Bejarano et al, 1996).

Applications

TTF-1 is useful in the investigation of metastatic adenocarcinoma of an unknown origin, since studies to date indicate that TTF-1 is exclusively expressed in adenocarcinomas of the lung and thyroid. This would be particularly useful in the investigation of pleural-based malignancies. The differential diagnosis between metastatic pulmonary small cell carcinoma and Merkel cell carcinoma may be facilitated with the combined use of TTF-1 and cytokeratin 20 immunopositivity, respectively (Byrd-Gloster et al, 2000). However, the role of TTF-1 in the distinction between pulmonary small cell carcinoma and extrapulmonary small cell carcinoma (eg bladder, cervix, prostate, parotid, thyroid and breast) is less than absolute (Kaufman & Dietel, 2000; Cheuk & Chan, 2001). Interestingly, TTF-1 is not expressed in other extrapulmonary neuroendocrine tumors (Agoff et al, 2000).

Comment

Antibodies to TTF-1 demonstrate an intranuclear staining pattern. Normal thyroid gland (follicle lining cells) and lung parenchyma (alveolar lining cells) serve as excellent controls. Antigen retrieval in EDTA at pH10.0 produces better results than at acidic pH.

References

Agoff SN, Lamps LW, Philip AT, et al. Thyroid transcription factor-1 is expressed in extrapulmonary small cell carcinomas but not in other extrapulmonary neuroendocrine tumors. Modern Pathology 2000;13:238–42.

Bejarano PA, Baughman RP, Biddinger PW, et al: Surfactant proteins and thyroid transcription factor-1 in pulmonary and breast carcinomas. Modern Pathology 1996;9:445–52.

Bingle CD. Thyroid transcription factor-1. International Journal of Biochemistry and Cell Biology 1997;29:1471–73.

Bruno MD, Bohinski RJ, Huelsman KM, et al. Lung cell-specific expression of the murine surfactant protein A (SP-A) gene is mediated by interactions between the SP-A promoter and thyroid transcription factor-1. Journal of Biology and Chemistry 1995;270:6531–6.

Byrd-Gloster AL, Khoor A, Glass LF, et al. Differential expression of thyroid transcription factor 1 in small cell lung carcinoma and Merkel cell tumor. Human Pathology 2000;31:58–62.

Chan ACL, Chan JKC: Pulmonary sclerosing hemangioma consistently expressed thyroid transcription factor-1 (TTF-1): A new clue to its histogenesis. American Journal of Surgical Pathology 2000;24:1531–6.

Cheuk W, Chan JKC: Thyroid transcription factor-1 is of limited value in practical distinction between pulmonary and extrapulmonary small cell carcinomas. American Journal of Surgical Pathology 2001;25:545.

Civitareale D. Onigro R, Sinclair AJ, DiLauro R: A thyroid-specific nuclear protein essential for tissue-specific expression of the thyroglobulin promoter. EMBO Journal 1989;8:2537–42.

Devouassoux-Shisheboran M, Hayashi T, Linnoila RI, et al. A clinicopathologic study of 100 cases of pulmonary sclerosing hemangioma with immunohistochemical studies: TTF-1 is expressed in both round and surface cells, suggesting an origin from primitive respiratory epithelium. American Journal of Surgical Pathology 2000;24:906–16.

Ghaffari M, Zeng X, Whitsett JA, Yan C: Nuclear localization domain of thyroid transcription factor-1 in respiratory epithelial cells. Biochemistry Journal 1997;328:757–1.

Goldstein NS, Thomas M: Mucinous and nonmucinous bronchioloalveolar adenocarcinomas have distinct staining patterns with thyroid transcription factor and cytokeratin 20 antibodies. American Journal of Clinical Pathology 2001;116:319–25.

Hecht JL, Pinkus JL, Weinstein LJ, Pinkus GS: The value of thyroid transcription factor-1 in cytologic preparations as a marker for metastatic adenocarcinoma of lung origin. American Journal of Clinical Pathology 2001;116:483–8.

Katoh R, Kawaoi A, Miyagi E, et al. Thyroid transcription factor-1 in normal, hyperplastic, and neoplastic follicular thyroid cells examined by immunohistochemistry and nonradioactive in situ hybridization. Modern Pathology 2000;13:570–6.

Kaufmann O, Dietel M: Expression of thyroid transcription factor-1 in pulmonary and extrapulmonary small cell carcinomas and other neuroendocrine carcinomas of various primary sites. Histopathology 2000;36:8–16.

Khoor A, Whitsett JA, Stahlman MT, et al. Utility of surfactant protein B precursor and thyroid transcription factor 1 in differentiating adenocarcinoma of the lung from malignant mesothelioma. Human Pathology 1999;30:695–700.

Ordonez N: Value of thyroid transcription factor-1 immunostaining in distinguishing small cell lung carcinomas from other small cell carcinomas. American Journal of Surgical Pathology 2000;24:1217–23.

Pelosi G, Fraggetta F, Pasini F, et al. Immunoreactivity for thyroid transcription factor-1 in stage I non-small cell carcinomas of the lung. American Journal of Surgical Pathology 2001;25:363–72.

Suzuki K, Lavaroni S. Mori A, et al: Thyroid transcription factor 1 is calcium modulated and coordinately regulates genes involved in calcium homeostasis in C cells. Molecular and Cellular Biology 1998;18:7410–22.

Whitsett JA, Glasser SW: Regulation of surfactant protein gene transcription. Biochemistry Biophysics Acta 1998;1408:303–11.

Zhang L, Whitsett JA, Stripp BR: Regulation of Clara cell secretory protein gene transcription in thyroid transcription factor-1. Biochemistry Biophysics Acta 1997;1350:359–67.

NOTES

Topoisomerase IIalpha

Sources/clones

Kamiya (monoclonal JH2.7), Novocastra (polyclonal, monoclonal 3F6).

Fixation/preparation

Applicable to fixed, paraffin-embedded sections following high temperature heat-induced antigen retrieval in EDTA at pH8.0.

Background

The phylogenetic antiquity of DNA topoisomerases indicates their vital function in the cell. The structure and maintenance of genomic DNA depend on the activity of these enzymes without which replication and cell division are impossible. DNA topoisomerase type II activity is required to change DNA topology and it is important in the relaxation of DNA supercoils generated by cellular processes such as transcription and replication. It is also essential for the condensation of chromosomes and their segregation during mitosis. In mammals this activity is derived from at least two isoforms, namely, topoisomerase II alpha (Topo IIalpha) and beta. Because of its essential role in cell replication, Topo IIalpha is the target for many drugs used for cancer therapy. Reduced expression of this enzyme is the predominant mechanism of resistance to several chemotherapeutic agents and a wide variation in the range of expression of this protein being noted in many different tumours. The immunostaining pattern of Topo IIalpha is similar to that of the cell cycling marker Ki-67 so that immunostaining of this protein has also been employed as a cell proliferation marker.

Applications

From the preceding discussion, it is not unexpected that the applications of this marker lie in its value as a predictor of chemotherapeutic response to enzyme inhibitors and in the determination of tumor cell proliferation. Increased Topo IIalpha immunostaining has been shown to correlate with recurrent colon cancers (Lazaris et al, 2002) and with chemosensitivity in ovarian and endometrial carcinomas (Koshiyama et al, 2001), and anthracycline-based adjuvant therapy in node-positive breast cancer (Di Leo et al, 2001). Topo IIalpha cell counts has been shown to correlate well with Ki-67 counts in meningiomas (Roessler et al, 2002; Konstantinidou et al, 2001), multiple myeloma (Wilson et al, 2001), adrenocortical tumors (Gupta et al, 2001 and pituitary adenomas (Saeger et al, 2001), and is a predictor of survival in patients with astrocytoma (Korkolopoulou et al, 2001), and ovarian cancer (Gotlieb et al, 2001).

Comments

While the use of Topo IIalpha immunostaining as a means to predict chemosensitivity to enzyme inhibitors is yet to be proven for a large range of tumors, detection of this protein has been shown to be a reliable substitute for Ki-67 as a cell proliferation marker.

Tonsils serve as suitable controls.

References

Di Leo A, Larsimont D, Gancberg D, et al. HER-2 and topoisomerase IIalpha as predictive markers in a population of node-positive breast cancer patients randomly treated with adjuvant CMF or epirubicin plus cyclophosphamide. Annals of Oncology 2001;12:1081–9.

Gotleib WH, Goldberg I, Weisz B, et al. Topoisomerase II immunostaining as a prognostic marker for survival in ovarian cancer. Gynecologic Oncology 2001;82:99–104.

Gupta D, Shidham V, Holden J, Layfield L. Value of topoisomerase II alpha, MIB-1, p53, E-cadherin, retinoblastoma gene protein, and HER-2/neu immunohistochemical expression for the prediction of biological behavior in adrenocortical neoplasms. Applied Immunohistochemistry and Molecular Morphology 2001;9:215–21.

Konstantinidou AE, Patsouris E, Korkolopoulou P, et al. DNA topoisomerase IIalpha expression correlates with cell proliferation but not with recurrence in intracranial meningiomas. Histopathology 2001;39:402–8.

Korkolopoulou P, Patsouris E, Konstantinidou AE, et al. Mitosin and DNA topoisomerase IIalpha: two novel proliferation markers in the prognostication of diffuse astrocytoma patient survival. Applied Immunohistochemistry and Molecular Morphology 2001;9:207–14.

Koshiyama M, Fujii H, Kinezaki M, et al. Immunohistochemical expression of topoisomerase II alpha (Topo II alpha) and multidrug resistance-associated protein (MRP), plus chemosensitivity testing, as chemotherapeutic indices of ovarian and endometrial carcinomas. Anticancer Research 2001;21 (4B):2925–32.

Lazaris AC, Kavantzas NG, Zorzos HS, et al. Markers of drug resistance in relapsing colon cancer. Journal of Cancer Research and Clinical Oncology 2002;128:114–8.

Roessler K, Gatterbauer B, Kitz K. Topoisomerase II alpha as a reliable proliferation marker in meningiomas. Neurology Research 2002;24:241–3.

Saeger W, Schreiber S, Ludecke DK. Cyclins D1 and D3 and topoisomerase IIalpha in inactive pituitary adenomas. Endocrine Pathology 2001;12:39–47.

Wilson CS, Medeiros LJ, Lai R, et al. DNA topoisomerase IIalpha in multiple myeloma: a marker of cell proliferation and not drug resistance. Modern Pathology 2001;14:886–91.

Toxoplasma gondii

Sources/clones

Accurate, American Research Products (1637–18), Biodesign (polyclonal), Biogenesis (polyclonal), Biogenex (GII-9), Chemicon, Dako (polyclonal), Fitzgerald (M26303).

Fixation/preparation

Applicable to formalin-fixed, paraffin-embedded tissue sections. Proteolytic enzyme pretreatment is essential before immunostaining. These antibodies are also applicable to cryostat sections and fixed cell smears.

Background

T.gondi is a protozoan parasite, which causes a mild and self-limiting infection in adults. Toxoplasmosis occurs in patients who eat raw or partially cooked meat, reflecting the widespread presence of this protozoan in animals used as food sources. Following gastrointestinal infection, active toxoplasmosis is accompanied by fever with enlargement of lymph nodes and spleen. The immune reactions cause the intracellular Toxoplasma to adopt a cystoid form in which they can persist for a lifetime. However, infections in immunocompromised patients may be fatal causing acute toxoplasmosis including toxoplasmosis encephalitis. Activation of a latent infection during pregnancy may lead to intrauterine transmission of the organism to the fetus resulting in spontaneous abortion, stillbirth or severe central nervous system damage.

The production of monoclonal antibodies against protozoa has been limited by the complex life cycles of these parasites. Clone GII antibody recognizes a tachyzoite membrane antigen of 30 kD. The polyclonal antibody (Dako) was raised against formalin-fixed tachyzoites of T.gondii isolated and purified from infected mice. This latter antibody does not cross-react with the following organisms: Cryptosporidia, Microsporidia, Histoplasma capsulatum, Candida, Blastomyces, Pneumocystis carinii, Entamoeba histolytica, Aspergillus, Cryptococcus neoformans and Mycobacterium tuberculosis.

Applications

Both tachyzoites (or trophozoites) and encysted bradyzoites forms of T.gondii are demonstrated with these antibodies. Infected Toxoplasma tissue including brain, lung, spleen and lymph nodes may be positively identified with these antibodies. This is particularly pertinent when examining tissue from immunocompromised patients, e.g. AIDS, where a high index of suspicion along with application of anti-Toxoplasmosis antibody may help arrive at a definite diagnosis.

Comments

The antibodies are best optimised using Toxoplasma-infected tissue.

References

Conley FK, Jenkins KA, Remington JS. Toxoplasma gondii infection of the central nervous system. Use of the peroxidase-antiperoxidase method to demonstrate Toxoplasma in formalin-fixed, paraffin-embedded tissue sections. Human Pathology 1981;12:690–8.

Kriek JA, Remington JS. Toxoplasmosis in the adult – an overview. New England Journal of Medicine 1978;298:550–3.

Luft BJ, Remington JS. Toxoplasmic encephalitis. Journal of Infectious Diseases 1988;157:1–6.

NOTES

Tyrosinase

Source/clone

Novacastra (Clone T311)

Fixation/preparation

A heat-induced epitope retrieval system is essential for antigen unmasking.

Background

Tyrosinase is an enzyme involved in the initial stages of melanin biosynthesis (Kwon, 1993). T311 is a murine monoclonal antibody generated to the tyrosinase recombinant protein (Jungbluth et al, 2000). On paraffin-embedded material, T311 revealed intense immunoreactivity confined to cells showing melanocytic differentiation. No immunostaining was present in unrelated normal tissues and tumors. Eighty-four percent of metastatic malignant melanomas were immunoreactive with T311 and showed predominantly a homogeneous expression (Jungbluth et al, 2000). Nevi showed intense staining at the junctional zone, while the dermal component revealed decreasing reactivity towards deeper areas (Jungbluth et al, 2000). Another study showed a sensitivity of 94%

for melanoma with a high specificity for melanocytic cells (Hofbauer et al, 1998). Immunopositivity correlated inversely with clinical stage with an exclusively homogeneous pattern in early stages of melanoma to a more heterogeneous pattern in later stages (Hofbauer et al, 1998).

In other studies, tyrosinase immunoreactivity has been demonstrated in approximately 85% of amelanotic metastatic melanomas, which is comparable to HMB-45 and melan-A (Kaufmann et al, 1998). In a study of conventional metastatic melanomas, 92% were immunopositive with tyrosinase (Miettinen et al, 2001). Tyrosinase is strongly expressed in virtually all epithelioid melanomas, but rarely expressed in the spindled variants (Iwamoto et al, 2001). Further, tyrosinase has been shown to be less useful in desmoplastic melanomas (Xu et al, 2002; Prasad et al, 2001). However, tyrosinase is the most sensitive marker for sinonasal melanomas and closely approaches the sensitivity of S-100 protein for oral mucosal melanomas (Prasad et al, 2001). Tyrosinase has also been demonstrated to be a sensitive and specific marker to

distinguish epithelioid melanocytic nevi from epithelioid histiocytic tumors (Busam et al, 2000). Tyrosinase has not been recommended for routine use in the diagnosis of renal and hepatic angiomyolipomas (Makhlouf et al, 2002). All four pigmented neurofibromas stained positive for tyrosinase were immunopositive (Fetsch et al, 2000).

Applications

Tyrosinase is useful in the diagnosis of both primary and metastatic melanomas. It is less useful in the identification of spindled melanomas, especially desmoplastic melanomas.

References

Busam KJ, Granter SR, Iversen K, Jungbluth AA. Immunohistochemical distinction of epithelioid histiocytic proliferations from epithelioid melanocytic nevi. American Journal of Dermatopathology 2000;22:237–41.

Fetsch JF, Michal M, Miettinen M. Pigmented (melanotic) neurofibroma: a clinicopathologic and immunohistochemical analysis of 19 lesions from 17 patients. American Journal of Surgical Pathology 2000;24:331–43.

Hofbauer GF, Kamarashev J, Geertsen R, et al. Tyrosinase immunoreactivity in formalin-fixed, paraffin-embedded primary and metastatic melanoma: frequency and distribution. Journal of Cutaneous Pathology 1998;25:204–9.

Iwamoto S, Burrows RC, Agoff SN. The p75 neurotrophin receptor, relative to other Schwann cell and melanoma markers, is abundantly expressed in spindled melanomas. American Journal of Dermatopathology 2001;23:288–94.

Jungbluth AA, Iversen K, Coplan K, et al. T311 – an anti-tyrosinase monoclonal antibody for the detection of melanocytic lesions in paraffin embedded tissues. Pathology, Research & Practice 2000;196:235–42.

Kaufmann O, Koch S, Burghardt J, et al. Tyrosinase, Melan-A, and KBA62 as markers for the immunohistochemical identification of metastatic amelanotic melanomas on paraffin sections. Modern Pathology 1998;11:740–6.

Kwon BS. Pigmentation genes: the tyrosinase gene family and the Pmel 17 gene family. Journal of Investigative Dermatology 1993;100:134S–140S.

Makhlouf HR, Ishak KG, Shekar R, et al. Melanoma markers in angiomyolipoma of the liver and kidney: a comparative study. Archives of Pathology and Laboratory Medicine 2002;126:49–55.

Miettinen M, Fernandez M, Franssila K. Microphthalmia transcription factor in the immunohistochemical diagnosis of metastatic melanoma: comparison with four other melanoma markers. American Journal of Surgical Pathology 2001;25:205–11.

Prasad ML, Jungbluth AA, Iversen K, et al. Expression of melanocytic differentiation markers in malignant melanomas of the oral and sinonasal mucosa. American Journal of Surgical Pathology2001;25:782–787.

Xu X, Chu AY, Pasha TL, et al. Immunoprofile of MITF, tyrosinase, melan-A, and MAGE-1 in HMB45-negative melanomas. American Journal of Surgical Pathology 2002;26:82–7.

Ubiquitin

Sources/clones

Accurate/Novocastra (FPM1), Biodesign (polyclonal), Biogenesis (242.9, polyclonal), Dako (polyclonal), Fitzgerald (polyclonal), Serotec (polyclonal), Zymed (UBI1).

Fixation/preparation

This antibody is applicable to formalin-fixed paraffin-embedded tissue sections.

Background

Ubiquitin is an 8.5 kD polypeptide found almost universally in plants and animals. The best documented function for ubiquitin involves its conjugation to proteins as a signal to initiate degradation via the ubiquitin-mediated proteolytic pathway (Jahngen-Hodge et al, 1992). Ubiquitin-mediated proteolysis is involved in the turnover of many short-lived regulatory proteins. This pathway leads to the covalent attachment of one or more multiubiquitin chains to target substrates that are then degraded by the 26S multicatalytic chains proteasome complex (Rolfe et al, 1997). Ubiquitin modification of a variety of protein targets within the cells also plays an important role in many cellular processes: regulation of gene expression, regulation of cell cycle and division, involvement in the cellular stress response, modification of cell surface receptors, DNA repair, import of proteins into mitochondria, uptake of precursors into neurons, and biogenesis of mitochondria, ribosomes, and peroxisomes (Ciechanover & Schwartz, 1994).

Applications

Ubiquitin immunostaining has be shown to be a highly sensitive and specific method for the detection of Mallory bodies, thereby making it a valuable tool in the study of alcoholic liver disease, adding objectivity to the diagnosis of alcoholic hepatitis (Vryberg & Leth, 1991). In the human spongiform encephalopathies, ubiquitin immunoreactivity has been demonstrated in a punctate distribution at the periphery of prion protein amyloid plaques and in a finely granular pattern in the neuropil around and within areas of spongiform change (Ironside et al, 1993). Analysis of the relationship of ubiquitin-positive dots and granular structures with pretangle neurons and neurofibrillary tangles suggested that the ubiquitin-positive structures are the result of degeneration and might be related to the initiation of neurofibrillary degeneration (Garcia et al, 2001). Ubiquitin-positive neuronal and tau 2-poisitive glial inclusions may prove to be a marker of frontotemporal dementia of motor neuron type (Forno et al, 2002). Ubiquitin has also been simultaneously present with GFAP in the cytoplasm and cell processes of tumor cells of astrocytomas (Galloway & Likavec, 1989). The demonstration of ubiquitin immunolabelling in both ductus efferentes and ductus epididymidis epithelia has concluded that ubiquitinated proteins are secreted into the epididymal lumen (Fraile et al, 1996). Ubiquitin expression has been demonstrated in the lung and adrenal gland in autopsy cases that died by fire accident (Shoji, 1997), suggesting that the adrenal gland reacts strongly to heat shock. Evidence of ubiquitin-positive myocytic intranuclear or cytoplasmic inclusions or positive-staining rimmed vacuoles in the setting of an inflammatory myopathy may be suggestive of a diagnosis of inclusion body myositis (Prayson & Cohen, 1997). On the therapeutic front, prevention of p53 ubiquitination (and subsequent degradation) in human papilloma virus positive cervical tumors should lead to programmed cell death (Rolfe et al, 1997).

References

Ciechanover A, Schwartz AL. The ubiquitin-mediated proteolytic pathway: mechanisms of recognition of the proteolytic substrate and involvement in the degradation of native cellular proteins. FASEB Journal 1994;8:182–91.

Forno LS, Langston JW, Herrick MK, et al. Ubiquitin-positive neuronal and tau 2-positive glial inclusions in frontotemporal dementia of motor neuron type. Acta Neuropathogica 2002;103:599–606.

Fraile B, Martin R, De Miquel MP et al. Light and electron microscopic immunohistochemical localization of protein gene product 9.5 and ubiquitin immunoreactivities in the human epididymis and vas deferens. Biology of Reproduction 1996;55:291–7.

Galloway PG, Likavec MJ. Ubiquitin in normal, reactive and neoplastic human astrocytes. Brain Research 1989;500:343–51.

Garcia Gil ML, Moran MA, Gomez-Ramos P. Ubiquitinated granular structures and initial neurofibrillary changes in the human brain. Journal of Neurological Science 2001;192:27–34.

Ironside JW, McCardle L, Hayward PA, Bell JE. Ubiquitin immunocytochemistry in human spongiform encephalopathies. Neuropathology and Applied Neurobiology 1993;19:134–40.

Jahngen-Hodge J, Cyr D, Laxaman E, Taylor A. Ubiquitin and ubiquitin conjugates in human lens. Experimental Eye Research 1992;55:897–902.

Prayson RA, Cohen ML. Ubiquitin immunostaining and inclusion body myositis: study of 30 patients with inclusion body myositis. Human Pathology 1997;28:887–92.

Rolfe M, Chiu MI, Pagano M. The ubiquitin-mediated proteolytic pathway as a therapeutic area. Journal of Molecular Medicine 1997;75:5–17.

Shoji T. Demonstration of heat shock protein, ubiquitin, in fire death autopsy cases by immunohistochemical study. Nippon Hoigaku Zasshi 1997;51:70–6.

Vyberg M, Leth P. Ubiquitin: an immunohistochemical marker of Mallory bodies and alcoholic liver disease. APMIS Supplement 1991;23:46–52.

Ulex Europaeus Agglutinin 1 Lectin (UEA-I)

Source

UEA-1 (Dako).

Fixation/preparation

Carbohydrates reactive with UEA-1 are generally active in formalin-fixed, paraffin-embedded tissue sections. Background staining may be reduced by the addition of 5% human serum to the anti-UEA-1 dilution buffer.

Background

UEA-1 is a plant lectin isolated from Ulex europaeus seeds (gorse seed) by affinity chromatography. The lectin is homogeneous containing 4.2% neutral sugar and 1.4% glucosamine (Horejsi, 1979). Its molecular weight is approximately 110 kD, comprising two covalently bound basic subunits. UEA-1 is specific to certain terminal α-L-fucosyl residues of glycoconjugates and also detects blood group H antigen (Pereira et al, 1978).

Applications

UEA-1 has been used successfully as a marker for endothelial cells. It has been shown to be more sensitive for benign vascular tumors than thrombomodulin or Factor VIII-related antigen (Yonezawa et al, 1987). In fact other workers have shown UEA-1 to be a more sensitive marker for endothelial cells of vascular tumors than Factor VIII-related antigen (Miettinen et al, 1983; Ordonez et al, 1984). UEA-I does not distinguish between the endothelial cells of blood vessels and lymphatics (Suthipintawong et al 1995). In some tissues Ulex lectin has demonstrated additional binding to epithelial structures (Holthofer et al, 1982). This latter immunoreaction has been exploited with UEA-1 demonstrating specific binding to collecting duct carcinoma of the kidney; enabling distinction from other types of renal cell carcinoma (Amin et al, 1997).

Comments

A study evaluating endothelial markers in well and poorly differentiated areas of angiosarcomas, it was found that CD31 and Ulex europaeus were the most sensitive markers staining both well differentiated and poorly differentiated ares of the tumors. Anti-FVIII-RA and CD34 did not stain undifferentiated malignantdothelial cells. Ulex europaeus and CD34 showed very low specificity (Poblet et al, 1996). It would appear that the use of UEA-1 is confined to identifying collecting duct carcinoma of the kidney. Benign vascular tissue makes appropriate positive controls for UEA-1.

References

Amin MB, Varma MD, Tickoo SK, Ro JY. Collecting duct carcinoma of the kidney. Advances in Anatomic Pathology 1997;4:85–94.

Holthofer H, Virtanen I, Kariniemi AL, Hormia M, Linder E, Miettinen A. Ul; ex europaeus I lectin as a marker for vascular endothelium in human tissues. Laboratory Investigation 1982;47:60–6.

Horejsi V. Properties of Ulex europaeus II lectin isolated by affinity chromatography. Biochima Biophysiology Acta 1979;577:389–93.

Meittinen M, Holthofer H, Lehto VP, Miettinen A, Virtanen I. *Ulex europaeus* I lectin as a marker for tumors derived from endothelial cells. American Journal of Clinical Pathology 1983;79:32–6.

Ordonez NG, Batsakis JG. Comparison of *Ulex europaeus* I lectin and Factor VIII-related antigen in vascular lesions. Archives of Pathology and Laboratory Medicine 1984;108:129–32.

Pereira ME, Kisailus EC, Gruezo F, Kabat EA. Immunohistochemical

studies on the combining site of
the blood group H-specific lectin
1 from *Ulex europeus* seeds.
Archives Biochemia
Biophysiology 1978;185:108–15.

Poblet E, Gonzalez-Palacios F,
Jimenez FJ. Different
immunoreactivity of endothelial
markers in well and poorly

differentiated areas of
angiosarcomas. Virchows Archives
1996;428:217–21.

Suthipintawong C, Leong AS-Y,
Vinyuvat S. A comparitive study
of markers for lymphangiomas
and hemangiomas. Applied
Immunohistochemistry
1995;3:239–44.

Yonezawa S, Maruyama I, Sakae K,
et al. Thrombomodulin as a
marker for vascular tumors.
Comparative study with Factor
VIII and Ulex europaeus I Lectin.
American Journal of Clinical
Pathology 1987;88:405–11.

VEGF (Vascular Endothelial Growth Factor)

Sources/clones

Oncogene Research Products (VEGF antibody-3, monoclonal), R&D Research, Minneapolis (MAB293, clone 26503.11), Santa Cruz Biotechnology (VPF/VEGF, used for immunofluoresence staining with fresh frozen tissue), Santa Cruz Biotechnology (polyclonal VEGF, reacts with the 165, 189 and 121 amino acid splice variants of VEGF).

Fixation/preparation

These antibodies are applicable to paraffin sections. A heat-induced epitope/antigen retrieval system for proteinase digestion is recommended prior to the immunohistochemical procedure.

Background

Vascular endothelial growth factor (VEGF) is a dimeric 46-kD, endothelial cell specific, glycosylated, heparin-binding cytokine. It has both angiogenic and vascular permeability factor functions (Dvorak et al, 1991). VEGF exerts paracrine effects by binding to specific tyrosine kinase-receptors on vascular endothelial cells (Terman et al, 1992). It may also exert autocrine effects by stimulating tumor growth (Liu et al, 1995). Hence, VEGF is one of the most potent, highly specific angiogenic factors.

VEGF expression has been investigated in two fairly large series of carcinomas: 59% (n=91) of epidermoid lung carcinomas (Mattern et al, 2996) and 51% (n=230) of breast carcinomas (Toi et al, 1995) examined immunohistochemically were found to have VEGF expressing carcinoma cells.

VEGF is synthesized by both tumor and normal cells and acts specifically on endothelial cells. VEGF stimulates and induces migration and proliferation of endothelial cells. Hence, VEGF is a useful marker of tumor angiogenesis.

Cytoplasmic immunoreactivity for VEGF has been demonstrated in 42% of melanomas, but not in atypical compound melanocytic nevi, cellular blue nevi or Spitz nevi (Bayer-Garner et al, 1999). Further immunoreactivity for VEGF was related to tumor thickness and to the absence of regression. Hence, although VEGF is not a useful prognostic indicator for malignant melanoma, it may be useful in discriminating between melanoma and benign melanocytic lesions.

VEGF immunoexpression was also not found to be a prognostic marker for head and neck squamous cell carcinomas (Salven et al, 1997). However, tumor-associated inflammatory cells showed high levels of VEGF expression in all carcinomas studied, suggesting a possible role in tumor angiogenesis.

The immunohistochemical localization of VEGF (comparable to the localization of VEGF mRNA) was expressed in all thyroid tumors (Katoh et al, 1999); including all types of thyroid carcinomas (including papillary, follicular, medullary and anaplastic) and follicular adenomas. In contrast in the normal thyroid, VEGF was identified in epithelium of isolated follicles. It was concluded that the histological type of thyroid tumor may determine the vascular pattern through a paracrine mechanism involving VEGF.

The characteristic vasculature and edema of sclerosing stromal tumors of the ovary has been demonstrated to be associated with the expression of VEGF (Kawauchi et al, 1998).

In the prostate gland, VEGF expression was confined to the basal cell layer in benign glands (Kollerman and Helpap, 2001). In high grade prostatic intraepithelial neoplasia, immunolabelling was no longer confined to the basal cell layer, but was seen in all neoplastic secretory cells. All carcinomas were immunopositive for VEGF. Hence, there was a trend for increasing immunolabelling intensity with increasing cellular dedifferentiation. Kollerman concluded that VEGF may have an important role in the process of malignant transformation and tumor progression (Kollerman and Helpap, 2001).

Strong VEGF immunoexpression in malignant chondrocytes was confined exclusively to high-grade chondrosarcomas (Ayala et al, 2000); interestingly showing a strong correlation with intracartilaginous vessels. Acquisition of these patterns of vasculature may be associated with metastatic potential of cartilage tumors.

Application

A definite diagnostic role for VEGF in surgical/cytopathology is yet to be established. It may be useful in distinguishing between melanomas and melanocytic nevi. VEGF immunoexpression may also be predictive of potential metastasizing cartilaginous tumors. VEGF expression correlates with vascularity, metastasis and proliferation of tumors and may therefore prove to be a useful prognostic marker.

References

Ayala G, Liu C, Nicosia R, et al. Microvasculature and VEGF expression in cartilaginous tumors. Human Pathology 2000;31:341–6.

Bayer-Garner IB, Hough AJ, Smoller BR. Vascular endothelial growth factor expression in malignant melanoma: prognostic versus diagnostic usefulness. Modern Pathology 1999;12:770–4.

Dvorak HF, Sioussat TM, Brown LF, et al. Distribution of vascular permeability factor (vascular endothelial growth factor) in tumors: concentration in tumor blood vessels. Journal of Experimental Medicine 1991;174:1275–8.

Katoh R, Miyagi E, Kawaoi, et al. Expression of vascular endothelial growth factor (VEGF) in human thyroid neoplasms. Human Pathology 1999;30:891–7.

Kawauchi S, Tsuji T, Kaku T, et al. Sclerosing stromal tumor of the ovary: a clinicopathologic, immunohistochemical, ultrastructural, and cytogenetic analysis with special reference to its vasculature. The American Journal of Surgical Pathology 1998;22:83–92.

Kollerman J, Helpap B. Expression of vascular endothelial growth factor (VEGF) and VEGF receptor Flk-1 in benign, premalignant, and malignant prostate tissue. The American Journal of Clinical Pathology 2001;116:115–21.

Liu B, Earl HM, Baban D, et al. Melanoma cell lines express VEGF receptors KDR and respond to exogenously added VEGF. Biochemical & Biophysical Research Communications 1995;217:721–7.

Mattern J, Koomagi R, Volm M. Association of vascular endothelial growth factor expression with intratumoral microvessel density and tumour cell proliferation in human epidermoid lung carcinoma. British Journal of Cancer 1996;72:931–4.

Salven P, Keikkila P, Anttonen A, et al. Vascular endothelial growth factor in squamous cell head and neck carcinoma: expression and prognostic significance. Modern Pathology 1997;10:1128–33.

Terman Bi, Doughner-Vermazen M, Carrion ME, et al. Identification of the KDR tyrosine kinase as a receptor for vascular endothelial cell growth factor. Biochemical & Biophysical Research Communications 1992;187:1579–86.

Toi M, Inada K, Suzuki H, et al. Tumor angiogenesis in breast cancer: its importance as a prognostic indicator and the association with vascular endothelial growth factor expression. Breast Cancer Research and Treatment 1995;36:193–204.

Zymed Laboratories. Polyclonal rabbit anti-VEGF (data sheet)

Villin

Sources/clones

Accurate, Biodesign (ID2C3), Biogenesis (20/24), Chemicon (15E2), Immunotech (ID2C3), Serotec (ID2C3).

Fixation/preparation:

HIER is required for fixed paraffin-embedded sections. Fixation in Carnoy's solution or methacarn preserves immunoreactivity. The antibody is also immunoreactive in fresh cell preparations and frozen sections.

Background

Microvilli increase the absorptive surface of epithelial cells by as much as 20 times. They comprise a highly specialized plasma membrane of a thick extracellular coat of polysaccharide and digestive enzymes and a core comprising a central rigid bundle of 20–30 parallel actin filaments that extend from the tip of the microvillus down to the cell cortex. The actin filaments are all oriented with their plus ends pointing away from the cell body and are held together at regular intervals by actin-bundling proteins. Besides fimbrin, which occurs in microspikes and filopodia, the most important

bundling protein is villin, which is found only in microvilli. Like fimbrin, villin cross-links actin filaments into tight parallel bundles, but in a different actin-binding sequence and is capable of stimulating the formation of long microvilli in cultured fibroblasts which do not normally contain villin and have only a few small microvilli.

Villin, a 95 kD, Ca^{2+}-regulated actin binding protein is found in absorptive cellsthat develop a brush border such as those of the small and large intestines, ductal cells of the pancreas and biliary system, and cells of the proximal renal tubules. Villin is also found in undifferentiated normal and tumoral cells of intestinal origin in vivo and in cell culture so that its expression is seen in cells that do not necessarily display microvilli-lined brush borders (Robine et al, 1985).

Applications

Villin has been employed as a marker of gastrointestinal tumors particularly those from the colon, stomach and pancreas, all such tumors staining positive in one study (Bacchi & Gown, 1991). Gall bladder and hepatocellular carcinomas were also demonstrated to express villin

(Moll et al, 1987). A subset of non-gastrointestinal tumors including some adenocarcinomas of the ovary, endometrium and kidney were also positive (Moll et al, 1987; Bacchi & Gown, 1991). About 30% of signet ring cell carcinoma of the lung were positive (Merchant et al, 2001) and rare lung adenocarcinomas were also positive but no staining was observed in breast carcinoma and mesothelioma. The presence of villin in renal carcinomas is variable and is frequently seen in clear cell and chromophilic tumors but not in chromophobe cell tumors (Moll et al, 1987). Villin also appears to be expressed in the tubular and glandular areas of better differentiated tumors and is not observed in sarcomatoid renal carcinoma, leading to the suggestion that villin may be a potential grading marker (Grone et al, 1986). Its expression in renal carcinoma suggests that they display proximal rather than distal tubular differentiation. It is also observed in the glandular areas of Wilm's tumor (Droz et al, 1990). Recently, villin immunoexpression was shown in 85% of gastrointestinal carcinoids and small cell carcinomas of the lung and in 40% of lung carcinoids with a characteristic apical membraneous staining pattern (Zhang et al, 1999). Villin has also been demonstrated in Merkel cells, highlighting their microvilli (Toyoshima et al, 1998).

Comments

Villin shows apical localization but may also be seen in the basement membrane area surrounding tumor nests (West et al, 1988). Clone ID2C3 shows reactivity with human, porcine and chicken villin.

References

Bacchi CE, Gown AM. Distribution and pattern of expression of villin, a gastrointestinal-associated cytoskeletal protein, in human carcinomas: a study employing paraffin-embedded tissue. Laboratory Investigation 1991;64:418–24.

Droz D, Rousseau-Merck MF, Jaubert F, et al. Cell differentiation in Wilm's tumor (nephroblastoma): an immunohistochemical study. Human Pathology 1990;21:536–44.

Grone HJ, Weber K, Helmchen U, Osborn M. Villin – a marker of brush border differentiation and cellular origin in human renal cell carcinoma. American Journal of Pathology 1986;124:294–302.

Merchant SH, Amin MB, Tamboli P, et al. Pulmonary signet ring cell carcinoma of the lung: Immunohistochemical study and comparison with non-pulmonary signet ring cell carcinoma. American Journal of Surgical Pathology 2001;25:1515–9.

Moll R, Robine S, Dudouet B, Louvard D. Villin: a cytoskeletal protein and a differentiation marker expressed in some human adenocarcinomas. Virchows Archives B Cell Pathology including Molecular Pathology 1987;54:155–69.

Robine S, Huet C, Moll R, et al. Can villin be used to identify malignant and undifferentiated normal digestive epithelial cells? Proceedings of the National Academy of Sciences USA 1985;82:8488–92.

Toyoshima K, Seta Y, Takeda S, Harada H. Identification of Merkel cells by an antibody to villin. Journal of Histochemistry and Cytochemistry 1998;46:1329–34.

Zhang PJ, Harris KR, Alobeid B, Brooks JJ. Immunoexpression of villin in neuroendocrine tumors and its diagnostic implications. Archives of Pathology and Laboratory medicine 1999;123:812–6.

Vimentin

Sources/clones

Accurate (V9, J144, Vim-13.2), Amersham, Biodesign (V9), Biogenesis (Vim-01, LN6), Biogenex (LN6, V9), Boehringer Mannheim (3B4, V9), Chemicon, Dako (VIM3B4, V9), Enzo, Immunotech (V9, V3260), Medac, Milab, Novocastra, Oncogene (V9), Pierce (ZSV5), Serotec (J144), Sigma (LN9), Zymed (ZSV5, ZC64).

Fixation/preparation

Most antibody clones currently available are immunoreactive in fixed paraffin-embedded tissues and HIER enhances immunostaining.

Background

Vimentin is a 58 kD protein which has been purified from a variety of sources and has been shown to form homophylic filaments with an average diameter of 10 nm. Its name is derived from the Latin word *vimentum*, which means arrays of flexible rods. Similar to the other intermediate filaments, vimentin is a protein monomer of highly elongated fibrous molecules with an amino-terminal head, a carboxyl-terminal tail, and a central rod domain. The latter consists of an extended α-helical region containing long tandem repeats of a distinctive amino acid sequence motif called the hepatad repeat. This central rod domain shows a striking sequence homology between intermediate filaments of different species and an even more marked homology of as high as 30% between cytokeratin, desmin, glial fibrillary acidic protein, neurofilaments and vimentin of the same species. Immunohistochemical staining revealed vimentin filaments as part of a wavy network of filaments in the cytoplasm of fibroblasts, associated with both nuclear and plasma membranes. It has been suggested that vimentin, like other intermediate filaments, serve as modulators between extracellular influences governing calcium flux into the cell and nuclear function at a transcriptional or translational level and may thus have a role in gene expression. Vimentin filaments can be precipitated as juxtanuclear whorls following treatment of cells with colcemid or vinblastine.

Applications

Vimentin is the most widely distributed intermediate filament and is expressed in virtually all mesenchymal cells and also by most other cell types in culture (Lane et al, 1983). With the widespread application of intermediate filament analysis to human neoplasms, it soon became apparent that although individual cell types and their corresponding tumors generally express a single intermediate filament class, several neoplasms may express more than one intermediate filament class (Azumi & Battifora, 1987). In many instances, this coexpression of one or more intermediate filament class occurs in a predictable manner and may be employed as diagnostic discriminators. Vimentin expression, traditionally accepted to be class specific for cells of the mesenchyme, can be co-expressed with cytokeratin in a number of epithelial cell types and their corresponding tumors. These include the endometrium, thyroid, gonadal epithelial cells, renal tubules, adrenal cortex, lung, salivary gland, hepatocytes and bile duct. Furthermore, there is increasing evidence to suggest that a variety of high grade epithelial tumors may acquire the expression of vimentin intermediate filaments (Leong, 1991). Vimentin expression has been described in carcinomas of the skin (Iyer & Leong, 1992), urinary bladder, breast (Raymond & Leong, 1989), prostate (Leong et al, 1988), gastric mucosa (Takemura et al, 1994), and uterine cervix. Several report have indicated a correlation of vimentin expression with high tumor grades in breast carcinoma (Raymond & Leong, 1989; Heatley et al, 1993; Domogala et al, 1994; Koutselini et al, 1995) and ovarian epithelial malignancy (Nakopoulpou et al, 1995). One report suggested that vimentin expression was a poor prognostic marker in node-negative breast carcinoma (Domogala et al, 1990) although this has not been confirmed (Seshadri et al, 1996). Expression of vimentin in epithelial tumors also corresponds to change in cell shapes and forms form epithelioid to fibroblastoid or spindle forms so that vimentin is regularly expressed in spindle cell carcinomas. Remodelling of vimentin cytoskeleton correlates with increased motility of promyelocytic leukemia (Bruel et al, 2002) and a decrease and redistribution of this protein was observed in aging Kupffer cells (Sun et al, 1998).

Many tissues in embryos and fetuses, including surface ectoderm, neural groove and brain, gut mucosa and musculature, and renal tubular epithelium, display coexpression of vimentin with another intermediate filament during their developmental stages before being replaced by the intermediate filament protein specific for the mature tissue type (Goel et al, 1997). Vimentin is expressed in epithelial cells in vitro, culture preparations, cell

suspensions and in exfoliated and metastatic cells in body fluids, suggesting that altered cell-to-cell contact and changes in cell shape may account for this apparent aberrant expression. Studies of cell cultures of mouse parietal endodermal cells led to the hypothesis that the acquisition of vimentin may be related to reduced cell-to-cell contact and the ability of epithelial cells to survive independently.

Immature muscle fibers contain desmin and vimentin and mature fibers lack vimentin. Regenerating muscle fibers react with anti-vimentin antibodies and more intensely for desmin than mature fibers. The detection of vimentin has therefore been applied to identify muscle regeneration especially in cases of infantile spinal muscular atrophy and the high incidence of reactive fibers in some congenital and early onset disorders may indicate developmental arrest (Bornemann & Schmalbruch, 1993).

Comments

Due to variability of fixation and HIER, vimentin has been used as an internal control or reporter molecule to assess the quality of antigen preservation and the uniformity of tissue fixation in fixed paraffin embedded tissue sections (Battifora, 1991).

References

Azumi N, Battifora H. The distribution of vimentin and keratin in epithelial and non-epithelial neoplasms. American Journal of Clinical Pathology 1987;88:286–97.

Battifora H. Assessment of antigen damage in immunohistochemistry. The vimentin internal control.

American Journal of Clinical Pathology 1991;96:669–671.

Bornemann A, Schmalbruch H. Anti-vimentin staining in muscle pathology. Neuropathology and Applied Neurobiology 1993;19:414–9.

Bruel A, Paschke S, Jainta S, et al. Remodelling of vimentin cytoskeleton correlates with enhanced motility of promyelocytic leukemia cells during differentiation induced by retinoic acid. Anticancer Research 2001;21(6A): 3973–80.

Domogala W, Lasota J, Dukowitz A. Vimentin expression appears to be associated with poor prognosis in node-negative ductal NOS breast carcinoma. American Journal of Pathology 1990;137:1299–1305.

Domogala W, Striker G, Szadowska A, et al. P53 protein and vimentin in invasive ductal NOS breast carcinoma – relationship with survival and sites of metastases. European Journal of Cancer 1994;30A;1527–34.

Goel A, Gupta I, Joshi K. Immunohistochemical analysis of human embryos and fetuses. An insight into the mechanism of subversion of antigenic differentiation in neoplasia. Archives of Pathology and Laboratory Medicine 1997;121:719–23.

Heatley M, Whiteside C, Maxwell P, Toner P. Vimentin expression in benign and malignant breast epithelium. Journal of Clinical Pathology 1993;46:441–5.

Iyer PV, Leong AS-Y. Vimentin expression in poorly differentiated squamous cell carcinomas of the skin. Journal of Cutaneous Pathology 1992;19:34–9.

Koutselini H, Markopoulos C, Lambropoulou S, et al. Relationship of epidermal growth factor receptor (EGFR), proliferating cell nuclear antigen (PCNA) and vimentin expression and various prognostic factors in breast cancer patients. Cytopathology 1995;6:14–21.

Lane EB, Hogan BLM, Kurkinen M, Garrels JI. Coexpression of vimentin and cytokeratins in parietal endodermal cells of early mouse embryo. Nature 1983;303:701–4.

Leong AS-Y. The expression of vimentin in epithelial neoplasms. Progress in Surgical Pathology 1991;12:31–48.

Leong AS-Y, Gilham P, Milios. Cytokeratin and vimentin intermediate filament proteins in benign and malignant prostatic

epithelium. Histopathology 1988;13:435–42.

Nakopoulpou L, Stefanaki K, Janinis J, Mastrominas M. Immunohistochemical expression of placental alkaline phosphatase and vimentin in epithelial ovarian neoplasms. Acta Oncologica 1995;34:511–5.

Raymond WA, Leong AS-Y. Vimentin – a new prognostic parameter in breast carcinoma. Journal of Pathology 1989;158:107–14.

Seshadri R, Raymond WA, Leong AS-Y, et al. Vimentin expression is

not associated with poor prognosis in breast cancer. Journal of Clinical Oncology 1996;67:353–6.

Sun WB, Han BL, Peng ZM, et al. Effect of aging on cytoskeleton system of Kupffer cells and its phagocytic activity. World Journal of Gastroenterology 1998;4:77–9.

Takemura K, Hirayama R, Hirokawa K, et al. Expression of vimentin in gastric carcinoma: a possible indicator for prognosis. Pathobiology 1994;62:149–54.

V

Vimentin

NOTES

Vinculin

Source/clone

Novocastra (clone V284, NCL-VINC), Sigma (hVin)

Fixation/preparation

This antibody is applicable to both frozen and paraffin sections. A high temperature antigen unmasking technique is recommended for the latter system prior to the immunohistochemical procedure.

Background

Vinculin is a cytoskeletal protein of 117–130 kD. Its gene is encoded on chromosome 10q11.2-qter (Weller et al, 1990). It is involved in the indirect binding of intracellular actin filaments to extracellular fibronectin. Vinculin is widely distributed in tissue with expression especially where smooth muscle actin and fibroblasts attach to the extracellular matrix (Burridge et al, 1980). Therefore, vinculin is a cytoskeletal protein associated with membrane actin-filament-attachment sites of cell-cell and cell-matrix adherens-type junctions. Hence, as an adhesion-associated protein, reduced or altered expression of vinculin has been associated with the acquisition of an invasive or metastatic phenotype in malignant transformation of cells (Lifschitz-Mercer et al, 1997). These workers demonstrated that the level of vinculin immunoexpression in low malignant, non-metastasizing squamous epithelial lesions was similar to that observed in normal squamous epithelia. In contrast, squamous cell carcinomas which are invasive and possess metastatic potential, immunolabelling for vinculin was negative or weak; concluding that vinculin immunoexpression in tumors arising from stratified squamous epithelia may be predictive of the metastatic potential (Lifschitz-Mercer, 1997).

It was previously reported that vinculin was distributed in renal tubular epithelium (Rahilly et al, 1991). Recently, a study of renal tumors revealed that immunoexpression of vinculin helps delineate renal neoplasms with a collecting duct system phenotype such as chromophobe-type renal cell carcinomas (Kuroda et al, 2000).

Applications

The use of vinculin immunoexpression in diagnostic surgical pathology is somewhat limited. It may have a predictive role in the biological behavior of tumors of squamous epithelial origin and may also be useful for the identification of renal tumors with a collecting duct phenotype.

The staining pattern of vinculin is membranous. Normal skin is a useful positive control.

References

Burridge K, Feramisco JR. Microinjection and localization of a 130K protein in living fibroblasts: a relationship to actin and fibronectin. Cell 1980;19:587–95.

Kuroda N, Naruse K, Miyazaki E, et al. Vinculin: its possible use as a marker of normal collecting ducts and renal neoplasms with collecting duct system phenotype. Modern Pathology 2000;13:1109–14.

Lifschitz-Mercer B, Czernobilsky B, Feldberg E, et al. Expression of the adherens junction protein vinculin in human basal and squamous cell tumors: relationship to invasiveness and metastatic potential. Human Pathology 1997;28:1230–6.

Novocastra Laboratories. Vinculin (data sheet).

Rahilly MA, Salter DM, Fleming S. Composition and organization of cell-substratum contacts in normal and neoplastic renal epithelium. Journal of Pathology 1991;165:163–71.

Weller PA, Ogryzko EP, Corben EB, et al. Complete sequence of human vinculin and assignment of the gene to chromosome 10. Proceedings of the National Academy of Sciences of the United States of America 1990;87:5667–71.

VS38

Sources/clones

Dako (VS38c)

Fixation/preparation

The antibody is reactive in paraffin-embedded sections and staining is enhanced by heat-induced antigen retrieval.

Background

VS38 was shown to detect a protein similar to the p63 protein. The latter is a non-glycated, reversibly palmitoylated type II transmembrane protein, which is found in rough endoplasmic reticulum. VS38 was originally described as a marker of neoplastic and non-neoplastic plasma cells (Turley et al, 1994).

Applications

It is now recognized that the protein detected by VS38 is not exclusive to plasma cells but serves to distinguish plasma cells from other lymphoid cells because of their high secretory activity (Banham et al, 1997). It has been recommended for inclusion in a panel of antibodies for the immunostaining of bone marrow trephines fixed in common fixatives including Bouin's solution (Gala et al, 1997).

VS38 immunostaining has been reported in neuroendocrine tumors and in melanocytic lesions, frequently positive in primary and metastatic melanomas and in a case of clear cell sarcoma of soft tissue (Shanks & Banerjee, 1996) and caution should be exercised when using this marker to identify plasma cell lineage. VS38 is also immunoexpressed in osteobalsts and stromal cells of bone tumors (Sulzbacher et al, 1997).

Comments

There is a need for a specific marker of plasma cell differentiation as a variety of neoplastic cells can display plasmacytoid features, and the converse, that is, poorly differentiated plasma cells and plasmacytoid cells can be difficult to recognize morphologically. In a recent study of endometritis, it was found that besides labeling plasma cells, VS38 also stained epithelium and stromal cells of the endometrium. In contrast CD38 produced strong labeling of plasma cells and not the other endometrial components, suggesting that CD38 may be a more specific marker of plasma cell differentiation (Leong et al, 1997).

References

Banham AH, Turley H, Pulford K, et al. The plasma cell associated antigen detectable by antibody VS38 is the p63 rough endoplasmic reticulum protein. Journal of Clinical Pathology 1997;50:485–9.

Banerjee SS, Shanks JH, Hasleton PS. VS38 immunostaining in neuroendocrine tumors. Histopathology 1997;30:256–9.

Gala JL, Chenut F, Hong KB, et al. A panel of antibodies for the immunostaining of Bouin's fixed bone marrow trephine biopsies. Journal of Clinical Pathology 1997;50:521–4.

Leong AS-Y, Vinyuvat S, Leong FJW-M, Suthipintawong C. anti-CD38 and VS38 antibodies for the detection of plasma cells in the diagnosis of chronic endometritis. Applied Immunohistochemistry 1997;5:189–93.

Shanks JH, Banerjee SS. VS38 immunostaining in melanocytic lesions. Journal of Clinical Pathology 1996;49:205–7.

Turley H, Jones M, Erber W, et al. VS38: a new monoclonal antibody for detecting plasma cell differentiation in routine sections. Journal of Clinical Pathology 1994;47:418–22.

Sulzbacher I, Fuchs M, Chott A, Lang S. Expression of VS38 in osteoblasts and stroma cells of bone tumors. Pathology Research and Practice 1997;193:613–6.

V

VS38

WT1

Sources/clone

Dako (polyclonal 6F–H2 directed to the amino terminus of the protein), Santa Cruz (C-19 raised against an 18 aminoacid peptide at the carboxyl terminus of the human WT1 protein; F-6 raised against the amino terminal 180 amino acid domain of the WT1 protein).

Fixation/preparation

Both antibodies are applicable to formalin-fixed paraffin-embedded tissue and immunoreactivity is enhanced by heat-induced antigen retrieval in citrate buffer followed by 0.4% pepsin digestion.

Background

Wilms' tumor gene (*WT1*) is a tumor-suppressor gene located on chromosome 11p13 (Pelletier et al, 1991). The Wilms' tumor gene encodes a protein (WT1) that is expressed in the developing fetal kidney and urogenital tract, the developing spleen and in fetal coelomic lining cells, including mesothelium (Pritchard-Jones et al, 1990; Park et al, 1993). WT1 is also expressed in mature benign mesothelial cells and may play a role in the malignant transformation of certain cells (Walker et al, 1994; Langerak et al, 1995). Using noncommercial anti-WT1 antibodies, studies have demonstrated discriminatory expression between mesotheliomas and adenocarcinomas with strong differential nuclear staining in mesotheliomas and cytoplasmic or no staining in adenocarcinoma (Kumar-Singh et al, 1997). Using a commercially available polyclonal antibody to WT1, a recent study demonstrated strong WT1 nuclear staining in 75% of mesotheliomas with absent nuclear staining in primary pulmonary adenocarcinomas (Foster et al, 2001). However 86% of pulmonary adenocarcinomas demonstrated cytoplasmic staining. Hence, nuclear staining for WT1 was shown to be highly specific for mesothelioma and in the appropriate clinical setting, can be a helpful adjunct in the distinction between adenocarcinomas and mesotheliomas.

A recent study using antibody clone 6F-H2 demonstrated WT1 with varying degrees of immunoreactivity in 93% of ovarian serous carcinomas (Goldstein et al, 2001). Ovarian mucinous neoplasms and pancreaticobiliary adenocarcinomas were negative for WT1. Nevertheless, many more non-Mullerian carcinomas need to be studied with the WT1 antibody before its width of immunoreactivity is completely understood. In the normal female genital organs, WT1 expression has been recognized in ovarian surface epithelium, inclusion cysts, and tubal epithelium, but not in cervical or endometrial epithelium (Shimizu et al, 2000).

The desmoplastic small round cell tumor (DSRCT) is a highly malignant neoplasm usually presenting in the abdomen of adolescent males. This neoplasm has been characterized with a translocation involving the Ewing's sarcoma gene on chromosome 22 and the Wilms' tumor gene *WT1* on chromosome 11, producing a fusion gene with expression of the DNA binding area of WT1. In an early study, four cases of DSRCT showed strong immunostaining with an anti-WT1 antibody (Charles et al, 1997). Subsequently, WT1 immunoreactivity using clone C-19 was confirmed in 13 DSRCT which showed strong nuclear staining (Hill et al, 2000). In contrast, all 11 cases of EWS/PNET were negative with

WT1 antibody. Another study also demonstrated WT1 immunoreactivity in all 15 cases of DSRCT examined (Barnoud et al, 2000). These workers also confirmed WT1-positive nuclei in 71% nephroblastomas and negative staining in EWS/PNET.

Applications

In the appropriate setting, WT1 (within a panel of antibodies) may be helpful in the distinction between adenocarcinomas and mesotheliomas. WT1 appears to have a high sensitivity and specificity for DSRCT and is therefore useful for differentiating from EWS/PNET. WT1 has a strong predilection for ovarian serous tumors, which may be helpful in differentiation from other Müllerian neoplasms and their metastases. However, further investigation in this area is warranted.

Comments

The nuclear antigen is sometimes associated with cytoplasmic staining. However, in the absence of nuclear staining, cytoplasmic staining should be regarded as spurious or may represent cross-reactivity with an epitope unrelated to WT1.

References

Barnoud R, Sabourin JC, Pasquier D, et al. Immunohistochemical expression of WT1 by desmoplastic small round cell tumor: a comparative study with other small round cell tumors. American Journal of Surgical Pathology 2000;24:830–6.

Charles AK, Moore IE, Berry PJ: Immunohistochemical detection of the Wilms' tumour gene WT1 in desmoplastic small round cell tumour. Histopathology 1997;30:312–4.

Foster MR, Johnson JE, Olson SJ, Allred DC: Immunohistochemical analysis of nuclear versus cytoplasmic staining of WT1 in malignant mesotheliomas and primary pulmonary adenocarcinomas. Archives of Pathology and Laboratory Medicine 2001;125:1316–20.

Goldstein NS, Bassi D, Uzieblo A: WT1 is an integral component of an antibody panel to distinguish pancreaticobiliary and some ovarian epithelial neoplasms. American Journal of Clinical Pathology 2001;116:246–52.

Hill DA, Pfeifer JD, Marley EF, et al. WT1 staining reliably differentiated desmoplastic small round cell tumor from Ewing sarcoma/primitive neuroectodermal tumor. American Journal of Clinical Pathology 2000;114:345–53.

Kumar-Singh S, Segers K, Rodeck U, et al. WT1 mutation in malignant mesothelioma and WT1 immunoreactivity in relation to p53 and growth factor receptor expression cell-type transition, and prognosis. Journal of Pathology 1997;181:67–74.

Langerak AW, Williamson KA, Miyagawa K, et al. Expression of the Wilms' tumor gene WT1 in human malignant mesothelioma cell lines and relationship to platelet-derived growth factor A and insulin-like growth factor 2 expression. Genes Chromosomes and Cancer 1995;12:87–96.

Park S, Schalling M, Bernard A, et al: The Wilms tumor gene WT1 is expressed in murine mesoderm-derived tissues and mutated in a human mesothelioma. Nature and Genetics 1993; 4:415–20.

Pelletier J, Schalling M, Buckler A, et al. Expression of the Wilms' tumor gene *WT1* in the murine urogenital system. Genes and Development 1991;5:1345–56.

Pritchard-Jones K, Fleming S, Davidson D, et al. The candidate Wilms tumor gene is involved in genitourinary development. Nature 1990;345:194–7.

Shimizu M, Toki T, Takagi Y, et al. Immunohistochemical detection of the Wilm's tumor gene (WT1) in epithelial ovarian tumors. International Journal of Gynecological Pathology 2000;19:158–63.

Walker C, Rutten F, Yuan X, et al. Wilm's tumor suppressor gene expression in rat and human mesothelioma. Cancer Research 1994;54:3101–6.

SECTION 2
Appendices

Appendix 1

Selected antibody panels for specific diagnostic situations

Appendix 1.1 Bone/Soft tissue – Chondroid-like Tumors

	CK	Vim	S100	EMA	CEA	GFAP	CD57
Chordoma	+	+	+	+	+	–/+	–
Parachordoma	+	+	+	+	–/+	–/+	–
Chondroblastoma	+	+	+	+	–	–	–
Chondroid chordoma	+	+	+	+	–	–	–
Myxoid chondrosarcoma (chordoid sarcoma)	–	+	+	–	–	–	–
Mesenchymal chondrosarcoma	–	+	+*	–	–	–	+
Clear cell sarcoma	–	+	+	–	–	–	–

*chondroid cells

Appendix 1.2 Brain – Metastatic Carcinoma vs Glioblastoma vs Meningioma

	CK	EMA	VIM	GFAP
Metastatic carcinoma	+	+	–/+	–
Glioblastoma	–	–	+/–	+
Meningioma	–/*	+	+	–

*Secretory meningioma may be focally keratin-positive

Appendix 1.3 Childhood Round Cell Tumors

	LCA	VIM*	CK	DES	MSA	CD99	Myogen	MYOD1	NSE	SYN	FLI-1	Chgn	NF
Hemato-lymphoid Tumor+	+/–	+	–	–	–	–/+	–	–	–	–	+/–	–	–
Neuroblastoma	–	+	–/+	–	–	–	–	–	+	+/–	–	+/–	+
Ewing's Sarcoma	–	+	–/+	–	–	+	–	–	–/+	–	+	–	–/+
PNET	–	+	+	–/+	–/+	+	–	–	+	+	+	–/+	–/+
DSRCT#	–	+	+	+	+	–/+	–	–	+	+	+	–/+	–
Rhabdomyosarcoma	–	+	–	+	+	–/+	+	+	–	–	–	–	–

PNET – peripheral/primitive neuroectodermal tumor
* Vimentin labeling shows up the cytoplasm, which is often not visible on H & E stains
+ lymphoblastic lymphoma is positive for terminal deoxynucleotidyl transferase (TdT)
#DSRCT – desmoplastic small round cell tumor, stains positive for WT1 which is not identified in the other tumors considered in differential diagnosis

Appendix 1.4 Gastrointestinal and Aerodigestive Tract Mucosa - Basaloid Squamous vs Adenoid Cystic vs Neuroendocrine Carcinoma

	HMWtCK	CEA	S100	Chgn	SYN
Basaloid squamous carcinoma	+	+	–	–	–
Adenoid cystic carcinoma	–/+	+*	–/+	–	–
Neuroendocrine carcinoma	–	–	–	+	+

*Confined to luminal aspects of gland-like spaces

Appendix 1.5 Gonads – Germ Cell Tumors versus Somatic Adenocarcinoma

	PLAP	αFP	HCG	CD30	CD117	CK	EMA	Vim	hPL
Seminoma	+	–	–*	–	+	–*	–	+	–
Embryonal carcinoma	+	+/–	–	+	–	+	–	–	–
Yolk sac tumor	+/–	+	–	–	+	+	–	–	–
Choriocarcinoma	+/–	–	+	–	–	+	+	–/+	+
Somatic carcinoma	–/+**	–	–/+	–	–	+	+	–	–

*Occasional trophoblasts may be positive.
**Mullerian tract, breast, gut and pulmonary tumors may occasionally be positive

Appendix 1.6 Granulocytic sarcoma versus lymphoma versus carcinoma versus plasmacytoma

	CD45	CD38	CK	NE	CD15*	EMA
Granulocytic sarcoma	+	–	–	+	+	–
Lymphoma	+	–	–	–	–	–
Plasmacytoma (poorly differentiated)	+/–	+	–	–	–	+
Carcinoma	–	–	+	–	–/+	+

*Other markers of granulocytic sarcoma include neutrophil elastase, myeloperoxidase, lysozyme, CD34, CD68.

Appendix 1.7 Intracranial Tumors

	GFAP	VIM	CK	NF	CR
Astrocytoma	+	+	–/+	–	–
Oligodendroglioma	+	+	–	–	–
Ependymoma	–	–/+	+ (surface)	–	–
Neuroma/neurocytoma	–	–	–	+	+
Schwannoma	–/+	+	–	–	–/+
Metastatic carcinoma	–	–/+	+	–	–

Appendix 1.8 Liver – Hepatocellular Carcinoma vs Metastatic Carcinoma vs Cholangiocarcinoma

	CEA	AFP	CK7	CK19	VIM	Hep Par 1	Albumin
Hepatocellular carcinoma	+*	–/+	–/+	–/+	–/+	+	+/–
Cholangiocarcinoma	+	–	+	+	–/+	–/+	–
Metastatic carcinoma	+/–	–	+/–	+/–	–/+	–	–

*Staining of canaliculi in hepatocellular carcinoma by polyclonal CEA

Appendix 1.9 Lung – Clear Cell Tumors

	CK	VIM	Chgn	SYN	HMB45	S100
Carcinoma with clear cell change	+	–	–	–	–	–
Clear cell tumor ("sugar" tumor)	–	–*	–	–	+	–*
Renal carcinoma, metastatic	+	+	–	–	–	–
Carcinoid	+	–	+	+	–	–

*Rare cells may stain positive

Appendix 1.10 Lymph Node – Round Cell Tumors in Adults

	CD45	CK	VIM	S100	HMB45	Melan A	MiTF
Melanoma	–	–	+	+	+	+	+
Carcinoma	–	+	–	–/+	–	–	–
Lymphoma	+	–	+	–	–	–	–

Appendix 1.11 Undifferentiated Round Cell Tumors

	CK	S100	CD45	Des	FLI	CD99	HMB45	Mart-1	Myogenin
Small cell carcinoma	+	–	–	–	–	–/+	–	–	–
Melanoma	–	+	–	–	–	–	+	+	–
Lymphoma	–	–	+	–	–	–/+	–	–	–
PNET	–/+	–	–	–/+	+	+	–	–	–
DSRCT	+/–	–	–	+/–	+/–	–/+	–	–	–
Rhabdomyosarcoma	–	–/+	–	+	–	–/+	–	–	+
Poorly differentiated synovial sarcoma	+	+/–	–	–/+	–	+	–	–	–

PNET – peripheral/primitive neuroectodermal tumor; DSRCT - desmoplastic small round cell tumor

Appendix 1.12 Mediastinal tumors

	CD45	CK	EMA	PLAP	CD99
Thymoma	–	+	+	–	+*
Lymphoma	+	–	–	–	–/+
Germ Cell Tumor	–	+	+	+	–

*staining of associated small lymphocytes that also stain for CD1a

Appendix 1.13 Nasal Tumors

	VIM	CK	S100	HMB45	NF
Neuroblastoma	+	–	+(SC)	–	+
Melanoma	+	–	+	+	–
Carcinoma	–/+	+	–/+	–	–

SC = supporting stromal cells and areas of ganglineuromatous differentiation stain positive

Appendix 1.14 Pelvis – Metastatic Colonic Adenocarcinoma vs Ovarian Endometrioid Carcinoma

	VIM	CEA	CA-19.9	CA-125	CK7	CK20
Colonic adenocarcinoma	–/+	+	+	–/+	–	+
Ovarian endometrioid carcinoma	+/–	–	–	+	+	–

Appendix 1.15 Perineum – Prostatic vs Bladder vs Rectal Carcinoma

	CK7	CK20	PSA	PSAP	CEA
Prostatic carcinoma	–	–/+	+	+	–/+
Bladder carcinoma	+	+	–	–/+	+
Rectal carcinoma	–	+	–	–	+

Appendix 1.16 Peritoneum – Myxoid Tumors

	SMA	Des	S100	Col IV	CD34
Myxoma	–	–	–	–	–
Myxoid neurofibroma	–	–	+	+L	+
Myxoid liposarcoma	–	–	+	+C	+
Myxoid fibrosarcoma	–	–	–	–	–
Myxoid leiomyosarcoma	+	–/+	–	+L	–/+
Aggressive angiomyxoma	+	–/+	–	+F	–
Angiomyofibroblastoma	+	+	–	+F	–/+
Low grade fibromyxoid sarcoma	+/–	–	–	+F/–	–

C = circumferential; F = fragmented, thin; L = linear, continuous.

Appendix 1.17 Pleura – Mesothelioma vs Carcinoma

	LMWCK	HMWCK	VIM	EMA	αSMA	CEA	CR	CD15#	Ber-EP4	WTI	B72.3
Mesothelioma**	+	+	+	+*	+/–	–	+	–	–	+/–	–
Secondary carcinoma	+	–	–/+	+	–	+	–/+	+	+	–	+

*Circumferential, with long microvilli; EMA may be substituted with HBME-1 which also highlights the characteristic microvilli
#Can be substituted with other myelomonocytic markers, e.g. LN1 (CDw75), LN2 (CD74), Mac 387
LMWCK = low molecular weight cytokeratin
HMWCK = high molecular weight cytokeratin including CK5/6
**mesotheliomas also stain for N-cadherin. In contrast carcinoma stain for E-cadherin and not for N-cadherin

Appendix 1.18 Retroperitoneum - Renal Cell Carcinoma vs Adrenocortical Carcinoma vs Pheochromocytoma

	EMA	VIM	CK	Chgn	SYN	S100	Mart-1	CR	Inhib
Renal carcinoma	+	+/–	+	–	–	–/+	–	–	–
Adrenocortical carcinoma	–	+	–/+	–	–/+	–	+	+	+
Pheochromocytoma	+	–	+	+	+*	+*	–	–	–

*sustentacular cells

Appendix 1.19 Retroperitoneum – Vacuolated/Clear Cell Tumor

	Vim	CK	S100	GFAP	CEA
Chordoma	+	+	+	–/+	–
Colonic adenocarcinoma	–/+	+	–	–	+
Renal cell carcinoma	+	+/–	–/+	–	–
Myxopapillary ependymoma	+	+/–	+/–	+	–

Appendix 1.20 Skin – Adnexal Tumors

	CK20	S100	EMA	CEA	GCDFP-15	SA	CD15	Chgn	NF	LYS
Squamous carcinoma	–	–	–	–	–	–	–	–	–	–
Eccrine tumor	–	+	+/–	+/–	–/+	+/–	+/–	–	–	–
Apocrine tumor	–	–	+/–	+/–	+	+/–	+/–	–	–	+
Sebaceous tumor	–	–	+	–	–	–	+	–	–	–
Pilar tumor	–	–	–	–	–	–	–	–	–	–
Merkel cell carcinoma	+	–	+	–	–	–	–	+	+*	–

*Merkel cell carcinoma often shows juxtanuclear whorls of neurofilaments and/or cytokeratin

Appendix 1.21 Skin - Basal Cell Carcinoma vs Squamous Carcinoma vs Adnexal Carcinoma

	EMA	BerEP4
Basal cell carcinoma	–	+
Squamous carcinoma	+	–
Adnexal carcinoma	+	+

Appendix 1.22 Skin – Pagetoid Tumors

	LMWtCK	HMWtCK	S100	CEA	VIM
Melanoma	–	–	+	–	+
Paget's disease	+	–	–/+	+	–
Bowen's disease	+	+	–	–	–

Appendix 1.23 Skin – Spindle Cell Tumors

	CK	VIM	CD34	CD31	αSMA	S100	HMB45	Leu7	DES	CD99
Spindle SCC	+	+	–	–	–	–	–	–	–	–
Melanoma	–	+	–	–	–	+	+	–/+	–	–
AFX	–	+	–/+	–	–	–	–	–	–	NK
DFSP	–	+	+	–	–	–	–	–	–	NK
PNST	–	+	–/+	–	–	+/–	–	+/–	–	+
Smooth muscle	–/+	+	–/+	–	+	–/+	–/+	–	+/–	–/+
Kaposi's Sarcoma	–	+	+	+	–	–	–	–	–	NK
Angiosarcoma	–/+	+	+	+	–	–/+	–	–	–	NK
Glomus tumor	–	+	–	–	+	–	–	–/+	–/+	–
Hemangiopericytoma	–	+	+	–	–	–/+	–	–/+	–	+/–

AFX - atypical fibroxanthomas
DFSP - dermatofibrosarcoma protuberans
PNST - peripheral nerve sheath tumor
SCC - squamous cell carcinoma
NK - not known

Appendix 1.24 Soft Tissue - Epithelioid Tumors

	CK	VIM	EMA	CD34	CD31	DES	αSMA	CD57	S100	CD99	Mart-1
Metastatic carcinoma	+	–/+	+	–	–	–	–	–	–/+	–/+	–/+
Synovial sarcoma	+	+	+	–	–	–*	–	–	–	+/–	–
Epithelioid sarcoma	+	+	+	+/–	–	–	–	–	–	–	–
Angiosarcoma	–/+	+	–	+	+	–	–	–	–	–	–
PNST	–*	+	–/+	+/–	–	–	–	+/–	+/–	–/+	–
Leiomyosarcoma	–/+	+	–	+/–	–	+	+	–	–	–	–
Melanoma	–	+	–	–	–	–	–	–/+	+/–	–	+

*Occasional cells stain positive
PNST - epithelioid peripheral nerve sheath tumor

Appendix 1.25 Soft Tissue - Spindle Cell, fasciculated

	SMA	MSA	Des	ScA	S100	Col4
Fibromatosis	+/–	+/–	–/+	–	–	+F
PNST	–	–	–	–	+	+L
Fibrosarcoma	–/+	–/+	–	–	–	–/+F
Leiomyosarcoma	+	+	+/–	–	–/+	+L
Spindle Cell rhabdomyosarcoma	–	+	+	+	–	+L
Synovial sarcoma	–/+	–/+	–	–	–/+	+C

PNST – peripheral nerve sheath tumor
F = fragmented; L = linear continuous; C = circumferential, around groups and individual cells.

Appendix 1.26 Soft Tissue - Myxoid Tumors

	S100	SMA	MSA	Des	EMA	CK	CD34	CD99
Myxoma	–	–	–/+	–	–	–	+	NK
Aggressive angiomyxoma	–	+	+	+	–	–	–/+	NK
Angiomyofibroblastoma	–	+	+	–/+	–	–	–/+	NK
Myxoid neurofibroma	+	–	–	–	+	–	–/+	NK
Neurothekoma	+	–/+	+/–	–	+	–	–/+	NK
Chordoma	+	–	–	–	+	+	–	NK
Myxoid Lipoma/liposarcoma	+/–	–	–	–	–	–	+/–	–
Myxoid chondrosarcoma	+/–	–	–	–	–/+	–/+	–/+	–
Myxoid MFH	–	–/+	+/–	–	–	–	+	–/+
Myxoid leiomyosarcoma	–	+	+	–/+	–	–/+	+/–	–/+
Botryoid embryonal RMS	–	–	–	+	–	–	–	–/+
Myxofibrosarcoma	–	–/+	–/+	–	–	–	–	–/+

MFH – malignant fibrous histiocytoma; RMS – rhabdomyosarcoma; NK – not known

Appendix 1.27 Soft Tissue – Pleomorphic Tumors

	VIM	DES	S100	MSA	ScA	HMB45	CK	MYOD1	Myogen
Rhabdomyosarcoma	+	+	–	+	+	–	–	+	+
MFH*	+	–	–/+	–/+	–	–	–	–	–
Melanoma	+	–	+	–	–	+	–	–	–
Carcinoma	–/+	–	–	–	–	–	+	–	–

*MFH – malignant fibrous histiocytoma may express Factor XIIIa

Appendix 1.28 Extraskeletal Myxoid/Chondroid Tumors

	S100	Cam 5.2	CK7	CK19	EMA	CEA	MSA
Myxoid chondrosarcoma	+	–	–	–	–	–	–
Chordoma	+	+	+/–	+	+	+	–
Parachordoma	+	+	–	–	+	–	–
Mixed tumor	+	+	NK	NK	+	–	+/–
Myxoid liposarcoma	+/–	–	–	–	–	–	–

NK = not known

Appendix 1.29 Stomach – Undifferentiated Spindle Cell Tumors

	CD34	SMA	MSA	S100	Chgn	SYN	CK	CD117(*ckit*)
LyMo/LyMSa	–/+(weak)	+	+	–/+	–	–	–/+	–/+
GIST	+	–	–	–	–	–	–	+/–
PNST	–	–	–	+	–	–	–	–
GAN	+/–	–	–	–	+	+	–	–

GIST = Gastrointestinal stromal tumor. This term is used for spindled tumors, which do not show evidence of myogenic or neurogenic differentiation, morphologically and immunophenotypically.
GAN = Gastrointestinal autonomic nerve tumors. Presence of amorphous extracellular collagen or skenoid fibres is often present and ultrastructural examination may be necessary to confirm the diagnosis of this aggressive tumor.
LyMo/LyMSa = leiomyoma/leiomyosarcoma; PNST = peripheral nerve sheath tumor.

Appendix 1.30 Thyroid carcinomas

	34BE12	Vim	Thy	Chgn	SYN	CEA	Cal	TTF-1
Papillary carcinoma	+	+	+	–	–	–	–	+
Follicular carcinoma	–	+	+	–	–	–	–	+
Medullary carcinoma	–	–/+*	–	+	+	+	+	–
Metastatic carcinoma	–/+	–/+	–	–	–	–	–	–/+

*Vimentin expressed in spindle cells of medullary carcinoma

Appendix 1.31 Urinary Tract – Spindle Cell Proliferations

	CK	EMA	Des	MSA	SMA	S100	Myog
Inflammatory Pseudotumor	–	–	–	+	+	–	–
Leiomyosarcoma	–/+	–	+/–	+	+	–/+	–
Spindle Cell carcinoma	+	+	–	–	–	–/+	–
Rhabdomyosarcoma	–	–	+	+	–	–	+
MFH	–	–	–	–/+**	–/+**	–/+	–
Neurofibrosarcoma	–	–	++*	–/+*	–	+/–	–
Malignant melanoma	–	–	–	–	–	+	–
Post-operative spindle cell nodule	–/+	–	–	+	+	–	–

*Triton tumor
**reactive myofibroblasts

Appendix 1.32 Uterine cervix – Endometrial versus Endocervical Carcinoma

	Vim	CK20	CK7	CEA	ER
Endometrial carcinoma	+/–	–	+	–/+	+
Endocervical carcinoma	–/+	–	–	+/–	–
Colonic carcinoma (metastatic)	–/+	+	–	+	–

Appendix 1.33 Uterus – Trophoblastic Cells

Trophoblastic cell	1st Trimester		2nd Trimester		3rd Trimester	
	HCG	HPL	hCG	hPL	hCG	hPL
Cytotrophoblast	–	–	–	–	–	–
Intermediate Trophoblast	+	++	–/+	+++	+	+/++
Syncytiotrophoblast	++++	+	++	+++	+	++++

Percentage of cell staining for the respective antigen: + = 1–24%; ++ = 25–49%; +++ = 50–74%; ++++ = >75%

Appendix 1.34 Uterus – Immunophenotyping of Syncytiotrophoblasts in Trophoblastic Proliferations

	hCG	hPL	PLAP	SP1	CK	VIM
Partial mole*	+ diffuse	+/++ diffuse#	+/+++ diffuse#	NK	+++ diffuse	–
Complete mole	+++ diffuse	+/++ focal#	+ focal	+++ diffuse	+++ diffuse	–
ChorioCa	+++ diffuse	+ focal	+ focal	NK	+++ diffuse	–
Implantation site IT, placental site tumor trophoblastic tumor[a]	+++ focal	+++ diffuse	+++ diffuse	+++ diffuse	+++ diffuse	+++ diffuse
Chorionic-type IT, placental site nodule and epithelioid trophoblastic tumor[b]	+ focal	+ focal	++++ diffuse	NK	++ diffuse	++ diffuse

IT = intemediate trophoblast
NK = not known; + = weak; ++ = intermediate; +++ = strong staining; # = expression increases with advancing pregnancy
In the 1st trimester, the pattern of expression of hCG in partial and complete moles is very similar. Similarly, the immunophenotypic profile of hydropic abortus and partial moles is very similar to that of normal pregnancy in the 1st trimester.
[a]stains strongly for alpha-inhibin and Mel-CAM (CD146); [b]stains for alpha-inhibin and weakly and focally for Mel-CAM (CD146)

Appendix 1.35 Brain Intraventricular Tumors

	PLAP	EMA	CK	CEA	Chgn	Syn	S100	GFAP
Ependymoma	–	–/+*	–/+*	–	–	–	+	+
Choroid plexus tumors	–	+	+	+/–	–	–	+	–/+
Subependymoma	–	–	–	–	–	–	+	+
Subependymal giant cell astrocytoma	–	–	+	–	–	–	+	+
Pilocytic astrocytoma	–	–	+/–	–	–	–	+	+
Central neurocytoma	–	–	–	–	–/+	+	+/–	–/+
Pineal tumors	–	–	–	–	–/+	+	+	–/+
Germ cell tumors	+	+	+	+	–	–	–	–
Colloid cyst	–	+	+	–/+	–	–	+	–/+
Meningioma	–	+	+/–	–	–	–	–/+	–

*surface staining only

Appendix 1.36 CNS Small Cell Tumors

	EMA	CK	Chgn	Syn	S100	GFAP	CD45	HMB45
Metastatic carcinoma	+	+	–	–	–	–	–	–
Malignant lymphoma	–	–	–	–	–	–	+	–
Metastatic melanoma	–	–	–	–	+	–	–	+
Medulloblastoma	–	–	–	+	+/–	+/–	–	–
Hemangiopericytoma	–	–	–	–	–	–	–	–
Plasmacytoma/myeloma	+	–	–	–	–	–	+/–	–
Pineocytoma/pineoblastoma	–	–	–/+	+	+	–/+	–	–
Esthesioneuroblastoma	+/–	+/–	+	+	+/–	–	–	–

Appendix 1.37 Tissue-Associated Antigens in "Treatable Tumors"

Lymphoma/leukemia	LCA (CD45)
Germ cell Tumor	PLAP
Breast carcinoma	GCDFP15
Thyroid carcinoma	Thyroglobulin, TTF-1
Prostatic carcinoma	PSA, PSAP
Trophoblastic tumor	HCG, HPL, Mel-cam
Rhabdomyosarcoma	Des, MYOD1, Myogen, Myoglob*
Ewing's sarcoma / PNET	CD99
Neuroblastoma	NF
Neuroendocrine Tumor	Chgn, SYN

Key: Chgn = chromogranin; Des = desmin; HCG = human chorionic gonadotrophin; HPL = uman placental lactogen;Myogen = myogenin; Myoglob = myoglobin; NF = neurofilaments; PLAP = placental alkaline phosphatase; PSA = prostatic specific antigen; PSAP = prostatic acid phosphatase; SYN = synaptophysin.
*low sensitivity

Appendix 1.38 Epithelial Tumors Which May Coexpress Vimentin Intermediate Filaments*

Thyroid carcinoma

Endometrial carcinoma

Adreno-cortical carcinoma

Ovarian epithelial tumors

Gonadal tumors

Salivary gland tumors

Renal cell carcinoma

Choroid plexus tumors

Breast carcinoma

Prostatic carcinoma

Ependymal tumors

Lung carcinoma

Hepatocellular carcinoma

Pheochromocytoma

Adamantinoma

Primitive/peripheral neuro-epithelial tumor (PNET)

*Any carcinoma, when sufficiently dedifferentiated, may coexpress vimentin; these tumors show this property with some regularity.

Appendix 1.39 Mesenchymal Tumors which may Coexpress Cytokeratin

Angiosarcoma

Leiomyosarcoma

Chordoma

Chondroid Chordoma

Chondroblastoma

Synovial Sarcoma (monophasic and biphasic)

Epithelioid Sarcoma

Mesothelioma

Meningioma

Malignant Peripheral Nerve Sheath Tumor*

Malignant melanoma**

Anaplastic Large Cell Lymphoma Ki-1

Dendritic cell sarcoma

*glandular component
**only in cryostat sections

Appendix 1.40 Tumors which may co-express three or more intermediate filaments

Astrocytoma	GFAP, Vim, CK
DSRCT	Vim, CK, Des, NF
ES/PNET	Vim, CK, Des
Leiomyosarcoma	Vim, Des, CK
Pheochromocytoma	CK, NF, Vim
Rhabdomyosarcoma	Des, Vim, CK
Pleomorphic adenoma	CK, Vim, GFAP
Endothelial cells	Vim, CK, Des
Teratoma	CK, Des, GFAP, NF, Vim
True mixed tumors (including Mullerian tumors)	CK, Des, Vim
Mesothelioma	CK, Des, Vim

Key: ES/PNET = Ewing's sarcoma / Primitive peripheral neuroepithelial tumor; CK = cytokeratin; Des = desmin; GFAP = glial fibrillary acidic protein; NF = neurofilaments; Vim = Vimentin.

Appendix 1.41 Abbreviations to antibodies and their sources

αFP = α fetoprotein (Dako)

bcl-2 (Dako)

BerEP4 (Dako)

CA-125 (Signet)

CA19.9 (Signet)

CD15 = LeuM1 (B & D)

CD31 (Dako)

CD34 (Oxoid)

CD57 = Leu7 (B & D)

CEA = carcinoembryonic antigen (Biogenex)

Chgn = chromogranin (INC)

CK = broad spectrum cytokeratin (clone MNF116 – Dako; AE1/3 – BMA; bovine keratin – Dako)

CK19 = cytokeratin 19 (Novocastra)

CK20 = cytokeratin 20 (Dako)

CK7 = cytokeratin 7 (Dako)

Col IV = Type IV Collagen (Dako)

CR = Calretinin (Zymed)

DES = desmin (Dako)

EMA = epithelial membrane antigen (Sera Lab)

GCDFP-15 = gross cystic disease fluid protein-15 (Signet)

GFAP = glial fibrillary acidic protein (Dako)

Hep Par 1 (Dako)

HCG = human chorionic gonadotrophin (Biogenex)

HPL = human placental lactogen (Dako)

HMB45 = melanoma-associated antigen (Dako)

HMWtCK = high molecular weight cytokeratin (34BH11 – Dako)

LCA = CD45, leukocyte common antigen (Dako)

LMWtCK = low molecular weight cytokeratin (35BE12 – Dako)

Mart 1 (Melan A) = melanocytic marker (Dako)

MSA = muscle-specific actin (Enzo)

MYOD1 (Novocastra)

Myogen = myogenin (clone F5D – Dako)

NE = neutrophil esterase (Dako) p30–32 = p30–32 glycoprotein (clone MIC2 – Dako; O13 – Signet)

PLAP = placental alkaline phosphatase (Dako)

PSA = prostate specific antigen (Dako)

PSAP = prostatic acid phosphatase (Dako)

S100 = S100 protein (Dako)

SA = salivary/amylase (Biodesign)

ScA = sarcomeric actin (Dako)

SMA = α-smooth muscle actin (Sigma)

SYN = synaptophysin (BMA)

TTF-1 = thyroid transmission factor-1 (Dako)

VIM = vimentin (Dako)

B & D – Becton Dickinson, Mountain View, California, USA

Biogenex – Biogenex Laboratories, San Ramon, California, USA

BMA – Boehringer Mannheim, Sydney, NSW, Australia

Dako – Dakopatts, Santa Barbara, California, USA

ENZO – Enzo Biochem, New York, USA

Novocastra – Novocastra Laboratories, Newcastle-Upon-Tyne, UK

Sera Lab – Sera Lab, Sussex, UK

Sigma – Sigma Chemicals, St Louis, Maryland, USA

Signet – Signet Laboratories, Dedham, Massachussetts, USA.

Appendix 2
Antibody Panels for Lymphoid Neoplasms

Appendix 2.1 Useful Markers in B-cell Neoplasms
Ig light chain restriction (IgK, Igλ)
CD20
CD79a
CDw75 (follicle centre cells)
CD45RA (neoplastic follicles)
bcl-2 (neoplastic follicles)
CD43 (neoplasms derived from small B cells)
CD5 (neoplastic B cells)
CD10 (CALLA) (follicle centre cells)
bcl-6 (follicular lymphoma, some diffuse B lymphomas)

Appendix 2.2 Useful Markers of T-cell Neoplasms
CD3
CD5
CD4
CD8
CD45RO
CD1 (precursor T-cells)
TdT (precursor T-cells)
CD7

Appendix 2.3 Markers of Reed Sternberg cells*

CD15

CD30

Vimentin

Fascin

CD40

CD45 -ve

CD20 –/+

CD3 -ve

EMA -ve

ALK -ve

*surrounding small lymphocytes are T-cells with CD4+, TIA-1+

Appendix 2.4 Useful markers of Monocytes/macrophages

CD45

HLA-DR

CD15

CD21

CD68

α-1-AT

α-1-ACT

S100 -ve

Appendix 2.5 Markers of Myeloid Cells

CD34

CD15

Lysozyme

Neutrophil elastase

Myeloperoxidase

CD99, CD43, CD68 and CD117 may also mark

myeloid cells

Appendix 2.6 Useful Markers of Natural Killer- (NK) cells

CD8

CD57

CD56

HLA-DR ±

Appendix 2.7 Markers of Langerhans Cells and Interdigitating Reticulum Cells

CD1

HLA-DR

CD54 (ICAM)

S100

CD45

CD68-

Appendix 2.8 Markers of Follicular Dendric Cells

CD35

CD21

S100

HLA-DR

Fascin

α-1-AT

α-1-ACT

Appendix 2.9 Panel for Small Cell Lymphomas

	CD43	CD5	CD23	Cyclin D1	CD10	CD38
SLL-BCLL	+	+	+	−	−	−
MCL	+	+	−	+	−	−
MZL	+/−	−	−	−	−	−
LPL	+	−	−	−	−	+
FL	−	−	−	−	+	−

SLL/BCLL = small lymphocytic lymphoma/B-cell lymphocytic leukaemia; MCL = mantle cell lymphoma; MZL – marginal zone lymphoma; LPL = lymphoplasmacytic lymphoma; FL = follicle centre cell lymphoma.

Appendix 2.10 Classic Hodgkin's Disease vs Lymphocyte Predominant Hodgkin's Disease vs T-cell/histiocyte-rich B-cell Lymphoma

	Classic HD	LP-HD	T-cell/histiocyte-rich B-cell lymphoma	Anaplastic Large Cell Lymphoma (ALCL)*
CD15	+	–	–	–
CD30	+	–	–	+
CD20	–	+	+	–/+
J-chain	–	+/–	–/+	–
Vimentin	+	–/+	–/+	+
CD45	–	+	+	+/–
EMA	–/+	+/–	+/–	+/–
CD3*	+	–/+	+	+/– (ALCL cells)
TIA-1*	+	–	+	– (ALCL cells)
CD57*	–	+	–	– (ALCL cells)
CD20*	–/+	+/–	–	NA

HD = Hodgkin's disease, LP-HD = Lymphocyte predominant Hodgkin's disease; EMA = epithelial membrane antigen;
*background small lymphocytes, in LP-HD CD57+ lymphocytes form rosettes around L+H cells.
*ALCL cells immunoexpress ALK protein. Most commonly T cell phenotype, sometime "null", rarely B cell phenotype

Appendix 3
Antibody Applications

Antibody	Useful diagnostic applications
α-Smooth Muscle Actin (α- SMA)	Smooth muscle, myofibroblasts, myoepithelium, leiomyosarcoma
α-1-anti-chymotrypsin	Macrophages/histiocytes and a variety of other cells
α-1-antitrypsin	Macrophages/histiocytes and a variety of other cells
α-feto-protein	Yolk sac tumours, hepatocellular carcinoma
ALK protein (p80)	Anaplastic large cell lymphoma with t(2;5)
Amyloid	Subtypes of amyloid
Androgen receptor	Prostatic cancer
Anti apoptosis	Apoptotic cells
Bcl-2	Follicular lymphoma versus reactive follicles, possible prognostic marker
Ber-EP4	(epithelial glycoprotein) Some adenocarcinomas, negative in mesothelioma
β-HCG	Trophoblastic cells and tumours including choriocarcinoma
CA125	Serous cytic tumours of the ovary and various adenocarcinomas
Cadherin	Putative marker of epithelial differentiation, absent in lobular carcinoma of the breast, possible prognostic marker
Calcitonin	Medullary carcinoma of the thyroid
Calretinin	Mesothelioma
Carcinoembryonic antigen (CD66)	Polyclonal antibody stains hepatocyte canuliculi, various adenocarcinomas but absent in mesothelioma
Catenins	Associated with E-cadherin
CathepsinD	Prognostic marker in breast cancer
CD1a	Langerhan cells, Langerhan cell histiocytosis
CD2	(Frozen sections only) Pan-T-cell marker
CD3	Mature T-cells, T-cell lymphoma
CD4	T-cell helper subset
CD5	T-cells, Mantle zone cells, small lymphocytic lymphoma B-cell type
CD7	(Frozen sections only) Immature and mature T-cells and nature killer cells
CD8	T-cell suppressor subset
CD9	Both B and T cells and their corresponding neoplasms
CD10 (CALLA)	Follicular centre cells, follicular centre lymphoma, Burkitt's lymphoma, myoepithelial cells

Antibody	Useful diagnostic applications
CD15	Reed-Sternberg cells, neutrophils, various adenocarcinomas
CD19	(Frozen sections only) B-cell lymphomas
CD20	B cells and B-cell lymphomas
CD21	B cells and follicular dendritic cells and their corresponding tumours
CD23	Small lymphocytic lymphoma, B-cell type
CD30	Reed-Sternberg cells, Ki-1 lymphoma, embryonal carcinoma
CD31	Endothelial cells and tumours
CD34	Endothelial cells and tumours, leukaemias, gastrointestinal stromal tumours
CD35	Follicular dendritic cells and follicular dendritic cell sarcoma
CD38	Plasma cells
CD40	Reed-Sternberg cells
CD43	T-cells, macrophages and often co-expressing B-cell lymphomas
CD44	Various isoforms, possible prognostic marker in various tumours
CD45 (leukocyte common antigen)	Almost all haematolymphoid cells and progenitors
CD45RA	Mantle zone B-cells, T-cells, reactive versus neoplastic follicles
CD45RO	T-cells, macrophages, granulocytic precursors
CD54 (ICAM-1)	Monocytes, endothelial cells, T-cells and B-cells
CD56 (NCAM)	Natural killer cells and corresponding tumours, neural tumours
CD57	Nerve sheath tumours, natural killer cells
CD66 (CEA family)	Various adenocarcinomas, bile cannuliculi of hepatocellular carcinoma, negative on mesothelioma
CD68	Macrophages and cells rich in lysozomes
CD74 (LN2)	B-cell lymphoma, some T-cell lymphoma, Reed Sternberg cells
CDw75 (LN1)	Follicular lymphoma L&H cell
CD79a	B-cells
CD99 (p30/32^{MIC2})	Ewing's tumour/PNET
CD103 (HML-1)	Memory B-lymphocytes and intraepithelial lymphocytes
CD117 (*c-kit*)	Haemopoietic progenitor cells, gastrointestinal stroma tumours, mast cells
c-erb B-2 (Her-2/*neu*,Herceptest™)	Breast cancer prognostic marker, predictor of treatment response
Chlamydia	Chlamydia (all species)
Chromogranin	Dense core granule in neuroendocrine differentiation
c-myc	c-myc
Collagen Type IV	Basal lamina
Cyclin D1 (bcl-1)	Mantle cell lymphoma
Cytokeratins	Cytokeratins
Cytokeratin 1/10 (34βE12)	Squamous cell carcinoma, loss of basal cell staining in prostatic carcinoma
Cytokeratin 5/6	Mesothelioma, squamous cell carcinoma
Cytokeratin 7	Carcinoma subset
Cytokeratin 20	Gastrointestinal tumours, transitional cell carcinoma, Merkel cell carcinoma

Antibody	Useful diagnostic applications
Broad spectrum cytokeratin (AE1/3, MNF116, polyclonal Antibovine)	Cytokeratins
Cytomegalovirus (CMV)	Cytomegalovirus
Cytotoxic Molecules (TIA-1, Granzyme B, Perforin)	Cytotoxic cells including NK cells and cytotoxic T-cells
DBA.44 (Hairy cell leukaemia)	Hairy cell leukaemia
Desmin	Skeletal and smooth muscle tumours
Desmoplakins	Follicular dendritic cells and tumours, epithelial cells (fixation sensitive)
Epidermal growth factors (TGF-α, EGFR)	Squamous carcinomas, possible prognostic relevance in various carcinomas
Epstein-Barr virus (LMP)	Latent membrane protein of EB Virus
Epithelial Membrane Antigen (EMA)	Some carcinomas, meningioma, Ki-1 lymphoma, plasma cell tumours, microvilli staining in mesothelioma
Epstein-Barr virus (EBR1)	(insitu hybridisation) EB Virus infection, Hodgkin's Lymphoma, post transplant lymphoproliferative disorders
Estrogen Receptor (ER)	Prognostic marker in breast and other carcinomas
Factor VIIIRA (Von Willebrand Factor)	Endothelial cells, megakaryocytes
Factor XIIIa	Dermal dendrocytes, dermatofibroma, atypical fibroxanthoma
Fas (CD95), Fas-ligand (CD95L)	Apoptotic cells
Ferritin	Bone marrow iron stores, low sensitivity for hepatocytes
Fibrin	Glomerular diseases
Fibronectin	Adenoid cystic carcinoma of salivary gland and breast
Fibrinogen	Glomerular diseases
Glial Fibrillary Acidic Protein (GFAP)	Gliomas
Gross cystic disease fluid protein-15 (GCDFP-15, Brst-2)	Breast, salivary, sweat gland tumours
HAM 56	Macrophages/monocytes
HBME-1	Membrane staining of mesothelioma cells
Heat Shock Proteins (HSPS)	Possible prognostic marker in various tumours
Helicobacter pylori	Helicobacter organisms
HepPar1	Hepatocytes, hepatocellular carcinoma, mixed hepatocyte/cholangiocarcinomas
Hepatitis B Core Antigen (HBcAg)	Hepatitis B infection
Hepatitis B Surface Antigen (HBsAg)	Hepatitis B infection
Herpes Simplex Virus 1 & 2 (HSV 1 & 2)	Herpes infection
HLA-DR	B-cell lymphomas, activated T-cells
HMB45 (gp100)	Melanoma, nevus cells
HMLH-1	(Mismatch repair gene product) Hereditary non-polyposis colonic carcinoma (HNPCC) and sporadic colorectal carcinomas with microsatellite instability

Antibody	Useful diagnostic applications
HMLH-2	(Mismatch repair gene product) Hereditary non-polyposis colonic carcinoma (HNPCC) and sporadic colorectal carcinomas with microsatellite instability
Human Immunodeficiency Virus (HIV, p24)	HIV infection
Human milk fat globule (HMFG)	Microvilli on mesothelioma
Human Papilloma Virus (HPV)	Human papilloma Virus infection
Human Parvo Virus B19	Parvo virus infection
Human Placental Lactogen (hPL)	Intermediate trophoblasts, trophoblastic tumours
Immunoglobulins: IgKappa, Lambda, A, D, E, G, M	Immunoglobulin producing cells
Inhibin	Granulosa cell tumour, adrenal cortical tumours
Ki-67 (MIB1, Ki-S5)	Cell proliferation marker
Laminin	Basal lamina
Lysozyme (Muramidase)	Macrophage/monocytes, granular cell tumour
MAC387	Macrophage/monocyte
mdm-2 protein	Putative prognostic marker in various tumours
Measles	Measles infection, subacute sclerosing panencephalitis (SSPE) inclusions
Metallothioneins	Possible prognostic marker in various tumours
Microphthalmia transcription factor (MTF)	Melanoma and melanocytic tumours
Muscle Specific Actin (MSA, HHF-35)	Myoepithelium, smooth, skeletal muscle differentiation and corresponding tumours
Myeloperoxidase	Granulocytes and histiocytes and corresponding leukaemias
Myelin Basic Protein (MBP) ganglioneuromas	Nerve sheath tumours, oligodendro-gliomas, ganglioneuroblastomas and
MyoD1	Rhabdomyosarcoma
Myogenin	Rhabdomyosarcoma
Myoglobin	Rhabdomyosarcoma
Neurofilaments	Neurons and neuronal tumours
Nerve Growth Factor Receptor (NGFR, $p75^{NPR}$)	Nerve sheath differentiation
Neuron Specific Enolase (NSE)	Peripheral nerves, melanoma, neuroendocrine cells and tumours with neuroendocrine differentiation, testicular germ cell tumours
Neutrophil elastase	Granulocytic tumours, leukaemia
nm23/NME1	Possible prognostic marker, anti-tumour metastases
$p27^{kip1}$	Cyclin dependent kinase inhibitor, possible prognostic marker in breast and other tumours
$p21^{waf1}$	Tumour suppressor gene, possible prognostic marker
p53	Tumour suppressor gene product, marker of poor prognosis
p80 (ALK Protein)	Anaplastic large cell lymphoma with t(2;5)
p-glycoprotein (p-170, mDR-1)	Chemo-resistant marker, bile cannuliculi

Antibody	Useful diagnostic applications
Pancreatic hormones (insulin, somatostatin, vasoactive intestinal polypeptide, gastrin, glucagon, pancreatic polypeptide)	Various hormone secreting tumours
Parathormone	Parathyroid tissue and tumours
Parathyroid hormone related protein (PTHrP)	Squamous cell carcinomas, cholangiocarcinomas, negative in hepatocellular carcinomas
Pituitary hormones (ACTH, FSH, HGH, LH, PRL, TSH)	Hormone secreting pituitary tumours of different subsets
Placental alkaline phosphatase (PLAP)	Seminoma and other germ cell tumours
Pneumocystis carinii	Pneumocystis infection
Pregnancy specific β-1-glycoprotein (SP1)	Placental cells and tumours as well as various other carcinomas
Progesterone receptor (PR)	Prognostic marker in breast, endometrial, ovarian and meningial tumours
Proliferating cell nuclear antigen (PCNA)	Cell proliferation marker, fixation sensitive
Prostate Specific Antigen (PSA)	Prostatic carcinoma
Prostatic Acid Phosphatase (PAP)	Prostatic carcinoma
Protein Gene Product 9.5 (PGP 9.5)	Neuroendocrine differentiation
PS2	Estrogen inducible protein
Rabies	Rabies infection
Retinoblastoma Gene Protein (Rb, P110RB)	Tumour suppressor gene product
S100	Melanoma, Langerhan's cell, Shaun cells, neural supporting cells
Serotonin	Subset of carcinoid tumours
Simian virus 40 (SV40T antigen)	Cross reacts with JC viral inclusions in polymorphonuclear leukoencephalopathy (PML)
Spectrin/Fodrin	Linked to E-Cadherin and [beta]-catenin
Surfactant (POA, apoA1)	Non-small cell carcinomas of the lung
Synaptophysin	Neuroendocrine differentiation
TAG-72 (B72.3)	Various adenocarcinomas
TAU	Neurofibrillary tangles
Terminal deoxynucleotidyl transfer (TdT)	Lymphoblastic lymphoma
Thyroglobulin	Thyroid follicular cells
Thrombomodulin	Lymphatic and vascular tumours, mesothelial cells and mesothelioma
Toxoplasma gondii	Toxoplasma infection
Thyroid transcription factor-1 (TTF-1)	Thyroid and lung carcinomas
Ubiquitin	Mallory bodies, astrocytomas

Antibody	Useful diagnostic applications
Ulex europaeus agglutinin-1 lectin (UAE-1)	Endothelial cells, various epithelial tumours
Villin	Adenocarcinoma subset, especially gastrointestinal carcinomas
Vimentin	Sarcomas, lymphomas, co-expressed with cytokeratin in some carcinomas
VS38	Plasma cells, neuroendocrine differentiation, some melanocytic tumours
Wilm's Tumour Gene Product (WT1)	Desmoplastic small round cell tumour, mesothelioma, Wilm's tumour, endometrial carcinoma, ovarian surface epithelial tumours

Suppliers

Suppliers

Details provided are, to the publishers' best knowledge, correct at the time of publication.

Abbott Laboratories Diagnostic Division
http://www.abbottdiagnostics.com

Accurate Chemical & Scientific Corporation
http://www.accuratechemical.com

Advanced Immunochemical Inc.
http://www.advimmuno.com

American Diagnostica Inc.
http://www.americandiagnostica.com

American Qualex
http://www.americanqualex.com

American Research Products Inc.
http://www.arp1.com

Amersham Biosciences
http://www1.amershambiosciences.com

Amgen
http://www.amgen.com

Ancell Corporation
http://www.ancell.com

Applied Biosystems
http://home.appliedbiosystems.com

Beckman Coulter
http://www.beckman.com

Becton Dickinson
http://www.bd.com

Bioclone Australia Pty Ltd
http://www.bioclone.com.au

BioDesign Inc.
http://www.biodesignofny.com

Biogenesis
http://www.biogenesis.co.uk

BioGenex Inc.
http://www.biogenex.com

Biomol Research Laboratories Inc.
http://www.biomol.com

Bio-Rad Laboratories Inc.
http://www.bio-rad.com

Biotech Italia
http://www.biotechww.com

Biotest AG
http://www.biotest.de

Biotest USA
http://www.biotest.com

BMA Biomedicals AG
http://www.bma.ch

Biosource International
http://www.biosource.com

Caltag Laboratories
http://www.caltag.com

DakoCytomation
http://www.dako.com

Enzo Biochem Inc.
http://www.enzobio.com

Euro-Diagnostica
http://www.eurodiagnostica.com

Exalpha Biopharmaceuticals
http://www.exalpha.com

E-Y Laboratories Inc.
http://www.eylabs.com

Fitzgerald Industries International Inc.
http://www.fitzgerald-fii.com

Gen-Probe Inc.
http://www.gen-probe.com

Harlan Sera-Lab Ltd
http://www.harlanseralab.co.uk

ICI
http://www.ici.com

ICN Biomedicals Inc.
http://www.icnbiomed.com

Intracel Corporation
http://www.intracel.com

Lab Vision Corporation
http://www.labvision.com

Mallinckrodt Chemicals
http://www.mallchem.com

Novocastra Laboratories Ltd
http://www.novocastra.co.uk

Oncogene Science Inc.
http://oncogene.com

Oncogene Research Products
http://www.apoptosis.com

Organon International
http://www.organon.com

Oxoid Ltd
http://www.oxoid.com

Paesel + Lorei GmbH & Co
http://www.paesel-lorei.de

Pharmingen
http://www.bdbiosciences.com/pharmingen

Pierce Biotechnology
http://www.piercenet.com

Research Diagnostics Inc.
http://www.researchd.com

Roche Applied Science
http://biochem.roche.com/

Sanbio B.V.
http://www.sanbio.nl

Santa Cruz Biotechnology
http://www.scbt.com/

Serotec Ltd
http://www.serotec.oxi.net

Sigma-Aldrich
http://www.sigmaaldrich.com

Signet Laboratories Inc.
http://www.signetlabs.com/index.asp

Thermo LabSystems
http://www.thermolabsystems.com

Thermo Shandon
http://www.shandon.com

Vector Laboratories
http://www.vectorlabs.com

Zymed Laboratories Inc.
http://www.zymed.com

NOTES

NOTES

NOTES

NOTES

NOTES

NOTES

NOTES

NOTES